FROM
HEAD
TO
HEART

LUCY DAVIS

AN INSPIRATIONAL JOURNEY FROM CORPORATE
BURNOUT TO SPIRITUAL WARRIOR

"The longest journey you'll ever make is the journey from the head to the heart."

LISSA RANKIN

This First Edition published in 2023

www.lucydavis.com
Instagram: lucydavis2222
facebook.com/lucydavisintuitivetransformation

Copyright © Lucy Davis 2023

The moral right of Lucy Davis to be identified as the author of this work has been asserted in accordance with the Copyright, Designs and Patents Act of 1988.

All rights reserved. No part of this work may be reproduced, stored in an information retrieval system (other than for purposes of review) or transmitted in any form or by any means, electronic, mechanical, photocopying, recording or otherwise, without the express permission of the publisher. Any person who does any unauthorised act in relation to this publication may be liable to criminal prosecution and civil claims for damages.

This book is sold subject to the condition that it shall not, by way of trade or otherwise, be lent, resold, hired out, or otherwise circulated without the publisher's prior consent in any form of binding or cover other than that in which it is published and without a similar condition including this condition being imposed on the subsequent purchaser.

A CIP Catalogue of this book is available from the British Library

ISBN 978-1-7392156-0-6

Cover design and text layout by
chandlerbookdesign.com

Printed in Great Britain by
TJ Books, Padstow, Cornwall

MIX
Paper from
responsible sources
FSC   FSC® C013056
www.fsc.org

To my beloved grandad, Peter Noye.

Grateful every day that you choose me to be your granddaughter this lifetime.

For the words of wisdom that awakened my soul in your dying days and that have been the catalyst for this book.

*I miss your human daily.
Thank you for encouraging me to go live life.*

I love you to the moon and stars, always x

CONTENTS

Thank You	1
Prologue	5
PART ONE – FROM THE HEAD	7
Distractions	*46*
Emotional Trauma	*81*
Delusion	*128*
PART TWO – TO THE HEART	147
Dis-Ease!	*163*
Mirroring	*229*
Straddling Two Worlds	*275*
Unfortunate Accidents	*344*
Synchronicities and Signs	*385*
PART THREE – THE JOURNEY HOME	413
Epilogue	609
About Lucy Davis	611

Thank You

Rik Arron. What can I say? Without you, this book would not be here in black and white. You saw something in me, my story, and this journey. You kindly offered to help me get this story out into the public domain, with the most precious gift of all – your time. You welcomed me into your family's life for ten months – week in and week out – selflessly dedicating precious hours until this masterpiece was produced.

You have become a friend, a brother, and a very important part of my life, and for that, I feel incredibly lucky. I am so grateful to you for the offer you made, the patience you have shown, and the incredible support in getting this done. The tears, goosebumps, the jaw-dropping moments are now out there for everyone to see what we have been doing behind closed doors. I know your girls will be so proud of you, not only for this, but the imprint you leave generally in this world.

Too soon to talk about book two? Never change, you are amazing. Love you Rik, thank you x

Dad. What a journey we have been on over the years. From daddy's girl to not speaking, to, thankfully, now an incredible relationship. We have had to have conversations that people would never dream of a father and daughter having, all of which have bought us closer together than ever. I am grateful for all we have been through this lifetime. It has been a privilege to be your daughter.

Here's to many more experiences to come. I love you x

Mum. Thanks for bringing me into life form this time around. I know I have tested you to the max over the years, from that little girl who used to round up the troops and climb over the back gate at school, to the woman I have become, as I stepped out of the norm and into my authentic self.

I am so grateful you have held space for me to do this, even though I know it has never made sense to you. I appreciate everything you have done and continue to do for me. I promise to make you proud. I love you x

Mark. I could not have asked for a better stepdad than the one I received when you came into my mum's life. It's been challenging for you to take on all that you did, and what people will read about in this book. So many would have walked away. You didn't, and for that, I am so grateful. The angels were looking down on Kirsty and I the day you arrived.

You reminded me how to be grounded, patient and logical – things that at 16 were not really in my makeup. I hope you realise how appreciated you are. I love you x

Kirsty. Sis, one of my biggest teachers to date. I am so grateful to you and for you. It's been a wild ride over the years. Thank you for trusting me in your times of need. I hope this book reminds you of a few precious moments you may have missed when they unfolded. I love you x

Ricky. I know I have said thank you to you a thousand times for the journey we have experienced together over the last 9 years. I also know you have completely underestimated the impact you have had on my journey. I am trusting this book will go some way to showing you how powerfully intuitive you have been, guiding me from that first smart-arse comment all those years back.

Thanks for being in my life. It's been a journey. Here's to the next chapter.

Kyle. A huge, heartfelt thank you, from me to you. You gave me hope when there was not one ounce left inside of me. You restored my faith in men when quite easily it could have gone the other way. Your patience, vulnerability and love changed my life. I am forever grateful to you for reminding me how to heal my heart. This journey would not be where it is, if it was not for you.

Donna. I know you only just entered my life towards the end of this book, but my goodness did you make an impact. My soul sister, colleague, and best friend. I thank you for all your support over the years. The amount of weird, channelled messages I have shared, and you have never once judged. You held space and smiled whilst they unfolded. I am grateful every day to you, for travelling the UK and the world on this part of our human experience together.

Thanks for being the bright shining star you are. Love you x

Katrina. Like the little whirlwind you are, you arrived, and my goodness have we created some storms since. Thank you for helping guide, unpick, and put the pieces of the puzzle together. It's been a pleasure to travel with you. Here's to the next chapter. Love ya girl x

Bela and Gabi. And last, but by no means least, my Little Beans – Gabi and Bela. One day, I hope you will realise how precious you are. You came into my life at a time when I was totally disconnected from the family. I missed those first three years of your lives; however, thankfully, we have been able to make up for it since. I trust you will both remember to stay in your light, rather than get disconnected – like your older sister did.

You are such special gifts to the world. I thank God every day for your existence. I love you to the moon and stars x

There are so many other people who have left an imprint on my life, it would be impossible to list you all here. You know who you are and I thank you with all of my heart for sharing this journey with me. I'm so grateful that we got to meet again this lifetime and to help each other grow and learn.

Thank you.

Lucy
xox

A note to whoever reads this book. Thank you for agreeing to be here at this time and for taking precious moments to read this book. Every situation, circumstance, and event on this journey has been written purely from my perspective and from my memory and recollection.

Prologue

If you happen to live near to where I live, in the early hours of the morning, you might see a lone figure running the paths and trails of the nearby nature reserve. She moves swiftly across the forest floor; sprinting up hills and darting along the hedgerows. And then you might catch her barefoot along the beach, chasing the waterline and then basking in the light of the sunrise.

More often than not she appears to be excitedly talking to herself. Many of the locals think she's batshit crazy, but she's not.

I know this because that lone figure is me.

Every day for several years now, I have done my morning 10km run and then, walking back home, I've gone online to speak live to my audience of tens of thousands of people from all over the world, on one or other of my social media platforms.

I don't always know what I'm going to talk about and I don't always know what I've talked about after I'm done because the messages come through me. Afterwards, I'll receive hundreds of responses from people who have felt moved, touched and very often even healed by the words that came out of my mouth.

Sounds weird, right?

It is. For sure.

It wasn't always this way, though.

In fact, my life couldn't have been further away from that very possibility.

And if you come with me on this journey now, I'll explain how this all came to be.

PART ONE
FROM THE HEAD

1

I was on top of the world.

Sitting on a sun lounger in a beautiful, five-star hotel in Dubai immersed in the sunshine. This is the life, this is what it's all about! This is living the dream.

I remember it all, that specific feeling. I can picture the exact sun lounger I was sat on, its position around the pool, and the incredible view I had of the surrounding pool area. The sun was still high in the sky, it was late afternoon and the high temperatures were just starting to drop.

At this time in my life, in 2013, I was working for CLS – a major financial institution, and it was in that era when they gave every employee, over a certain level, a BlackBerry device so they were contactable – in the event of something happening whereby they required your support. It would ring and beep constantly as emails, calls and texts came in. It was always going off! When you agree to work for CLS, you tend to hand them your soul in exchange for your salary. It's handed over to the person in question willingly, though. We know what we're getting into. I had chosen to give them my life. They contacted you whatever and whenever, and to be honest, you just got on with it! I was cheeky about it; if I was going to be contactable by work, then my friends and family could also contact me on that phone whilst I was out of the country, so that I wouldn't get charged. So there were even more reasons why it was constantly beeping and making noise.

I had flown to Dubai with one of my best girlfriends and one of my guy friends. We were notorious for taking trips whenever we could. I was a wanderer at heart, the gypsy spirit of the group, and thankfully, I had people who would regularly wander with me; and we could afford to do it. Another friend, from my hometown of Bournemouth, had flown over to Abu Dhabi to see some of his family and he had taken the journey through the desert to come and meet us in Dubai, so there were four of us in total that day.

We were sat by the pool, chilling and chatting. We had been swimming and having fun, setting ourselves up for the evening ahead. The sun had started to go down, although in Dubai it was still very hot.

I sat there soaking up the last bit of sun, reflecting on this perfect day, when my BlackBerry started ringing. It had been a glorious sunny day and I'd already been out in the sun for several hours, so I had that nice sun-kissed feeling. I thought about how my mum, having had a skin cancer scare, wouldn't be impressed by the colour I had gone in such a short space of time. I looked at the phone and no surprise it was my mum. I wondered what she might want, being that she knew I was away, but then I remembered that she was taking my grandad to the hospital, and she was probably calling to give an update. We were a very close family, and I adored my mum and my grandad.

I answered the phone, "Hey Mum, how are you?"

She said, "Are you okay?"

"Well, that's a random question. Of course, I'm okay. I'm in Dubai and the sun's shining. What's not to be happy about?"

"Are you sat down Lucy?" she said firmly. "Are you with someone?"

And I was, I was sat on my sun lounger and I thought – *Oh fuck*!

We were only in Dubai for the Easter weekend. Two days of annual leave for a six-day trip, that's a good exchange rate. My heart sank. It felt like black storm clouds had instantly formed over my head because I knew what was coming. I suddenly felt really cold.

And then she said to me, "Today at the hospital, they have given grandad 12 weeks maximum to live."

My mind went into instant overdrive – *I still have a few days left in Dubai and grandad's only got 12 weeks. Three days is too long. I live in London. He lives in Bournemouth.*

There was so much noise in my head, that I wasn't listening to what my mum said after that. I was caught up in my own world and my own story. I kept thinking – *How on earth are we going to get through the next 12 weeks? What on earth are we going to do without him? How on earth will my mum cope with having no parents?*

My mind kept spinning.

In previous years, my grandad had been diagnosed with Idiopathic Pulmonary Fibrosis. To my limited understanding, from what had been shared with me, the oxygen taken into his lungs was essentially causing scar tissue, making it extremely challenging to breathe. I remember someone describing it to be like a honeycomb effect. So his lungs were getting increasingly solid with scar tissue as time went on. From diagnosis, it's expected that you will survive no more than five years. Long term, his lungs would make it so challenging that he would not be able to breathe anymore.

I immediately started going into strategy mode, it's what I did best. It's what I did for a living, after all! Getting organised, sorting shit, attempting to control everything. I started thinking about what we can do to help him get through this, and how can we all make it as pleasant for him as possible. *Were there any other treatments? Did we need a second opinion?*

I felt that huge black cloud forming ever greater over me. That once glorious evening sunshine was now a shadow of doom and gloom. I wasn't sure how I would get through the next couple of days. I didn't want to be there. I wanted to run away. I wanted to be at home, right there and then!

We had ended up in Dubai for this trip as the winter had seemed exceptionally long in the UK that year. We all needed some sunshine and some fun, together. We all worked really hard; my girlfriend was a media lawyer, my guy friend was an Executive Director at JPMorgan, and I had recently become a Director. If truth be known, we all worked hard at our partying too, we knew how to have a good time together. Even though we were all so different, it somehow worked beautifully. We travelled as much as we could together; as soon as we had a few days, we would plan something and jet off – Paris, LA – you name it. And when we travelled, we did it in style – five-star hotels, airport lounges, upgrades, and all whilst collecting our air miles and points. We lived a very busy, materialist existence. Let me be honest; splashing out bought me happiness back then.

Just a few weeks earlier, I had returned from a three-week Christmas trip, and this was very typical of the life that I led at that time. I had more money than I knew what to do with. I had a very extravagant lifestyle with lovely cars, an amazing home, and eating in the best restaurants with exceptional wine. I worked hard, and I played even harder, although that didn't come without its fair share of sacrifices.

My mum did everything she could to keep us in a decent lifestyle. When my dad left the home, she earned just £11k a year, and she used that to bring up two teenage girls. At sixteen years of age, I made a promise to my mum that I would never rely on a man to survive – and my goodness did I honour my word! I worked my butt off! I gave everything I had to become independent! Not receiving handouts from my parents has made me determined and focused.

I watched my parents and deemed my level of success based on their values. My mum's number one value is security. My dad's number one value is financial abundance. He worked so hard when we were growing up that we barely saw him. Their two very different approaches were my benchmarks for success and abundance, and I am so incredibly grateful that they were.

These values had led me into an incredibly fortunate situation where abundance was the norm for me. I loved nice handbags, shoes, and clothes, and I loved to spoil people. If it were someone's birthday, I would make sure that for that day, they felt like a King or Queen. That feeling of wishing to help people never went away. I loved to see the smiles on their faces.

I once had a friend from Bournemouth come to stay with me in London one February. I had just been paid my bonus at the end of January, and she had come up for my birthday. We went shopping in Shepherd's Bush, London. I treated us to lunch, and then, out of nowhere, I decided to buy a Mulberry handbag and a Louis Vuitton bag, all within about three minutes of each other. It felt so good! My friend's jaw almost hit the ground as I splashed out extravagantly. This friend of hers from sleepy Bournemouth had just splashed out more money in three minutes than she probably earned in a month. Looking back, it was not classy at all. I was caught up in this world of zeros. Money meant nothing, really. It was just something I was lucky enough to have plenty of.

And yet, here I was, in a posh hotel in one of the wealthiest countries in the world, and I'm going through this experience where my material world was about to collapse.

2

For me, my life has always been about polarity, and when I look back, here I was on this sun lounger in this beautiful five-star resort, everything being brought to us by staff, nothing was too much effort, and yet it all means nothing to you, when you are about to lose the one thing that was truly important, family.

At this time in my life, I was not speaking to my dad. My grandad, since my nan had passed, had actually fulfilled that father role for me. I shared things with him that I would likely never have shared, even with my dad. This man – my grandad – meant the whole world to me.

The second I put the phone down, I burst into tears after talking to my mum and doing my best to hold it together for as long as I could. There was an overwhelming release. My friends saw me and came over and said, "Oh my God, is everything okay? What's happened?"

"My grandad is dying," was all I could say.

"Oh babe," she said and put her arms around me. "Is there anything we can do?" And, for whatever reason, I decided to truly step into my pity party at that moment – *Oh my God, my world is falling apart. Why is this happening to me?*

I'd gone in an instant from *I've made it* to *Oh my god, this is awful, poor me*.

I felt like a wave had just come crashing down on me, and I was struggling to come up for air.

Then, almost in an instant, my corporate training kicked in, and because I'm sat around the pool in a beautiful five-star hotel, and people are walking around looking amazing, I didn't want to sit there blubbing, so I did my best to hide it. Corporate Lucy doesn't show emotions, and God forbid she should show anyone she's weak.

What was interesting, looking back, is that all of the staff disappeared now; it was as if nobody was coming to ask if I wanted something like they had been doing all day. All of a sudden, it felt like – *You've got to sit with this girl, you've really got to feel what's going on here, and you've got to make some clear decisions as to what it is that you're going to give your focus to and what you're not.*

I sat on this sun lounger in the middle of paradise, surrounded by people, yet I had never felt so lonely. It was like a portal of emotions had opened right under my sun lounger, and I had to decide if I was brave enough to do anything about it.

After another hour of sitting outside, I headed back to my room. I walked through the hotel in a haze. Back in the room, I just paced up and down the large bedroom in a trance.

My friends did their best to jolly me up for the evening. We were due to be going on a big night out, as it was one of our last nights. I didn't want to go and have to pretend everything was okay, but then

I also didn't want to be on my own. At that time in my life, I was not comfortable being on my own. I was always with people, always busy. I would always distract myself with something or other. If I ever knew I was going to be on my own for a night, I would always search for someone who was free to do something. And that particular night, I was scared that if I was left alone, I might start crying and never actually stop.

In my attempts at getting ready, I couldn't stop crying. I would feel like I was doing okay, hold it together, then my eyes would start watering, and then the tears would start flowing again. I kept trying to put mascara on, but it would just run down my face. My eyes became sore and irritable. I did my best to pull it together, though. I looked at myself one last time in the mirror and thought – *God, you look like shit. What are you doing this for?*

In the taxi on the way to the club, all I wanted was to get out. I wanted to scream! I was in terrible turmoil. I should have been appreciating where I was, but I fucking hated it. I hated the taxi; I hated the brightness of all the lights. I was just looking to find holes in everything. I felt like screaming at the top of my lungs and letting it all out. But I didn't. I just did what Lucy Davis did best – kept a tight lip on it and pretended everything was okay.

We arrived at our destination, Buddha Bar. The hotel the club was in was big, bright, loud, busy and full-on. As we walked into the club, it was dark and a huge contrast to all the bright lights that we had come in from. There were lots of what I would call "call girls" in the bar, dolled up, looking absolutely incredible, but blatantly working the room. There is a lot of wealth in Dubai, so of course, there would be a lot of sex and alcohol – it follows the money.

The loud music echoed and reverberated around inside my head in a horribly trippy way. Normally, the music in a club would lift my energy, but on this occasion, I felt as if my energy was being suppressed even further; it actually felt as if I was going into a dungeon and having all of the life sucked out of me. I had a lot of heavy emotions going on inside. It felt like the darkness was pulling me into a vortex and saying – *We've got to take you down even further because you're not quite there yet.*

I stayed at Buddha Bar for an hour or so, but I was hurting too much, and I wanted to go to bed. My girlfriend was looking to catch up with a guy from back home that she'd met on a dating app or something, and I was in no mood to be wing-woman that night. My good friend from Bournemouth was happy to leave with me – what a diamond. He tried to keep my spirits up in the taxi on the way back, but I was tired; my heart hurt, my eyes were sore, and I felt like a bloody mess. He still told me I looked beautiful, even though I clearly didn't – but that's the kind of friend we need in our lives.

When we got back to the hotel, we sat on the balcony for a while and talked, and then I told him I needed to go to bed, so he left me to it. I took my makeup off, jumped into bed and fell asleep immediately. Unfortunately, a few hours later, I was woken by my friend returning to the room and bouncing off the walls after one too many shandies.

I don't remember much of the next day. I woke up, and my initial reaction was it had all been a bad dream, but that wasn't the case. It was real. I was heartbroken. My friends were hungover and feeling delicate, so I sat by the pool and grabbed the last bit of sunshine before our journey home.

In the early hours of the morning that next day, we flew home. Before the flight, I messaged my mum and told her that as soon as I got back, I would sort everything! We would figure out how this was all going to work over the next twelve weeks. I mean, they could be wrong about grandad, right? They could have made a mistake? I had already done that whole internal dialogue thing. In my mind, I had been rehearsing the conversation with my boss about my grandad and possibly working from home or taking time out.

On the plane home, despite it being an overnight flight, I decided to sit and drink wine and eat whatever food they were providing for us. I couldn't bring myself to watch a movie or talk, so I kept spinning around in my mind everything that was going on. My grandad was going to die. What on earth would life be like without him? I was also worried about my mum; she had lost her own mum years earlier due to pancreatic cancer. Interestingly, my nan had also been given around 12 weeks to live. She passed just days before her and my grandad's fiftieth wedding anniversary. So for my mum, this was her last parent. She would be an orphan. This was tragic! I just couldn't imagine it.

After a couple of drinks, my mind seemed to work even faster than normal. The combination of everything that had gone on was total sensory overload, and I couldn't switch off. I started to feel like I couldn't cope. So what's the best thing to do? Work. And that's what I did for the rest of the flight.

3

Hours later, we got off the plane, working our way steadily through customs, then picking up our baggage. I said goodbye to my friend; she was doing her own thing and going her own way. I got a taxi back home on my own. I got in the car, and I put my head back and breathed. The driver asked me, "Good trip?"

I looked at him and smiled inanely. The rest of the journey was a total blur. All of a sudden, I was at home.

I walked to the front door with my enormous suitcase; I don't travel light. It was about seven-thirty in the morning, and so there was a real hustle and bustle as people headed to work, but here I was, standing on the roadside with my luggage, looking up at my apartment, and wondering what was about to unfold.

I lived in a top-floor apartment, which meant navigating two flights of stairs with my bags. At the bottom of the stairs, I looked up and thought — *That has got to have all been a nightmare.*

I somehow lugged everything upstairs and shut the door behind me without even bothering to lock it. I dropped my bags, went to my bedroom and threw myself on the bed, lay there like a starfish, and sobbed my heart out. I sobbed and sobbed and sobbed because all of a sudden, I was on my own; I didn't have to keep up appearances, I didn't have to be strong anymore, I didn't have to do any of those things. I just let go, and I knew that I needed to allow all of this to take place before I spoke to my mum because I knew that if I was to get upset, my mum would be upset. And, of course, I had to keep up appearances! I was the strong one. I wanted to be the support for us all. When my dad left back in 1995, I was the fixer. I was the one that held the family together.

It felt as if I laid there for an eternity; it was probably only an hour or two.

I was supposed to be logging into work from home. Normally, I was one of those studious members of staff that would land from holiday and log on straight away and work, so I didn't need to take it as an extra day of annual leave, but not today.

I spoke to my boss and explained to him what was going on because, for me, that was my priority. I needed to know that I had a level of flexibility to do what I was going to need to do. God love him; he was so kind and empathic. Prior to this, I had judged him as weak. I had selfishly and ruthlessly thought that he would never help me get where I needed to get to in my career. At this moment, when I needed it most, I was truly humbled by his kindness. He told me to take whatever time I needed and to keep him in the loop. He was actually a really decent family man who had been totally screwed over by the company; always overlooked because he was one of those genuine workers that deliver and never moan. I often wonder where he is and what he's up to. Whatever it is, I hope it's somewhere he is truly valued.

After speaking to my boss, I called my mum to tell her what the plan was. My mum was in the middle of renovating a bungalow at the time, and it was an absolute shit show; they were pretty much gutting it all. For my mum, her home is her pride and joy; she's a bit of a perfectionist where the home is concerned. She has always wanted everything to be "just so."

I said to her, "Right, I've spoken to my boss, and I've agreed to stay in Bournemouth for three or four days of every week."

My mum said, "You can't do that. We're doing the house up! Where are you going to stay?"

I remember thinking at this point, a big juicy – *Fuck you!*

I had been stressing for the last few days after she had dropped this bombshell about grandad on me while I was on holiday – which, let's be honest, probably could have waited. And here she is now, saying I couldn't even stay there.

Fuck you very much!

Thankfully, one of the guys who had been with me in Dubai had an apartment in Bournemouth and he lived in London, so he gave me a set of keys and told me to come and go as I please. So, even in the worst moments, when even my mum was being a pain in the arse, I always had somebody that had a solution. This apartment in Bournemouth was a beautiful synchronicity.

I went to work as normal on Wednesday and Thursday of that week, then at the end of Thursday's working day, I said goodbye to everyone and told them that I'd see them again on Monday, before starting the long journey home. My first stop was Wimbledon to get packed up at my apartment; then I aimed to leave after rush hour to set off on the hour-and-a-half journey home to Bournemouth.

I had decided that driving down on a Thursday night was a better option – the M25 motorway on a Friday evening was always chaos, and traffic jams really pissed me off, so this would hopefully mitigate that potential situation.

I jumped in my Mini Cooper convertible – a little beige number with a black roof. I loved that car – my good friend Mickey had nick-named it Pepper, and it just stuck. I started the drive down to Bournemouth, and I began saying prayers out loud – and this is me who didn't believe in God at that time. I kept repeating over and over – *Please make this as painless as possible. Please let me spend as much time with my grandad as possible. Please let him know that I love him. Please let him not see my fear that he's not going to be there, please.*

I was praying without knowing what I was doing. I did that the whole way down from Wimbledon to Bournemouth. I don't remember the journey itself. I don't remember if the roads were busy. I don't remember anything. It felt like I was being driven. I just instinctively prayed.

The only other thing I thought about when I wasn't praying, was my nan – my grandad's wife. She had passed several years earlier, and I had held her hand when she died; it was something I will never forget. She was diagnosed with pancreatic cancer in the January of 2003. She died eight weeks later. She very bravely made a decision that she was not going to have treatment. Everybody thought she was off her head, except me. I thought she was so brave. I wished she'd had treatment, I was not ready for her to go, but I respected that she did not listen to anyone else; she stood her ground. The more I think about it, the more I realise I am like her. She was such a straight talker, she would sort shit out, and take no-nonsense. In the last four weeks of her life, she said some interesting things. She would sit on her bright orange crimson couch, like she was surrounded by sunset, and we would talk. Often my grandad would hear the conversation and leave the room, joking about us talking crazy nonsense again. We would often speak about life after death. Whether it was a thing or not. I truly believed that there had to be something. I couldn't get my head around why we would go through all of this, for nothing. She agreed with me. My nan was deeply spiritual; my grandad was the absolute opposite. One particular day, she said, "I will get you a message to you. I promise you, I don't know how I will do it because I don't know how it's going to work, but I will get you a message." And I believed her, I really did.

I kept saying to her, "Yes, please, get me a message. I'll do whatever it takes to receive it"

I sat with her, thinking – *You are a miracle. The fact you can be so calm, you've literally surrendered your life because you don't want to have radiation treatment and chemotherapy.*

Essentially she said to us, "I'm going."

Not long after that, she died.

When I eventually arrived in Bournemouth, it was dark. I had never been to my friend's apartment, so I found myself crawling along the road looking for it. When I was given the address, I had never quite connected the dots that it was on the road directly opposite the cemetery where my nan's ashes had been buried all those years earlier. I continued my slow kerb-crawling, trying to not look too weird to anyone who may have been watching. Eventually, I stumbled across the property. It looked a bit dark and creepy, especially with the cemetery across the road.

I parked up and left my bags in the car, so I could open up, switch on all of the lights and hopefully realise I was creating a huge drama in my mind. Walking in, I felt cold, really cold. Of course, nobody had been there for a while, so the heating hadn't been on, but my coldness was more than that. I think it was the fear inside of me, the fear of being in the place on my own, the fear of being opposite my nan's ashes, the fear of my grandad about to pass.

I went to my car and grabbed all of my stuff in one trip. I looked like something out of a comedy sketch – everything stacked high and balanced precariously. Anything to avoid two trips.

Once I had collected my things, I sat in bed with my laptop. I was hungry, but I didn't want to hang around in the kitchen, so I finished up a little bit of work to try and get ahead of the game for tomorrow. Tomorrow would be the first time I saw my sweet grandad since the trauma of the prognosis.

4

The next morning I woke up early, set my laptop up on the desk and logged onto work. It was before 7 am when I went online. I had agreed that I would be taking some time out during the day to spend time with my grandad, but I didn't want people to think I wasn't working at all. The fear of other people's opinions of me was still very prominent.

I got into the shower and accidentally scolded myself that morning. *Typical.* I dried off, got dressed and then messaged my mum and asked what would be a sensible time to get to grandad's house. I wanted to be respectful as I knew he had regular care coming in to help, as he wasn't able to navigate things as quickly as he used to be. He was such a proud man. He always wanted to be showered, dressed and have brushed his teeth before he saw visitors. My mum suggested around 9.30 am, so I reworked my meetings and did a few hours' work, and then I got into my car and headed over.

The sun was shining that morning. It was just starting to feel warm. The birds seemed to be singing extra loud that day. The hustle and the bustle of the university students and traffic was prevalent. I wondered how many of the people that were out and about had huge stuff going on for them also. I mean, you never know, do you?

Once again, I don't remember the journey to his house that day. I drove with the roof down and immersed in the sunshine, but then I also felt guilty for wanting to be happy in the sun. I very much felt my nan was with me that morning.

My grandad lived in a lovely little bungalow on a hill, in a place called Northbourne. Whenever I went there, it took me back to such fond memories of my childhood. I pulled up outside his bungalow. I sat in my car for a moment and looking up at the house and thought – *Can I really do this? Am I really strong enough?*

It had only been two or three weeks since I had last seen my grandad. I had witnessed his struggle to walk and breathe back then, but now because we had an end date, it all seemed so much more serious. How does anyone carry on knowing that information? Do people give up knowing they maybe only have 12 weeks to live?

Sitting there at the wheel of my car, outside his house, I felt the guilt of why I hadn't spent more time with him. Why hadn't I been going there every week rather than every two or three weeks, when I already knew he was poorly? Why on earth had I been so selfish? Really, what had all the partying and socialising been for? What's life without family? So many sabotaging thoughts surfaced. I felt so guilty, so ashamed.

I sat in the car for about five minutes. I knew he had seen me out of his bedroom window because that's what he did. I looked in the rear-view mirror and there were tears in my eyes and I thought – *Right Lucy, compose yourself, pull yourself together, sort it out.*

I eventually got out of my car and walked through the black iron gates, up the drive and towards the door. I rang the doorbell and heard a voice say, "Come through the back door." I walked down the side of the house and in through the back door, and I was greeted by a lady. He didn't have full-time carers at this time, but he had carers popping in regularly to make sure he was okay and to check if anything needed doing for him.

My grandad was such a proud man, and he was always immaculate. I walked into the lounge, where he was sitting in "his" chair – every grandad has a chair, right? He looked at me with his soft, kind eyes as if to say – *I'll be alright.* I went over to him and leaned in for the biggest squeeze, "How are you feeling?"

"I'm fine," he said.

Typical man, and typical proud grandad – I thought.

"Are you really fine, though?" I asked him. I looked over to the side of his chair, and there was an oxygen tank with wires that were going up his nose. He was clearly not fine. He was keeping up appearances, probably because it gave him strength and dignity. That was what was so beautiful about my grandad. He was so protective of his family, he put a brave face on it all. He never moaned. For as long as he could, he would keep a smile on his face.

On that first visit, I asked him if he would like me to make a cup of tea. He wouldn't have it!

"No way, you're not taking that away from me. I'm capable! I make good tea. I'm going to be making it." He said, and he went off to make a cup of tea. He shouted back, "D'you want a biscuit with that?"

"Go on then, I'll have a cheeky biscuit with you."

That was important to him, a cup of tea and a biscuit. It was how the family unit would always come together, it was an important part of life.

We sat there that day and talked about all sorts. I asked him so many questions, "How are you really feeling, Grandad? Are you okay? Are you up for going for a walk? Would you like to sit in the garden? Is there anything I can do for you?"

He just kept repeating, "I'm alright. I'm alright."

The carer came in a couple of times to check on him before leaving, but otherwise, it was just a normal day.

It didn't feel like he was dying.

So brave. So honourable. He must have been in pain. He must have been scared shitless. But you would never have known it by the way he composed himself.

Those first few weeks, I kept saying to my mum, "Are you sure he's as sick as they say?" I just didn't see it in him, he was either a bloody good actor or at this point, he was doing okay!

It was around week four of me visiting on a Friday that there was suddenly a huge shift in him.

I developed something of a routine over those weeks. I'd go in for a few hours during the day. I would then go back and finish work, and then I'd pop back to his house again in the evening. Sometimes we would have fish and chips, or on many occasions, we all made dinner. And then, on Saturday and Sunday, I would do the same. I spent as much time as I could with him over the days I was down in Bournemouth, without taking away his freedom. I would go over at least twice a day on Saturdays and Sundays, and then I would go back to London for the week.

I did that for the first four weeks, and then he had to go for a check-up at the hospital. By this point, he was using his oxygen a lot more. The doctor, at that meeting, said to my mum that my grandad was deteriorating a lot more quickly now. It was a devastating blow for all of us. This is when the downward shift started to become clearly noticeable.

I spoke to my boss and asked if I could stay in Bournemouth for an extra day a week to spend more time with the family due to his condition deteriorating. My boss was incredible, he was very supportive. I was so glad I had these conversations with my boss, and I had asked for help. Looking back, it was probably the first time I had ever vulnerably let someone into my life and asked for support. Sounds weird, maybe, but it was true. I was tough, I had it together, I would fix it myself!

At this time, my grandad stopped answering the door himself. More often than not, he just sat in his chair. He had no energy. He had no breath in him. He was starting to lose that sparkle. My heart ached so much for him, especially when my uncle Michael had to start coming over to shave him, as he could no longer do it himself. He was such a proud man, I imagine it really pained him to have started to lose his way like this and to be more and more reliant on other people. It was terribly sad to watch such a beautiful soul crumble from the inside out – despite his best efforts to fight it.

By this point, he had a live-in carer. She was great fun and straight-talking, which I know was good for my grandad. She took no-nonsense, which kept him fighting, I feel. What also shifted, though, was this quiet, safe sanctuary that we had created over the past few weeks had now become busier, with more and more people popping in and out in order to help and spend time with him. Interestingly, despite the presence of more people being around, about six weeks before he died, all of a sudden, my grandad started opening up to me, in a big way.

5

On one occasion, I pulled up outside the house, I had been chatting to my mum on the drive over, and she had warned me to prepare myself for what I was going to see. I parked my car further up the road, so I couldn't be seen, and I cried and cried.

Eventually, I pulled myself together and went into the house. As I walked into the room, my heart broke. All of a sudden, this very familiar space looked so different. Oxygen tanks and tubes everywhere. I'm not sure I hid the emotion too well as he looked up with his kind eyes and said, "Alright, duck?"

I looked at him and I just thought – *Oh, fuck, this is it? This is the slippery slope. It's really happening.*

I smiled at him, "Grandad, let me make you a cup of tea."

"I'll do it, " he replied.

"No way, you will not. I'm here, I'm your granddaughter, I'm in charge today."

He laughed at me as I walked out of the room. I stood in the kitchen composing myself, the carer noticed, so she came over and asked if I was okay. I thanked her and stood there breathing deeply.

I composed myself and went back into the room with the cups of tea. I would normally have sat on a couch across the room from him, but on this day, I decided to pull a little stool over to sit as close to him as possible. I plonked myself down next to him and picked up his hand. I must have known, intuitively, because that's when it happened. The moment he started to open up.

He looked me in the eyes and said, "Are you happy?"

I looked back at him and smiled, "Of course I'm happy. What do I not have to be happy about?" To lighten the moment, I made a joke, "You're my grandad, of course, I'm happy."

He looked at me with his beautiful grey eyes, and he said, "No, but are you really happy?"

Those words pierced through my heart into the depths of my soul. I wanted to sob, but I held it together.

As if by magic, the Sun appeared in the living room where we were sitting. It felt like we were on a stage, and all of a sudden, there was a spotlight shining on us. It felt as if he was looking deep into my soul asking the most profound of questions. Questions my grandad just would not ask! I said to him, "Grandad, I have got so much to be happy about. I've got an amazing career, incredible friends, and a wonderful family." But, in truth, I knew I was justifying the fact that I was fucking miserable. I was justifying everything. He saw straight through me, I could feel it. I was embarrassed.

He asked again, "But are you really happy? Are you really doing what you want to be doing?"

I sat there in disbelief, contemplating. At this point in my life, I was not in the slightest bit "spiritually" aware. It popped into my mind, though — *Could this be my nan talking to me through grandad?*

My grandad was not normally somebody who pried. If you asked for his advice on something, he would give it, but never without invitation and he would never push it further than that. This conversation, though, was piercing my soul with this questioning, which he'd never ever done in my life before.

I just sat there holding his hand and thinking — *I'm going to cry in a minute, I am going to get overwhelmed. This is not about me! Pull it together!*

So I toughened up. He was on his deathbed. I was not willing to play the victim! I had to fight it, but my victim mode was kicking in big-time.

He then continued on this path, "Lucy, you are the light. You are the sunshine. I've always called you my sunshine, now it's time for the world to see your light. It needs your light."

At this point, I'm starting to think – *My God, these drugs are good.*

A huge part of me wanted to listen to the stuff he was saying, but there was this other part of me that was rationalising it all – *These drugs must be amazing because this is not him at all! Who is this?*

And no matter which way you look at it, whether you believe it or not, the whole time it was my grandad, it was him in his true essence. It was his kind, beautiful face looking at me. It seemed like all of his wrinkles, his age and his suffering had disappeared in front of me, and there was just this timeless wisdom coming from him. It was like nothing I had ever witnessed before. It was so strange.

It seemed he just knew that, with the time we had left together, he had to pierce whatever bravado and armour I'd been wearing. He kept coming back at me, "But do you really love your job?"

"Grandad, I get paid so well, they've given me the flexibility to be here with you now. Of course, I love my job."

But, inside I was thinking – *I fucking hate it. I hate it! Get me away from it!*

In truth, there was nothing more that I hated than having to go to that place, sit at that desk and be told what to do by those twats! My boss's boss at the time was a total arsehole; I will never forget him pulling me into an office when he was over from America on one occasion, he had a go at me purely because I was a woman! He told me I would never make it because I was a woman, and I just thought – *Fuck you!*

I had been miserable for a long time, but I hadn't wanted to admit it to myself. In that moment, though, sitting there with my grandad, it was bringing all of my shit up to the surface. It was bringing every insecurity that I'd ever had right up into view. My beloved grandad was making it all come up and it was extremely uncomfortable. Quite frankly, I did not like it – at all! It made me feel hot and cold, it made me feel vulnerable – something I was not used to feeling! I felt as if I was a little girl again, and although I was in the comfort and the security of my grandad, I was raw. This was real, and he just kept going.

Then, as quickly as he started, he stopped! It was as if he was now going to let me sit with all of it to ponder and feel it. And then, just like that, we were back talking about really random things, like my nan's dog, Tessa, that had passed away.

It was all so weird. It was everything all at the same time, every polarity you could imagine colliding inside me. I hated him at one point, and yet loved him so much. I was angry with him for invoking all this stuff, and yet so utterly grateful at the same time. It was like being in a washing machine, on the spin cycle with the door open. Not a nice feeling.

Knowing what I know now, I can see that he was channelling. He was bringing in much-required messages. He was the conduit to help awaken my sweet soul. Back then, though, I did not have a clue. As far as I was concerned, this was crazy talk between my grandad and me.

This had been an early morning visit. What a trippy start to the day. I went home to do some work with my mind spinning. God knows how I focused that day. When I went back later, I took him his favourite caramel shortbread mini treats with chocolate on the top, he loved them. God love him, it was rare he ate anything sweet, but for these, he would always make an exception. He smiled as I handed him the box, then instantly started again, "You do realise you are here to shine the light for people Lucy, don't you? Do you think your current job helps you shine the light for people?"

I started to think – *Far out, here we go again, this is nuts.*

I really didn't want to hear it, but I knew that I either had to run away and have nothing to do with him for the next few weeks until he passed, or it was time to face up to this stuff.

I asked him outright, "Grandad, where is all this coming from?"

And he said, "What do you mean, where is it coming from? I want to know that my granddaughter is happy."

In a second, he normalised it. It actually really pissed me off that he could be so rational when all of this weird stuff was coming out of his mouth. Even to this day, when I discuss it with my mum she asks, "Are you sure that happened?" She knows it did, though, because she witnessed it on several occasions.

The conversation took an even stranger turn when he started to talk to me about men, a subject he would never have spoken to me about. My grandad had been amazing with me following a miscarriage I once had, and men were not a taboo subject at all, he just let me make my decisions. On this day, though, he said to me, "You know, you deserve somebody that's very special."

I was in a pretty weird place with relationships at that time, and so I said, "Well, I'm sure I'll get there, Grandad. I'm sure everything will work out the way that it needs to be."

He replied to that, "Just make sure you always realise and remember that you are the light the world needs to see. You are the light, you are the sunshine and don't settle."

It was hard to take in.

What a day. What a head fuck.

But then, bizarrely, life carried on. I did my best not to think too much about what we had discussed. You could say I happily distracted myself.

About a week later, I was in another situation with him in his lounge. All of a sudden, he started telling me about his time in the army, and the fact that he had been a boxer. This was so interesting to me because firstly I had never heard anything of the kind until this point, and secondly I had recently fallen in love with boxing.

"Grandad, why have you never told me this? How did you never tell me that boxing was a massive part of your life?"

The shift within him must have made him feel that now was a safe time to share these stories. He continued to share more and more over the coming weeks. He shared things that he'd never shared with anybody else. He shared stories of how promiscuous he had been before he met my nan. He told me about his bad gambling habit and how my nan had taken herself and the kids away from him until he sorted himself out, and he did, he never gambled again from that time onwards. The odd bet on the horses here and there, but he never allowed it to take hold again.

All of this was revelation after revelation. It was so strange to me because my grandad was an angel sent from above. Everything he shared, I needed to hear. He was essentially telling me the things that I would need in my life to come, such as that you could clear an addiction. Although I didn't realise it at the time I was addicted to partying, taking recreational drugs, drinking alcohol and generally distracting myself. I was addicted to it every single weekend.

He was showing me through his story – the fact that he'd used sex as a tool, the fact that he'd been addicted, the fact that he'd found in my nan his perfect partner; it was as if he was saying to me – *Everything is possible for you.*

Looking back, it was profound.

During that precious time, we truly were inseparable. We were closer than ever before, and we had a beautiful bond between us. Everyone could see it.

At about the eight-week period, I was now working from Bournemouth for three days a week, but he was deteriorating very rapidly. The more he deteriorated, the more he would share, and the closer we would get. I started to feel that he was handing over all this infinite wisdom, and although it still didn't make any sense to me at that time, and I didn't yet know what to do with it, I somehow knew it would end up being important. It was so beautiful. It was like I was living in a magical storytime with my grandad.

At around the nine-week mark, I walked into the house, via the back door one day and said, "Hi Grandad." All I heard from his bedroom was, "Oh God, she's here."

I playfully said, "What are you talking about? That's not very nice." When I walked in, I realised it was because he was still in bed, he hadn't been able to get up that day. And that was the real start of things deteriorating rapidly.

He hated this. I could see it in his eyes. He was so ashamed of himself. He was so proud. He was always dressed, ready and waiting in his chair, no matter what. And so I said, "Well if you're not going to come and sit with me in the chair today, I'm going to come to you." And I climbed on the bed with him. From that moment onwards, he didn't ever put on a show for me again.

Sadly, in those last few weeks, he told me he was scared about dying. He told me that he didn't want to go. He just wasn't ready. I became extremely protective of him. Other members of the family, or friends, would share their views on what should be done, and grandad would look to me with a knowing glance. They were not in tune with him anymore. People would suggest he needed to be kept moving and helped onto his zimmer frame. In my head, I was thinking – *What the fuck are you on about? He can't do any of that stuff anymore, stop it!*

In the eleventh week, for Father's Day of 2013, we decided to have a big, family barbecue because we knew it would be his last. All the family gathered together – there were loads of us. It was busy, but in a good way. My grandad looked over his brood in awe. He sat in his chair with his oxygen, just watching what was going on, with tears in his eyes. I kept an eye on him all day. All of his favourite humans were around him. It was very special. I couldn't imagine how it must be feeling knowing that this was going to be the last time this was going to happen in his life.

One of my uncles, who had been in denial about his prognosis, came over and said, "Come on dad, let's get you out of that chair. Let's get you outside."

With that, my grandad looked at me with this heartbreaking look on his face.

My uncle was not aware of the panic on my grandad's face, so he hoisted my grandad out of his chair. It was awful. He couldn't do anything. And my grandad bravely spoke up at that point and said, "I can't do this." At this point, my uncle was now on the floor trying to move my grandad's feet, and then the penny dropped for him. My uncle broke down because he realised where things were really at.

The look that my grandad gave me, I will never forget, for as long as I live. Every time I think of that look in his eye, I feel so sad for him. At that moment, he was a scared little boy, who just wanted to be protected.

I shouted at my uncle that day, I told him that what he did was not appropriate, I was furious with him. My mum and stepdad calmed me down. I just didn't know how he couldn't see what was going on! My uncle did later apologise for his actions.

After the Father's Day barbecue, my grandad went to bed and he never got out of bed again.

When I said goodbye to him that Sunday evening, I was sure it would be the last time I ever saw him, I felt that would be the night he would just think – *I've seen my family and now I'm good to go.*

I kissed him on the forehead and said, "Night grandad, I'll be in tomorrow." I sobbed all the way home.

The next morning, I called my mum, fearing the worst and was really shocked to hear that he was still with us. I went to the house and the whole family was there. It felt imminent. There were medical people coming in and out, starting to administer the diamorphine. There was that really pungent stench starting to form. It's a horrible smell. There is absolutely nothing quite like it – and not in a good way.

I didn't really know what I was doing that day, but I was intuitively guided to do certain things. I asked him if he was warm enough, I opened up the windows because I thought that if he's going to pass we don't want his soul loitering, we want him to go to my nan and be free. I sat there holding his hand and chatting to him. My older sister was a mess, she couldn't handle any of it at all, bless her heart.

I'd come to terms with some of the strange discussions we had had a few weeks earlier and so inside I was thinking – *Grandad thank you so much for reminding me that I'm the light. Thank you so much for telling me about your boxing in the army and for reminding me of the fact that good people still exist.* He really was the most amazing person because he always held space for me and never judged.

My mum was talking to him about memories from when she was a child. It was beautiful, all of us sat around sharing stories, and letting him be in a place of peace. He couldn't speak back but he would squeeze my fingers or move a little bit from time to time.

On the Monday evening, we all said goodbye, certain, once again, it would be the last time we would see him. The carer insisted we go home and get some rest and she promised to call us if anything happened.

No call came that night.

I called my mum in the morning and asked, "Is grandad still here?"

And she said, "Yes he is. I don't know how he's done it, but he's still here at the moment. Just prepare yourself, Lu."

I made my way over and as soon as I walked in, I noticed the smell had become even stronger. All the windows and doors were open, to allow the airflow. I walked in and said, "Hey, Grandad." I took up my seat next to him, held his hand and started chatting away to him, chewing his ears off about absolutely anything that popped into my mind. As I sat holding his hand, I got this really intense feeling that he was going to pass. It was weird, I had a knowing, but I didn't know how I knew. I kept chatting to him and letting him know that it was okay.

When everyone had left the room, I leaned forward and whispered in his ear, "If you know that it's time for you to go, then please go to Nan. We're going to be okay, I promise you. We will never forget you."

My mum, my uncle, and my stepdad were in the other room. My stepdad popped his head in the door and told me that the three of them were popping out; they were going to pick something up and they would be forty-five minutes or so. I said goodbye to them from my grandad's bedside. It was just my sister, my other uncle, and the carer left in the house.

It was silent now.

My sister was on one side of me. I was holding my grandad's hand as we heard the car pull away. And then my grandad sat up, gasped his last breath of air and with that, he was gone.

I feel in my soul, to this day, that he waited for my mum to leave, before he chose to go. The busyness, the noise had all stopped. He surrendered, and he went.

It was so powerful and heartbreaking, all in one moment. We all cried like babies.

What's even more strange was that my nan and my grandad had passed away in exactly the same room, in exactly the same position, holding my hand, just over 13 years apart.

6

As expected, after my grandad passed, the house was a very sad place to be. My older sister and I were inconsolable; we sobbed as we hugged. My uncle wrapped his arms around both of us, stepping instantly into the lead man of the family role. The carer held safe space for us to grieve, doing whatever she could to make the situation better.

Suddenly, my uncle panicked and realised he needed to call my mum and his brother. They had only been gone a matter of minutes when grandad passed. I knew it was going to break my mum's heart, that he had passed while she was away. I wasn't sure how she would handle it. My uncle made the dreaded call, he was really stepping up into his role as the senior male in the family, following in my grandad's footsteps. Through the phone, we could hear my mum's trauma, it was terrible. My uncle said they would be back in a few minutes.

The carer went off and started to make some calls to get things organised. I had never considered the process of what happens when someone passes. There's so much to deal with straight after a heartbreaking, life-changing event – the paperwork, the calls, the organisation. Thank goodness for the carer who took care of the practical aspects while we sat, holding my grandad's hand.

Despite knowing for twelve weeks that my grandad was going to pass, it did not make it any easier when it actually happened. The pain was unbearable. I had always wondered whether it was better to know and to be able to plan the last days and weeks, or if it would be better to be unexpected. A few years down the line I would test that theory out for real.

When my grandad passed, I felt a presence leave the room. Of course, my family thought I was crazy. I knew my grandad had not really been there physically since the Sunday of Father's Day. However, something must have been hanging around, as I'll never forget the feeling I had, like a cold shiver, and someone gently brushing on my arm. I imagined this was his soul going to my nan, who would be waiting.

When my mum arrived back at the house, there was a huge, second wave of upset. She walked in the room to find her dad lying there, gone. I could see the guilt on her face that she had not been there when her dad had decided to cross over. It was clear to me that he had waited for her to go out for him to be able to leave, but it certainly was not the time for that conversation. She was devastated, naturally. She kept saying, "I should never have gone out." My mum was the 'apple' of my grandad's eye. They had such a special relationship. Over the years, all of the three brothers had typical sibling 'beef' with my mum because she was so special to my grandad, being the only daughter.

For a while, we stayed in his room. We wanted to remain close to him, connected in whichever way we could. It felt as if an hour or so may have passed when someone suggested putting the kettle on. Here in the UK, generally, when things become challenging, the kettle gets put on. There is a really beautiful feeling of community within a family when the kettle is boiled and a fresh cup of tea is in hand. It's almost like our armour. We can make any necessary decisions when the family comes together around tea.

It was the first time in a while my sister or I had left his room, we had loyally stayed by his side the last few days, holding his hand, since it happened. We meandered into the lounge where the rest of the family were. Mum had made us all fresh tea. I sat and stared into the empty space where my grandad would normally have been perched. It was weird. It was eery. I missed him so much. I wanted him back. He'd only just gone.

As we drank tea, everybody started sharing stories. I sat and listened to some of the amazing stories, shared by his children. I was not ready to share any of the stories we had shared together in those past recent weeks. They were private stories between my grandad and me. I could feel a shift in the room whilst the stories were being shared. I feel talking about him kept our spirits up that day. It made us feel he was still there, and we were still connected, that he had just gone to the toilet or something. From time to time, we had a little giggle, sharing some of the lighter moments that had happened in the recent weeks, but the heartbreak in the room was prominent. He was a truly, deeply, loved man. I am certain to this day, he was sat in that room with us – a smile on his face, a few tears in his kind, beautiful eyes, watching over his loved ones.

Death is such a weird thing. The physical body is gone, and there's that nagging pain of knowing you will never see them again in that physical form. And yet, there had to be something, something more. There's just no way we would go through all of this, for there to be nothing else, right?

That afternoon felt like being on a surreal, emotional rollercoaster. It was such a contradiction, it felt good that my grandad was no longer suffering, but selfishly, I wished to have him back for just one more conversation. It had been really horrific watching him struggle and take those last few breaths.

Before we knew it, it was maybe four or five o'clock in the afternoon. Things were being cleaned and put away. Discussions started up about who had to call who, and what jobs people would be organising over the coming days. I wasn't quite ready for such practicalities at this point, so I chose to leave. I felt a strong desire that I needed to be on my own and process everything that had gone on over the previous eleven and a half weeks.

I got in my car, drove up the road a couple of hundred meters to get out of sight of the house, stopped, and sobbed like a baby. I had wanted to be strong and hold it together for my mum. I wanted to make sure that she was okay and I didn't want her to see her baby crying at this time. I have no idea how long I sat there crying before I pulled myself together to drive back to my friend's place.

When I got home that night, I wrote my boss an email bringing him up to speed on my grandad. I received a really lovely email back from him. I thank my lucky stars that God had sent this guy to me at that time. Looking back, it was probably a little weird that the only thing I did that night was email my boss, but I must have wanted attention from somebody, and for them to tell me everything was going to be alright; my grandad, the one person I really needed at that time, was no longer there. So, I guess it was my boss who was my go-to person in that moment.

That evening was horrific. I was alone in the house, opposite the cemetery where my nan's ashes were. I felt so uneasy. I felt like there were things around me. I would suddenly feel something cold by my neck and get those little bone shivers, but there would be nobody there. Was I driving myself crazy with this, or was it really happening?

The next morning, in typical Lucy style, I woke up as if nothing had happened. I knew I needed to dust myself down, get my shit together and support my mum and my sister. I also needed to check in with work. I was almost clinical – as if I had allowed the emotions to flow, then quickly thought – *Oh God, I can't be doing that again.* That was the way I knew how to cope back then. You hear people say, "Show up like you weren't crying the night before," and I was going for that independent, strong woman kind of vibe. I thought nobody needed to know that yesterday my heart was completely broken into a million little pieces. Today I'm tough, I'm strong and I'm back.

Truth be known, though, tough as I was on the outside, on the inside I wasn't strong at all. I was actually super sensitive. Believe it or not, at this period in my life I was truly poor at communication, especially when it meant articulating how I was feeling personally. I would close down, lash out verbally – anything to distract from having to be vulnerable and let people know I was hurting. My coping mechanism was – be tough, be strong, hold it together!

I truly believed at this time, that method had never let me down.

I stayed down in Bournemouth an extra couple of days after my grandad passed. I wished to be around to support my family. I also knew I would not get disturbed or encouraged to go out in

Bournemouth. No one knew I was even there, so I was able to process everything that had gone on, before going back to my life in London.

On the way back to London, my best friend, James, called and suggested I meet him in Clapham to celebrate my grandad's life. As much as I did not feel like celebrating, I also did not feel like being alone, and I definitely felt like getting pissed. As soon as I got back, I dumped the car and my stuff at my apartment, spruced myself up a little bit, for the first time in weeks, and headed to Clapham. James was a very dear friend, we had become very close since the early days of clubbing back in Bournemouth. We had been through so much together and knew we could rely on each other like a brother and sister. He was always the first one to pick me up, and me him. He tragically passed in 2016. God rest his sweet soul.

On the short walk to the station, a couple of my girlfriends called me, so they came to join us also. We stood outside a bar in Clapham, the sun was shining and it was a glorious hot day. There were moments of emotion, and moments where I felt guilt for laughing and joking with my friends. We did a lot of toasting to my grandad. Long story short, I got pissed. Totally and utterly pissed.

I had a great time that day. After the initial upset, I held it together quite well. It got to the point, after several hours, where one of the girls suggested that we go and get something to eat because, in her words, "Lucy's getting really pissed." To be fair, we were all getting rather well-oiled, over-confident and quite loud by this point, but in typical Lucy fashion, I declared, "Nah eating is cheating, let's just carry on." I had that real masculine bravado thing going on and I felt like – *I can handle it, don't you worry, I'll get through this no matter what.*

And I did.

7

At some point that following week, my family asked me to do a reading at the funeral, and, of course, I agreed. I felt it was my responsibility. Deep down, though, I was thinking – *Shit, I don't know if I can hold it together to do that.* Then I thought about it some more and realised that as they've asked me, and it's for grandad, I've got to do it.

What's really interesting, for some reason I wrote a poem. I'd never written a poem before in my life, and I have never written one since. I showed the poem to my mum and my uncle at first, to ask their opinion. They both burst into tears and said it was "absolutely perfect."

My sister got wind of this and asked to be involved too. I was only asked because everyone knew I would be able to hold it together, whereas my sister came with no such guarantees, so I suggested we read a paragraph each. This seemed to be a good compromise, and she was happy with that.

On the day of the funeral, before the hearse had even turned up at my grandad's house to collect us, my sister turned to me and said, "Lucy, I'm not sure I can read it." I reassured her it was fine, I would do it on my own, if I had to. I suggested she should come up with me and we would stand together, and then if she felt strong enough to read it she could, and if not, I would do it with her beside me.

When we got to the crematorium, it was busy. There were so many people there. It was absolutely freezing that day, for that time of year. Perhaps it was just me, the numbness and shock of it being the final goodbye.

I had driven my sister and my nephew to the cemetery. We had left early to escape the awful bit at the house when the cars turn up with the coffin. However, there is no avoiding that moment at the cemetery. I saw the hearse with the coffin pull in, and my sister and I broke down. It was a hideous sight. It was a level of emotion I was not used to. I'd been to funerals before, but this was something entirely different. I thought – *Oh God, I've got to hold it together.*

When I saw my mum, she was totally brokenhearted, it hurt me so much. Thankfully, my stepdad was there to help my mum. I looked around at the whole family and noticed the different dynamics, it was very interesting. One of my uncles was cracking jokes – that was his coping mechanism – other members of the family were quieter and more internalised.

The crowds had gathered by now, it was far busier than I had ever envisaged. Some people were outside, others were already in the waiting room.

Then we got the nod to go into the crematorium.

The service was absolutely beautiful. It was very apparent throughout, how very loved my grandad was. Everyone who spoke mentioned his beautiful energy. My stepdad and my uncle did short readings, and then we sang. Next up, my sister and I were called to do the reading. We walked slowly together up to the platform to do our bit. I took a deep breath and then started to read the first paragraph, which went okay. Then it was my sister's turn. She read one line and then the emotion got the better of her. She burst into tears and couldn't read anymore because she was sobbing so much. I had no choice but to carry on and read the whole thing. I got to the very last line of the poem, which read – *Grandad, you were the best, and how are we going to carry on this life without you* – and I broke down. I physically couldn't say those words. Everyone was watching me as I wept, there was silence in the room – it felt like everybody held their breath. Out of nowhere, my sister kicked into protective mode and took the paper from my hands. She finished the poem, in style. It was a real moment. I had really needed my big sister, and for the first time that I can ever remember in my life, she stepped up, protected me and got it done. I appreciate that might sound mean, but it's the truth. It was almost like she put an angel wing around me and said – *Don't worry, I've got this, we'll get through it*. So she held it together and spoke those last words, and the whole crematorium was in floods of tears because it was so beautiful and so heartfelt. They had witnessed a very special moment.

After we had finished, we returned to our seats and sobbed. We let all of the emotions out. The whole service had been extremely emotional. It was like a little whirlwind of magical energy had been building within the crematorium.

Just when you feel you cannot cry anymore, we got to the bit in the funeral where the coffin is dropped. It took my breath away, as it all suddenly seemed so final.

As we were leaving, we walked passed where grandad was, and put flowers down. We said our goodbyes and then left the room to go to an outdoor space, where people congregate. When we walked outside it was really hot, the sun was shining. It felt so weird to have gone from this sombre mood inside, with everyone crying and feeling sad, to outside where people are coming up and giving you hugs and making polite conversation. It felt like the outside world was calling us to move on with life.

We went back to my grandad's house, for the wake. It felt even weirder having all of these random people there, most of them he probably hadn't seen in bloody donkey's years either. He had become a bit of a bugger towards the end – he didn't really want to see people; I guess you could say he had great boundaries because essentially he didn't want to be around people that didn't mean anything to him.

I sat there in the corner looking at the chair where he used to sit, next to the stool where I had put myself for the last twelve weeks. There were moments that afternoon when I thought I saw him sitting there, and then I would look again and it would actually be somebody else. To be totally honest, I was quite judgemental and critical that day. I was really angry with these people because I was hurting – *Why are you even here? And why the fuck are you cracking jokes, don't you know my grandad has just died?*

Regardless of how I was feeling, I waited until the end because I wanted to support my mum, and I wanted to help her tidy up and sort things out. After we had tidied up, everyone sat down in total silence. We had done everything we needed to keep that stiff upper lip and get through it all. All of a sudden we were in an eery silence. It felt like we had reached the end of a road. Nobody wanted to talk, it was a time to retract and reflect. Out of nowhere, my stepdad – who is such a gorgeous man, and whose answer to everything, whenever there's a problem, is food – stood up and asked, "Does anyone want fish and chips?" And while everybody else thought it was a great idea, I just thought – *How the hell is that going to fix this?*

I knew then it was time for me to go, so I said my goodbyes and went.

I stayed down in Bournemouth just another day to sort myself out, and then I went back to London. And when I say that from that moment onwards I went back to business as usual, that's exactly what I did.

8

After my grandad passed and I had reflected, albeit briefly, about those precious last weeks we had spent together, I unconsciously decided to block everything out and go straight back to being the thriving, hustling, busy Project Manager that I had been before. Turning up early, leaving late, and immersing myself fully back into the party scene. On some level, I was trying to convince myself that the previous weeks had not happened, that they weren't reality. Looking back, I don't believe I was ready to handle the magnitude of what those conversations with grandad had meant or implied. My partying after my grandad's passing became much worse than it had been before. I made some decisions and choices in the months after grandad that would very quickly have a profound effect on my life, some good and a lot not-so good.

A month or so after the funeral, into the summer of that year, I went to the V Festival in Essex, determined to have an amazing time. I went to a lot of festivals back then and absolutely loved them. It was where I could truly let my hair down with my friends. All of us were doing pretty well for ourselves and worked very hard in our careers. This was our escape, though, it was our time to be anything we chose to be. No deadlines, no phones ringing, no conference calls. Just being with the people we loved.

On this occasion, my best friend, James, a.k.a Jimbo, decided to grace us with his presence. He was hilarious, no matter where we went or what we did – great fun to be around. Months earlier we had organised transport for a group of us to leave from my apartment in Wimbledon. We had all been in a group chat for months leading up to this event, so everyone knew exactly what was going on. The night before I got one of those typically famous Jimbo texts, "Okay, so I may have been talked into going out tonight, but I will 100% be there tomorrow morning.. no matter what. Do NOT leave without me." My best friend and I both joked that we would be shocked if he actually made it to us the next morning on time. And if he did, we placed bets as to whether he would have been to sleep or not.

The next morning, everyone had arrived and we were good to go, but there was no sign of Jimbo – as expected. We called him, texted him, called some more, and then we made a group decision – it was time to go, without him. We all loved him dearly, but he was consistently inconsistent. So, we set off for the festival. About an hour into the journey, my phone started ringing. It was Jimbo! He had passed out, woken up and realised he had missed us, and so he sweet-talked his Dad into driving him from South West London to Essex for the festival. Classic Jimbo!

Jimbo was a proper head-case, but in an amazing way. He was crazy yet also the kindest, most beautiful, sweet, loving soul you would ever wish to have in your life. We were family at the core. I always knew I could rely on him. Before we were about to go out and have a good time we would always hang up the phone by saying, "All aboard the crazy train – toot toot." That was one of our sayings.

When we arrived at V, the minibus dropped us off and we had the awful challenge of carrying everything to the campsite. To my fellow festival-goers, I admire you all, we have been able to navigate things that very few others have succeeded in. Thankfully, Jimbo arrived just as we were about to start the mission. He was totally off it, dancing around and ready to get straight back on it – bearing in mind it was only around 11am at this point.

Once we had navigated our way to the campsite, we started to get our space organised. This was going to be our home until Monday morning, so getting it sorted now before we got wasted was a must.

Once we were set up, we decided to take a walk around the festival site. It was always interesting to do this the day before the actual festival got started, to see what kind of crowd was there. The vibe was already starting to hot up, the weather was stunning, and it was forecast to stay that way the entire weekend.

That night we had a really good time. Great music, good friends, a bit of dancing, and lots of chatting. We stayed up until the early hours of the morning, but decided some sleep was necessary, so that we were ready to party the next day.

The next morning, I was up really early. It was a beautiful day, yet again, and so I sat drinking water and watched as the world started to wake up around me. With no sign of life in the tents around me, I went for a quick wash in the communal area – or what we would call back then a 'bird bath' – which was where we splashed a bit of water on ourselves to freshen. It was water, wet wipes, deodorant and done!

Once I was dressed and ready for the day, the others started to stir. I lit one of the BBQs so we could make bacon sarnies. I was a meat-eater back in those days. I joked with everyone that this would be our first and last meal of the day. As I cooked, the cans and bottles of booze got cranked open. It was about 9 am and we were turning up the heat on this party.

The gates for the festival opened at 12 pm, which is when the actual festivities started, so we set off in good time towards the gates – a decent walk away. In the queue, I started chatting to people, and make friends with all the security and the police. It freaked my friends out because they knew what contraband I had in my bra, but I didn't care. You never know when you might need their help, and anyway, it's nice to be nice.

Once in, we headed straight for the VIP tent. We had bought VIP tickets this year, so we got a premium experience and use of better facilities. It was a glorious day again, and there was loads of room to sit outside in the sun.

We were all starting to get our boogie on and have a good time. Everyone was beautiful. Everywhere you looked there were women with flowers in their hair, and guys with sunglasses on and their guns out. For some reason, when I went to festivals I drank pints of cider. I never drank it at any other time, but it was always a thing for me as soon as I crossed the festival line. Me and the girls had just ordered fresh pints from the bar, when I saw this absolutely stunning guy across the VIP area. He was tall, dark and absolutely gorgeous. I mean there were many gorgeous men there, but this one really caught my eye. I said to my girlfriends, as I nodded in his direction "Oh God, seriously, this soon?" We all started to giggle.

At this point, I had been single for a couple of years, after a breakup. I was dating and chatting to people but it had been at least two years since I was into anything serious. I was just starting to find my feet again and feeling ready to get back out there and date, but in reality, I had such a good group of friends that I didn't really make the time or effort to fit a man into my life. I liked this guy, though, there was something about the way he held himself, the way he walked, the way he looked. I could tell, even from this distance, that he was going to be trouble, but I kind of liked it. He was a flirt, you could tell, someone who had his eyes everywhere, but there was something raw that was attracting me to him.

I was telling my friend that I thought this guy was absolutely gorgeous, when all of a sudden she said, "Oh my god Lucy, he's coming over." Why is it that as soon as someone says that to you, panic kicks in, you feel you've got lipstick all over your face and teeth, and all of a sudden you're a sweaty mess? All these questions come up – What if they don't like me? What if they do like me?

He came over and started flirting. We chatted and then quite naturally began dancing. He pulled me in close to him and asked my name. He really was smoking hot. I saw the girls giggling and gossiping over their drinks. Those girls were my world; they only wished for my happiness – and vice versa. It had been such a shitty year all in all. I could feel their love as they could see I was finally starting to smile freely again.

After a while, one of the 'hot' guy's mates pulled me away from him. "Come on. Come and dance with me," he said. It was really weird. I wasn't sure if the 'hot' guy had sent this guy in to act as a block, or if this guy was just being a bit of an idiot. Either way, I decided it was not for me. To be fair, he was a good dancer. He was clearly a lot of fun too, as everyone was laughing and joking with him, but something felt a little off. I asked one of my friends if they could entertain the weird dancing guy for a little while so that I could take a breather. I moved away and went over to the bar to grab a bit of space. Whilst in the queue for the bar, the 'hot' guy followed me over and came to speak with me again. We blatantly fancied each other, and had this weird connection going on. During the conversation at the bar, he made a strange comment. It was something along the lines of – *It's a real shame because I think that you are perfect.*

I was confused, so I asked him, "What's the real shame?"

"Sometimes you've just, you know, you've got to step aside."

Now I'll be totally honest with you. By this point in the day, I was starting to feel a little bit off it. This guy was making no sense, and games were not really a thing I enjoyed; the last thing I needed was someone messing with my head.

"I don't know what the fuck you talking about, you're talking in riddles mate," I said very abruptly cutting him off. Thankfully, by this point I had been served, so I grabbed my drink and walked away. When I returned to the girls, they asked what had been going on. I said "He's a bit weird. Very hot, but weird. Next."

I got straight back on it and carried on dancing, and having a good time with my friends. Out of nowhere, the weird dancer guy appeared. He was constantly on my case, flirting, spinning me around. He grabbed me and asked, "Can we could meet up tomorrow?"

Now, I was at the festival with my friends to have a good time and not to be tied down. I told him, "Look mate, if we bump into each other tomorrow then we bump into each other tomorrow. Let's leave it at that."

There is no intent to blow my own trumpet when I say this, but whenever I was out and having a good time at these kind of things, I was like a honeypot to the bees, where men were concerned. I would get lost in the music, and lost in myself, and I'm guessing that would appear attractive to the opposite sex. On many occasions, the girls would laugh at how the men would congregate around me, and I would be blissfully unaware.

I decided that this was my turning point, this was where I was going to let my hair down and release everything that needed to be released and just frickin enjoy myself; step back into the Lucy that everybody knew. The good time, fun Lucy was coming back.

That night, I rounded up about 50 people, mostly strangers – who were all up for an after-party – and invited them back to our tents. It was amazing. We all sat chatting until about six in the morning. I was such a good time girl back then and this was great, I was in my element. It distracted me. I felt happy. I laughed. I was getting loads of attention. I was getting all of my needs met.

The next morning, with barely any sleep, I was back making bacon sarnies again. It was the only meal we had the day before and it would likely be the same again today. It was a role I had willingly stepped into. I loved to make sure everyone was okay, that they were fed and feeling good. As soon as I was done eating, I was offered a 'pick me up'. It was about 11 am, so I thought – *When in Rome, why the heck not? Looks like we are in for some fun today girls and boys.* About twenty minutes later, the party was in full swing. I started rounding up the troops and we headed over to the VIP area again, where we could sit and chill in the sun, whilst drinking beers.

From out of nowhere the weird, dancer guy from the previous day appeared. He was throwing lots of cheeky, cheesy chat-up lines at me. He seemed harmless – just a cheeky Jack the Lad kind of person, who wanted to fit in with us, so I introduced him to the squad and he joined the party.

I spotted the 'hot guy' from yesterday observing all of this from the bar. I smiled at him and he smiled back. I wondered what was going on with him. I tried to block it out, but it was starting to get under my skin. I decided to go over and speak to him, and have it out.

I walked over to the bar to buy a drink and he immediately came over to me and said, "Really, I'm gutted."

"What are you gutted about?" I asked him, impatiently, but he just wouldn't say. He just looked at me with his beautiful blue eyes and said, "I'm sorry."

Spoiler alert for a forthcoming story, but I found out about a year later that the weird, dancer guy had turned around to his mate – the hot guy – and said, "You can have any of the tens of thousands of girls here, but that one. You're not allowed that one." And for whatever reason, his mate had said okay, and granted him ownership of me, without any consultation with yours truly.

In that moment, though, in the VIP tent, I didn't know anything about this conversation. I just thought his behaviour was weird and it wasn't something I was prepared to nurture or chase, so I dropped it. I went back to my friends and explained to them what had happened, they agreed it was time to forget about that one.

The rest of the weekend was amazing, we all had the best time drinking, dancing and enjoying ourselves. My goodness, we had a lot of stories to tell off the back of that weekend. It was a really good time, loaded with very happy memories. I never realised this would be the last festival Jimbo and I would go to together.

When it eventually came time to leave the festival we hugged and said our goodbyes, and then went off in our different directions.

9

When I got home, I sat and for a while and thought about the weekend and then quickly snapped into practical mode. Back to work.

Within a few weeks, everyone from the festival had found each other on Facebook – including the weird, dancer guy. Oblivious to me he had exchanged details with one of my friends, Jackie, so we could all keep in touch. When later I asked her how they had found me, she said "You looked like you had such a good time with him, I thought you'd like to see him again." Thanks, Jackie.

A few weeks later, I was out in southwest London one night, with my good friend Anthony. We had been for a steak and a few glasses of red wine – as it was our favourite thing to do. We went to a bar near his place in Balham for a final glass before I hit the road back home on the Northern line to South Wimbledon. I had known Anthony for many moons. We had first crossed paths in Bournemouth years earlier, and become re-acquainted when I moved up to London. We became great friends and always had a good giggle together. He was a beautiful soul. At this point in my life, I could rely on him for anything, and vice versa.

I was nearing the end of my glass of wine when my phone started ringing. I didn't recognise the number, so I ignored it; I was slightly well-oiled and in the company of someone, so felt it rude to answer. Once we had said our goodbyes and I started the two-minute walk to the tube station, my phone rang again, so I answered it.

"Oy oy, how you doing hot stuff?"

It was weird, dancer guy, the cheeky chappy from the festival.

"How did you get my number?"

"Oh I asked Jackie, I told her that I'd had a proper laugh with you at the festival and so she gave me your number."

I thought — *I'm going to have to have a little chat with Jackie about giving my number out to complete strangers.*

But, over the next few weeks, I let my guard down with him because he made me laugh, and we started to hang out a little more. In the September of that year, I went on my first date with him. Very quickly, I realised there was something not quite right, there were so many red flags.

Oh my goodness, I paid the price for ignoring those warning signs.

Distractions

Isn't it interesting how at key times of stress in our lives, we reach for things to distract us from sitting in that moment and having to feel it?

I'm sure I can be bold enough to speak on behalf of most of us when I say sitting in that moment of hurt — like when a relationship breaks down, or a loved one passes — is not something we would choose for ourselves. If we had the option, we would most likely choose to bypass any of that; keep everyone we love alive and close to us always, and never have to experience loss or lack. However, that's not the way this human experience has been designed for us.

How would we remember abundance if we had not experienced a sense of lack? How would we recognise happiness if we had not felt what it is to feel sad?

These emotional experiences are what shape us and assist our evolution. Although, at the time of the experience it doesn't always feel that way. More often than not, it hurts — and we are taught from a young age to run away from pain, that it isn't good. This, though, is when we step into the world of distractions. Distractions have been designed as a test for us.

It is of primary importance that we acknowledge and recognise what distractions we have in our lives. Distractions are everywhere. In the consumer world we live, most of the material goods on offer are there to distract us from feeling. This is the harsh reality of how the human experience has been shaped for generations. I, me, mine. More, more, more. Distractions are often subtly wrapped in discussions with friends that can go something along the lines of, "let your hair down....you deserve it....oh it's just a bit of fun." And that's where the trouble starts.

At that time in my life, distractions looked to me like alcohol, drugs and sex. If I had a bad day at the office, I'd have a drink. If it was the end of the week, I'd have a drink. If it was a good day, I'd have a drink. When my grandad passed, my aim was to get as wasted as possible.

All harmless bits of fun, on the surface, but the truth of the matter was, I was doing it to stop my feeling of the bad day, or the loss and grief. Strangely, I was also doing it to celebrate too. Unconsciously, at every opportunity, I was blocking out my feelings. Notoriously alcohol and drugs, although they succeeded in temporarily blocking out feelings, inevitably led to feelings of loneliness kicking in at some point later on. That in itself becomes a good excuse to get connected with an ex or someone from the past, in order to feel less lonely. But, that would only start the cycle of guilt and shame the following morning, when I came to my senses and realised I didn't want to be keeping that kind of company.

This, my friends, is what I mean when I talk about emotional trauma. Experiences that have happened, but then cause you to run from those painful feelings, and look for distractions as a tactic to avoid feeling them.

Have you ever observed this pattern in yourself?

10

Not long after my grandad died, around the time of V festival, I kept getting an overwhelming urge that I had to go away somewhere on my own. It was not something I had ever done before. I had travelled all over the world with other people, or flown to various places on my own and met up with people once I was there, but I had never gone away all on my own for a proper holiday.

When I began telling people that I wanted to go travelling, everybody I told wanted to come with me. For some reason, though, I was absolutely certain in my gut, that I needed to do it on my own. It was just a passing thought at that time, though, I was busy working so I didn't really do too much about it.

Since I had hit 29, I had developed this overwhelming urge to travel again. I had gone off to Australia for a while when I was in my early 20s. I was in a relationship at the time, and my boyfriend Mark stayed back in the UK. He was supportive of my choice to travel, as it wasn't really his thing, and he gave me the space to live out my dream, which I loved him very much for.

The first time I landed in Sydney, I totally fell head over heels in love — not with a person, but with the place. Considering I had never been there before, it felt like home to me. I remember flying in and the pilot telling us to look to one side so we could see the Opera House and the Harbour Bridge. I was in awe of this place. It was everything I had wished England was; the lifestyle of being outdoors and on the beach really spoke to my soul. It was weird, I had grown up in a beach town, but the weather in England did not really offer what Australia did. That first trip cemented my love for the place, a love that would remain with me right up to the very moment of writing this book. I had no idea that it would feature so heavily in my life going forward. I just knew something about the place felt like home to me.

At that time, when I was 29, I was still working in JPMorgan, and climbing the corporate ladder. I felt very important in the shaping of the technology of the company at that time. Every time I would get the urge, the pull of Australia, I would shut it down telling myself — *You're too old to travel now*. I had really let society get into my head that I would not find my husband, settle down and have children if I went travelling. I thought that flying off to the other side of the world would not bring in the things I really wanted for my life.

I was lucky, though, that I had the opportunity to travel quite a bit with JPMorgan. I had been able to work from the Sydney office for a short stint, and they even offered me an opportunity to move there. I had been with the company for so long, and they would have willingly let me work across the other side of the world rather than lose my knowledge. I was scared though. I feared my friends would forget me. I feared my family would be so far away when things went wrong, and that I would not be able to make it back in time. I was essentially living for the 'what ifs', rather than listening to the truth in my heart and soul.

And so, I stayed in England. I prioritised other people's happiness above my own. I prioritised my fears over my love and my truth.

In September, not long after my grandad's passing, I was right back into the swing of work. I was travelling down to IBM in Portsmouth at least once or twice a week, and I loved it. I would head down on a Tuesday morning, stay overnight, and then head back home the following day. It was great to get out of the office, and also on a personal level, it was really convenient because I had some friends who lived in Portsmouth, so I got to spend time with them.

There was one evening specifically that will forever stay in my mind. We had been considering going out for a bite to eat, but one of the girls suggested going over to hers for dinner, and that she would cook. It sounded perfect to me. I was staying five minutes drive from hers, so it was super convenient, and it meant we could chat properly. It was the first time I had seen her after my grandad's passing. Interestingly, I had met this beautiful soul at V Festival the year before. We had had one of those magical moments whereby we met and clicked straight away, and then we were like glue from that moment on.

I arrived after work, a bottle of wine under my arm. I kicked my shoes off at the front door and made my way through to the kitchen, where she was cooking up a storm. She had prepared the dinner table. I grabbed the wine glasses, poured us an extra-large glass each and we got chatting. We went through the normal mundane conversations of work stuff, and then moved on to life stuff.

"How are you doing?" she asked.

I said, "Okay."

She nudged a little further, "No, come on, how are you really doing?"

I turned to her, more serious than I had ever been in all the time we'd known each other, and from nowhere I just said, "I have to get away. Babe, I absolutely have got to get away."

"Why?" She looked concerned.

"I'm stressed. I hate my job. I just don't love life at the moment. I haven't got over my grandad. I'm in a fucking mess."

"Babe, what are you going to do? Where are you going to go? Let me come with you," she responded.

"You know what? I've got to do this alone. For the first time in my life, I feel like I need to do something on my own. Otherwise, I feel I will not achieve what I need to do."

I didn't really know what I was talking about.

It was a dark September evening in England. At that time of year in the UK, it's starting to get a bit grimy, and a little bit cold. It was raining outside, and we could not help getting carried away chatting and dreaming about hot and sunny locations.

"Spain?" my friend suggested.

"Nah," I replied. I was thinking bigger, better, further away. Then it suddenly came to me, "Thailand! I've got to go to Thailand." I had been there a few times before and I loved it.

Moments earlier, my friend's housemate had returned home from work. She came into the dining area and joined us on the large bench for a glass of wine. "Lucy's going to go to Thailand," my friend shared excitedly.

Her housemate lit up, she said, "Oh my God, if you're going to Thailand, you need to go to this place called Tiger Muay Thai, you can have a holiday and do fitness at the same time. Lucy, with your love of boxing, you will love this place so much. I've been there a few times, you will meet amazing people. You have to go." She was so excited for me, she carried on, "I am so jealous at the thought of you going there. I know you like your boxing, so if you go there at least you've got something to distract yourself with, you're not going to be on your own then."

So, of course, impulsive me, I thought – *Fuck it*.

I got on my laptop there and then and booked it. I closed my laptop with a huge grin on my face. I had just booked a trip to Thailand, on my own. What was I thinking? However, in that moment, I loved it.

I loved this version of me who booked things without even having booked the time off work. *Fuck it, they'll honour it* — I thought.

I had booked flights and accommodation from London to Phuket, via Bangkok, plus a week's all-inclusive training at Tiger Muay Thai. I was set to leave in just over a month. I had searched out the best accommodation nearby and found a gorgeous little hotel called CocoVille. My friend's housemate had visited there and she said this hotel was lovely. It was about a 5-minute walk from Tiger Muay Thai and I would be very comfortable there. Of course, I had to book the best room in the hotel. I was delighted, on the spur of the moment I had taken action that had been calling me to do so for years.

For the first time since the sun-lounger in Dubai, just before my world fell apart, I felt content. In just a matter of weeks, I would be on my merry way to Bangkok, then on to Phuket. *Let the adventures begin* — I thought.

11

The next few weeks passed extremely quickly. There were things that kept me busy outside of work — getting currency, deciding what I needed to take, and getting in as much boxing training as possible. I had no idea what to pack. Even making simple decisions such as whether to take my boxing gloves or not was a challenge at that point in my life. When in doubt, overpack! Ladies, I'm sure you can resonate with that. I took so much stuff that I did not require, it was ridiculous.

The guy I had started seeing maybe a week or so before, had started to stress because I was leaving. He knew I had recently lost the man that meant the world to me, my grandad, so as much as he didn't want me to go, he knew I really needed to do this.

Before I knew it, I was standing at the airport with my bags beside me. I was completely and utterly alone, about to head off on my very first solo trip, where I would know absolutely no one. There would be no one there to greet me as I landed. No one to show me where I was going, or what I was doing wrong. That's when it hit me — *What the hell am I doing? This is insane.*

I was scared. I had all these little voices piping up — *What will you do if the plane crashes? No one will miss you. What if you get taken off somewhere like those horror stories you've heard about Thailand? What if you get involved in drugs? What if you get lost? How will you communicate, they don't speak English?* My mind was going absolutely haywire. I was alone in Heathrow Airport. I knew no one. There was only one thing to do. Get checked in, go through security, and then wine!

So that's exactly what I did.

I went to the nearest bar, got settled in with a huge glass of wine, and finally started to relax. The more I relaxed, the more people I seemed to attract to talk to. I had no idea at the time that spending time in airports was going to become one of my favourite things to do in the coming years. I met some lovely people that day.

I was two glasses of wine in, when I heard the call for my flight. *Oh my goodness! This is it, it's really happening, it's time to go.*

As I boarded the plane, I was welcomed by the most beautiful, smiley, happy faces I had ever seen In my life. I was flying Thai Airways for this trip. The plane was very purple, and I loved that. Once the doors closed, I knew there was no going back and so, again, I started to relax and enjoy the moment. The hostesses walked through the plane spraying this awful stuff through the air vents, it was horrible, it made you feel like you were drowning in chemicals.

The plane felt so gentle and quiet; I was used to the noise and chaos of the boisterous trading floor. I was able, for the first time in a long time, to just kick back in my chair and reflect on how hectic life had been since Dubai in April. That six-month period had been chaotic – all about other people and distraction, it had been about everything except me. In fact, it had always been like that. I had been getting wrecked and running away from it all; that had been my pattern for months, for years even! And, for the first time in a long time, I sat in my chair on the plane and thought – *Thank you God, I've made it here. I've got some time to myself. It's time for some peace.*

It was twelve hours later when the plane landed in Bangkok, and nothing could have prepared me for what hit me as I left the plane. That initial wall of heat hit me smack in the face. It was like a ball of absolute fire – hot, humid, and sticky. And then, as I walked into the terminal, there was this incredible smell, it was the smell of the orchids. It was overwhelming, in such a good way. Then there was the brightness of the purples and the pinks of the flowers. It was a totally amazing sensory overload. It was almost like I had walked into a wall of something so powerful, it took all of my attention to focus on just being there. There was a beautiful aroma of Thai food swirling around the place too, it was incredible. I loved the sight of the beautiful Thai women who stood there smiling and welcoming everyone off the plane, with their perfect makeup, their perfect faces and their perfect dresses.

I thought – *Oh my gosh, this is incredible. I am so glad I am here.*

It was at that moment that I first knew, deep within my soul that something huge was about to unfold. I could feel that I was changing my life by going on this trip. It felt like I had taken dark glasses off, and removed the storm cloud from over my head. All of a sudden, I had clarity. It was so bright and so vivid. It felt like I was seeing in colour again, for the first time in many, many years.

I had to catch a connecting flight to Phuket, where the Tiger Muay Thai gym was. I don't remember much about that flight, other than looking out of the window and seeing all these scattered islands everywhere and thinking the colours were beautiful. The flight was only about an hour and a half, and so as soon as we were up, we were coming down again.

That was when the fun really started.

Phuket was busy. It was hectic. It was crazy. The queues to get through customs were frickin ridiculous, and everyone was only talking in Thai. My fear started to pipe up again, out of nowhere. It had been so peaceful for the last seventeen hours of travelling, even in the chaos of Bangkok airport, and here I was almost home and dry, and yet the fear was here. *What the fuck am I doing? I don't understand the language. I'm here on my own. How am I going to get anywhere? I don't have a taxi. What if the hotel car doesn't come? How will I find them? I don't speak the language. How am I going to navigate my way? What the fuck am I doing?*

I was having an inner drama queen hissy fit in my mind. Thankfully, the hotel had organised a regular taxi to pick me up. As soon as I walked out of the terminal with my things, there was a guy with a massive sign saying Lucy Davis, Lucy – spelt Lusy. The guy who picked me up was such a sweetheart, he was lovely. He tried his best to talk to me. He offered me a bottle of water and said the word in Thai and I would say the English word – Water. We conversed like that as best we could, him in Thai and me in English.

The journey from the airport to where I was going was about an hour long.

"Is this where we go?" he asked once we got moving.

"I have absolutely no idea, I've never been here before," I tried to get him to understand, without success. I kept repeating, "Tiger Muay Thai, Tiger Muay Thai." It was my assumption that everyone in Phuket knew Tiger Muay Thai, so I kept repeating it in the hope we would eventually get there.

"Find Tiger Muay Thai and then we'll find my hotel," I encouraged him. I knew my hotel was just a few hundred yards down the road from where Tiger was.

Eventually, we came across it. The driver stopped so I could take a look and I remember thinking – *Oh God, what have I come to? What have I got myself into?* I had a vision in my head of what this was going to be like, and this wasn't it. It was just a series of wooden shacks with corrugated iron over the top, and while it looked kind of cool with oodles of boxing bags hanging up, I was used to nice, sophisticated, air-conditioned gyms; this was just sawdust, and grubby mats on the floor, open-air sides without walls, and it just had this bit of plastic pulled across the front. My initial thoughts were – *This is intense. What the fuck am I doing? I'm going to catch something here, for sure, some weird disease like rabies. Oh fuck Lucy, you're stuck here for 10 days. What have you done? You've really messed up.*

On top of the incredible melodrama that was rattling around inside my head, the taxi driver didn't appear to know where he was going, which was weird considering I believed he was the hotel taxi driver.

"Coco Ville, Coco Ville," I said, several dozen times.

"Ahh Coco Ville," he replied, the penny finally dropping, but then he started driving me down a little alleyway. It was dark, I couldn't see where on earth I would be staying. *Oh God, I'm staying in a shithole, surrounded by a shithole.*

I was throwing a proper princess tantrum inside.

Finally, he pulled into the entrance of a hotel, and it looked surprisingly nice. It looked civilised anyway. I breathed a sigh of relief. Finally, I had arrived, and I suddenly felt happy about it. I got out of the car and noticed the buddha statues, and some beautiful elephant ones too, dotted around the outside of the hotel. It really was truly beautiful. Yes!

The hotel reception was truly stunning, with open sides and tropical plants everywhere. It was a gorgeous space, which clearly also doubled up as a restaurant during the day. It had a beautiful wooden triangular arched roof, and there were huge wooden tables and chairs. In the middle of the reception area, there was a long, dark mahogany brown table with big wooden chairs, and there was a group of people sitting around the table laughing and playing games. I could hear the tropical wildlife chirping away in the background. What an absolute delight I had chosen.

I awkwardly rocked up to the reception area with my bags. I was tired and grubby from travelling all day and night, and sweating in the same clothes for 24 hours.

I made my way to the desk. There was an extremely beautiful woman behind it. She was immaculate and pristine, which made me feel even grubbier than I already did. The more I looked at her the more I just wanted to get in the shower. I didn't want to talk to anyone, I just wanted to get clean.

As she was copying my passport and taking my payment, I caught sight of an extremely attractive man sitting at the dining table having a laugh with friends. He was really frickin attractive. For the first time in a very long time, I felt embarrassed, I even blushed. Now blushing was rare for me. It took a lot for me to get embarrassed, but seeing this beautiful man, and knowing he was watching my moves while I stood there grubby as heck, I blushed. I tried my best to ignore him – easier said than done – when all I really wanted to do was stare at him. I just hoped and prayed that in the moody Thai lighting, and it being eleven o'clock at night, he couldn't see me properly.

After about fifteen minutes of sweating in reception, the lady finally handed me my room key, and she let me know that someone would carry my bags to my room for me. The room number was 222 – which didn't mean anything to me back then, even though my birthday is the 2nd of the 2nd. The reason I remember the room number is because I actually stayed in the very same room again, many years later.

The room was absolutely beautiful. I jumped straight into the shower and then climbed into bed and attempted to sleep. I did fall asleep for a little bit, but was suddenly, and annoyingly, wide awake – and it was really freaking early. Welcome to the world of jet lag;

I had never experienced it before. I made my best effort to go back to sleep, but failed miserably.

I figured it was time to get up and go for an exploration. I pulled open the door of my apartment and the heat hit me instantly again, only now it was even hotter. I heard a weird noise in the background, it was like a strange slapping sound. "Heh, heh, heh, heh."

What the fuck is that? I checked the time. *It's six in the morning!* And then it came again. "Heh, heh, heh."

I grabbed my flip-flops and headed off to investigate this noise. I walked through the hotel following the sound. "Heh, heh, heh, heh." It lead me down the street and to the neighbouring gym. What an incredible sight! I stood and watched in awe as all these people were hitting pads, boxing, kicking and sparring – at that time in the morning! I'll be honest, in my mind, I was thinking – *There is no way you will catch me doing that at this time of day. This is just way too much. You are on holiday, lighten up peeps.*

I watched for a bit and then went for a walk to explore the area some more. As I started walking, people were smiling and saying hello in English. I suddenly realised that everybody was speaking English, literally everybody. So my near breakdown the day before was slightly unhinged and totally unjustified. *Thank you, God.*

It's amazing what a bit of light does for a situation. Last night I had hated everything and wanted to go home, but this morning, when the sun was shining and everybody had a smile on their face, all the trauma and the drama disappeared.

I took a walk down the road, the five-minute journey to Tiger Muay Thai. I had heard this was the place to go. It had gained quite a reputation around the world, according to my friend, so although there was a gym on my doorstep, I had to go and check this place out.

I walked in and everybody there was immediately friendly. I asked if I could sit and watch for a moment, and they said no problem. Unbeknownst to me, the Thai trainers had different ideas. They were really playful and would flirt, "Oh, what's your name? Come training with me." It was hilarious. Thankfully, I am a pretty strong woman and can stand up for myself, so I played along with them.

I sat and watched for a while and then a couple of girls walked in. They made a beeline for me as I was on my own. It was lovely that they wanted to make me feel part of it. I started chatting to them; they were lovely girls from Australia. Although they didn't know each other prior to the trip, they both lived in Western Australia and had met on their travels. To my surprise, and as luck would have it, they were staying in the same hotel as I was. Someone definitely had my back. It was all coming together. Almost as if it had all been perfectly planned way in advance, rather than the spontaneous haphazard plans I had actually made.

After a while, I went back to the hotel to sit and relax by the pool. While I was sitting there another girl came along and asked if she could join me. It was so lovely to be surrounded by friendly women. This girl was from Australia too. We ended up chatting most of the day and sharing our stories of how we had ended up there. The sun was shining, we were sitting in our bikinis, there were palm trees all around, the sounds of frogs croaking and birds tweeting, and all the while drinking fresh baby coconuts. This was turning out to be my tropical Thai paradise.

Once again, I caught myself sitting there, on my sunbed thinking – *This is the life. This is the life I have been craving.* This time around, though, that statement felt very different to when I made it six months earlier. This time it wasn't from a material wealth perspective, like it had been previously. I had finally surrendered to what life really should be about – simplistic, ordinary, happy, peaceful, and with lots of joy and love. Finally, I had found the calm in my storm. I had found somewhere that felt like my true sanctuary.

A couple of days later, one of the Australian girls I had met invited me to join them on a night out to Patong.

I remembered Patong from a previous visit, "Are we going to the red light district?"

"Pretty much, yes," she replied.

Patong was such an interesting place. It was the polar opposite to the place where I currently was. It was bright, it was loud, it was brash, it was overloaded with bars, restaurants, nightclubs, and cheap market stalls selling knock-off gear. Patong was where people went to really let their hair down and get loose. I had been to Patong previously, just before the tsunami back in 2004. I have had a few events happen in my life, where I have stood there afterwards and thought – *Thank God, I must have been protected!*

I had been an absolute angel so far on the trip. Apart from the airport, I hadn't had one alcoholic drink, so I was determined to make up for it that night.

I put on a cheeky little black dress, which was dolled up by my standards. I'm not the kind of girl who takes hours to get ready. I shower, I put a tiny bit of makeup on, throw my clothes on and I'm ready for some fun!

Patong was not really my thing, but my goodness, I needed a good night out to let my hair down and blow off the cobwebs. As I walked out of my apartment, the extremely attractive guy that I had seen in reception on that first night when I arrived, walked passed me. He made some smart-arse comment, "You scrub up alright." I shot back with a cheeky comment of my own. He was clearly taken aback and commented about me having good banter. He leant in and kissed me, from absolutely nowhere. *Whooooa. What the fuck! What was he doing! Why me?* I had not anticipated that. He was gorgeous!

He let go of me and said, "When you get back after your night out, come and see me, this is my room."

"Okay," I said, having absolutely no intention of going back to his room, even though, my goodness, I wanted to. I had come on my period earlier in the day, so as much as I would really have liked to join him later, you could say I was saved by the bell.

I got to the hotel reception to meet the girls absolutely flabbergasted. *What on earth was tonight going to bring if that was what had happened and I hadn't even left the hotel yet?*

We had the best laugh that night. I got drunk, obviously. Actually, I got absolutely hammered. We drank shots with ladyboys. I ended up dancing around the pole in a bar. The Thai women loved it, they clapped, cheered and encouraged me on. A few years prior to this trip, I had been learning pole dancing in my hometown of Bournemouth. I had been quite good at it, until one day, I did a move wrong and ended up with a massive egg on my arm. It was so painful, so I stepped away from it after that. The pole in this bar, though, bought my inner stripper goddess back to life.

We ended up getting tuk tuks back to the hotel at four o'clock in the morning, pissed out of our heads. We were hanging out of them, and we had ladyboys coming up to us and cracking on to the boys that we were with. It was hilarious, hot, sweaty, innocent, drunken fun. It had been a while since I laughed like that.

When we eventually got back to the hotel, an hour later, at 5 am, I staggered back to my room. I walked passed the hot guy's room and I thought – *Should I? Shouldn't I? It's 5 am, he's going to be pissed if I knock, but at the same time he said to knock so is it rude not to?* I really wanted to knock on. So many questions for one little drunken mind. Thankfully, common sense kicked in, I remembered I had started my period and I would regret it in the morning, so I took off my shoes, quietly snuck past his room and took myself to my bed, alone. I laughed when I got into bed. It had been a long time since I felt that mischievous. Thankfully, my angel was looking after me that night because we all know what would probably have happened if I'd have gone into his room drunk.

The next morning, after just a few hours of sleep, and feeling extremely rough, I broke out of my room and threw myself into the pool outside my room – it was almost like my own private pool for the best part of the day. The hot guy appeared out of nowhere and cheekily asked, "So did you get a better offer last night?" I didn't know what to do with myself, I wasn't ready for that kind of conversation, especially as I was still feeling hanging – so I just said, "Maybe." And from that moment on, the banter started up between the two of us. That was it, our friendship was cemented in banter, and cheeky, smart-arse comments. I found out this guy was a professional boxer from Sydney. His name was Ricardo, but he was known as Ricky to his friends in Phuket.

He suggested we hit a few pads and worked on some technique. So, we did.

I was training with a guy, who fought Manny Paquiou back in the day, and Ricky was training in the ring next to me. One thing about Ricky, from the day we met, he always wanted to help, whether you asked for it or not. Despite his cheek and smart-arse banter, he was a kind soul, and a really beautiful human. I could see past the flirting and playfulness to this deep human, and I was intrigued to get to know him more. I felt that, much like myself, he too was totally lost. We ended up becoming really close and spent lots of time together from that point onwards. Within a day or so, I got over the regret of not going to his room – as attractive as I found him, I was thankful it had not happened. If we'd had sex that night I'm not sure we would have ever become as close as we did.

Several days later, my ten days trip was up. I was absolutely devastated to be leaving my friends, and all the connections I had made. I didn't want to say goodbye to Ricky either. We had become good friends and training buddies. He was the only one who had been able to keep me on my toes with banter. He was at the start of embarking on a worldwide trip, and so we discussed keeping in touch through Facebook. We talked about wanting to see each other again, but I didn't think we actually ever would. How many people have you said goodbye to on a trip and never even thought of them again, let alone actually seen them?

I was dating this guy back home, who, in truth, I no longer wished to be with. I hadn't actually wanted it from the start, but now my regret kicked in. I realised I had to be honest with him. It was unfair to be with someone who was never going to be your forever person.

And, at that moment in time, as we said goodbye, I didn't think I would ever see Ricky again.

However, the Universe had other plans.

12

Less than a couple of months after I returned from Thailand, in December, I was going away again. I had a right royal life at this time in my life. I would go on four or five holidays every year. That was my thing. This time, I was going to the Caribbean on a cruise with my best friend for three weeks, over Christmas and New Year. I would never normally have booked a cruise, but there's a very 'Lucy' story about how it happened.

The Christmas the year before, I was cleaning my apartment. I had this large ceramic sign on my shelf with a motivational quote written on it, I can't remember exactly what it said, but bearing in mind what was about to happen it would have been something heavily ironic like, 'Live your best life." I was cleaning around the house, going about my business, and the ceramic thing fell off the shelf and smashed on my nose, breaking both it and my nose. *Fuck, that really, really, really hurt.* In agony, and with blood everywhere, I looked in the mirror and that really didn't help me at all. I called my mum in hysterics, "Mum, I've broken my nose. My nose is straight, but it's moved across my face, what the fuck do I do?"

She calmly said, "Get yourself to the hospital, now. Call me when you have more information."

I looked in the mirror and saw I had a big cut across the bridge of my nose; the ceramic sign itself had actually split. *That's a nice little war wound* – I thought. I called my bestie, Jimbo, he only lived down the road, I thought he would be able to help me get to the hospital. In true Jimbo fashion, he dumped everything and arrived at my house within an hour, and then laughed his head off at the absolute state of me. He was crying as I told him what had happened to me, as he drove me in my car.

When I got to the hospital, typically, a super hot doctor came over to inspect my nose. Why is it that if you go somewhere looking hot to trot there is no hot guys in sight, but as soon as you rock up looking a mess, a superman lookalike appears and comes to your aide? The hot doctor looked closely at my lopsided nose.

It was decided that I needed to have immediate surgery on my nose to ensure I would be able to breathe properly. This was to take place just before Christmas. Typical!

I spent Christmas that year with my mum. Prior to the accident, I had arranged to go out for New Year's Eve, but clearly, I wasn't going to be going out looking the way I did. My best friend Catherine kindly offered to come over to my house, make us dinner, and have a few cheeky drinks to make up for the fact I had black eyes and a big cut on my nose. Of course, we got pissed that night.

Part way through the night, when we were both extremely well oiled, an advert came on the TV for a cruise. We sat for a minute or so, and then drunkenly talked ourselves into going on a boat! I didn't even like boats! Thankfully, Catherine and I were both in the fortunate position where we could afford to do whatever we chose to do, so we went online and we booked this beautiful two-week cruise around the Caribbean for the following Christmas.

We woke up the next morning and we both said – *What the fuck have we done? We're going on a fucking cruise, for God's sake!*

So then a year later, and that cruise was coming up. It had only been a few weeks since I had returned from Thailand, a trip that totally changed my life, and my perspective of life. I was hoping and praying that this cruise would be the timeout I needed to help me make some big decisions, and step forward with my life.

In mid-December, we started the journey to Fort Lauderdale, where we were picking up the ship. We checked into a stunning hotel for the night before we embarked on the cruise.

Boarding the ship was pretty special. They had a boarding party, and it was so much fun.

I was most excited for Christmas Day. We were visiting nine different countries on this cruise, but on Christmas Day we were going to Jamaica. From a very young age, I craved going to Jamaica because of the movie Cocktail. It had been one of my favourite films when I was growing up. It was that scene in the Dunn's River Falls that really got me. I'm such an old romantic at heart!

On Christmas Day, we got to the waterfall, and I was about to relive this moment of my childhood. I had always imagined doing this with a man, but Catherine would have to do. As it happened, a few days earlier, an extremely attractive guy had made himself known to me on the cruise. He was Canadian and drop-dead gorgeous, and lovely with it too. His dad had been doing his best to match us up from early on in the cruise, but I told him I had a boyfriend back home. They were such a charming family and they really looked after Catherine and I.

The waterfall was amazing. We had a blast that day, and took some hilarious pictures, which I will always treasure. I felt in that moment, that everything was perfect! Nothing could have changed my mood.

When I got back to the boat, I switched my phone on and received a call from my boyfriend. Out of nowhere, he called me a c**t. I was in shock. He told me I was a cheating c**t. Happy Christmas to you too! With the five-hour time difference, it was much later in the day for him, he was clearly drunk and not thinking straight. He became abusive and extremely vulgar. I thought – *How could he do this on Christmas Day, after the amazing day we have had?* Catherine overheard him on the phone, it wasn't difficult, he was shouting. She saw me in tears and told me straight that I should not put up with being spoken to like that. I could see she was heartbroken for me. I realised she was right. I put the phone down and made the decision that I would end the relationship as soon as I got home.

Then I switched my phone off. That was it. No more. No one deserves to be spoken to like that.

It was fate that she had heard him saying what he had said because I probably would have let him talk me back around the next day. Instead, I decided to get on with my holiday, and although I was devastated, I was not going to let him ruin another second.

Having made the decision to leave the relationship, that Christmas Day evening, me and my best friend got dressed up in our beautiful dresses. If there is one thing that is special about cruises, it's that you get to dress up every day, if you choose to. Later on, after a few drinks and a bellyful of food, Cat popped out of her dress in front of everybody, because she'd eaten too much. It was hilarious. I was laughing so much at her. It was just the tonic I needed.

Later that night, as we were walking through one of the casinos, the hot Canadian guy grabbed me and asked me to join him for a drink at the casino table. My friend Catherine gave me the nod. As if by magic, though, he said, "Oh, Catherine, I want you to meet my brother."

We had such a great night, we went in all the bars and nightclubs, and ended up hanging out by the swimming pool in the early hours of the morning. For the rest of the trip, the four of us became inseparable.

It was almost like Ricky had been brought into my life to remind me what life was supposed to feel like. And then this Canadian guy had come in from nowhere to do the same for me – all in a matter of weeks. At the same time, my actual boyfriend was being a dick. The Universe was pointing the way for me. It was becoming clearer.

My mind had been made up. It was time to be honest and step away from this unhappy, unhealthy relationship situation that I had found myself in. In truth, it had been a rebound relationship and a distraction off the back of the trauma of my grandad.

13

Arriving back in the UK at New Year, after everything that had gone on the year before, left me in a pensive and solemn mood. The words of my grandad were echoing around inside my head, and I started to reflect on my life, for the first time ever. I thought a lot about my childhood and my upbringing, and I began to find that my memories were not quite as accurate as I had imagined them to be.

We live our lives out and then create a story about that life as we go. When we cast our eyes back and look at that life with clarity, beyond the story we have created, we can often see a very different world emerge.

When I reflected on my childhood, I saw absolute perfection. I was happy and I felt very lucky.

Obviously, there were lots of things that happened that were not perfect, but they never took away from the fact that I truly believed my childhood was pretty much spot on.

When I was born, my mum and dad didn't have much money; I was certainly not born into wealth. My mum wasn't working, as my sister was two years older than me, but my dad made up for it. He was a doer. He was determined to create a life of abundance for us, and he worked harder and harder every year.

I don't remember much about my first few years. I have a few early memories – like letting the hand-break off the car and rolling down the hill when I was three – but not much else. I have a lot more memories from when I was five onwards, though.

Dad was doing really well, studying, working, and bettering himself constantly so that we would have more money. I never remember going without as a child. We were always clean, dressed nicely, and able to do fun activities without there being any concerns about money.

I was a carefree child. I was happy-go-lucky. Even from being a baby, I was always happy and always smiling. I never slept through the night, apparently – which says a lot about who I am now. My mum often tells people that I didn't sleep through the night until I was seven – whether that's actually true or not I don't know. She said I was an absolute nightmare – a beautiful one, of course.

I had invisible friends too, lots of them. No surprises there. I was always surrounded by them too, and always busy chatting to them; I never felt alone.

I loved to roll around in the grass, pick daisies, and hold buttercups under my chin. I loved the sunshine, and I loved life as a little person.

I also really loved animals, although admittedly I wasn't very good at cleaning them out or looking after them. I just wanted to hold them and play with them. It may also be no surprise to learn that I could talk to the animals.

I basically lived in a magical wonderland as a child. I relished every moment and filled it with wonder and happiness. I had an unshakable innocence and purity that the adult world had yet to erode.

My nan said, before she passed, that she could imagine me being married, living on a farm with a number of children and animals running around everywhere because I had such a beautiful connection to nature.

I was not one of those children who was scared of the dirt, quite the contrary, I was happiest when I was outside, rolling around in the dirt and connecting with nature. I didn't have an interest in day trips to buildings like churches or historic institutions. Whenever I got told I had to go somewhere like that because my sister was really into history and historic buildings, I'd have a hissy fit. I liked being outdoors and free.

My desire to be outside all the time was reflected in my schooling, and showed up on my reports; they said I was easily distracted and that if I applied myself I could achieve so much more. I wanted to be anywhere else other than at school. Most mornings when I was little, my mum would get me dressed for school and I would get undressed and get back into bed.

It's fair to say, I hated school.

I caused absolute riots at nursery. I would scream the place down, and cling on to my mum when she dropped me off. I would do anything to create a scene, in the hope my mum would take me home with her. My mum and the nursery staff quickly learned that there were two toys I really liked and that if they could distract me with those two toys my mum could sneak away before I realised she had gone, but when I did realise I screamed my head off. Funnily enough, I am just as easily distracted even all these years on. Apparently, a couple of hours later, I would settle and start playing with the toys and the other children. A couple of hours, though! That's a long time for a little one to be screaming and upset.

The first day that my mum walked me to the infant school, I caused absolute chaos. I cried hysterically again. I didn't want to be left there, and I clung, screaming to my mum's leg with all my strength until she ended up crying too. I just wanted to feel safe, and the school didn't make me feel like that. My mum somehow managed to prise me off her and throw me into school. I was forced to show up every day after that. There's no grace or dignity for parent or child in this. Our parents were forced to do this, they had no other option back then. That was just the process and nobody questioned it. There wasn't such a thing as homeschooling. You had to go to school, and if you didn't go then your parents got in trouble. Simple as that.

According to my mum, I did eventually settle in and was able to walk into school without tears and drama. This particular school itself was just a one-storey building, no upstairs or anything like that, but the outdoor area was okay and I liked that. They had climbing frame equipment and a concrete area where we did sports, and then there was a large field at the back.

One day, I was playing at the back of the field and I saw a gate. It was an oversized metal gate. Come to think of it, it was a bit like a bloody prison gate. It was maybe five feet tall, which was pretty huge to us little people back then. Standing there, I realised I could see my house across the road; I could actually see my front door. I went and found a couple of my friends and told them that I could see my house from the gate, and I pointed it out to them. The temptation of seeing my house but not being able to go to it, proved too much for me.

On one specific day, a few days after spotting the gate, I really didn't want to be at school. It was cold, it was boring and I wanted to go home. That day, I decided that I was going to climb the gate. I walked out across the playground, strolled across the field to the back gate, and somehow managed to clamber over it – bear in mind I was only 5 years old at this point. I jumped down the other side of the gate, somehow managing to land safely without breaking any bones. I guess children bounce a lot easier. I continued to walk towards my home, storming across the grass on the other side of the gate, and then innocently marching across the road. Thankfully, it was a quiet road that we lived on; we were at the very start of a cul-de-sac and so it wasn't too far for my little legs to go. Dangerous all the same, though.

I got to my house and rang on the doorbell. I've absolutely no idea how I would have reached it but I was a determined little thing and nothing was going to stop me. I could hear my mum on the other side of the door, likely looking through the peephole, but because I was so dinky there wasn't anybody she could see. When my mum eventually opened the door, wondering who was there, she looked down on the doorstep and there I was.

"Lucy, what the bloody hell are you doing here?" she shrieked.

I casually informed her that I wanted to come home, that I wasn't enjoying myself at school. My mum was mortified because she has always been somebody who does as she's told, and she really plays the game. My mum wouldn't dare to cause any attention to herself by doing anything rebellious – which is why she gave birth to me I guess, because I've got enough rebellion for the two of us. I think that day was my first instance of me being truly rebellious, but then five years old is pretty young for a rebel. What can I say? I just knew that I wasn't enjoying being pumped through the school system, and I guess my beautiful little soul was feeling – *Get me the heck out of here.*

Unfortunately, my youthful rebellion was short-lived and I was taken straight back to school. My mum told me I was not allowed to climb the gate again, not under any circumstance. I did, though – several more times. I think my mum found it really quite funny that first time, even though she would never have said that to me then, but now we have a laugh about it. It's a story that most of my friends get told, the first or second time of meeting my mum.

Another moment of rebellion during my school years came a little while later when my sister and I were at Hillview Infant School. We had moved from that house in the cul-de-sac which was near my nursery, and into another one. We moved around a lot when we were children. My dad worked hard and got promoted all the time; new bonuses and pay rises meant we could move into bigger and better houses, so that's what we did. I was sat in the main hall one morning for assembly. I'm sure most of you remember sitting on the brown wooden floors as a child, listening to the headmaster's daily nonsense. Back in those days, the hall was used as the gym, the dining room, and all sorts of things – it could be adapted at any time, depending on what needed to go on in that space at that time. Every morning, the headmaster would ask the pupils who were in attendance at assembly, "Does anybody have a birthday today?" And then whoever's birthday it was would put their hands up and they'd go up on stage where they'd get a badge to wear for the day, and also they would be given a single Smartie, as a birthday gift. I mean who gives one single Smartie?

On this particular day – when it was most definitely not my birthday, and of course, the teachers knew that – nevertheless, I put my hand up. My sister, who is two years older than me, was in the same assembly, sat there with all her friends, and was absolutely mortified. She has told me since that day she cringed so badly when she saw what I was doing, she went bright red and shrunk down embarrassed of her little sister, and told her friends that it absolutely was not my birthday.

It's fair to say from a young age I was determined, a rule breaker and extremely confident. If I wanted something, I would go and get it. The funniest bit about it, in my opinion, is the headmaster, said nothing. The teachers said nothing too. I really didn't care. I had my eye on a Smartie and I knew the only way to get one was to be bold. I tottered up on that stage, had them all sing to me, and I got my Smartie! I was really, really proud of myself standing up there.

In the car home that night, my sister told my mum, "Lucy told everyone it was her birthday. She got up in front of the whole assembly, it was so embarrassing." I remember thinking – *I don't get your problem. I got a Smartie.* It continues to make me smile at how utterly confident I was as a child. I was so happy-go-lucky, so carefree. I genuinely didn't give a damn what people thought about me. I felt so loved and so protected. Genuinely, I felt like I was invincible. It was never from malice or trying to push boundaries, I just knew what I wanted and was pretty good at figuring out from a very young age how to navigate that.

14

Regardless of school and other restrictions, I felt like I had won the lottery with the parents that I ended up with. I loved them so much, and felt I was very lucky to be born into the family that I was. It was a happy and abundant life.

My pets were the best part of my childhood, though. I had a white rabbit called Flopsy, he was a male and absolutely gorgeous. He was so friendly and lovely, I would pick him up and run around the garden with him and get him to chase me, and then I'd chase him back. We had such a beautiful connection.

Flopsy lived in a hutch in our back garden. We would check in on him before school, as soon as we got home, and before we went to bed. He was a bright white, dwarf rabbit, and so cute. One day, my dad went out to see the rabbit and it had died. It was rock solid and stuck in a strange position. He had apparently contracted myxomatosis – which is sadly common in rabbits. They can pass extremely suddenly. My dad was so worried about how we would react to the rabbit dying, we were very young and it would have been our first encounter with death, so he kept me away from the rabbit for a day. Without our knowledge, he went to a pet shop and discreetly bought another rabbit, exactly the same as Flopsy. My dad then took out the dead, original Flopsy and put in this new version – Flopsy 2 – in the hope we wouldn't realise. Of course, it wasn't even two minutes before we realised it wasn't the same rabbit. Yes, the new rabbit looked almost exactly the same, but not quite the same enough. It was a little bit smaller, and I'm almost certain this second one was female too, and not quite as chilled as the first one either.

Kids are super perceptive, they don't miss a trick. There is absolutely no point in attempting to fool children. They know. They know more than we know – especially the bright little buttons coming through since 2000.

We then got a guinea pig called Mopsy. Mopsy was black and brown striped and her stripes made her look like a brown and black zebra. Oh my goodness, she was cute, and as small as she was, she housed such a huge personality. She was like a mini-me. She was chirpy, confident, and loved a good chat, and she had the cutest hairstyle in the world. I absolutely idolised her.

Both Flopsy and Mopsy were my fur babies. We were joined at the hip – or the tail, in their case. I loved the rabbit because I could chase it, but the guinea pig made such cute noises and was so sweet. I would sit down on the grass in a dress and let Mopsy run around under my dress like it was a little tent. Oh, the beauty of the connection between child and pet. There is nothing like it.

At some point, I went to school one day and came home with another guinea pig. I didn't ask my mum or anything like that, and I've no idea why I was able to get a guinea pig from school, but I came home with one and this one we named Pickles.

So, unlike normal families that had cats and dogs, I had little things like the rabbit and the guinea pigs, and some fish too; then, of course, there were the horses.

Horses were a big deal to me at eight years old, and they still are. I was completely and utterly obsessed with horses. I had pictures of them all around my bedroom walls, and I would badger my dad every single day, "I want a pony. I want a pony." I drove him mad because some of my friends had horses from my school; it was constant harassment. Once I actually got to see them and ride them, my badgering took on a whole new level.

I totally fell in love with horses and horse riding. I had a few horse riding lessons at different places, and on other people's horses, before my parents found Green Cottage Riding Centre in Three Legged Cross, which is the place where my love for horses grew to a new height. I'm almost certain my mum and dad thought if they took me horse riding, it would get it out of my system – that when I realised there was grooming, mucking out, and cleaning tack, I'd get over it pretty quickly. Big mistake! Thankfully, my parents were amazing and this decision fuelled an absolute obsession. Horses became my number one thing.

I truly believe my interest and absolute love of those creatures is what kept me on the straight and narrow as a child. I formed a bond with the animals, and also with the people involved. I really felt like I belonged somewhere, for the first time in my life. They gave me peace, they gave me purpose, and they gave me the drive to get up in the morning.

The interesting thing about it was that I was also naturally very good at it. I was a very good rider, very quickly. I took to it at an incredible speed and, thankfully, I was taken under the wing of the owner, and her daughter, at the place where I was learning to ride. They must have seen something in me that made them choose to invest time and energy into me. I started getting invited to attend shows with the daughter when she was competing. I went to some incredible places over the years – Olympia, Horse Of The Year show, and the New Forest show. I would often be invited to travel away with them over the weekends, and I would actually sleep in the horse box. It was such an adventure.

Soon after, I started showing and competing the horses myself, which led to some amazing opportunities to ride horses that were not normally available to students from the school. That gave me a leg up on the journey, to the point where people started to know my name in those circles.

The belief in me, from these people, encouraged my parents to see how good I was and of the potential I had. I was more passionate about horses than I had been about anything in my life.

When I was about eleven years old they agreed to me loaning my first horse. I feel my dad was still probably hoping I'd grow out of it and get tired of it, but that just didn't happen.

My dad was amazing, he would drive me all the way to the stables on Saturday and Sunday mornings and then pick me up in the evening. The stables were a good forty-minute drive each way – which looking back, is an incredible thing for him to do, to give up an hour and a half on a Saturday and Sunday. It's amazing what my parents did for me, especially when it's highly unlikely that I ever even said thank you. We take so much for granted as kids. I guess parents get their thanks in seeing the joy on their children's faces.

I especially loved it when my parents came to watch me ride, bearing in mind neither of them had the slightest interest in horses. It was mainly my dad that came to support me, though. He was, and still is, very supportive of my dreams and passions. When I look back, it's amazing – the thought of him holding my horse as I would go and walk around the jumps before riding them, and manoeuvring the horse box. For someone who did not know anything about horses, he was amazing. My parents were actually very cool, and I never gave them enough credit when I was younger. So, Mum and Dad, thank you! I'm glad we picked each other this lifetime.

On school holidays, I would be at the stables from morning to night, every day that I was allowed. My dad would drop me there in the morning because the stables were only about fifteen minutes from where he worked. I'd spend the whole day there helping – mucking out, walking the ponies. I did anything and everything I could. I wanted to learn and to be a part of something. I shaped a whole existence through the horses, they were my true first love.

When I reached about 14, I was competing at a relatively high level, and out of nowhere, a lady offered me the most stunning pony to loan for free. She asked me to ride him, show him, and do as much jumping and eventing as I chose to do. He was young and they were looking for him to gain some experience. He was amazing. We had so much fun. We evolved together and gained confidence from each other. I had some wild experiences with that boy and I often think about him.

I have no idea where I gained this incredible ability to ride. I know I got my love of horses from my grandad, but no one else in the family rode. Horses gave me some of the best experiences of my life. They taught me, from a very young age, how to love unconditionally, how to appreciate all things conscious, and also how to communicate with a divine creation that can't physically speak.

Having loaned other people's ponies, I really upped the ante on my dad to buy me my own horse. I'm not sure why I was so determined to own one, I guess so no one could take it from me – which would have been heartbreaking. After a heavy-duty session of pleading, my dad finally said yes. I couldn't believe it.

The daughter of the riding stables offered to drive me around and help me look for the perfect pony. We went to several places, but were unsuccessful. Finally, though, we drove down to Dorset, and that was where I fell in love with a 14.2hh dark bay, gelding called Jack. He was absolutely stunning, he was everything that I could have wished for. Elegant and very handsome. I rode him, and jumped with him – as did my instructor – I just knew he was the pony for me. I was totally head over heels in love with him. My dad wasn't there that day, so we agreed to go back to see him once more and do a deal, and then get the vet to check him over.

On the second visit, though, we noticed he was a bit nippy in the stable. It raised concern because if he bit someone that could be dangerous. He was fine outside of the stable, but inside, he was not comfortable at all. We decided to get the vet to check him out, and see if there was something he was in pain with, something that could potentially be resolved. However, the vet informed us that his temperament was something we were going to have to live with. My heart was broken in two, just like that. My first ever heartbreak. I cried and cried. In the end, after a lot of huffing and puffing, we all agreed that because he was going to be in a yard where children would be, he wasn't right.

A few weeks passed. I had almost given up on looking for a horse, that heartbreak had been hard. I thought it would be better to face the risk of someone taking a loan horse away from me rather than go through the disappointment of searching for my own.

And then I met Harry.

Harry lived about twenty minutes from my house. I had travelled all over the South of the UK looking for a pony and this beautiful bay gelding was just twenty minutes away all this time. He was incredible, such a beautiful boy. When I went to view him, bearing in mind that I'd fallen in love with Jack previously and had gotten my hopes up, I was a bit nervous to meet him. I had already fallen in love with Harry from the images. He was the spitting image of Jack, just younger. Harry was only four years old, and so only a baby really. He'd only just been broken in about six months earlier, so it was a huge commitment to buy a four-year-old. It was not something I had ever thought about taking on; that was until I met him. He was calm, patient, excitable, lively – absolutely amazing. Within minutes of meeting him, I was in love with him; and interestingly, it was just my dad and I that went to view him so we agreed upon it right away.

He was the perfect pony. We had such an incredible experience together. Our first full season out showing together, we won it all. Every show or competition we entered, we would be called in first or second place. This was quite phenomenal for a brand new collaboration. This was where I truly learned the art of how effective the right partnerships could be. Way before any interaction with a human male, I had learned from these incredible conscious beings.

After about 8 months, we moved him from where he was to a new home. It was lovely – a busier yard where he had plenty to look at, and we had a cross-country course to bomb around right next door.

Whilst we were at this yard, things went up another notch. We would be travelling most weekends to events. I travelled the UK with the horses. This travelling gave me a sense of freedom and adventure that was poignant for what I would need in my adult life. It's amazing how, when you look back, it's all been divinely orchestrated to provide you with the skills that will enable you to succeed at your mission in life.

After my parents' divorce – a whole saga yet to come – it was not so easy to get out to the yard anymore. Although I was 16, I didn't have my dad running me around every weekend, taking me to shows – sadly I was barely able to see him at all – so we moved Harry much closer to our house. This was when things started to change with me. Up until this point, horses had been my world for over half my life, but I started to lose interest. I no longer had the social circle of the busy yard and that community of people to chat to and assist my growth. It was so confusing to me, as I loved him dearly, but in the months after my parent's divorce, I am embarrassed to admit Harry became secondary to other things in my life. I ended up selling him a year after their divorce. It absolutely broke my heart.

It's fascinating how trauma shows up in each of us. Following the divorce, I went on a path of self-destruction that I was unaware of, and as a consequence of that, I sold Harry. Looking back, years later, I was so angry that I went on a mission to self-sabotage my happiness, and horses at that point in my life were my happiness.

Many years later, my mum and stepdad went to a New Year's Eve party, and randomly – it's never random – they were sat at the same table as the people who had owned the stables where I had last kept Harry, before I sold him. They told my mum that Harry had been put down. The next day, and out of the blue, I received a call from my mum. It was a normal conversation at first, "Hi Lu, how are you? Happy new year."

"Yeah I'm good thanks Mum, how are you? Nice evening?"

"Harry's dead."

Just like that.

Then she followed up with, "They told me that he had laminitis and he had to be put to sleep."

I was in shock. "Oh no Mum, that was my baby."

"I thought it was best you knew," she continued, very matter-of-factly.

I was devastated at the news. It was like I'd lost my baby for the second time. It highlighted so much guilt, regret and shame. I had gone from being the most perfect owner to quite a shitty one – to say the least. I did not look after him like I could have done. I definitely didn't nurture him like I had done from the get-go. His needs were no longer my priority, and now he was gone. There was no time to say sorry. No time to make up for what I had done.

This was the start of having to live with the consequences of my actions.

And it hurt like hell.

15

One memorable day, when I was 8 years old, my dad dropped me off at the stables early. He always went to work super early, leaving home by about 7 am; which was no trouble to me, I couldn't get to the stables quick enough. In fact, I would have stayed there overnight if I could have done; if they would have had me I would have stayed there forever and never left.

I ran into the stables and had an amazing day. I did my first jump and made a huge amount of progress; I was so excited for my dad to come and pick me up so I could tell him. When he walked into the stables, he started chatting to the people who owned the place. I saw him before he saw me and I ran up to him, "Dad, dad, dad. You won't believe what I did today." I just wanted him to know everything that had happened, so I chattered away excitedly at a million miles an hour.

My dad was my absolute hero, he was like Superman, Batman and Spider-Man all rolled into one. He was just incredible. He's very kind, and also very driven — some would say cut-throat in business — but when it came to his children he was very loving and supportive of anything and everything we did. I idolised my dad and had him on the highest pedestal, but I was still a bit fearful of him, or rather I had a healthy respect for his authority. My mum would often threaten us with, "What will your Dad say?" It's interesting how parents play those games to gain control — good cop, bad cop — not realising how it impacts the children.

At that time my dad had a company car, it was a midnight blue Vauxhall Omega, it was really nice for its time and pretty much new. We were driving back in it that day from the stables and I was so excited, with non-stop chatter the whole way home; like kids do. Kids don't stop to ask their parents, "How was your day?" I would share intricate details with him about how a certain riding position worked and how I did this and how I did that. Most of the time he just nodded and said yes to show he was listening, but I really wouldn't have blamed him if he wasn't.

When we were a few minutes from home, my dad pulled up on one of the side roads, at the back of a tennis club. I thought it was weird; the house was less than a minute away in the car, I probably could run home in less than three minutes, even with my little legs at that time. We sat there for a moment, in silence, and then he turned the engine off. I wasn't sure what was going on. It was all a bit weird. He had never done this before. And then he looked at me and said, "Your mum is not happy with me."

I responded with, "Why what have you done?"

He told me that he'd been away on a business trip with his secretary. That meant nothing to me, I was eight years of age. I had no idea what he was talking about. And then he said, "And your mother thinks that something went on with me and my secretary." It just didn't make sense, I didn't know what he was getting at. What 8-year-old child can process any of that? It was when he said, "Mum's really angry with me." That's when I had a reaction. Someone was hurting my mum and I was angry about it.

I don't honestly remember what happened immediately after he told me this. The next thing I remember was when we pulled up on the drive, I opened the car door, ran through the side gate, in through the back door, through the kitchen, and straight passed my mum, who shouted after me, "Lucy, are you okay?" I kept on running. I ran straight up to my bedroom, slammed the door, and sat with my back up against the door with my head on my knees and sobbed. I got into that awful sob cycle where I couldn't catch my breath. I watched the tears drip from my eyes onto the carpet beneath me. I was heartbroken. I knew my mum was hurting. I didn't understand why or how, I just knew it was happening and I did not know what to do about it, or how to cope with it. So I just sat there and sobbed.

I heard my mum shout at my dad, "What the hell have you said to her?"

My mum came up and sat on the other side of my bedroom door. She attempted to get in and talk to me, but I wouldn't let her into my room. I feel parents know sometimes that their child needs a bit of space, but they also know that they need to be there for their child, and so she left me for a few minutes and then she gently nudged my little body with the door, without hurting me, and she edged her way in. When she came into the room, I looked at her with my eyes all red and puffy from the tears, I had snot dripping everywhere, and I said, 'Daddy didn't mean to hurt you?" And that was step number one of me becoming the "fixer" in many of my intimate relationships.

I cannot imagine how my mum dealt with what she had found out about my dad, as well as seeing her child breaking her little heart in front of her. All I know is how I felt and what that then led to.

My mum held me close to her while I sobbed. I was so angry. I was feeling all of these strange emotions that I wasn't used to. I was a happy-go-lucky child, none of this made any sense. Even though my mum was holding me, I felt so alone in my big bedroom. I was conflicted because I really loved my mum, I'd always been close to her, but up until that point, I was a daddy's girl. I was like his little shadow.

I sat and cried with my mum for ages before she eventually calmed me down and even coaxed me downstairs to have some dinner. From that moment onwards, though, I was a different child.

This situation was very interesting. I knew somebody had hurt my mum and I wasn't okay with that. I was very protective of my family. I didn't want anybody to hurt my family, but in this case, it was my dad that had done the damage. I didn't grasp the fact that my dad had cheated at that point. I didn't even know what cheating was, to be honest with you. I was 8 years old. I guess I felt there was a misunderstanding, some wires had got crossed or something like that. I just knew that it didn't feel good.

With what I know now, this is where so much of my later trauma came about – not trusting people, holding back in intimate relationships. That conversation with my dad completely blew my world apart.

The next day, though, I carried on as if nothing had happened.

Kids are resilient, or so we like to think. One day you go to bed crying, the next day you get up and you've forgotten about it. The thing was I clearly hadn't forgotten about it because it shaped the rest of my life.

16

After that, although we all carried on 'as normal', there was quite a lot of turbulence during the next few years, not just between my mum and dad, but also because we moved house yet again.

I never lived within walking distance of my school or my friends. I actually became quite envious of people who did. I really wanted to be near my friends. By this time, I was older and I had started to enjoy school, especially the social life, but it was a pain that we had a 20-minute car journey to get there, or for me to ever see my friends. I always had this envy of not being able to pop to my mate's house after school or at the weekend, or even just simple things like friends congregating in the cul-de-sac. Our house was beautiful, though, and we were very privileged; I guess it just goes to show we always crave what we do not have.

Another life-changing moment happened when I was doing my 11-plus exam. In the UK, this is an exam that you take when you are 10 or 11 years old to decide if you could go to a Grammar School or not. I was 10 years old when I took mine, it was just before my 11th birthday.

The exam was to take place in the large, wooden assembly hall. As we walked in, there were neat rows of individual wooden desks. Do you remember those single wooden desks where the tops would lift up, and people had carved their names in the wood? And how you would let your fountain pen ink seep out into the wood to mark it?

The room was laid out in a very military style and everyone had a specific desk that had their name and number on it, so the teacher could identify who was who. I walked into this exam feeling terrified. This was to be a real turning point. The hall seemed bigger than normal, and it seemed much colder than usual too. The desks were set up so you couldn't look at each other or each other's work — which, let's be real, we did all the time in the classroom. Everything seemed so big, so formal, clinical, and overwhelming. I couldn't see any of my classmates, and I just felt very alone.

At the front of the hall was a big stage, and there was a teacher sitting on the stage with a clock in front of them; they had a bell that would start and end the exam. It was so scary.

I really set myself up here, I'd always been carefree in exams up until this point, but this one bothered me.

To this day, there are certain things that I won't do because there are exams involved, and quite frankly, I think they're bullshit. Anyone can read and memorise a book. It does not mean they actually understand it or are good at it. It just means they can memorise stuff better than other people. I'll be honest, I never studied, not once; it never resonated with me. It just seemed pointless, a bit like the whole schooling system itself. The trouble with me was that I really wanted my parents to be proud of me. I wanted my teachers to be proud of me too. I knew that I was capable of going to Grammar School and doing great things, but this pressure was awful.

I sat at that desk, in my row, staring up at the teacher, waiting for the bell to go off. The teacher took his time explaining the rules, how the process would work, the length of time we were going to be there for, and what sounds to listen out for. It was horrible.

The bell sounded and echoed around the hall. The sound of everyone opening their papers and starting to scribble frantically was the only sound in the room. We must have been about 15 minutes into the exam, when a boy called David suddenly started kicking the desk. The next thing I knew, he fell on the floor and had an epileptic fit. There was a huge bang with the kick of the desk and then the fall. It was hideous. The silence of the room made it even more shocking. Everybody stopped, stared and looked. This poor kid had fallen on the floor, no doubt hurting himself on the way. He was thrashing about, clinging onto his tongue, frothing at the mouth. It was very, very scary to witness. It was the first time I'd ever seen anything like it; I thought he was dying. I didn't know what epilepsy was, I'd never heard of it, and I honestly thought this boy was going to die right there in front of us. He continued to thrash around on the floor. He could have badly hurt himself with the wooden chair, the wooden desk, or the wooden floor, and nobody was there to support him. Thankfully the teacher did get there in the end, but it was absolutely terrifying to watch.

They had to wait for him to come around to be able to get him out of the room safely, then they gave him water and waited until the ambulance arrived. All of this was happening with a bunch of 10 and 11-year-olds, going through an exam, watching. It just goes to show what pressure can do to people. It was a perfect example of if you push yourself too much, or if you are put under too much pressure, your body is going to have an outlet for it. It was scary. Nobody wanted to see that. None of us had heard about epilepsy. It wasn't something that got talked about.

The ambulance eventually came to get him and took him out of the room, and then the teachers just said, "Right, everybody take your seats, the exam is continuing now." Literally, just straight back to business as usual. Another mighty fine example of sweeping things under the table.

I have wondered how many others were impacted by that situation. Sadly, the next time I saw David, I was a bit scared of him, because nobody educated us or told us what epilepsy was all about, they just left us to deal with it, and I thought he might do it again in front of me.

I look back now and I think that was the moment when I decided to change. That was the moment where I got my head down and I buckled up. I started paying a lot more attention at school – I never revised for an exam again, though, but I decided that I would pay more attention and be more present. I was going to show up more, and I wouldn't let anything stop me from being the best I could be. That was my introduction to becoming competitive. I consciously decided – *Right! Enough of the messing around, it's time to be serious.*

And serious is what I became.

And to be honest with you, I don't even know why I did that exam because my parents later decided that I wasn't going to a Grammar school anyway. It had all been a waste of time.

Emotional Trauma

No child can go through life without going through some level of what I call 'emotional trauma'. We can have the most beautiful existence in the outside world — have an amazing home, good parents, an abundant life, and yet internally we may process things in a very different way to the actual experience. When we are young, we soak these experiences up like a sponge, sucking up all of the information from our outside world — a world that our individual souls have committed to navigate during this human experience. No child can go through what they perceive to be traumatic situations and it not change their life.

Trauma is a very triggering word in my experience, which is why I opt for it — to assist breaking people through as quickly as possible. Trauma can mean anything that has created an emotional response within you — which more often than not leads on to a reaction of some kinds. It could look like your mum not telling you she was proud of you. Maybe a feeling of not fitting in, or of not being wanted as a child. How about a very common one — not feeling loved? It can also mean much more obvious things such as abuse, abandonment, adoption, and divorce; the list is endless.

Most people shy away from acknowledging their traumas, as we have been convinced over the years that it means we are 'damaged'. Who wants to admit they are 'damaged'? It's better to convince ourselves we are good, even if deep down we know we are not. And in here lies the issue. We all have our own very individual journeys of discovery whilst we are here in this skin suit. It's our job to be open, vulnerable and recognise that trauma can be created from many different avenues.

It is truly shocking how we have been duped into believing that feelings and emotions are bad or weak. We have been taught the only way to survive is to be tough, compete and to fight. We have buried the the divine feminine elements of self healing, love, and nurturing, in place of a toxic masculinity. It is very important we recognise our patterns. We have all had things go on in our lives that have changed us from our core essence, and that's okay. It is our responsibility to decide if we choose to live from that damaged place, protecting our wounds and feeling like everything and everyone is a threat. Or, if we choose to step back into our truth, authenticity, love and vulnerability.

As a child, when we have no concept of what things mean, we make up the ending point in our head, which is normally premised from a feeling of not feeling safe, which then goes on to become trauma later on in life. The thing about emotional trauma, it's very rare it comes out as anything other than a scream, a cry or a physical feeling at the time it occurs. It transforms into trauma when we normalise it, ignore it, or attempt to work around it in our daily lives. Then over the years it gets compounded and blamed on hormones, diet, family, friends — when in reality, and most commonly, it's been created in exceptionally ordinary situations.

It's time for us to create greater awareness of our own traumas. If we could remember this, we would not project them forward onto our little people — which is why I now do what I do for a living. People are so scared of their children experiencing the same as they have, that they either become overprotective — and so the child rebels — or they pretend their traumas do not exist and then they both create a mirroring effect with one another, whereby we call in all that we would really like to avoid.

Please remember to encourage your child to live their life. You are not here to stop them experiencing what they came down here for. They are here on a mission of their own, just like you are.

It's our job to do the very best we can.

17

From what appeared to be out of nowhere, we moved house again. We moved from the house on the corner, the one down the road from the tennis club, to another house a couple of roads away, parallel to where we had lived. I mean who does that? It made absolutely no sense to me. My dad always appeared to have ants in his pants. The more successful he was at work, the bigger house he wanted. Success created movement for him; a trait I have mirrored to some degree over the years.

Very recently, my mum told me the story that she was out shopping for the day, when my sister and I were much younger. She was having a lovely time, but when she got home, my dad declared he had bought a new house!

"By the way Carol, I've bought a house."

She asked him, "What do you mean you've bought a house?"

"You remember we really liked that area? Well, I went down there and I bought the best house."

It was such a shame because the other house, before this random move, was beautiful. I loved all of the houses we lived in, for all different reasons, but this last one had been special. The house we moved into was haunted. Some extremely weird things happened in this house. It was this house where I felt much darker energy than I had ever felt before. I was extremely sensitive to energies as a child, but I switched it off as a result of some of the childhood incidents I have mentioned previously. In this house, though, it was hard to ignore what I was feeling.

Once we moved in there, things changed between my mum and dad, me and my sister. This was the first time I remember hearing my mum and dad arguing, and it became very common. My sister changed all of a sudden too. She had gone from being this deep, astute, kind, caring sister to someone who I no longer recognised. It was weird. Almost overnight she had gone from spending time with me to spending none at all. She was angry and distant, and always going out with her friends – sometimes not coming home at all. She just wasn't like my sister anymore. It's really weird when you are close to someone, then all of a sudden you aren't anymore.

It's challenging to get your head around it, especially when there seems to be no rhyme or reason for it.

At least I had a nice room in the new house. I had a cosy, single bed and a big mirrored wardrobe. I had a lovely window that looked out onto the back garden and I had a shelf with all my ornaments and trinkets on it. The walls were covered with posters of horses. My new bedroom was above the kitchen area, and one night I heard my parents shouting at each other, really going for it. I could hear the muffles through my floor. They were arguing about my sister, but I couldn't quite make out enough of what they were saying, so I went to the top of the stairs so I could listen in better. My sister would have been about 13 at this point, and I would have been 11. My sister became a hugely troubled energy which rippled through the family in a big way.

One night, I went to bed as normal, and woke up to a woman leaning over me. It was a much older lady, she wasn't causing any harm or anything like that. She was staring, almost endearingly at me. Of course, she wasn't a real woman, she was in spirit. It was absolutely terrifying. I screamed at the top of my voice. Eventually, my mum and dad came running into my room and calmed me down, but I truly believe that's where I decided to shut down my ability to see spirit, in all its glory.

Sometime later, after that event, my parents bizarrely shared another story with me about how they had been in bed together one evening, and in the middle of the night my dad had woken up, believing there was someone in the room with them, and he had started lashing out, assuming it was a burglar. When he switched the light on nobody was there. He was attempting to punch thin air, but he was absolutely certain there had been a man standing and watching them just moments earlier.

I'm not sure these were bad spirits as such, or just looking for attention. It was freaky, though.

On top of what was going on in our living space, there was a lot that would go on in the loft. There were blatantly spirits there that hadn't crossed over. For some reason, these spirits would really antagonise my sister. Now, what we didn't know at the time, but we found out later, was that my sister had done a ouija board with her friends from school. They had done this when she was around

13 years of age, and right around the time when she just switched into being someone totally different. Like with any energy work, a ouija board can potentially bring in some dark energies, especially if you are not protected. I honestly believe that this is what changed my sister. Something from that day forward was able to manipulate her down some extremely challenging roads.

So this house was a really shitty move by all accounts. We had weird stuff going on in the loft; I'm seeing spirits, my dad is seeing spirits, my sister is being manipulated by spirits, and generally, we're all feeling totally freaked out. To make matters even worse, my parents were arguing more than ever. This house was doomed. It was really like something you see in a horror movie where everything keeps going wrong.

The change in my sister upset me the most. She shifted from this very deep, thoughtful and extremely creative person, to this person who was distant, moody, and lacking in any communication skills. If she wasn't out and about, all she would do was sit in her room listening to techno and trance music at full volume. It was like one night she went to bed as one person, and the next day she was a totally different person. She started seeing a boy, he was slightly older than her, and she started spending more and more time with him. She was completely smitten. I had no idea why, I could not see it at all. My sister and I have extremely different tastes in men, thank God.

One day, that I remember very clearly, my sister was arguing with my mum about wanting to go out. She tended to go for my mum because I guess we both perceived she was the pushover out of both our parents. There is always one in every family who you know you can get away with a tiny bit more than the other. In our family, it was mum. My mum was holding her own with my sister this time, though – putting her foot down and saying absolutely not. It became a fierce argument. My dad had to get involved and he said she was absolutely not to go out. She stormed off to her room, which was on the first floor, opened up the window and jumped out. Somehow, she was unhurt, but we should have known at that point that something wasn't right with her.

After all of the toxicity in this house, especially my parents fighting so much, they decided to buy yet another house to do their best to sort things out. I was so happy to be moving on, so much bad stuff had happened in the years we lived in the haunted house. There were happy memories too, but few and far between.

What was very interesting about the haunted house was that we found out, years down the line, that the next person to move into that house just dropped down dead. When I heard that tragic story, it confirmed for me that there was clearly something going on with that house. There were trapped energies or entities there that needed clearing.

By the time we sold that house and moved out, I was 15 and my parent's relationship was over. They made all the right noises about how this new house would be for us all, but the reality turned out to be something very different.

18

The new house was actually a bungalow and it was absolutely stunning. It was much more semi-rural than we had ever lived before. Although it was on a relatively busy road, our closest neighbours were a good distance away, and we were predominantly surrounded by trees and woodland. The plot itself must have been about a third of an acre, with a huge sweeping gravel drive out the front of this extremely pretty bungalow. It had been newly built and we had plenty of space to play around in.

Despite the obvious demons in the previous house, my sister really didn't want to move. Where we were had been convenient for her, socially. A little bit too convenient maybe. This new house was about 30 minutes away from Bournemouth town centre, buses were only one every hour and it would take an hour to get there. This was not ideal for either of us and our social lives. My sister had started driving and she passed her test first time, which was amazing. My parents bought her a little navy blue car that she would bomb around in, and this gave her a new level of independence, and the chance to get 'out of the sticks' – as she would call it.

At some point during the move from the old house to the bungalow, my parents decided it was time to stop living in a loop, to stop hurting each other, and put an end to all of the destruction that had been going on, and so they chose to separate. I don't have any memory of when that decision was made. My mum told me recently that they made the decision to divorce after the documents had been exchanged on the new property, but not being able to pull out of the sale, we moved there as a family. Very quickly, though, my dad moved out and pretty much disappeared.

I have absolutely no recollection of being told about the divorce. My whole adult life I believed he just went, but when I asked them recently, they both confirmed that they sat me down and told me.

It just goes to show how easily children can block out moments of trauma. What's even more fascinating is in all the years of work I have done on myself, at no point have I been able to recall that conversation. My mum said I did not handle it very well. I was a daddy's girl and heartbroken he was leaving.

My dad was never very good at talking, unless it was about business. He shut down feelings and emotions as quickly as they came up. His discomfort with his feelings made it an impossibility for the words to come out, even when he was coming from a place of love.

I was extremely sad when we moved, and that my dad was only around for a very short time before he left us. And when he did leave, he just disappeared and ran away. I didn't speak to him or see him for many months. His running away from a difficult situation, mirrored a pattern that I began to live out in my life. Whenever things got tough, I would just pack my things, book a flight and bugger off abroad until I felt okay to return. You could call it distractions.

Within a relatively short period of time, one of my mum's friends set her up on a date with her ex-boyfriend – a very generous thing to do. That guy was Mark, who is now my stepdad. Someone was clearly watching down on my sister and I when Mark came into our lives. He has been absolutely amazing over the years and a true stepdad. He is totally the opposite to my dad where communication is concerned. Mark is very open, he wears his heart on his sleeve and communicates clearly what he is thinking, and feeling. Over the years he has had to put up with a lot. Honestly, the guy deserves a medal.

The first time I remember my mum going on a date with Mark was when she was pottering around the bungalow all dolled up and looking amazing. I told her she looked pretty and she said she was going on a date with a guy called Mark. I was excited for her to be moving on. She deserved to be treated better than she had been, but it still broke my heart that she was going out with someone other than my dad. It's a really weird feeling when your parents split up. You are under the illusion when you're young that your life will stay the same, and your parents will always be there. Then, one day, you wake up and one of them is no longer there. And eventually, someone else comes along and fills their space. I do truly believe communication is key through any shifts like this. I would never want people to stay together if they made each other unhappy, but when there are others involved, in particular children, then communication is absolutely vital.

It was quite fun having my mum out on the dating scene with her new fella because it meant she loosened up with my sister and I. Leading up to my 16th birthday, I kept asking for a party. We were living in the bungalow that was in the middle of nowhere and so a party wouldn't affect any neighbours. Unexpectedly, she said, "We'll see." Which meant yes, in my head. Luckily, though, Mark was keen to whisk my mum away for a weekend, and so that was it, it was set! Party at mine for the sweet 16! The only deal was that my sister Kirsty had to be there to oversee everything. Done deal!

In the week or so leading up to the party, everyone at school was buzzing. It was all anyone was talking about. I was at an all-girls school, but we managed to invite some of the boys from the boy's school too. Game on!

A group of us – the 'party committee' – arranged everything. We decided what was going to happen, we set all the times and arranged how people would get there and get back home again. We discussed the music, the theme – you name it, we let our imagination run riot. It was amazing, we were so excited to have this beautiful big house to ourselves, and there was plenty of room for us to go wild outside too.

The whole build-up was part of the excitement, and we thought it was going to be the best thing that had ever happened. At that time of year, especially from New Year to half term, it was always boring. It was cold and miserable, so this was something to really look forward to.

Before I knew it, the party was upon us. Mum and Mark had planned to go away on the Friday night, and they would be back on Saturday at some point. When they were about to set off, my best friend and I were watching them load the car up, willing them out of the house. They gave me a kiss, told me to have fun and that they would be back the next day, and then, off they went. They jumped in the car, started the engine and drove across the gravel drive. As they pulled off onto the road the car gave off a little wheel spin. That was the sound that signalled — *Let's get this party started!*

We cranked up the music, and people started arriving. It was buzzing. My sister was in her room, doing her own thing with her boyfriend. That's all they would normally do anyway, just hide out in her room. We knew she was there if we needed her, but aimed to have a good time without her assistance. We cranked up the tunes and just started causing absolute mayhem.

Steadily, more and more people turned up. The girls arrived first, and then the boys turned up — fashionably late, as was typical of them. There were crisps and snacks on the go, and more importantly vodka. Everyone that turned up brought their own booze too, the really cheap stuff too — 20 20, Hooch, Smirnoff Ice and bottles of Southern Comfort! Everyone had been warned that we were miles away from anywhere, and we couldn't get supplies very easily, so they came fully equipped to party.

It makes me laugh to think of the parents that must have willingly gone out and bought their children alcohol to send to the house with them. Some people bought cigarettes, and there was even some pot going around.

We got wrecked. That was the mission going into it, and I'm pretty certain everyone succeeded, with honours. Most of the time, we were outside the front of the house, where the security lighting lit us up perfectly. Thinking about it now, it must have been absolutely freezing on a February evening, but I don't remember that even being a consideration that night.

My sister would check in occasionally, but she just said for me to get on with it, and do whatever I had to do; so we did. As the night went on it got messier and messier. My very best friend was absolutely off her rocker that night. She was someone who if she was drinking, she was drinking to get drunk. That night, though, the concoction of alcohol and pot — which we weren't very used to — blew our socks off. Believe it or not, I was the most sensible one at that party that night. I guess I had a level of responsibility as it was my house, and alcohol wasn't yet my thing — although, I gave it a good go.

It was actually that night that I started smoking cigarettes. I thought it looked cool holding a cigarette, but the taste of it was actually disgusting. I was determined to make myself like it. It took about two years to really embrace the taste and by that time I was addicted to nicotine. You have to admire my persistence, though.

It got to near the end of the night, and some of the parents had started to come and pick their kids up. There were no mobile phones back then, and so you had to arrange a time for your parents to pick you up and you had to leave whether you were ready or not. I looked around outside at all the debris – the cigarette butts, the glasses and the general mess. It was a disaster. There was broken glass everywhere. Things had been smashed inside and outside the house, people had been puking in the gravel and in the flowerbeds. Inside, there was alcohol all over the floor and crisps and chocolate had been trodden into the carpet. I think my mum would have expected some mess following a 16-year-old's party but this was a whole other level of destruction. It hurt my head to even consider having to deal with it. I was hoping that my sister and my best friend, who was staying over, would help me out in the morning.

The entire night, my sister had been safely tucked away in her bedroom, away from the noise and the destruction. When she started to hear people saying goodbye and cars pulling off the drive, she emerged from her room. She didn't look good. I wondered if she was upset, or maybe she had an argument with her boyfriend, or something like that. She asked, "Lu, are you alright? Is everything okay?"

I looked around the house and said, "Kirst, look at the state of this place, you're going to have to help me tidy this."

"Screw you," she said playfully. "This is your party, you deal with it." Which, to be fair, was true. She had not as much as set a foot outside her room, so it wasn't really up to her to sort the mess out. I was pretty certain that beyond her bravado, when push came to shove the next day, she would help.

As we were chatting, I noticed she looked vacant and troubled. Although I had a bit to drink, and so wasn't functioning at my very best, I knew in my heart something was going on. I asked her outright, "Kirst, are you alright?"

She looked surprised that I had been so blunt, and then she looked really sad. She said to me, "Lu, promise me if I tell you something, you won't tell mum and dad, or Mark?"

"Of course, I won't tell mum anything, you know that," I said. I could tell something was weighing extremely heavy on her heart. I felt it.

At this stage of our lives, my sister and I had become quite distant. There wasn't much of a relationship between us, which was sad as we had once been extremely close. Since she started dating this particular guy, it seemed she had become bored and irritated by the family. It saddened me because she was another of my heroes; that's the story of my life. I idolised her. I wanted to be just like her when I was little. I wanted us to be able to go out and party together when we were older. I imagined her helping with boys, and helping me choose what to wear. And because I was never a girly girl, I hoped for advice and guidance with makeup and stuff like that. I desperately wanted to be part of my sister's life. I had often imagined us getting to the age where we could both legally go out, and because there were only two years between us, we'd have so much fun and get into so much trouble together. I really thought my sister would be my best friend.

Despite the distance that had grown between us, what came next completely shocked me. It stunned me to the core and subsequently turned my world upside down for many years to come. We were standing in the hallway, just inside the front door, looking out onto the drive. There was no one else around at this time, everyone had gone. She looked me straight in the eye and said, "Lucy, I'm addicted to heroin and crack."

It's fair to say that those were the last words I heard and then everything else went silent. My mind switched off, those words kept ringing in my ears. I must have misheard her. There is no way. My heart broke into a million little pieces, right there and then. Even now my heart sinks when I say it out loud. *How on earth had this happened? How the heck am I not going to tell my mum?* My mind was spinning. Nothing made sense. I felt physically sick. I was waiting for her to tell me it was a joke, but that never came. It was horrific. This is serious shit!

How would I tell my mum? That thought kept running through my mind. I had made a promise to my sister and there was no way I could break it. She would never trust me again. I was one of those people who once I made a promise I will see it through, I will honour that promise, but this was my sister, my big sister. And heroin? Who the hell ever spoke about heroin? Where on earth do you have to go to get hold of heroin? It was a dirty, dangerous drug. Everything that I'd ever heard about it was dirty. And crack? I didn't even know whether it was better or worse.

It felt like a scene in a movie where everything's going on around you and it's just a complete blur. I needed to process it, but I just didn't know how to do it. *I'm not equipped for this. I'm 16 years of age. This is my 16th birthday. I want my mum!* The one time I really needed her, I had sent her away.

I don't really remember much of anything else that she said to me, but I do remember her begging me to keep my promise and not to tell. I just kept repeating to her, "Okay, I promise, I promise. I promise." My mind just didn't know what to do. How could I not tell my mum? I would never forgive myself if God forbid something happened to her and I knew. How would I live with that?

"You're the only person that can help me get better Lu, the only one."

I was broken. I heard those words and that became my mission. The fixer, the rescuer in me was activated.

As soon as I could get away from her, I ran to my bedroom, and in the same scenario as my 8-year-old self when my dad had upset me, I slammed the door and sat with my back to it and I sobbed my heart out. I needed someone, anyone to be there for me at that moment. My best friend was nowhere to be seen. Where the hell was she?

I was on my own dealing with this stuff and I didn't have a clue what to do. I mean, how do you deal with that? I was sixteen years of age, and in an instant, through all this chaos, I had changed into a full-blown adult. It felt like this was the turning point in my childhood, and this was the moment where it ended. It sounds dramatic, but that's how it felt.

All I could think when I sat behind that door crying was the words she had said to me – *You're the only person that can help me get better.* I really took that on board.

By this time, it was getting really late. My mum was due back the next morning, so not only did I have to deal with this awful revelation on my own, but somehow I had to tidy up the house and the garden too. The pressure in my head felt intense, it was like I'd done drugs myself and the room was closing in on me and chasing me down. It was awful.

I probably got about an hour or two of rest that night because I was so devastated. I also had this overwhelming worry about my sister. I kept going into her room to make sure she wasn't dead. I didn't know enough about those drugs, but from what I did know, I thought that if she was meddling with this stuff then she could die on me. It was horrible. I could tell she had been smoking stuff in her room because it absolutely stank.

I was tired, I was scared, and I felt utterly helpless.

I went to try and find my best friend to see what had happened to her, and that's when I found the absolute carnage that she had created. She had climbed into my mum's bed, absolutely hanging drunk and stoned, and ended up puking all over the bed and all over herself. *Oh, my God! As if there isn't enough to deal with right now, I've got to sort her out too, and she's a fucking mess!*

I went into full-on panic mode trying to sort out whatever I could. I knew I was going to have to be honest with my mum and admit it all just got out of hand. I started collecting everything I could and filling bin bags and loading up the dishwasher. I dragged my best friend out of bed and made her help me.

I was processing constantly. My mind was unravelling and creating massive worst-case scenarios that would probably never happen, but that's what I did in order to cope. I was overthinking everything, creating massive internal dramas. Poor me. Everything had gone so wrong. This was supposed to be fun and just looked at what had happened. *Why was I never capable of just having fun? Why could things not just go peacefully and smoothly?*

When my mum and Mark got back, I was all alone. My best friend had been picked up, and my sister, Kirsty, had gone out. I very much doubt she wanted to deal with seeing my mum and Mark, especially after the revelation she dropped the night before.

I did manage to get the house looking much more ship-shape before my mum got back, but I had to break the news about the bed to her, which went down like a lead balloon. The mess itself became irrelevant very quickly as I attempted to navigate triggering my mum into action, without breaking my promise to my sister. Very soon after she walked in the door, I said to her, "I'm worried about Kirsty." I didn't say anything more than that, I couldn't say anything more than that. What I needed was for them to take action and keep an eye on her. I carried on with whatever I was doing, but thankfully it was enough of a push for my mum to go into her room and start checking out what was going on in there.

Within about a week my mum had found some aluminium foil that my sister had used for her drugs, which then led her to find all the paraphernalia and the evidence she needed to confront my sister.

I never broke my promise. I really did the best I possibly could to honour my word. I know my sister believes I did break my promise, and that breaks my heart, even now, all these years down the line.

She was so angry with me. She possibly still is.

And although it hurts, thankfully people did find out. Thankfully they got her the help she required and into rehab. And although, admittedly, it took years and years before she actually became clean, at least I knew people were aware of what was going on and that she could get the help she needed.

19

After the chaos and trauma of my 16th birthday party, and finding out that my sister was a drug addict, I took the ironic path of then taking recreational drugs myself. In my mind, I justified the difference between what my sister was doing and what I was doing; the drugs I did were party drugs.

So, not wanting to do things by halves, I became the ultimate party girl.

I remember the exact moment when I turned my attention from light use of alcohol to party drugs. I was in a club called The Venue at Tower Park in Poole. My cousin and I had first started going there after my parent's divorce because it was the only place we could get in as 16-year-olds. The main reason we could really get in there was because my cousin was seeing one of the security guards, but that's another story.

Tower Park was a leisure complex, essentially. It had an actual water tower at the very top of it and before it was turned into a leisure estate it used to just be open fields. Over the years, they had turned it into a big complex with a large supermarket, a cinema, bowling alley, ice skating rink, a couple of restaurants and a bar. It very quickly became the place where those of us who went to Poole and Parkstone Grammar would hang out. It was the kind of place you would probably go to on a Saturday afternoon with your kids; then at night, it became a completely different place.

The nightclub there, The Venue, was huge. It was above the cinema and a bar called Colonnades. You had to queue up along the outside of the bar to be able to get in to the club, and once you reached the front of the queue, you would get asked for identification to prove you were old enough. Luckily, we never got hassled because of the security guard my cousin was seeing. Looking back at pictures of when I was this sweet 16-year-old, they are hilarious. What a sight! I looked so much older than I was. I had big hair that I would always spruce up, and massive boobs. I found if I wore a low-cut top, the security guys wouldn't even bother looking at my face, just my legs and boobs. I got away with a lot because of those boobs. I don't know what ever happened to them, though, as I don't have them anymore!

I would go there every Friday night with my cousin. I was always close to her growing up, but when my parents split up, we became much closer. I grew up so much in a really short space of time hanging out with my cousin. I was a really innocent little girl until my parents split; the horses had helped me to maintain that innocence. Before long, my friends from school got wind that I was going clubbing, so they asked to come along, and soon enough we had a bit of a Friday night crew. And by Friday, I mean every Friday night, without fail. We would turn up, flirt our way in — by this time, we were all on first-name terms with the door staff — and we would get drunk, dance, have fun, and then stagger home. Such innocent times.

On one of these Friday nights, I got chatting to a guy. I was well oiled. I'd had a few bottles of cheap alcohol, even though I still didn't enjoy alcohol at this point. This guy was extremely attractive. Apparently, he was a really good football player, or so I was told, and you could tell he looked after himself. He enjoyed a few drinks, but footie was his priority — and clearly women too. He introduced me to his friends. They were all lovely and they really welcomed me into their group. This group of friends were people who would take, what I would call 'party drugs' — like a pill or a bit of speed. My friend and I were chatting to these two lads, thinking that we were the bee's knees. I had on a little skirt, with heels and my boobs hanging out.

One of the lads came over and asked if my friend and I wanted to share a pill. We looked at each other with stars in our eyes and thought – *Fuck it! Why not?*

And just like that, it started.

He handed the pill over and told us to go to the toilet and break it in half, so we could share it. He gave us his water and sent us on our way. We felt so naughty, but excited at the same time. At no point did I stop to consider my sister, my mum, and all of the trauma from a few months earlier. This was my fun, this was my life, I'll do what I choose!

We went into the toilet, sneaked into a cubicle, and broke the pill in half. We looked at each other, did a 'cheers' with our drinks, and dropped our first-ever half a pill. We had no idea what to expect.

About twenty minutes later, my friend and I had huge smiles on our faces. We were moving much more freely to the music; it felt as if it had got louder, and the vibrations coming through the floor were more intense. It felt good to close your eyes and move, and that was it. I fell in love with ecstasy.

I danced the whole night long. I love to dance anyway, but that night I danced until the bitter end. My friend had to peel me out of the club at the end because I was having the best time. I was chatting to everyone, laughing, smiling and non-stop dancing; I finally felt like I belonged. I had a whole new level of confidence. I felt beautiful. Everybody wanted to talk to me, and to hug one another. I had so much to say to people. I loved everyone. It was almost like this divine goddess, that had been hiding inside of me, just bloomed.

Once they had eventually dragged me out of the club, discussions of an after-party started. Of course, there was no way we were going home. We had made a whole new circle of friends. They were our new best friends and we all loved each other. We were staying together, forever!

We trundled out of the club, and all of a sudden the cold hit us, especially as we were dripping with sweat from dancing non-stop for hours. We went back to a guy's house, and the party continued. Everyone was smoking weed and drinking. I didn't fancy doing any of those things. I just wanted to keep chatting and dancing. Then, all of a sudden, I started coming down. I didn't feel happy and chatty anymore. I just wanted to go home. I sat there silently, though, as

I didn't want to call a taxi and actually have to speak to someone. Suddenly, everything became a bit of a drag. The fun of the night had started to fade. I mentioned to my friend that I was ready to go and she agreed. We probably should have just gone back to hers after the club, if we were honest.

In a bizarre decision, my friend and I actually walked back to her house that night. We walked down the road with our shoes in our hands. Our pupils were like saucers. We laughed and chatted all the way home to keep each other going. We reminisced our way back through the evening. We were loving that moment, the fresh air, and being sixteen, and young, free, single, and off our boxes.

And quite honestly, that was the start of the party life for me.

To bring in some context, this was 1995. The UK in 1995 was the centre of the world for music and partying. The whole music and club scene was alive and booming.

Every single Friday night we would venture out to a night at The Venue called The Heritage. The Heritage, was much more deep house. We would go in, meet up with our crew, and 'neck' whatever we could get our hands on. Twenty minutes later, it would be party time; all night in the club and then on to the afterparty.

That turned into my life for a very long time. Every weekend for years, without fail. I would tell my mum I was going to stay with my friend, and then we would go out on the Friday and party until the Sunday. It was so much fun at the time, although the Sundays weren't great – having to deal with parents' questions on a comedown; and it wasn't as if I could answer them honestly either.

It started with half a pill, then very quickly I upped the ante and started taking whole pills. Back in those days, a pill was a few quid, they were very affordable, much more so than alcohol. Quite often we were given them for free. If one of the guys thought you were cute, or maybe he had a chance with you, he would pop one in your hand and hope it sweetened you up. Looking back on it now, I wonder what was I thinking. Anything could have gone wrong, and for many other people, it did.

We would start the night off with a half or even one, enjoy that journey, then when the effect wore off, we'd just take another half or one, to get high again. And that's what we did. We chased the high. I can only speak on behalf of myself when I say this, but I don't think anything ever compared to the very first one I did. Don't get me wrong, I had amazing nights after that, but nothing quite like that first high. I guess that's how they get you, you constantly chase that first ever high you experienced.

As time progressed, I would do a pill and very little would happen. I'm not sure if they were dud pills, or if my body had got used to them. Whichever it was, I would take another one. I'll never forget, a few of us drove up to London one night to go to an event that was on. It was in the heyday of my partying, where we would jump in a car on a Saturday afternoon, drive somewhere, then go out partying and drive home after we stayed somewhere for the night. One of our other friends had got us on the VIP list at this club. Walking in, we felt so cool and so sophisticated – we thought we'd really made it. Of course, we all had pills on us to take that night. It was a standard thing. I took one and as it started to kick in, I told my friend I didn't feel good. It was the most horrible experience I had had to date. It felt awful. I was seeing all sorts of weird things. I felt paranoid and really wanted to leave, but I could not do anything about it. I couldn't walk properly. I felt like the marshmallow man. I couldn't see properly. Everything was morphing into one another. It was totally freaking me out. Then to make matters much worse, I looked to the deejay for some sanity and I saw loads of military men standing in front of him. It was like I was on a battlefield and everyone was armed and ready, other than me. I started thinking – *Oh my God, what the fuck is going on?*

I freaked out. That was the first and last time I did ketamine. I had no idea what was in the capsule I had taken, but it turned out it was ketamine. It was horrible, it was dirty. That was my introduction to how bloody evil people could be in that world. Ketamine by all accounts was a lot cheaper than a bit of ecstasy, so they often cut it into things to bulk it out. Horrendous!

I'll be honest, it did not stop me doing ecstasy, though.

I am actually embarrassed to say this, but being as brutally honest as I possibly can be, things got so out of hand with my drug taking that one night I took thirteen pills. I don't know how I'm even still here to tell this story. I just kept going... and going... and going. The scary thing about it was, I remember my sister had told me that people had called her "cane-head" at one point in her journey, and here I was, absolutely mirroring her, without thinking about the potential implications. We had all heard of people dying from taking half a pill, but that didn't stop us at all. The irony of all ironies, I was doing this as a way to deal with the fact that my sister had just told me she was a drug addict; sabotaging myself but with the cheap justification that it wasn't hard drugs, it was just party drugs!

I was teetering on the edge of the darkness. I had a drug addict for a sister and I thought she might die — and my mum's heart was breaking over this. I now came from a broken home. I had no idea where my dad was, or if I would ever see him again. There was a new man in my mum's life. I lived miles away from my friends, and I wanted to blot it all out and dull it all down. Some people might have chosen food, or they might lash out at people in anger, some maybe even used sex as their tool of sabotage. My choice was to get off my head. I thought — *For the next seven hours, I'm going to pretend that I don't have any problems whatsoever, and I'm going to dance.*

It was a total contradiction. I was putting on the facade that I was happy and joyful — and this is where my name LucyLove came from — all those years ago, everyone used to call me LucyLove because I was always the person chatting to people and looking after them, and sprinkling love wherever I went. In reality, though, behind closed doors — and what people didn't see — was that I was really traumatised by everything that had been going on. I was miserable deep down inside and for a few hours, the drugs made me feel special.

After a number of years of doing this, though, I stopped enjoying it. I stopped going clubbing, which meant naturally gravitating away from doing pills. I might do one or two a year when I went to a festival, but they did not feature regularly in my life like they had done. I was really proud of myself for growing out of them.

However, then cocaine entered the frame.

People might find it weird to hear, considering I am such a huge chatterbox, but cocaine used to shut me up and stop me talking completely. That's so weird for me. I'm a talker. I'm a communicator. People would give me coke and after the first line I'd be all right, but after the second line I didn't want to talk, let alone have the capacity to do it. I would sit, listen and then I would get it in my head that I wanted to go home and be on my own. The great irony of me doing coke was that it was suppressing the positive thing that people knew me for. When something transforms your personality that much, it's not a good thing. To be perfectly honest with you, I didn't enjoy doing coke at all. I didn't like the way it made me feel, but at the same time, I really couldn't stop myself from doing it. I would say no, no, no...and then when the first lines got racked up, I'd jump in. I had absolutely no willpower, not an ounce of it – every pun intended. I did it to fit in. I did it so I wasn't the odd one out.

It got quite out of hand with my friends and me – and we were all as bad as each other. It only took one of us and we were all in. We would go out for dinner and then half an hour after we had finished, everyone would be saying – *Fancy a cheeky one?* It didn't ever make sense to me – we had bellies full of amazing food, but hey, lets do a line!

Looking at it now, I empathise with anybody who finds themselves in a situation where they feel that they need to do drugs, drink alcohol, or whatever their tool of choice is because they are running away from something in themselves. I definitely was. I never judged my sister for her choices, I understood that she had her reasons too. I just wanted to rescue her.

The big turning point for me came when my friend Mickey died.

20

Mickey was a guy I had met when he helped my sister get clean. I loved him for that reason. I loved my sister more than anything; I would have done anything to get her well and this man had helped, so I was forever grateful to his sweet soul. The huge irony of it all was that he was actually a coke dealer, yet he helped her get clean.

A friend of mine had got to know him, and on one occasion she invited me over to join them. He knew I was Kirsty's sister, so straight away he loved me. He was so protective of me and I really cared for him like a big brother. Whenever I spent time with him he would make me laugh so much. He was a real character. A cheeky, cockney chap whose heart was so pure. He was just lost and misguided. He was a true salt of the earth character. We would have some of the most profound conversations when we were together. He always said I should get into the government. He just saw something in me that I could never have seen in myself.

"Lucy, you need to run to become an MP," he would say. "We need somebody that gets it in government. You'd be perfect!"

"Mickey, seriously? I'm never going to get into government. They're all crooks," I would say back to him.

"Yeah, but we change it from the inside out," he would reply.

When I look back now, his wisdom was phenomenal. He was such a beautiful soul, despite his troubles.

When he was taken, it probably saved my life.

The way it all played out was terrible. Mickey always used to get his coke from London, and that's why everybody loved it so much; it was pure and clean. He would drive up to London – which is where he was originally from – source the coke and drive it back down to Bournemouth. This was a weekly occurrence and not a one-off thing. He must have been being watched by the police for a while, or maybe somebody had given his name to get a lighter sentence because on one occasion he got stopped by the Police on the M27 near Bournemouth. During a short search, they found the drugs, and he was immediately remanded in custody due to the amount he was in possession with. He was found guilty for possession with intent, and immediately sentenced and sent down to Dorchester Prison. The sad part of the story is, he never made it out of there alive.

I was still living in Bournemouth at the time, so Dorchester wasn't that far away to drive. One of my best friends and I got a visitation order and off we went. We took a cheeky little mid-week drive to Dorchester to see our pal. I'd never been in a prison before and I don't wish to go in another one either. Although, I am really glad I went through the experience to see him, as it was the last time I saw him alive.

We walked in and it was filthy and drab. We were checked thoroughly wherever we went. You're not allowed anything on you at all because they fear you could give something to the prisoners. We were so innocent the two of us, we had no clue what we were doing. We were surprised that we had to give up everything and give all of our details to be put in the system. It was bloody scary.

They eventually let us through the big gates to get to the visiting area. Mickey came in. We were not allowed to hug, or anything like that – the guards watched us like hawks. We sat across the table from him and chatted. We bought him up to speed on what was going on.

He filled us in on what had happened, and how on earth he had ended up in there. He was convinced someone had grassed him up. Despite the heavy chats, we did also have a good old laugh.

I asked him, "How are things going in here?"

"Alright," he joked. "There's definitely a few people in here that don't like me though," he replied, ominously.

'Is there anything you need me to do? Is there anything you need us to get for you?" I asked innocently.

Very quickly, though, time ran out and we had to go. He was given 18 months, so was due to be out in around 9 to 12 months; we said goodbye and hoped to see him soon.

A few weeks later, I woke up and saw a post on a friend's Facebook page that said, "I'm devastated at the news of Mickey." Naturally, this alarmed me, it was the first I had heard of it, so I called his mum – we'd become quite close and I figured if anyone's going to know what's happened to Mickey, it would be her. As soon as she heard my voice, she broke the news that he had been found dead at the bottom of the stairs in the prison.

Instantly, I just knew he'd been murdered. I had no way of actually knowing it, there was just a feeling inside of me. My gut and my intuition just told me. I didn't say anything, though, I felt it would be totally disrespectful to come out with my thoughts to his mum. Then all of a sudden, she came out with it, "Lucy, something is not right about this." Clearly, she felt exactly the same as I did. She had made the trip from London down to the prison to try and get to the bottom of it. She was a tough woman, a true East End cockney, well-seasoned at dealing with her troublesome children. She took absolutely no shit when it came to her family. She went to the prison and requested they showed her the photographs because they had to take photographs for evidence. She said from the position he was found in, there was absolutely no way he would have fallen naturally in that way. At the same time, because this happened in prison, we were never going to get the absolute truth about what had happened. She knew in her soul, though. Never doubt a mother's intuition.

Had he not warned me when we had seen him, I probably would never have thought anything untoward had happened, but he had specifically said there were a few people in there that really didn't like him. He was an older guy. In his early 50s at this point, very confident and forthright in his opinions. He would not be scared to call someone a dick if they were being a dick. And of course, in an environment like that, I imagine it would not be well received.

Sadly and ironically, I missed his funeral. I had booked a trip to Thailand with my partner many months earlier, so I was out of the country. I was devastated that I couldn't physically be there. It seemed so unfair. I arranged to do lots of special things from Thailand; I floated things on the water for him and lit a lantern and said some prayers, which is what they do over there when people pass.

With Mickey gone, everything changed. Besides the fact that when he went to prison the decent coke supply got cut off, I started taking massive steps back from that scene. I decided that because Mickey was not there — and I really trusted Mickey — I didn't want to go and buy something off a random person. I had plenty of time to feel into it whilst I was away in Thailand. I mentioned it to my boyfriend a few times, and he really didn't like the whole coke thing at all. I thought — *Something's got to change.*

And, admittedly, it wasn't an overnight thing, it was more of a gradual process. However, in as many weeks as it took me to get into the drug scene, it took me to get out. I got to the point where I just didn't want it. I didn't even care that my friends were doing it, I just didn't want to be involved in it anymore. It no longer resonated with me. And so, as a result of my choices, my circle of friends changed. We were no longer aligned with one another and people started to fall away.

21

At around the time of my 16th birthday party, my sister's addiction revelation, and my wild partying, I met the boy who would become my first proper boyfriend. The boy who I truly handed my heart over to.

I was living in the house where my birthday party had taken place, the one which was more rural and off the beaten track. All of my friends were still in Bournemouth, so they were a long way away from me, a good 30-minute drive, or an hour on the bus. My social circles were so limited at this point in my life, so I decided to get a job closer to home, so I could be part of something.

I had been working as a chambermaid in the Royal Bath Hotel. I'll be honest, I loved it. I have some hilarious stories about things that went on in that hotel. When I was there it was a 5-star hotel. It was a sought-after place to stay, in an amazing location close to the beach. However, it soon went downhill when they built a shoddy entertainment centre that blocked part of the views of the beach. The hotel never recovered after that.

When we moved house, it was no longer easy for me to get there on a Saturday morning, as it was about an hour's journey on a bus. Now, no disrespect meant, but at 16 years old, there was no way I was going to travel an hour on a bus to go and clean people's bloody bedrooms. I'm not even sure the buses ran that early on a Saturday, and I started work at 7am! At first, I stayed at my friend's house, who was one of the gang I went out with on a Friday night. We would go out, get totally off our heads, and then rock into work the next day and just deal with whatever came up. Then we would go home at two o'clock in the afternoon and sleep. We did that for a few months and then it became too much hard work, so I applied for a job at my local Tesco.

I thought it would be nice to meet some friends who were on my doorstep. I saw it as an opportunity to go and create a new social circle. There were loads of people who worked at Tesco that were at college or university and so I knew I'd meet some cool people around my age. I worked two evenings a week and also a Saturday. Occasionally, I could get a Sunday shift, which was exciting because it would be paid double time.

I knew I would get the job when they were interviewing me, I could just feel it. I could really picture myself working there. It felt really grown up to me. It had an office feel to it, but just with a big shop underneath, and you got to make your own coffee and help yourself to food. You even got a discount when you shopped there.

When I started, I predominantly worked on the deli counter. The reason they put me on there was because I was so friendly and chatty. Customers would always comment about my smile and how I brightened their day. People would specifically come in on the days I was there for a chat! Thankfully, my prayers were answered about meeting new friends. I started working with a girl called Becky, who was the same age as me. Becky became my best buddy for many,

many years, and I absolutely loved her. She was like the sister that I didn't have at that period of my life, and we became inseparable.

I thought she was amazing. She shared that she had been bullied at school, and so she was somewhat traumatised by that. I believe I brought her out of her shell over the years and helped her grow. She became really confident, and even now, in her present life, she's thriving and has an amazing career. I'm not blowing smoke up my own arse, but I don't think she would have done some of that if I hadn't been pushing her. I'm sure she would admit that herself. It was such a beautiful friendship.

One week they changed my days, and when I was at work that day, I saw this really cute guy. He was working in the cold section of the store – you know, the cheeses and the milk. I used to really dislike being in that section because it was so bloody cold!

On this night, we were in together for the duration of our shift. I walked into my section and bumped into him. He said, 'Hi', and so I shyly said, 'Hi'. He introduced himself as Phil, I said my name was Lucy, and then we went off in our own directions. We had one of those interesting smile exchanges as we walked off. Becky was watching. She could tell I liked him. She brought me up to speed on him because she went to the same school. She told me that he was a good footballer and that he had a really pretty girlfriend. I remember thinking – *Oh well, never mind, at least he's a nice bit of eye candy* – and I just closed it down straight away. From that night on, we hit it off, though. Just a bit of harmless, flirty fun. I would catch his eye and then quickly turn away – it was real teenage stuff. We would bump into each other again and again in the back corridors between the fridges and the storage – and we would have a little chat. He asked me where I was from and how I came to be working there and stuff, and I asked him bits about his life. I saw him every Saturday after that. He became a beautiful part of the Tesco scenery. In my opinion, he was perfect. He was good-looking, a bit moody, and he clearly had a bit of a chip on his shoulder. To me, that was perfect.

One night, we were closing up, I was due to get picked up and he was also waiting for a lift. We were having a chat and he said, "Do you fancy coming to The Academy with Woody and I on Friday?" I knew Woody, because he worked there also, so I said, "Well, if Becky can come too?"

"Yeah, sure don't worry about it. We'll drive, we can all go together."

I hadn't even asked Becky yet, but I called her when I got home all excited, "Becky, you've got to meet me at 8:30 on Friday. Be ready. I'll get changed in Tescos and we'll go out from there."

"Oh my God, where's this come from?" she asked. We were like little kids. This was really exciting. We were going to be picked up by some boys, driven to a club and then spend the night dancing with them. And not just any boys, but Phil!

We walked into The Academy, and the music was pumping. I was buzzing because I was there with this really frickin smoking guy. However, that bubble burst very quickly when we arrived because he said, "I'll be back in a minute. I've just got to go and do something." He gave me a kiss on the cheek, and I was taken aback by that, and then he went off. Becks and I went to the bar to get some bottles of horrible, cheap booze. We were ready to get the party started, and then I saw Phil go over to a really beautiful girl.

I asked Becky, "Who's Phil talking to?"

She said, "That's his girlfriend."

And I thought – *Oh God.* I can't lie, my heart broke a little bit at that moment. I had to pull myself together. I had a big swig of my drink and just thought – *So what, we're just friends.* Becky and I hit the dance floor and just started to have a good time. We were dancing and chatting, and then several boys started to come up to us and chat. A guy came over and started flirting with me, then out of nowhere, Phil appeared and said, "I hope you don't mind if I butt in," and he grabbed me by the hand and took me upstairs.

I said to him, "What are you doing? Your girlfriend's here."

He sat me down on a bench – I'll never forget it – the music playing in the background seemed to elevate the moment, there were people up on the stage having a great time, it felt like they were cheering us on. Phil looked at me and he said, "I've just broken up with her. I hope you want to be with me." My heartbreak from earlier turned very quickly into delight. Then we kissed. It was perfect. He was perfect. I'll be honest, in that moment, I had absolutely no consideration for his poor girlfriend who had just been dumped. From that moment on, that was it.

We were together for five years.

I know every first love is special and maybe I remember mine through rose-tinted glasses, but I truly believe what we had was magical. He was well out of my league. When he said he wanted me, I felt as if I had won the lottery. I knew I wanted him from the first moment I set my eyes on him, but I just didn't see what he might see in me. Later on, those insecurities would play a big part in completely destroying our relationship.

The first few years of us being together were amazing, though; we were inseparable. Then, as we got a little older, 18 years old, and we were doing our A-Levels, it was understood that we were both going to go to University, and we were really open and honest about it. And, of course, I would support him doing that, and he would support me doing whatever I wanted to do.

One day, he decided that he was going to follow in his sister's footsteps and go to Aston University, which is in Birmingham. I was very supportive of it, but I had decided to stay on in Bournemouth and do something else for that first year when he was going to be in Aston. He was really supportive of that too – well essentially, he had a year to be a single lad at university. We were very comfortable with each other, and there was lots of trust – although I imagined university life would probably bring some temptations for him. I didn't worry, though, I trusted.

That September, he went off to Aston and I stayed behind, doing my own thing. We spoke as often as we possibly could. I would go up there to visit him whenever I had the chance, and I got to know his flatmates in the halls really well. We had such a good time when we were together, but it was during that period that my insecurities started coming up. He wasn't just down the road anymore. I couldn't be with him in five minutes when I felt sad or when I had something really exciting to share with him, and I didn't like it. I think this was a throwback to the separation I felt when my dad left.

When I passed my driving test, I gained more freedom. My mum laughed at me when I told her my maiden voyage would be the three-hour trip to Birmingham. It didn't phase me at all. I just did it. I'm certain that's why I'm so confident driving to anywhere now. Even at that young age, I was a Wanderess! I just cracked on, and I did it because I wanted to see him.

I could see Phil was enjoying himself. He was out drinking and partying and associating with girls that I didn't know. I don't think he cheated on me, but the past baggage from my dad was coming up and slapping me around the face. In order to cope with it, I started overcompensating by going out for drinks all the time with the boys from work. A heavily competitive edge kicked in. Looking back, it was the first time I really stepped into my masculine energy and to being driven by my toxic ego traits. I was very competitive anyway, especially in sports, Phil was too. We already had that little bit of edge and competition, having to get better exam results than each other. So I figured that if I didn't know what he was getting up to, I would just go and get up to my own stuff.

I really have to give him so much credit. He was so patient with me. He was so supportive and no matter what he did or said, I will always be grateful to him for the support he gave me over the years with my sister. He was my rock. He did not deserve my insecurities being spewed all over him, and me being a real bitch at times. I remember one phone call, he was in his halls, I was on the phone to him and I was just being hard work for the sake of being hard work. It wasn't like I even had a point, I was just being difficult because I could be, and I wanted to piss him off. I naively didn't realise that if anything was going to push him to someone else, it would be that kind of behaviour!

The following year, I actually joined him in Birmingham. I decided to go there to be with him, rather than go to other places that I probably should have gone to in order to get the best experience out of university. I prioritised being with him over my own choices. He never asked me to, but I decided he was more important than me and my happiness.

Being in Birmingham together wasn't great, though. We spent time together and we got on, but it wasn't like it was back in Bournemouth. It felt like we had spread our wings and really started moving away from each other.

I was really popular at university, particularly with the boys. I became really good friends with the football and rugby teams. I was adopted as part of their crew, which shows where my energy was at that time. There was this one night, Phil had pissed me off in one way or another, and all the rugby boys were going out, so I decided to join them with a couple of the girls that I knew. That night I drank eleven pints of Stella. I wasn't a big drinker then at all, so you can imagine the state of me. On top of that, I barely ate at university. My diet was not particularly good. I wasn't that easy to feed, so I barely ate.

I was tiny at this point, maybe 6 stone maximum. There are pictures from then, and I look ill. I got absolutely steaming that night. All the lads folded me up into one of those massive tumble dryers in the laundromat. I couldn't get out because I was laughing so much, and they were laughing so much. At one point they really couldn't get me out, it was so funny, but not funny all at the same time. Imagine having to call the fire brigade out because I was trapped in a bloody tumble dryer. My future kids will be so proud!

The more I hung around the lads, the more I liked it. There was this one guy in the rugby team, he was a really big guy with fair hair, and he really took a shine to me, he was like my protector. And he kept saying to me, "When are you going to finish with your boyfriend for me?" And, even though he wasn't my type – I'm more of the leaner footballer type – it made me realise that I was attractive. I started to get confident that there were many men who liked what I looked like, and they wanted to spend time with me.

There was another guy, Laurie, he was a footballer, and absolutely gorgeous. He had dark brown hair and really, really piercing blue eyes. I remember thinking – *You're dangerous*. He was so lovely and calm, and so good-looking, charismatic and charming. A dream basically. This was where things started going really wrong between Phil and I because I all of a sudden I was thinking – *Fuck you, if you're not going to give me attention, I'll go get it elsewhere.* This was when my sabotaging of relationships really began. I started pushing away the people that loved me rather than being vulnerable and letting them know how I was truly feeling.

We went on like that, Phil and I, for a while. I ended up going back to Bournemouth and within a few months of me being back home, I met a guy in a leisure centre who was absolutely gorgeous. He was called Mark. He was everything I liked. He was a semi-professional football and a semi-professional golfer; absolutely gorgeous, and, dangerously, he liked me too. All the girls threw themselves at him, and by all accounts, he was a bit of a player. Once again, I thought he was out of my league, and I had him on a bit of a pedestal. When he asked me out, I thought he was joking. All my friends warned me not to go anywhere near him because he was such a well-known lad about town. I couldn't help myself and I said yes, even though I was still with Phil – albeit the relationship was hanging on by a thread.

I honestly went on the date innocently. I know that sounds like a whole heap of shit. How can a date be innocent? But truly, Mark intrigued me. There was no way I would do anything. Interestingly, I did end up spending time with this person, and I really enjoyed it. He bought something out in me that I had been lacking. Most importantly, he was interested in me, Phil wasn't anymore. It ended up with this guy, who was a complete player, saying to me, "I want to be with you."

We ended up kissing, and I broke up with Phil. I completely broke Phil's heart. I shattered it into a million pieces and his friends hated me for it. I wasn't fair, I wasn't nice. I didn't do it the right way. Phil was very angry with me. He had heard on the grapevine that I was dating this guy called Mark, and I remember him screaming at me and shouting at me, and I just said, "No, it's not true. No, it's not true." But, it was.

I'll be honest, I wanted the security of Phil. I loved him, we'd been together so many years, we just forgot we needed to invest in each other. However, I was so drawn to Mark, I wanted him too. He was everything that I had ever wanted, and we were amazing together.

The truth of the matter was I was really meddling with people's hearts and minds because, selfishly, I had discovered that I was attractive to guys all of a sudden. I never anticipated when I met Mark that first day, that he would be my second love – and we would also be together for 5 years.

22

Mark and I had a great relationship. He was amazing. He was so kind and understanding, and a general all round great guy. We had a very intense relationship. We would spend as much time together as possible. We were passionate, loving, and full-on. It was amazing.

One day, a little while into our relationship, I was in the shower at my mum's house where I was living and I started to feel faint. I had to hold onto the side of the shower because I felt so unsteady on my feet. Soon after that, I fainted. I had never fainted before in my life. Something was off, something felt weird. I had been doing some really bizarre things leading up to this day. I never ate spreadable cheese, however for the two weeks preceding this I couldn't get enough of it. It makes me feel sick to think of it even now. I had thought this was a bit weird, but that was it. Nothing more, nothing less.

After I fainted, I booked myself an appointment to go to the doctor. He asked me lots of questions which I answered honestly. He ran a couple of observation tests, then suggested we did a urine test and a pregnancy test. I said, "No way, that cannot be the case, I haven't missed a period." He informed me all of the signs and observations pointed to me being pregnant, but he was happy to be proven wrong. Then I was sent off to do the pregnancy test.

I came back to his office and he asked me to think that if I was pregnant how far gone I thought I could be. I thought about it but had absolutely no idea. I was on the pill and I hadn't missed a period, so it couldn't be very long. He looked at me and said, "Lucy, you are definitely pregnant and I think you are a lot further down the line than you think you are."

Oh shit.

He gave me some cards and some numbers to call. I walked back to my car, got in and put my head in my hands – *What the fuck am I going to do? How the fuck am I going to get through this?*

Everything was spinning around at a million miles an hour. Normally my first port of call would be my mum, but she had her hands full with my sister, so I just sat there and I thought – *What am I going to do? I cannot have a baby, I cannot give my baby away.* Every possibility was unthinkable. I just wanted to disappear, to not be there.

I had no idea what to do, so I called Mark. He came to get me, and to talk to me. He was amazing. He could easily have said I was on my own and done one, but he didn't. He said he would stand by me whatever I decided, and he just empowered me to make the decision. He said, "Whatever it is Lucy, we will make it work." And I trusted him. He was so honourable. Quite honestly, I wish I had never had to go through it, but there is no one in this world that I would rather have had to have that conversation with. For the first time in many, many years, I had to be vulnerable and let someone look after me.

I thought about it – well that was all I thought about. I was only 21, and he was 20. I thought that if we had a child now, that would be our lives ruined. He was a very talented footballer, and an exceptional golfer. I did not want to destroy his life, by a mistake we made. I would never forgive myself for ruining his life because I really did love him. It was so sad we had to go through this.

The timing was dire also! My sister was probably the worst she'd ever been in her life with the drugs. I had recently had to pick her up from a drug dealer's house, she was so out of it when I got her home, we put her in the bath, and all of her hair was falling out. She was so skinny and grey, just pure skin and bones. So my sister, it seems, is dying in front of me, my mum's not coping at all, and the doctor had now said to me, "You've got to make a decision immediately about what you want to do with the baby because if you want a termination, it has to be done by 12 weeks." I had no time at all to decide what to do, and I've got to speak to my boyfriend, talk it over and make a decision. *Shit! What a mess, Lucy!*

This was in typical Lucy fashion. Everything happened all at the same time. Multiple fires burning concurrently.

I was feeling guilty on so many levels. I found myself in a situation where the only way out of it, or the only thing that I could see, was to have a termination. Just that word sends shivers down my spine. I don't judge anyone who has gone through it, I just never thought I would. I was always so careful, I really was. I took my pill religiously, not knowing I was super fertile – and Mark was too, by all accounts. Thankfully, both Mark and I were in a position where we could pay for it privately, so it could be done very, very quickly.

After much turmoil and angst, I made the decision for us both. The day after I found out that I was pregnant I booked in for a termination. I didn't allow myself time to think about anything – what the termination process would be like, or how it might impact my body in the long term. I didn't ask my mum for her help or support, because she had her hands full with my sister. I didn't have anybody to speak to about it. I was a young 21-year-old kid making a huge, life-changing decision for me and this other person, let alone the baby. I was absolutely mortified by it all. I never anticipated how much I would hate myself for it, or whether Mark might hate me for it, but I knew it was what I had to do. And I stand by it. At that time, it was the right thing to do. I would never, ever, want to make that decision again.

After I made the decision and told Mark, we made a phone call. They told me to go in immediately to be scanned. Mark came with me.

The place was only about 30 minutes drive from where I was living at the time. We pulled up outside this place, I looked at this building and I remember thinking that this is just awful. I was devastated. How on earth have we ended up here? It wasn't just the building itself, which was horrible, it was thinking about what went on inside this place that was really the most shocking bit of it all.

I kept saying to Mark, "I can't do it, it's a baby."

He kept reassuring me, "I've got you. Don't worry. We'll be okay, Luce."

He held my hand whilst we sat there, and he asked a lot of the questions on my behalf because I just couldn't bring myself to do it. Once we had the initial discussion, they took me off to a room to give me a scan to see how far gone I actually was. We were both absolutely mortified to be told that I was eleven and a half weeks. Thankfully, at that moment in time I didn't realise how developed an eleven-and-a-half-week-old baby was. I was so ignorant back then. When I think about it now, even though I have forgiven my younger self for it all, it still breaks my heart. I had thought back then that it was fine up to twelve weeks. At no point did I ever comprehend it was a living thing inside of me that had a heartbeat, and that knew what was going on. They told us we had no choice but to get the procedure done the next day. So we booked and paid to go in the next day.

That evening, the day before I was now due to go in for the procedure, my mum asked me to 'babysit' my sister. My sister had reached a whole new level of self-destruction – stealing and getting into a lot of trouble. I was being aloof as I didn't want to tell my mum that I was going for a termination. I said to her, "I'm sorry Mum, I can't do it, I'm busy."

My mum started yelling at me, telling me I was selfish. I get it, I really do get it now, but back then, I didn't. She was hurting, she was doing all she could to protect her baby and her other baby was being awkward. The more she spoke, the more I bubbled up underneath – I was hormonal as well. She kept going on and on, "Why would you have to do this? I'm going to have to leave your sister on her own."

I ended up getting to the point where I couldn't take it anymore and so I just screamed out, "Because I'm having a fucking abortion." And of course, that stunned the whole household. My sister started crying, my mum was crying, and to top it all off I was crying too.

I snapped! I thought I was strong enough to do this on my own and with Mark, but I wasn't! I needed people to understand. My mum was upset that I hadn't told her, she said she would have helped me, but I hadn't wanted to burden her. It was just an absolutely horrific situation. I've never felt so alone in my entire life.

I stormed out the house, slammed the door and I went for a walk to get my head together because I couldn't process what was going on. I hadn't wanted to tell my mum at all, and most definitely not in such an angry way.

The next morning, Mark came and picked me up. I was fasting because I had to be put to sleep that day, so I was really ratty and grumpy with him, and, trust me, I let him know I was pissed, I even said I wouldn't be here if it wasn't for you. I was venomous towards him that morning, I really was, and it was so undeserved because he was amazing. He didn't deserve to be treated like that – at the end of the day it takes two to tango. Mark, if you ever read this, I'm so sorry.

When we arrived at the private clinic, they said Mark wasn't allowed to come in with me. I was devastated. I wanted him to sit with me and hold me until I went in.

They took me into this cold, extremely clinical room. They closed this green curtain around me and told me I had to put on this horrible green gown and that I would be expected to walk down the corridor on my own, to the operating unit. It was like walking the Green Mile. Literally, green everywhere.

When I got to the room I needed to be in, everyone was really sweet, they were smiling at me and giving me reassuring looks and gestures. The room was so clinical and cold, though. *What the heck am I doing here? How did it come to this?*

There were all these machines and implements, and I realised that I had no idea what they were about to do. I do not actually think I asked – which in hindsight was probably wise.

They told me to lie down, they put the intravenous line in. I went off really quickly. It was the first time I had ever had an anaesthetic.

When I came round, I was all alone. I wanted Mark to be there. I kept asking the nurse when I could go home but they had this rule that after a general anaesthetic they made you have a cup of sugary tea and a sandwich. The sandwich looked horrible – a pasty-looking cheese and tomato thing. I sweet-talked one of the nurses into putting my sandwich in the bin so I could go home, I bargained with her that I would have a biscuit and the tea, and amazingly she binned the sandwich. She really looked after me and she told her matron that I had eaten the sandwich, and so Mark was allowed to come in to take me home.

He walked in and I sobbed. I felt so guilty. As a precaution to stop me falling pregnant again, the hospital advised me to change my contraceptive pill, as I had been on a contraceptive pill when I had fallen pregnant with Mark. I willingly did this as I did not want to go through this again, ever in my life. However, once again the Universe had different ideas. Within three months, I had fallen pregnant again on the pill; highlighting how fertile I was. Mark and I agreed what we could not, and would not, terminate the pregnancy.

Just weeks after finding out I was pregnant, I had my first miscarriage. No sooner had I got over the shock of finding out I was pregnant, I was devastated to experience loss again. This is when a new self sabotaging pattern kicked in – the guilt, the resentment, and the shame that I felt for going through that termination, I believed resulted in this punishment. I blamed myself and my selfish actions for creating this physical trauma.

To be honest, I felt guilty about this for years and years. I carried that guilt with me right up until I was 36 years old.

To think about it now is weird because I would have a 22-year-old child. I trust that everything happens for a reason and that child is now one of my biggest supporters. I was in no way equipped to be a mother then. I was just a kid myself.

23

After I left university, I went back home to Bournemouth to look for a job. I didn't have any idea what I wanted to do yet. I hadn't enjoyed what I'd done at university, and no clear career path was making itself known to me.

As a young girl, I had said to my mum that all I want to do was help people, and quite rightly she said to me, "Sweetheart, that's wonderful but you do know that being a nurse doesn't pay very well?" I had already decided that my version of success was through money, and that came from my dad and so I quickly shut down the idea of helping other people. He had money, I always saw him as abundant financially. We always had nice things. Both mum and dad had nice cars, and we were always moving houses. That was my early perception of success. The fact that he was rarely there for us as kids didn't seem to alter my perspective on thinking him 'successful' – because I knew he was working really hard to give us a nice life. It was all about the material stuff.

I decided that I was going to follow in my dad's footsteps. I didn't even really know what he did; I knew he was a qualified accountant by trade, but even that didn't mean much to me. All I knew was that I wanted what he had and I was going to get it.

Whenever I would drive down the dual carriageway into Bournemouth from the Airport, we would drive past this incredible glass building. I remember that building being there my whole life, although I later found out it was only built in 1984. I loved that building because it looked like a massive greenhouse, and it fascinated me. I wondered what went on in there. It appeared somewhat mystical and magical. When we would drive past it, I would always think – *I'm going to work there one day.*

A few months after I got back to Bournemouth, I saw an advert in the back of the local paper and said to my mum, "Where's Chaseside? What does that mean?"

She replied, "Oh, you know where the motorway is? It's the big glass building just behind there. It's owned by Chase Manhattan Bank."

I was so excited, "Oh my God, I need to go there." I didn't care if I got the job or not, I just had to go there and see what it was like inside that building.

At the time, I was working doing some admin for a life insurance company, nothing meaningful, so I got my CV sorted and I became totally obsessed with this opportunity. I was going to get that job! This was for Chase Manhattan Bank, for God's sake. An American bank in Bournemouth! It was an amazing chance for me. The way I thought of it at that time was – banks made money, and if banks made money, then I'm going to be successful, and then my mum and my dad will perceive me to be successful.

So I applied, and I got an interview.

On the day of the interview, I had absolutely no clue what I was doing. I hadn't bothered doing any research, I didn't do any research back then. I mean, looking back, who goes to an interview, knowing nothing about what the company does, let alone the role I was being put forward for? Somehow, though, I always managed to get away with it.

I came off the slip road from the dual carriageway and turned into this incredible estate surrounding this enormous glass building. As part of the deal for Chase Manhattan to set up in Bournemouth, they had to build lots of new homes for the staff to relocate, and also a leisure centre that was called "The Littledown", as a form of entertainment, something for the people to do. It was huge, all of it. I kept on driving until I came up to a security barrier and some traffic lights. It was very official, all high-level security. I spoke to the security guy, he checked the list for my name, and when he found it, he ushered me through the barrier. It was really exciting. I'd never been into anything like this before. Even when you got through the barrier, the place was so huge that you had to drive for about half a mile along a grass-lined driveway. I eventually got to the car park and it was rammed, almost every parking space was filled. This was when it hit me how big this company was. I eventually found a visitor's space, parked my car, took a deep breath and started walking toward reception. I couldn't help but be in awe of how big it all was.

The main building, the huge glass greenhouse, was nestled amongst a landscape of lush greenery and plants, and with beautifully manicured paths and hedges leading away from it to guide the staff from one building to another. It was simply stunning. As I approached the reception area, reaching out above my head was a futuristic walkway stretching from one building to the other, presumably so that people didn't have to get wet in the rain when walking between buildings. I thought – *This is what I'm looking for!*

I stepped into the reception area and looked around. The entire space was massive. I sheepishly approached the lady on reception and gave her my name. She was really lovely, and told me to take a seat. I sat down and looked around, and it was absolutely magnificent. There was glass everywhere, and huge high ceilings. There were flower displays, plants and trees all around. It was magical. And the glass wasn't just normal glass, it was a green colour, so it all amplified a rainforest vibe. There were so many people walking past too, a constant flow, and I noticed very quickly that there were many attractive men. *Yes! This is good. I feel like I've gone to heaven.*

After a while, a gentleman came down and introduced himself, he took me through the security turn-styles, and as we walked we had a nice chat. He walked me to the interview room where there was another person waiting for us both. It was a typical interview setup, I sat across the table from them whilst they fired questions at me. I was so young, so naive and so full of life, everything was exciting. In my head, I just thought I was going to be paid a fortune here because this is the big time. Even just sitting in the interview I felt like I had made it.

The interview lasted thirty minutes maximum. I wasn't sure how it had gone because the guy just walked me back down and he said, "Thanks, we'll be in touch." I was certain I hadn't got it. I started to re-run the interview in my head and began chastising myself for saying stupid things. However, I was so honest with these people, I was totally myself, and they obviously loved it because later that afternoon they called me and said, "If you're interested, we're interested."

That was when the fear kicked in. *Holy shit! I got it!* Of course, my ego jumped in and started to create problems and tried to sabotage the excitement. Why couldn't I just enjoy it, without creating things that could go wrong?

Chase Manhattan Bank, before they would even discuss your contract, required you to be drug tested. Now of course, as you well know, naughty Lucy was up to plenty of mischief at this time. So I started panicking. Obviously, I wanted the job, I didn't want anything to jeopardise it, and I would do whatever it took, but at the same time, I was in shit because this was a Tuesday and the weekend before I had been off my box.

They asked me to make an appointment to go to an external place to get drug tested, via a urine test. I desperately needed to know how long the drugs stayed in your system for. This was the pre-internet days and so the only people I could ask were the people who had either sold the drugs to me or taken the drugs with me – not exactly the most reliable sources. They all said for coke and pills it was usually about two days. Weed was much longer but I didn't smoke weed back then, it sent me bat shit crazy and made me really paranoid.

No class B's for me then, I was all about the Class A's and for once, that was a really good thing.

Everybody said to drink lots of water beforehand and I should be okay. When they called me, I booked an appointment for the week after just to be on the safe side. I decided to lock myself away for that week and not speak to anyone. I set my intention, without knowing that's what I was doing, and I focussed — *I have got to get this job for the sake of my family.* My mum, God bless her, was earning £11.5k a year at this point. She was supporting my sister and I on that, God only knows how. I knew this was my opportunity to help. I knew that I could take some of the burden off her, not that she ever asked for it or even wanted it, but I wanted to start stepping up and levelling up to be my own person. First, I had to pass that bloody drug test, though. I'll be honest with you, I even considered sending somebody else to do the drug test for me; I was prepared to cheat my way through if I had to.

I went to this drug test place and was so nervous. I turned up there, sat outside in my car, holding on to the steering wheel and talking myself round — *I can do this! I can do this!* I drank loads and loads of water. All week I had been really good, I had been exercising loads to try and get the drugs out of my system. I walked in and the lady was so lovely. She checked my name and my ID — so I would have been up Shit Creek if I had sent somebody else in my place. She explained what they were going to do, asked me a few questions and then I had to go off and do a urine test.

I brought the sample back to her and she tested it there and then in front of me. Thankfully I was clear! I was so happy and relieved I started dancing around the room. She said, "Oh wow, you're happy."

I said, "This is the biggest opportunity I've ever had in my life." That's how I viewed it. This was my chance. I had decided that I wasn't going to be like other people, just doing whatever they could do to get by, and no disrespect to what my mum was doing, but she worked as a secretary for an estate agent and they treated her like shit, she got paid minimum wage, and I didn't want to be like that. I wanted to be more like my dad. I wanted to be able to afford nice things.

After everything I had been through with my parent's divorce, I said to my mum at the ripe old age of 15, "I am never going to rely on a man for money, ever." It was such a bold statement. I was so pissed off with my dad for leaving, and I was upset for my mum because she had such shit money. My mum was so proud that she would never have asked for help. I remember sitting there in the bungalow with her one day and I just said, "I will commit to it now. I will never rely on men for money." And of course, that was a massive part of my bullshit story. I honoured my word. I was loyal to that statement to the bitter end until I was about 36, and there are still elements of it that will come up from time to time because I had it almost printed on my DNA cells.

I asked the lady at the drug test place if I could have a hug, and although she said yes, she looked at me as if I was crazy. She must have sent the results off straight away, because within about two hours I had a phone call from Chase Manhattan Bank, offering me £21.5k a year, plus perks. At that time, it was ten grand a year more than my mum was earning. It was huge! This was my first proper job and I got £21.5k a year, private health care, and I would be receiving bonuses. They had a scheme whereby if you were ranked in the middle to upper section of your grade, you would get a bonus. I saw the pound signs light up. I started allowing my imagination to run wild – I could change my car, I could give my mum some money, I could buy a house. This was it! I had made it! And I had not even started yet.

24

Besides the money, the social aspect was exciting me immensely. I was going to be surrounded by hundreds of people my own age, or close to it. Lots of new faces that I had not met before. I was excited for the fun, and I was excited for the parties I had heard about.

On my first day, though, I was petrified. The reality of the situation set in. I had no idea what I was doing, I had no idea if my team were going to be nice. What if I was really rubbish at my job? To top it all off, when I arrived at reception they informed me I would be on a half-day induction, so of course, I felt the pressure even more. There were lots of people starting that day too – some temporary staff, and others like myself who were going in permanent.

The induction was boring but not as daunting as I had thought it would be. At lunchtime, a guy came to collect me to take me to my office. On the walk, I asked him whether he liked working there and how long he had been there. He was nice, he had good banter, and he gave me a mini tour on route, which settled my nerves no end. I had absolutely no idea what I was going to do in this office, everything they had said to me at the interview made no sense – they used words like derivatives, reconciliation, and confirmations. All I knew was that whatever I had turned my hand to in the past, I was able to conquer. Why would this be any different?

He lead me into the office, and immediately I thought – *Oh no! What have I done?* It was massive. People as far as you could see. It was an open-plan office and there must have been 200 people in there, easily. My heart sank. I had never been around that many people in that small amount of space before. It was overwhelming. I felt a sense of panic rising up in me. I don't feel that the guy picked up on my panic, though, as he smiled very sweetly and took me to my team and introduced me to everyone. After making polite introductions, my supervisor told someone to take me for lunch over in the canteen. That person ended up becoming my sidekick for quite a while. We bonded over the fear of first days, and celebrated the joys of not knowing what we were doing.

The work was boring. Really boring. It didn't make any sense at all. I learnt very quickly how to do it, and I ended up being very, very good at it. Everything I looked at had lots of zeros after it. It felt like it was a made-up world that I was living in. *Who on earth had that amount of zeros? How did that amount of money even exist? How does it make sense?* I questioned it all. I carried on doing it, though, even without the answers – like a good little girl.

I truly believe working at Chase Manhattan is the reason I have always had a good relationship with money. I got used to seeing all of the zeros and the millions and billions on the screen. After a while, these numbers did not make me bat an eyelid. To me, one hundred million was like a tenner. I was working with powerful companies that were doing huge trades between them. The monies being spoken about as a profit in a single trade were more than most people would earn in a lifetime. I know now I was being shown how corrupt the system was, but at the time I had absolutely no idea. It was fascinating, and equally horrifying, how much pressure was involved in this environment.

By the time I had been there about a year, I was starting to become a bit of a shining star. I was very communicative, I appeared to be able to get the best out of anybody. I was one of those people that if somebody was not pulling their weight, being awkward, or just not showing up, they would send me to talk to them. I had a beautiful way with people. All of a sudden, after a bit of love, they would start pulling their weight. It was just really nice to be trusted in that way. Seeing what I was capable of, they put me through supervisor training and earmarked me as a star of the future. One day, my boss said to me, "We would like to take you to the London office for the day Lucy, would you be interested?" I said yes immediately. My ego was straight on it, 'Oh, check me out.' My shoulders were back, I had the strut, I was IT. Nobody else in my office was going, I was the chosen one.

A few days after that initial conversation with my boss, we travelled up to London together. We met at the train station in the morning to get a 6 am train. I sat there with him talking and holding my own, asking lots of questions. I had his undivided attention for two hours there and two hours back, so I used this opportunity to present myself as the perfect employee. I wanted what he had. I wanted the next pay rise. It was clear that they had already recognised my good work, and my work ethic, but I wanted them to know deep in their souls that I should be their first and only choice for promotions.

We got off the train at Waterloo and headed over to the London office which was in the vicinity of Bank and Liverpool Street stations. From the outside, the building looked like a spaceship. It was spectacular; even more so than the Bournemouth site, which was the head office of the UK and maybe even Europe at the time. I walked in and the interior took my breath away even more than the exterior.

The trading floor was on the second floor of the building. There were eighteen floors in total, so it was low down in the grand scheme of things; to ensure people's presence on the floor as much as possible throughout the working day. We got off the escalator and walked into the trading floor, and it hit me like a hurricane. It was sensory overload like I had never experienced before. My eyes literally popped out of my head. My supervisor was laughing at my excitement. I was in awe of it all – the noise, the commotion, the people signing and shouting at each other. I was like a child at Christmas – wide-eyed and opened-mouthed.

There was a particular area in the middle of the floor that caught my attention. It had different letters and numbers in lights that would flash on screens. Now I know that to be the different FX rates from around the world, but I didn't know that at the time. The entire experience was absolutely incredible, and totally inspiring. That was when I set the intention – *I'm going to work here one day! I have got to get myself to be one of them.* I needed to be around this. It was fast. It was loud, it was bright. It was colourful. It was full on, and it was exactly what I would like for my future. This was it!

That was where my big dreams came from, and my desire for more, more, more. I saw these people in their sharp suits, looking amazing. The women had the most incredible shoes, and for someone who had a shoe fetish back then, it was the icing on the cake. I never thought I would be in such a professional role; I guess through my younger years I always felt I would be with horses throughout my career. Here I was, though, in an environment for snappy suits and stunning heels. I wanted to be a part of it all. I saw the money, I saw it as literally dripping off them, and I wanted to get me some of that. I'll be honest, my ego came online massively. I wanted what other people had.

It made my life in Bournemouth seem so sleepy.

Eventually, we left the trading floor and went off to another one of the offices for some meetings. I could not get the trading floor out of my head. I was in the room listening to people talking, but my mind was on the trading floor. *How can I get there? What can I do? Who do I need to be around? How am I going to navigate this situation? Who's going to introduce me to the right person to make this happen?*

This was a massive deal. It was there, that day, and that introduction to the trading floor that flicked the switch in my brain to become hungrier for success than I ever had been before and to become increasingly money driven.

On the train back to Bournemouth, my boss asked me how I felt about the day. I could not hold back anymore. I told him, "I've got to work there, I tell you now I'm going to do whatever it takes for me to be involved in that. I would just love to spend more time in London." I could see he was impressed with my excitement. He looked on and said, "Okay, if you want to spend time in London we can organise that. Maybe once a fortnight or once a month? How would that suit you? That's what we could do if you are keen?" I could have kissed him right there and then. I had no idea prior to this moment how catastrophically one single day could change your whole life.

Soon after that came the next little golden carrot to be dangled in my face, and encourage me to become even more driven. I had been ranked as one of the top people in the team that I was in, which meant they gave me a nice bonus. Bonuses were paid out based on a percentage of your salary. It was something that, although we half expected to get, when we actually got the letter that stated the amount we were getting, it felt amazing, like money for nothing. It was usually given mid-payday between our January and February salary. It worked as a sweetener to wipe our minds from the previous year's hard efforts, and to get us ready for the next year. Trust me, nothing came easy in that place. Every penny we earned, we had to work hard for it. It's true what they say, the salary is the price they pay you to give up on your dreams.

Not long after the bonuses were paid out, my boss – who had been my biggest fan – moved into a different role within the company. A new department had been created in the Bournemouth office and he was moved into a management role. I was really happy for him, but devastated for myself at the same time. Although he truly deserved it, we lost a good one that day.

25

I missed my old boss. He had been such a great help to me at the start of my career. I really hoped that his replacement would be just as good, but that is when 'The Witch' arrived.

I probably shouldn't use the word witch, it's an injustice. Witches were and are amazing – though that is a story for another time, and another book maybe. The woman boss who came in after my other boss absolutely hated me. There were many of us she didn't like, but she appeared to dislike me even more, possibly because I had been doing so well under my previous boss. And where he totally had my back, this woman went after me at every opportunity. It was cringeworthy. All of my colleagues and the other supervisors and managers noticed it, and consistently asked what her problem was.

It's fair to say at Chase Manhattan they hunted out their prodigies and groomed them to become the next leaders, and I had been that chosen person, up until this point; and she didn't like it at all.

At some point, Chase Manhattan was taken over by JPMorgan and so I was then working for one of the biggest corporate entities on the planet.

Over the course of the next seven or eight months, the management team started having discussions with our team about moving certain functions of the business to India, to reduce costs. This was the first time I really learned JPMorgan's mission was about efficiency, streamlining and making profits for their shareholders. I had never seen this side of the business before, but it was cut-throat. This was the initial push in migrating things over to India, that led to many business functions and departments following suit. The perception was that the stuff we were doing in our office was an easy function to hand over. I must admit, it probably did seem easy, but in reality, it was bloody difficult. I don't think any of us appreciated it ourselves until we started training people to take the function back, and then we realised how challenging the work we did was.

The Witch – as I will continue to call her, although the grim reaper probably would be a better name – was in charge of selecting a pool of people who were going to be staying on to run the business alongside the Mumbai team. It was also her responsibility to decide who would be 'put at risk', which basically meant got rid of. I felt really uncomfortable with this process. I knew this woman absolutely despised me, but everybody kept reassuring me I would be fine, as I was the golden child.

Guess what? I was right! My job got put at risk. One of the top performers put at risk! All I could think was – *Fucking bitch!*

On the day the news was due to be communicated, we all had 15-minute slots booked in, for her to tell us our destiny. We all had letters that were handed to us when we walked in, then we were given an opportunity to discuss what was inside the letter. When she told me I was being put at risk, although I knew it was coming, I was pissed off! I stormed out of the room!

In my anger, my ego piped up and I thought – *Fuck you. I'm not going to do the testing on the new system. I'm not going to be training these people that come over from India. Why the fuck should I help you?*

The great irony was that everybody was being given to me to train. All of the problems that were being identified were being thrown at me because I was damn good at my job, and yet here she was getting rid of me! I had a real chip on my shoulder from this point onwards. It was my first rejection in this company, and I didn't like it. I was furious. I went on the warpath. I wanted blood. If I'm going down, she's going down with me! I didn't know how to deal with rejection. I'd been rejected from my dad, and this was my first experience of professional rejection.

My mind went off on one. I worried I might never get another job again, so I decided not to do any work the rest of that day and that I was going to search for a job on the JPMorgan intranet system. They had a great intranet system, where they would share any jobs that were available within the company, anywhere around the world. It was actually amazing. If you wanted to move to America or Australia, you could search out all the relevant jobs and apply for them. It was set up this way to retain talent. If they thought you were the best fit for the team, you would get a chance at the job by going through an interview process. It was as simple as that, wherever you wanted to go they sorted it. I went on to the job site and I was searched for anything in the Bournemouth area.

A massive part of me wanted to use this as a good excuse to go abroad, but I was nowhere near brave enough for that yet, so I stuck to looking at different jobs in Bournemouth. I stumbled across a couple of roles. There was one in particular I was drawn to, it was a role in technology. I had never had any experience in technology, but I heard that in that department you had a higher level of promotion. I made my mind up, I wanted that job!

I heard back shortly after I sent my application that I had been successful and I got an interview.

The interview took place at Chaseside, in a beautiful listed manor house building that was part of the land before they built the modern glass office building. It felt very special and important. The technology teams had much bigger budgets than the business teams did. This whole experience was proof that technology was where I should be based.

Lady luck must have been shining down on the day of the interview because later that day I got the job offer. *"Fuck Yes!"*

I went up to The Witch and told her I had been offered a new role. I was smug as you like! I was so happy that I had been able to navigate this traumatic situation for the best. I was buzzing. The role that I was in was a Senior Professional level; the job I had just landed was an Associate level, which meant I was getting another big promotion. The Witch was spitting fire because she was an Associate too. She had desperately tried to get rid of me and in doing so I had gotten a promotion to the same level as her. She was fuming, it was written all over her face, and that's when the fun started. The technology team wanted me to join them within a month, but The Witch wanted to keep me for three months. She knew she needed me to train everyone – and yet not enough to keep me on in the team! I ended up having to have some tough conversations with the HR Department because I figured if I was that important that she needed to keep me on then why was she getting rid of me? I felt she wanted to sabotage my success and I wasn't going to let her. After some hardcore negotiations, we came to an agreement of six weeks, so everybody was happy – apart from The Witch, of course.

I felt so amazing the day I actually left that building. It was another big step for me, professionally and financially. I had gone from £21k a year up to £25k in that first year, and now I had been told I was going to go up to £35k a year. The Witch had done me a massive favour.

Divine justice! Thank you!

Delusion

That's the interesting thing about emotional trauma, because no one talks about it or even admits that it is there, it festers away behind the scenes and then uses everyday situations, circumstances and experiences to attempt to grab your attention for you to remember, and then maybe do something about it. Every choice your human makes, takes you closer to getting reconnected to your soul.

We will often find ourselves really excited about something, but then when the reality happens, it's not at all like we expected and we end up going through a transformational experience – for better or for worse – that shapes us and our onward journey.

Let's take my parents' divorce as a really good example. My dad was my hero. I idolised him from a very young age. When my parents got divorced, it felt like he left me. This is trauma. I made it about me from this point forward, as it hurt me. I created a story in my mind that went something like, 'Any man I love will leave me' or 'Even if a man loves you, he'll leave you'. This is when the trauma response kicks in, 'I must protect my heart at all costs. I will not allow that to happen again'.

At any point in my life – whenever I felt that physical feeling of loss, abandonment or heartache in relation to a man – I would run away, or push them away, and create a situation in my head that would mean they couldn't get close enough to me to hurt me again. None of these men were my dad, but I projected that feeling of abandonment onto anyone I met who posed a threat, and I chose to relive that initial pain over and over, because I had never dealt with that initial trauma.

At no point in my life did anyone that I would call a safe-guarder — my parents, family, or teachers — you know, those people who you hold in high regard to keep you safe; none of them ever shared anything with me about emotional trauma. It's not something my friends ever spoke about either, so up until I figured this out for myself, in my mid-thirties, I had no idea that every decision I had been making was creating more trauma responses off the back of the initial trauma.

I trust you are keeping up and the activations are being felt in your sweet soul.

The human experience is designed to test you. Your soul is placed in the womb of a portal that will transport you into this lower level of consciousness; knowing that all of your memories, as to why you wanted to come through, will be wiped away within the first seven to ten years of being incarnated. Mainly we come through with karma to heal, or experiences we maybe did not close out in previous incarnations, and we all pick a time at which we have committed to finally remembering.

It is extremely easy to get swept up in the current of life. It is even easier to become a victim to the circumstances you find yourself in, leading you to compound those already existing traumas into something that you then find challenging to break yourself free from.

How do you break yourself free from something people do not talk about?

Can you look back at some of the experiences that you have been through so far and see the gold?

Can you see why you had to go through it?

What have you learned from it?

26

I had to move over to one of the other buildings for my new job. I felt so grown up. It was much smaller than what I had become used to whilst working at Chaseside, but I really loved it. There was one girl in my team who I got on really well with immediately, she was lovely. We ended up becoming good friends over the years. It was nice to have some female company as it was predominantly men within the technology team.

I didn't understand very much of what we were doing when I took on the role. They showed me the back-end systems, which were quite impressive. It was where the code was written. I remember thinking – *Nah, my brain is not made for this.* Thankfully, there was a guy in the team that took a bit of a shine to me. He helped me so much, he patiently explained everything so clearly, and he showed me all that I had to do. With his mentoring, I actually became a very good coder.

In all honesty, though, I hated the role. I didn't enjoy it at all. I knew it was a powerful stepping stone for me and it would open other doors.

Within about nine months of being in that role – and bearing in mind it probably took me a good four months to get to grips with coding – out of the blue, my manager asked for a meeting with me. I really liked this guy. He had a bit of look and feel of my dad; I called him my work dad. He was tall and dark, just like my dad, and he had that Mediterranean look, just like my dad did too. He was kind, compassionate, funny and quirky as heck. He was a really good guy, and I liked him a lot. We entered the meeting room and he invited me to sit down and then he asked, "How are you settling in Lucy?"

"Really great," I said.

"That's good, I'm glad you are happy. I must say, I have been watching you and I think you'd make a really good Project Manager. Is that something you would be interested in?"

I didn't know what to say and so I just said, "Oh wow, that's so nice."

In truth, I did not know what a Project Manager was, and I wasn't that fussed to find out. As long as it was more money and there were promotion prospects, I was not bothered about the semantics.

"That sounds fun," I said, "What does that entail? What have I got to do for that?"

"Basically, you'll get a team of people, you'll lead them and coordinate deliverables on our most important projects." And that was it, just like that, I was in. I tried to remain cool but inside I was thinking – if I get to talk – which I'm good at – and I also get to lead, then just tell me where to sign. I'm all over it. Of course, what I was really thinking about was the money. More money! It was time to start rubbing my hands together as I was on the cusp of more promotions and more pay rises. Bring it on!

My boss informed me that he'd sent a proposal over to his boss regarding this new role and would come back to me as soon as he could. He was excited, though, which really rubbed off on me. I was starting to get completely carried away in the moment with this opportunity.

A couple of days later, the main boss came down to Bournemouth from the London office to have a chat about it. He was a really friendly, super confident man, with an extremely strong vibe. He was contagious. His energy made me feel as if I could achieve absolutely anything. He bowled over to my desk in front of everyone – which of course raised some eyebrows – and said, "Lucy, hi. My name's Jim." He put his hand out to shake mine, "It's lovely to meet you, Lucy." I couldn't help but recognise how much charisma this man had. He was strong, assertive and extremely articulate. People liked him. I liked him. He had a big personality. "Do you mind if we have a chat?" he asked, and he beckoned me forward with his hand. This guy knew what he wanted and how to get it.

I was slightly overwhelmed by all of this, I mean a top dog Managing Director of JPMorgan wanted to speak to me! Little Lucy, who felt like she had blagged her way from nowhere into this role.

Jim took me into a private meeting room on a different floor of the building. We sat chatting for a while, getting to know each other. He asked questions about me, my family, my current situation, and my interests. He then went on to ask me about my goals, the vision I had for my life, my drive, my passions and where I really wanted to be.

I told him very confidently, "I'm going to be working on the trading floor. I have to work on the trading floor in London. Will you support me to do that? Or will I have to go somewhere else to achieve it?"

I was so confident with what I wanted. I wanted the money, the cars, the homes, the status. I wanted success. I wanted to be known for being the girl that made it in a male-dominated world.

I affirmed to him, "I am going to be the woman that shows all of the women that they can do it." He could see that I was a strong, determined, young woman who was ready to make her move. This was a time when there was a push for diversity, and the drive to get women in male-dominated environments was at an all-time high. Boxes needed to be ticked with the Human Resources departments. A willingness to promote women in technology was rife, and here I was, giving it to him on a plate. He joyfully said to me, "Right Lucy, we're going to put you on some courses and we're going to get you into that role of Project Manager as soon as possible. I think you could be very big in this company." That was music to my ears, all I needed to hear. "You have my full support. I will be your mentor from here on, Lucy!" My ego was absolutely loving it. A Managing Director, my mentor! Wow!

I knew in my core that I was going to be important. I had always known that I had something important to bring to the world. I had thought at one point it would be caring for people, but as a Manager, within a Global Investment Bank, I'd certainly be caring for lots of people.

I stepped into the Project Manager role almost immediately after that conversation. Through all of the heavier and more negative sides of working in the Investment Banking World, working with Jim was different, he always stuck to his word. He really did look after me. He was a fantastic mentor. He had done exactly what he had promised he would do. Now it was my time to deliver. It was time to show him, and all the other people who believed in me, that they had picked the right girl for this fantastic opportunity.

I became a sponge, I took it all in and learnt so much. I was really good at what I did. Looking back, I think I must have been calling on some form of ancient wisdom because I found myself commenting and adding valuable information, and then wondering where on earth those words had actually come from. There were so many extremely talented people in that organisation and I felt they would never accept me, or hear my opinions, but they really started to value what I had to say. One thing I have always done is ask bloody good questions. This was a strength. I could listen to plans and ideas, and then throw in some questions that no one had considered, and those questions always then moved things along in a more positive and effective direction.

I was naturally good at organising, so project management came very easily to me. I was really bloody good at multi-tasking too. I was also naturally very good at connecting with people. There were people in the development team who were good at technology but not good with people. Technology is an interesting place to work, there are a lot of interesting characters and some difficult people. Thankfully, I was one of the few people who could get through to these kinds of people. I would go over and sit with them at their desk and engage with them. I always started out talking to them about their lives because I had a genuine interest in that. I won most of them over and ended up having some incredible connections with these people. As I grew in confidence, their confidence in me grew. They learned to trust me and believe in me. They loved it when I vulnerably went to them and asked for help. I could see them almost puffing their chests out to assist and protect.

One of the people that I really clicked with was a guy called Steve. He shared my birthday, the second of the second. He was older than me, though, but we always used to joke about being 'birthday twins, darling!' He was the most quirky, stubborn, obstinate man you would ever meet. I can say all these things about him because we still speak to this very day, and I know he will read this and smile, knowing it's all true. I absolutely adored him. We were the most bizarre pairing, but what a team. He even trusted me enough to kick his butt to get on a dating app, which is where he met his now-wife. At work, though, he was a pain. He was awkward with everybody. He didn't want to help people. He didn't really like people. He was great at his job, though, it he knew exactly what he had to do and just wanted to be left alone to do it, in his own damn time. When we started working together, he started to soften and to become more open. On many occasions, people would send me over to speak to him as they couldn't get anywhere with him. I'd always get what I wanted from him, without any hassle.

That's what my gift was to the technology world, I never went steaming in there, clapping my hands and making demands. I would get to know my team. I would find common ground with them, learn how they liked to be communicated with, and recognise how I could get the best out of them, with as little disruption as possible. And that's how I went on to be a very successful, results-driven, Project Manager at JPMorgan.

27

Very quickly they migrated me from working on the smaller projects and started giving me much bigger ones. I went from small monthly changes to multi-million-pound projects, re-engineering entire technology systems. It was a really intense period of time. I was working really hard and getting recognised for it too, but I was the living, breathing example of 'work hard, play ten times harder'.

During this period of time, I was partying very hard. It was getting quite intense and it had started to take over my life. All of this was happening around the time that my dear friend Mickey passed. Thankfully, I had reached the point where I knew I had an addiction problem and I had to take action. I had to get the heck out of Bournemouth and fast too, if I wanted to be okay. I was troubled. I was in a really bad way. No one would have known it at the time, though because I was completely functioning. God knows how, but I was a machine. I could go out all night, and then go to work as if nothing happened. I don't know how I did it and how I got away with it. As much as I loved Bournemouth, everyone around me was partying hard. It didn't matter what day of the week it was, there was always an excuse to get wasted, and I couldn't see a way out of it, I just couldn't say no. I had absolutely no self-control and discipline. I was sabotaging everything I loved, and risking it all. And for what?

And that is how the matrix works, this is the way of the world.

I had gone from being a successful and driven girl, passionate about making a difference. And now I had become entangled in the toxic masculine energy of the world all around me, and I had become addicted to money, promotions, and then getting off my head. I really didn't like the person I was becoming and to compensate for that, I was doing way too much coke at the weekends. I had completely forgotten who I was. I was completely misaligned, and the drug taking made that even more amplified, but it also took the edge off.

I knew something had to change. I knew if I did much more coke, I would not live to tell the tale. One day, out of nowhere, I walked into the office and said to my boss, "You're either going to let me go to London to work, or I'm going to quit." I didn't ask for more money or make any other demands, I just needed to get out of Bournemouth and go to London, and fast. My boss could see I was serious, and after dropping this unexpected bombshell on him, he said, "Leave it with me for a couple of days. There's obviously quite a lot we need to talk about here."

He must have got straight on the phone to the big boss because the very next day Jim was back at my desk again, "Hello, Lucy."

"I'm guessing you want to talk to me," I said.

"You're spot on. Come on, I'll take you for coffee."

That day, for that conversation, he took me out of the building to chat over a coffee, at a place down the road. It wasn't a formal meeting room setup, he just wanted to have a chat, an open conversation, almost a heart-to-heart. When we sat down it became very apparent he was looking at this situation more as if I was his daughter rather than his employee. We ordered the drinks, took a seat and he turned to me and asked, "Lucy, what's this about? What's this really about? Do you have stuff going on that you're running away from?"

I sat there and thought about what he was saying, it was so lovely that this man, who normally only ever gave a shit about success, actually really cared and was just trying to understand where I was coming from. He gave me a safe space to be open, honest and vulnerable in return – something I had not really been used to in my time working there, trying to keep up with the boys. Obviously, I didn't tell him I was taking coke; I had not lost the plot completely. There is most definitely a time and a place for that, and this was not that time. I didn't want to leave the company, just the town. I let him know that I felt stale, I felt low, I wasn't excited to go to work anymore, I felt drained and needed to get out of Bournemouth because things were getting too much. I told him I needed to go to the big bad city, see the lights and experience it all.

Jim was amazing – in situations like this, he always was. He turned to me and said, "Well, then that's what we'll do. We will get you to

London. How quickly can you move?" It was literally just like that, instant. In truth, though, I hadn't really thought that far ahead, so it caught me off-guard. I had a house that I owned, so it wasn't as convenient as renting a place and giving a month's notice. However, very quickly, we agreed to a date and I got my arse in gear.

This was it! I was going to London! And I was so excited by the thought of it.

28

Instantly, I got my passion back; everyone else in the office not so much. Most of them were devastated I was leaving because I was the one that would organise the nights out, I was the one that got us all together, I was the one that would keep everything really fun and playful. However, I knew this was my opportunity to go up to London and to shine and show people what I was made of. Innocently, I didn't even consider at this point the idea of getting paid more money but there was a massive difference at that time between Bournemouth salaries and London ones.

I spoke with the HR team a lot. They helped me work out the logistics of how things would work. I agreed to stay at my dad's for the first month, as he was living in Weybridge, Surrey. I assumed he'd be okay with it, although I hadn't actually reached out and asked at this point. How could he refuse his youngest daughter, though? I was almost certain he'd love to have me back in his life, although it had been a long time since we had lived together. I must admit though, the thought of it felt weird. He barely knew me as an adult, and then there would be the small issue of my new stepmother to contend with.

Despite having a lot to sort out, six weeks later I relocated to London. It's amazing how much you can do when you set your mind to something. During one of the conversations I was having with HR, in the six weeks leading up to my move, they casually dropped in that they were going to double my salary. I was shocked. Having a little hissy fit about needing to get out of my hometown due to my partying had got me my salary doubled overnight. And, yet again, I found myself feeling into that same old feeling of – I've really made it now.

It was so exciting on that first day in London. I had to get the train in, then I had to walk to the office through the early morning London commuters. Somehow, it felt extremely grown up to be doing this.

I was a little nervous when I arrived at the office. My desk was positioned right outside of the big boss's office. I'm not sure if he felt he needed to look after me after that conversation in Bournemouth when I had asked to move, or if he just intended for us to be working closely together. Either way, I was there sitting at my new desk, in the London office; my new home.

In all my excitement, my ego kicked in. I really started bigging myself up inside, and I developed an over-inflated sense of worth. I made myself out to be this important person. Although I knew there were tens of thousands of people that worked for JPMorgan, I truly believed I mattered, I didn't realise at this point that I was just a number in a huge pool of people. Even after my earlier experience with being put at risk, I naively believed this company had a heart and actually cared about me.

As would be expected, with more money came more responsibility; with more responsibility came bigger projects, which meant longer hours, and harder deadlines. Within a month of being at my dad's, I had found a gorgeous apartment in Wimbledon Village that I moved into. I need not have bothered, I was working such long hours I was rarely ever there.

Within a few months of being in London, I was given a brand new project to work on. It was huge. I was told this would be the one to get my name up in lights and get me recognised by all of the top management people. Looking back, I can see they were just massaging my ego and stringing me along. This project was going to re-engineer the whole backend of JPMorgan's settlement system and make it more efficient. I was told that this was as big as it gets. I looked at the brief and thought – *Yikes! I don't know how I'm going to do this.* And then I gave myself a little pep talk – *I'll do it, though, and I'll do it well. I'm good at my job, I've got a good team around me. We can do this!*

One thing I must reiterate about JPMorgan at that time, the people were prolific. There wasn't anyone that was a joke. There were a few lazy people but they very quickly got rid of those types. Generally, the people were phenomenal – the quality of their work, and the way their brains worked was amazing. It was so inspiring.

I feel grateful to this day for being able to work so closely with such highly intelligent people.

Working on this project, though, was really heavy going. I quickly found myself working from seven in the morning until seven at night, then getting home and working until eleven at night, sometimes as late as two o'clock in the morning. There were many occasions when I didn't leave the office until the early hours. It was a merry-go-round that you dare not step off for fear you may not be able to get back on again. You would get on it, do some intense work for a long period of time, then you would have to take some time out and go on holiday to sort yourself out, just to stop yourself from burning out. I was getting the money, I was being paid a lot to do what I did. I could afford the holidays and the time out, so it was all okay – or so I thought.

I was often sick during these times. I was constantly getting tonsillitis, chest infections, bronchitis, laryngitis, and I was on antibiotics at least once a month. I would have to work from home whilst recuperating, there wasn't really such a thing as a sick day. I was completely stuck for a few years in that cycle. Looking back, I was addicted to it. I thought I loved it. I thought I loved the pressure, the intensity, the going out and drinking after work. I didn't do many drugs when I was in London, but then I also didn't exercise or look after myself, at all. I had no idea that the food I ate was causing me issues with my hormones, my digestion and my immune system. Quite frankly, I had absolutely no clue about anything back then.

I remember there was one specific, and poignant, weekend, though. It was a release weekend, which meant we were deploying some technology from the testing stage into what we called production. It was a big deal; the first of many releases for this big project. It was causing a lot of stress as it was the first time we had ever done it on this huge project. There was a massive amount of pressure on me for things to go smoothly, which they rarely did on a release weekend. We had done a lot of work for this. We had prepped for this, and tested it over and over until we were sick to our back teeth of it. There was a lot of focus and scrutiny from senior management within our department for this weekend, and apparently even the big, big boss – good old Jamie Dimon – was watching. We were under the spotlight. It had to go well, there was no choice.

I was living in my apartment in Wimbledon Village, a beautiful part of the world, truly stunning. I had been working crazy hours leading up to this release, preparing for it, getting all the plans organised, getting it signed off – you could not do anything in that world without it being signed off, it was a bureaucratic nightmare. That Friday, I went to work at seven in the morning, knowing it was going to be a big weekend; we had a lot of last-minute checks to do. I went in early to make sure everything was okay, and so that I could leave at a reasonable time to get home later that day. The releases were going to start being run by about 7 or 8 pm UK time, so I wanted to be home and online as the magic started to happen. As soon as I arrived, I had a meeting with one of the bosses that I was working with and I went through everything with him, in minuscule detail.

The whole day was really full on after that, I had back-to-back meetings across several different time zones around the world. Everyone wanted a piece of me, but there was never enough of me to go around. I didn't even get time for lunch that day – although it wasn't rare that I worked through lunch when I was working in corporate. It was a false economy really because I needed to keep my energy up, and food would have done that. One of the bosses got to the point where he said, "Right, let's take some time out, let's go get some food because we've got a really big weekend ahead, let's go to the pub." And I just thought – *How the fuck can we go to the pub when there's so much to do?* I thought I'd rather go home earlier than go to the pub. So they all went off to the pub leaving me to carry on with what I was doing. It was a theme. I would quite often 'take it for the team' and stay behind. I didn't know how to say no.

I stayed on and had conversations with other teams making sure my project plan was there, making sure they all had a copy and that it was safe, just in case, for any reason, I couldn't get online at the weekend. This was my job. Cover all bases as if the worst catastrophic event was about to happen. There was so much that could go wrong, and it usually did, so I had contingency plans for my contingency plans.

It got to about seven o'clock that evening, I sat in my chair with my head back and my arms slumped by my side. I wondered how on earth we had got through that day. One of my bosses who was working with me on this project, a good friend of mine, came over to my desk and we both just sat at the desk, chatting about the weekend ahead because he was going to be online supporting me, thank goodness. We were the dream team working together. It was essentially just the two of us who were going to be supporting the work over the weekend and directing everybody to the plan. He was like a Tasmanian devil. You would send him in and watch as he would ruffle everybody up, but cause all of these little shifts and reactions in people to get the job done. He was magical at doing that, it was his strength. People knew they wouldn't want to find themselves on the wrong end of him. I had witnessed him shouting at people across the room and down the phone, really ripping them to pieces. I always thanked my lucky stars I was one of his chosen ones.

It got to be about nine o clock and most people had left. I had some extra stuff to add to the plan, so I chose to stay on and do it before travelling home. I ended up staying there until 11.30pm that evening; and my apartment was about an hour's journey home from the office. Normally, I would have got the last train, but because it was so late they called me a taxi. By the time the taxi had come and driven me home, it was about one o'clock in the morning!

As soon as I got home I logged on, and although I wasn't asked to, I just did it. I had exceptionally high standards of myself, I was so loyal to the company and I would do anything for them, at any cost – even my health and wellbeing. I hadn't eaten all day, so I sat there at two o'clock in the morning finally eating something, looking at my laptop, as I was fast approaching 24 hours of being online.

Of course, as soon as I logged on there was an issue taking place. So I jumped straight on the chat, "Hi guys, it's Lucy, I've just got home from work and I'm going to help you get through this issue and then we'll get some rest afterwards." Of course, the issue ended up running until about nine o'clock in the morning; I'd been up over 24 hours working, with just an hour off, which was to travel home. What a start to the weekend!

I called one of the girls in the UK and I told her she needed to take over for a bit while I got some rest, otherwise, I was going to be useless to everybody all weekend. She was cool with that, so I headed to bed.

That rest only lasted for about an hour and a half. I woke up not knowing where the heck I was and started to panic as to what may have been going on whilst I was dozing. I decided to get up, make a cup of tea and then log in, just to check everything was going ok.

Once again, there was a massive fire going on, so I jumped in, took control and told them I'll help them sort it. And because I was so close to it, I managed to get it sorted. Again, though, I found myself working all through the Saturday until about two o'clock in the morning on the Sunday. It was at this point I recognised what a shit show it was. I wasn't thinking straight, I kept feeling like I was going to make some silly mistakes. I handed over to my boss and let him know, "If you need me, call me, I need some rest."

About two hours later, after I had a little bit of rest, my BlackBerry started ringing and I thought – *Fuck off!* I was getting irate by this point, it was the frickin weekend, and I was missing out on spending time with friends, and my partner. I hadn't had any decent sleep at all, I had barely eaten and all I wanted to do was cry!

I answered the phone and yet again there were fires happening everywhere. It was just chaos taking place again. It seemed as soon as I stepped away, the shit would hit the fan. So, of course, I jumped back onto my laptop and started guiding them, talking them through everything until we got it sorted. I ended up doing that until the early hours of Monday morning.

There was so much that went on that weekend. Everything failed, connections dropped, databases wouldn't work, literally, everything that could go wrong did go wrong, and it wasn't through lack of planning. We had planned, and then planned for that plan failing, and planned again just for good measure! When in the early hours, everything finally seemed to be standing up, I eventually went to bed.

My alarm woke me up at five o'clock on the Monday morning, so I could get to work for seven, and I was furious. I was absolutely seething – *Fuck you, I'm not going to work today. I'm not prepared to do it. I need some time off. This is fucking ridiculous. Who the fuck do you think you are?* Bearing in mind this was all my own doing. I had chosen to work the hours. I was the one that could not say no. However, I was looking for someone to take the blame. Someone I could have a go at.

To get to work I had a fifteen-minute walk to the train station, then from Wimbledon to Waterloo it's a twenty to twenty-five minute trip, and then it was a twenty-minute walk from Waterloo over to the embankment, which is where I was based at that particular time. So, it was a good hour trip on a good day – which actually isn't too bad for working in London. The trains, though, were hot, and the people smelt. It was just bloody horrible and with having had no sleep, I felt awful, like everything was closing in on me again. I was getting quite furious with people, through no fault of their own, purely because they got on the same train as me.

By the time I walked into the office, having wound myself up all the way, I had decided that I'd had enough. I just can't do this anymore. And in that moment I was done, and I was sure to tell my boss in no uncertain terms.

Now I don't know whether, if the train had been empty, I would I have had this kind of reaction, or it was the whole set of circumstances that led to it. I was tired. I was ratty and wanted to run away. You know, typical Lucy fashion. I wanted to run away and get as far away from these dickheads as possible. I know they paid me good money, but nothing is worth what I had to do that weekend. And it was at that point, I really recognised that I had sold my soul to the devil.

That very day, I started looking for a new job outside of JPMorgan. At this point, I had been there for nine years. It was a long time to be in one place, especially in that industry. I was tired, frustrated, and I didn't feel I was getting the recognition I deserved. Truth be known, if you want people to value you, staying in one company is not the way to achieve it.

A soon as I put my CV out, I was approached by BNP Paribas, another Investment bank, only this one was French. They invited me for an interview, offered me more money and gave me the promotion that I wanted, and so I went in and I quit my job. JPMorgan immediately offered to give me more money than BNP Paribas had offered. They promised me a promotion and lots of other things to stay, but I was done. Well and truly done. That weekend had broken me. I was no longer the same person. I'd been there nine years, I was tired and I just didn't want to be there anymore. No amount of money could make me choose to stay. I had given them everything, literally everything. My boyfriend at the time had mentioned I preferred work to him. We had a discussion once and I said if you're actually asking me to choose between my job and you, I've got to choose my job. I still had the attitude from when I was 16, that no fucking man is going to hold me back. I don't need his money! I was seriously cutthroat. I had no consideration for how my truths landed. I was lost in the pursuit of money back then because that's what I was conditioned to believe. I had to do it alone! I had to show the girls that they could do it too.

29

At that point in my career, I only needed to work a month's notice due to the level that I was. Before I knew it, I was out the door from JP and starting my new role at BNP Paribas. What a shock to the system it was. It was like chalk and cheese. Everything I thought I wanted, I got at BNP Paribas. I could rock in at eight o'clock in the morning and go home at half past five. It drove me potty, though. It was so slow. I was used to the cutthroat of the fast life. With this role, I was forced to slow down, which was something I had not known for nine years. It was really quite challenging to be able to do that, I needed to retrain and regulate my body

I only lasted thirteen months working at BNP Paribas. The only reason I lasted that long was so it did not look so bad on my CV. I couldn't handle it, I had been programmed and indoctrinated by one of the best banks in the world. I missed the fast-paced, heavy expectations I had become used to. I'd been trained to be tough. I had been trained to have exceptional standards and expectations. And this was so different.

Looking back on it there were some beautiful things about BNP Paribas that I didn't appreciate at the time. They used to send me to Paris every week on the Eurostar to do work with the French team, and that was an amazing opportunity. Travelling in that first class section, with all of the lovely things that entails – wine on the way, the beautiful food – it was a really wonderful experience.

My boss from JPMorgan, the big boss, the real confident one, Jim, called me up one day and asked for a chat. He had moved to a new company and said, "I want my superstar back." I was interested immediately. I was unhappy where I was, but obviously had to play the game and play it cool. "You need me to join your team? Tell me the money we're talking about and I'll have a think about it." It was always about the money with me. The other thing that mattered to me at this point was that I felt ready to become a Director. Jim knew how to work my ego. He offered me the role as a Director, plus £30k a year more. He gave me everything I wanted and more. He knew exactly what he was doing when he reached out to me because he knew he wanted to build a team under him that he could really trust so that he could take his foot off the gas, that was the whole point of him leaving JPMorgan at that stage of his career.

So I quit BNP Paribas as soon as I could and rejoined Jim, my mentor, the one person that had believed in me wholeheartedly from the get-go. This move, though, was where things started to shift. My body started to play up even more than it had been over the previous years. I had been having a lot of tests, and I'd had several minor operations, but this was different. I was inflamed and I was hurting. I didn't have any energy. I couldn't focus like I used to, and I just didn't really enjoy the chase of it anymore. My periods were all over the place. My stomach had so many issues. My hair was falling out, I was carrying a lot more weight for no reason I could think of. I booked in to see my doctor regarding my irregular periods, and to go through a few other things that had been going on with me over the years. I'd had quite a few issues with my womb, fibroids, growths, sporadic periods, all the women's stuff. And at this point, aged thirty-three, I was going through a really nasty patch of it. She really urged me to consider a full hysterectomy, bearing in mind I had no children at this point, and this was without having done any scans. I'm still shocked to this day that this suggestion was said so off the cuff. I walked out of the doctor's, furious. I called my mum, and sobbed down the phone at her. I couldn't even speak properly. She was on the other end of the phone asking, "What the hell is going on? What's happened to you Lucy? Are you okay?"

This was the first time in my life where I looked at a GP and thought – *Fuck you!*

I didn't realise it at the time, but there were going to be many more times I felt this way.

As well as my body starting to give me trouble, I had been getting these inner urges to go travelling again. I had been getting them for a good few years at this point, but I always managed to ignore them as my rational mind kept telling me that I should have children, settle down and get married. However, in this new role, I just couldn't shake the feeling. At this period in my life, I was having about five holidays a year, so it wasn't like I wasn't getting my needs met where travel was concerned, but there was something else that was pulling me. I felt calls to wander and explore. I'll be honest, I thought I was going mad, and every time I spoke to my mum about it, she confirmed that yes, it sounded like I was actually going mad.

So, for the time being, I settled for taking as many holidays as I could each year to stave off the inner calling to travel properly. I would set my heart on a destination and see which of my friends wanted to come with me, and in that way I got to travel the world, staying in the best places, having fun with my friends.

And that is how I came to be sitting on that sunbed in Dubai, when I got that fateful call from my mum, and my life would be changed forevermore.

PART TWO
TO THE HEART

30

I landed back from the Caribbean in January 2014 to extremely harsh weather, knowing I had to deal with a whole heap of shit.

I had spent fourteen days jumping around different Caribbean islands, all little paradises in their own special way. Enjoying different experiences daily – food, fun, and connections; the best bit of it all was that I got to do it all with my best friend in the whole wide world. I absolutely adored her, she was incredible. We had both been through our own amount of strife over the years since we first met, but the bond and friendship we had was super special.

As we had been leaving the cruise, and I was attempting to navigate my massive suitcase, I had on this beautiful little red boob tube dress. It fitted perfectly on me. I loved that dress. I was manoeuvring my enormous suitcase at the same time as saying goodbye to people when the dress burst open and fell down to the floor! I was mortified! Rather than drop my suitcase and bags, I stood there stunned with my lacy pants and strapless bra on. There was nothing else to do but laugh my head off as I pulled the dress back up and start walking off the ship. It was too late, though, everyone noticed. Thank God I even wore underwear that day because back then I didn't always. Catherine was wetting herself. It was karma from when I had laughed at her when the same thing had happened to her earlier on the trip.

On the plane on the way back, we reminisced about all the incredible things that we had done – like walking up the Dunn's waterfall in Jamaica, kayaking in Grenada, spending time on the Island of St Lucia, and of course the gorgeous Canadian man that had made an appearance, a welcome distraction for Christmas.

Despite my recent holiday bliss, my life back home was far from blissful, and there was a lot that I needed to sort out. Life was such a contradiction. I was going to have to deal with my relationship fallout, and then face going back to work.

When we get off the plane it was horrific. The cold weather and the rain hit us like a slap across the face. The airport was busy because it was the post-Christmas return leg. Everyone seemed depressed, moody, tired and jet-lagged. We trudged our way through customs, and then, on the other side, said our goodbyes. Catherine was going off in a totally different direction to me; she was going to Essex and I was going back to Wimbledon. It was emotional. We had been inseparable for the last few weeks; laughing from first thing in the morning, until last thing at night. It was going to be a shock to both of our systems being alone and back at work.

In the taxi home, the driver wanted to chat, I didn't. I was distracting myself by thinking about the extremely attractive man from Canada. I hadn't taken any of his details to be able to keep in touch with him because I knew I had shit to sort out back here, and keeping in touch with him would really not help anything. It was a cute little holiday thing.

The day after I got back from the trip, I could no longer avoid the conversation with my boyfriend. He knew I was back, and he had called me and acted like nothing had happened, which annoyed me even more.

"I need to have a chat with you," I mentioned, during our conversation.

"You're going to finish with me, aren't you?" he replied aggressively, confirming once again my decision was the right one.

"No, no," I lied. "It's just a few things I think we need to iron out," I lied again because I knew if I didn't there would be an argument over the phone, and I couldn't face that at the time. Interestingly, all of my previous relationships had ended off the back of some big show down. I mean, this one was worthy of that too, but I wanted to try to walk away with ease and grace.

The next day, he came over and we had the conversation. I ended it. I told him I wasn't prepared to put up with that kind of behaviour anymore. I deserved better than to be spoken to like that. He didn't take it well, I didn't care.

Looking back, this relationship had been about me recognising my worth, and realising that I deserved more respect. For the first time in my life, I set clear boundaries. It felt incredible. It was very empowering.

I felt good being freshly single again. It was a little weird because I used to text and talk to him a lot on the phone, so there were gaping holes of time I needed to fill. So, I went back to work and kept my head down, attempting my best to get through miserable January.

Midway through January, Mr. Canada managed to find me on good old Facebook. He worked in recruitment in Canada, so he was basically a bloody good detective at finding people. When I got the message from him, I was quietly happy. He had gone to all this effort to hunt down the chick from the cruise. It made me feel special and gave me a much-needed little ego boost. This gorgeous, kind, lovely man had pursued me – the secret sauce for what all women want. It gave me something to focus on and distract myself with.

31

Towards the latter end of January, another very welcome distraction arrived. I got a message in my Facebook inbox from Ricky – the gorgeous guy who I had met in Thailand. It was so lovely to hear from him. We hadn't really spoken since I left in October. He had tagged me in a few pictures, I had liked a couple of his pictures, and I'd made a few cheeky comments, and vice versa, but this was a private message to me; proper contact. It was very nice to receive it. He was excited and wanted to share some of what had been going on with him. He also wanted to hear all about what I had been up to. He was in South America and it sounded like he was having the time of his life, experiencing so many different things whilst on his travels. I'll be honest, I was a little envious, but I was happy for him. Despite him being a total stranger, I felt this sense of freedom when I spoke to him. We were deeply connected and it was different to anything I'd ever felt before. It was like being back with someone I'd spent many years with. We ended up chatting for a few days on and off, then he asked me if I fancied going over to South America to meet him. Now me being me, I was constantly looking for the next escape from work and to go on a journey. I didn't need to think twice about getting myself on a plane and going somewhere, and this was going to be no different. At no point did I consider how well I knew him, or whether I would be safe. There was none of that in my head. It was just an absolute yes! With bells on. There was not even any playing hard to get – I'm embarrassed to say. It rolled off my tongue the instant he asked. There was blatantly unfinished business between the two of us; and to visit a place I had always been scared to go to, with someone I was extremely attracted to, what is there to question, or play hard to get about?

At that time, I had fear around South America, though, as my head was filled with the visions and stories that were all over the mainstream media – the drug lords, the shootings, the crime. I perceived that everyone got shot over there, and it was an extremely poor place, loaded with drugs. That was the image that I had in my head, completely fabricated by the media, films and documentaries. On top of that, I didn't speak Spanish, so another reason not to have gone there. Ric suggested meeting in Ecuador, and it really ticked all of the boxes. When he then proposed we went to the Galapagos Islands together, I was packing my bags straight away. This was a once-in-a-lifetime trip. I knew it was going to be a big deal. This magical place that I had seen over the years through David Attenborough programmes, I knew I had to go there – and going with him was going to be a beautiful, unexpected bonus.

We agreed to go at Easter because I could get a few weeks off work then. I would fly to Guayaquil in Ecuador, spend a few days there, and then I would fly to Quito to meet him. We planned to do some stuff in Quito, before heading off to the Galapagos Islands together. Our intent was to go on a cruise so we could explore a few islands. Now when I say cruise, I do not mean a cruise liner. It was more like a tiny little boat that you live on, to enable access to the islands without causing too much damage to the environment around the islands. On my way home, I was going to stop off in Miami for a few days to just chill out on my own. And that was it – decision made. Flights were booked and it was time to see what was about to unfold next.

All in all, it had been a successful start to the year. Mr. Canada had found me, completely unexpectedly, and Mr. Australia and I had booked a trip!

I allowed myself to run away with these feelings of happiness. I had needed a distraction from work and all that was going on in my personal life, and Ricky was a very welcome distraction. I couldn't help but smile at what was unfolding. I wondered if I had gone back to his room in Thailand that night, whether we would have been making these plans at all. I had regretted not going back there at the time because of the way things had panned out, but now it seemed that patience was what was required. I guess wondering about it was irrelevant – I didn't go back to his room that night and yet here we were planning this trip. So who cares about the past? I nipped those unknowingly sabotaging thoughts in the bud and carried on feeling happy and a little bit smug that I was about to get another opportunity to spend some time with him.

32

Not long after planning that trip with Ricky, my womb issues started picking back up again. Since my early twenties, every few years I had issues in the form of intermittent bleeding between my periods. The first signs would be some pain and discomfort, then I would start to lose a lot of blood. Off the back of that, over time, I would step into anaemia and all that comes with significant blood loss. I had come on my period as normal after the cruise, then over the course of the next few weeks, it just didn't stop. With this condition, it's not just the inconvenience that is the issue – although when you are going through a super plus tampon and a super plus towel in about an hour, it can be challenging – it was the fatigue, the dizziness and the physical symptoms that created the most distress. I could not do anything. I was drained just walking to the train station.

After about a week of this constant bleeding, I booked in with my doctor, but having experienced this since my early twenties, I knew the way that this was going to go. After an initial appointment with the doctor, I got a referral letter to go private, and within a few days, I had an initial consultation with a specialist, and he advised that I would have to go in as a day patient for tests. Off the back of the tests, it was shown that the lumps were back in my womb, which would require yet another operation. It was always so inconvenient when this happened. I never knew why they could not tell me what caused it. It was always just a case of, "Yes they are back, now we must operate." How can putting someone to sleep be easier than identifying the root cause of the issue? This was the point when I started to recognise that the medical profession had very little understanding about true health. I guess we are all just winging it, attempting to figure out life in this human vessel, even those, perhaps especially those, who have gone to university for many years to study how to 'fix' the body.

The whole situation was a major inconvenience, to say the least, and to top it off, it was around the time of my birthday. I had organised a big birthday party and this bleeding had not been part of the plan. My birthday is on the 2nd of February and anybody that knows and loves me knows that birthdays are the king, the queen, the prince and the princesses in my world. I love a good birthday celebration. I am very passionate about birthdays. I truly believe that everybody's Earth day needs to be celebrated and celebrated hard. It's a celebration of you, and the day you decided to incarnate and come through into this incredible physical vessel that you are inhabiting right now. So for me, it was a big deal that my birthday was going to be clouded by this womb issue.

In 2014, the second day of the second month was on a Sunday. Perfect! We can have a huge party on Saturday night, and see in my birthday in style. We could start at mine, go out, and then head back to mine for the after-party.

At the time I was living in a really beautiful apartment over two floors. It was very central, on the high street, and, conveniently, there were restaurants and bars across the road. It was a little bit too convenient at times; very dangerous for a party girl like me. To top it off, there was a nightclub about a fifteen-minute walk from my house. I had lots of people saying they were going to come. People coming up from Bournemouth, from London, and even the girls from Portsmouth planned to come. My house was going to be busy, to say the least.

A number of the girls came to my house earlier in the day, before the party. The plan was to take our time to get ready. I was an easy-going party girl, it only took me an hour to get ready, from start to finish – I never really got into the whole five hours to get ready thing – but it was fun to be with the girls. It took my mind off my womb. None of the girls knew. Only my best friend had any idea as to what was going on with me.

Everybody got absolutely smashed at my house, before we even left for the club. I could tell tonight was going to be a very messy one. We were all hanging out in my big kitchen, chilling with drinks, and chatting. The music was pumping and we were all getting in the mood. The mission for the evening was to let our hair down in style.

Eventually, it was time to leave the house. We staggered to a bar first, and very quickly it got chaotic. We were doing Jaeger bombs, tequila shots, the lot. Whilst everyone was getting tanked, a random guy started chatting me up, so in typical Lucy fashion, I invited him and all his friends to come and join us in the club in the VIP section I had booked.

The club was absolutely rammed by the time we got there and the queues were massive. It was a freezing February night. As VIPs, we went straight to the front of the queue, and, thankfully, they let us all in without checking how smashed we were. We were escorted to our area within the VIP section, where we were met with massive bottles of vodka, humongous bottles of champagne, mixers and ice. It was about to get even messier than it already was.

I had been quite emotional during the day because of the bleeding and everything that was going on with that. I was doing my best to have a good time, and put on a brave face but I was very emotional. I had done a lot of crying earlier on in the day, and my eyes were feeling sore.

To be truly honest, I was scared. I didn't know what was going to happen. I didn't know if I would have to have this operation, which I'd already had done twice before. I did not want to be put to sleep. I wanted to find out what the root cause was, but the doctors just fobbed me off. Doctors don't know, it's as simple as that. A couple of years before this issue, I'd had the same problem, and my doctor said the only treatment would be a full hysterectomy. Who would say that to someone who had not even had children yet? I had to really fight to get the operation done rather than them doing the full, horrendous procedure that they were recommending. I was frightened back then that while I was under general anaesthetic they would do something to me. You just don't know, let's be real about it. Nobody knows what's going to happen to them. In my early twenties, I had woken up from my first operation, and they had put a marina coil inside me. I never asked for it. They never asked my permission, but this is what happened. So that's why I had a certain level of fear around hospitals.

For a few years, the coil assisted in appeasing the symptoms of bleeding and stopped the growths recurring. However, with the suppression of my hormones, topped with fake hormones being released from the coil, my body was a mess. I would get massive boils on my face from time to time, and they were so sore and painful. It was a tale tell sign on the outside, that something significant was wrong internally. I think now that anything being inside you for years is not right. Nothing should be suppressing your 'normal' bodily functions, such as the production of hormones, or your periods. We have been led to believe our body expelling blood, sweat, mucus, or puss is all an inconvenience that must be stopped at all costs, but the reality is it's your body's way of communicating to you what is going on with it.

After 4 years of the coil being inside me, it was time for another one as it no longer worked, and so the cycle was in place. Their mentality was to just keep on replacing it. There was never any talk about getting to the root cause of it or figuring out why this was happening in the first place. It was just blanket, sweeping statements. The fewer questions asked, the better.

Back at the birthday party, it went off. It was totally crazy. I was distant, a bit emotional and barely drinking, which made everything seem ten times worse. I was doing my best to enjoy it, but, with hindsight, I should have cancelled it. I couldn't, though, I didn't like to let people down. People had travelled down, they had hotels booked, and I would have felt bad. I prioritised them over myself. Not being able to say no is another trauma response – I hasten to add.

Everyone else was having a great time at the party. People were standing on the chairs dancing and singing and causing utter carnage. I noticed people disappearing off to the toilets in pairs, it just didn't stop. I was not really a fan of doing coke when I was out. I was always paranoid someone would catch me, or it would fall out of my nose or something. I was the exception – I hasten to add – most people loved it.

One of the funniest things that happened that night, and it made me giggle a lot, was one of my very dear friends was stood up looking at the deejay, and it was almost like he just fell asleep standing up. He was so drunk, he just hit the deck. He was okay, though, he picked himself up and he was fine, a bit confused. It ready made me laugh. Very quickly the bouncers came along, plucked him from the VIP section and threw him outside. Within about half an hour of each other, four of the other boys got kicked out. As all the boys were staying at my house, it seemed like the perfect time to call it a night and head home.

We all trundled out of the club. It felt good to be leaving that environment and to go back to my safe space, although the carnage would likely continue there.

And it did. It went on for hours.

I got to the point after about two hours of being home that I couldn't take any more of it. My head was spinning and people were starting to piss me off, so I made my excuses and went to bed. Luckily my room was on the top floor, the furthest point away from the kitchen – where everyone was hanging out – so I got away with it. My best friend was amazing, she sorted everything out downstairs for me – she put people to bed, sent people off in taxis, and came in to check that I was okay. We sat in my room, chatting and putting the world to rights. We reminisced about the Caribbean and we spoke about my impending trip with Ricky. At that moment, there was no one I would rather have been with. She was amazing. We had been through so much together over the years. We had laughed, cried, and had our fair share of ups, downs and heartbreaks. She was a much-needed rock during those dark moments, and for that, I will be forever grateful to her.

In truth, I lost a lot of blood that night. That was the harsh reality of this situation. Whenever it surfaced, I would end up losing a lot of blood due to my body believing it was on a constant period. It was never an easy time. These were pretty serious issues. Life almost always had to go on hold for me, due to the sheer amount of blood I lost. At times, I could not dare to even leave the house because it was flowing so significantly.

33

A week or so after the party I ended up in hospital. I had to have an operation to get my womb back to normal, without all the lumps and bumps that were causing the problems. Thankfully, they never cut me open, they were able to go up the vaginal passage and get everything sorted that way. There are a lot of women out there that have to be sliced open every time. It breaks my heart for them. It's such a huge recovery from an operation like that, let alone all the additional trauma that comes from being cut open and having to be stitched up.

The operation went well.

I then focused all of my energy on getting myself back on track to be able to go on the trip to South America. It was so important to me to get away, and actually, that's a very important pattern in my life.

I was very consistent in the pattern that if something went wrong, I wanted to leave. I would rather avoid the conversation, the trouble, the drama and just extract myself from the situation than actually sit there and have to have challenging conversations or deal with the emotions and feelings that were surfacing.

It was a very big part of my journey back then. I was not prepared to use my voice. I would use it in anger. I would use it in hurt. I would use it in guilt and frustration, but I would never say to somebody what I wanted, or how I wanted it, or anything like that. The thought of being vulnerable and actually asking for help seemed weak. Of course, there was a direct correlation between that and what was going on in my womb, with my digestion and my immune system. A couple of years earlier, I had also been diagnosed with an under-active thyroid. The thyroid is part of our endocrine system, along with the womb. What you tend to find is that people-pleasers, those who will not stand in or speak their truth, have issues with their thyroid. It's to show you clearly that you are required to use your voice. The reason my thyroid was flaring up was that I wasn't speaking my truth. The reason my womb was flaring up was that I was resentful and I felt guilty – not only because I had been promiscuous at various points throughout my life – but because I was holding on to a lot of shame, guilt, resentment and anger from my dad leaving my mum, let alone my own antics of cheating on somebody. There is a lot of shame, guilt and resentment held in our physical vessels from the traumas we create and hold onto when we behave like this.

Very interestingly, a few years later, I met a lady in a vegan restaurant in Manchester, when I was with my assistant doing a seminar up there. She had overheard the conversation we were having about this topic, and she said to me, "I hope you don't mind. I overheard your conversation. I would be really interested to speak to you about it." We got talking that night. It transpired she was a GP, and her sister-in-law had been diagnosed with cancer in her womb. She was very, very poorly and by the time we spoke, in a hospice somewhere local to where we were eating. I asked the lady some questions about her sister-in-law, as instantly when she started talking I was intuitively guided to look at whether the lady had cheated at some point. What transpired was that her sister-in-law had indeed cheated on her husband and although her husband had forgiven her, she hadn't, she couldn't forgive herself, hence the manifestation of the cancer in the womb. In just a couple of questions to this lady, I knew she had cheated and there was a huge amount of forgiveness required to be able to unlock her from this prison of dis-ease she had put herself in.

As the years have passed, my gifts of discovery have come online much more. Without asking too many questions, I have the ability to get to people's traumas relatively quickly, in order to assist their breakthroughs. This GP was amazed. I truly hoped from that moment on that she would take what I had shared and implement it through her practices.

The epiphanies that I have witnessed since I went through all of those issues with my body have been incredible, and actually, I look back now and I can see it as a blessing, although it certainly didn't feel like it at the time. The threat of somebody taking away your womb and the discussions of what they might need to do with your thyroid are awful. They were heightened as my nan had to have her thyroid gland removed and my mum had been on medication for that for her whole adult life, pretty much. Even scarier, though, was when I recognised the ancestral trauma in my mum's family down the line of females. My nan, great nan, and my mum all had to have their wombs removed. I believe it went back further than them too. There was a female ancestral line within my family that had these issues. It was a really, really big deal that thankfully I chose to take on and deal with once and for all. Igniting my passion for the physical vessel is what led to my awakening. Without any of these challenges, I would not be here telling this tale of what is possible.

At the point in my life where I had this surgery, I had just turned thirty-five. I had been holding myself back from travelling for years to focus on my career, find a husband, and have a child and settle down. However, no matter how much energy and focus I gave that, I was absolutely no closer to it. I had just come out of a toxic relationship. I was single. I hated my job. I felt lost. I didn't like what I saw when I looked in the mirror. I partied to fit in and make myself feel better. Rather than admit I was lonely and unhappy, I just kept on going.

Towards the latter end of February, my mum and stepdad came to see me and we went out for a late birthday lunch. I decided to use this as an opportunity to test the news on my mum that I was going to do something about getting out of my job. My mum knew I wasn't happy.

My mum is very connected to my sister and I. She plays her intuition down, but it's real and she's good at it. I was feeling the pain. I was feeling the hurt from my womb issues, my weight was fluctuating, my thyroid wasn't working properly. I had also had a recent breast cancer scare, when I had found a lump in my left breast. I was really starting to spiral downwards at this point, and very much in victim mode. I couldn't see a route out. I haven't even mentioned some of the other health issues I had, because as significant as they were, they paled into insignificance with everything else going on. I used to get tonsillitis, laryngitis, bronchitis, and chest infections almost every month. I was on antibiotics every single month, for at least a week at a time, without fail. It was so clear my body was screaming at me that something was not okay, but I had no idea how to connect the dots. I knew something was not right, but I didn't know how to do anything about it, and neither did anyone else. What I was looking for was just not mainstream.

What I did keep hearing, though, and what I did keep remembering, was my grandad's face and his words – "Are you happy? Do you love your job? Do you want to be where you are?" As much as those words often played out inside my head, I did not know what to do with them, so I would just brush them aside and keep my eyes firmly on my next escape, which in this instance was to meet Ricky in Ecuador.

This trip meant the world to me. It was what kept me going through all of these tough moments. I thought I could figure out all the health stuff when I got back.

When I told my mum and my stepdad that I was considering taking some time off of work to figure out who I was and what I wanted. My mum's face was a picture. She said, "You are 35 years of age Lucy, when are you going to settle down? Don't be so ridiculous!" And I get it, I really do. She asked me, "Why do you feel this need to keep exploring? What is wrong with you?" I knew it was coming, but I had to speak my truth. It was the beginning of my evolution and she didn't like it at all. My stepdad was a little bit more excited for me, although he attempted to hide it, so as not to piss my mum off. More often that not he was the mediator between my mum and I. My mum was very driven by security and he appreciated I was driven by freedom. He got my desire to travel and be a little bit different from the rest. He was always diplomatic, whereas my mum was more emotional. Seeing my mum's face and hearing her concerns and feelings made me question myself. She suggested I was being selfish, she mentioned that my sister was still not in a good way, and she even said to me, "What if something happens to your sister whilst you're away?" It was heavy stuff. To be fair, she was under a lot of pressure with my sister, and for me to add to it by disappearing off would not help her. What I was planning to do was totally alien to my mum. She had met my dad, got married, had kids, and all when she was exceptionally young. She never really travelled, she didn't really have a desire to. She still lives in Bournemouth, where she was born, where she went to school, and where she grew up. She never left. For me, though, I went to University in Birmingham. I went to London as soon as I possibly could. I would go on holiday four or five times a year. It just wasn't in me to be sitting still and settling. I know it frustrated the heck out of my mum. She wanted me to be normal, just like her friend's children were perceived to be. The thing is, I was never normal. I didn't want to be. And, most importantly, this was about saving my life.

I mentioned to my mum the stuff that grandad had said to me on his death bed. Her response was, "Oh, nonsense, he was on his deathbed." She normalised it as if it was not anything important. No one seemed to get it. I knew deep down that I was here for a big reason. I had just forgotten up until now. I knew on some level that my soul was saying to me, 'Lucy, it's time to wake up'. It makes me get emotional even now when I think about it because that's what my grandad was doing, he was saying to me, 'Lucy, it's time to come out of your slumber and shine your light for the rest of the world to see.'

All of this was taking place in the February, the year after he passed. Only eight months down the line from his leaving us. All of a sudden the shifts had started occurring. I was questioning everything that I had previously just accepted. Signs and synchronicities became normal to me. I would see numbers like 111, 222, 1111. Really weird little things would start coming up and into my mind, strange visions too. I would think something, and someone would speak it and vice versa. People would say stuff to me, and I would say, "Wow, how did you know I needed that answer?" It was like I had wiped the sleepy dust from my eyes and was starting to see a little more clearly, with a little extra colour. Something was starting to shift within me. There was an energy that was starting to stir. The beast was being awoken. She was so pissed off with being held in victim mode, she was so fed up of allowing these monstrous health issues to keep holding her back. There was a newfound warrior within that was waking up. A warrior that was feeling love more than ever before, and who cared more than she ever anticipated. I began to reflect and see so much more. It hit me that when I was a little child I never got sick, then from the age of sixteen onwards, I was always sick. If it wasn't my throat then it was my chest. If it wasn't my chest it was my skin. My body started communicating, letting me know I had wandered too far from my path, but I had absolutely no idea yet who they had sent me down here to be.

After that awkward conversation with my mum, I mentally started preparing myself to go on the trip with Ric. I was proud of myself for being honest with my mum. I didn't have to disclose everything to her, and I'm kind of surprised that I did. Previously, I did anything to keep the peace. I would let people walk all over me rather than deal with conflict or drama. I never wanted to let my mum down, she had been there for me since my dad left, and I was in total awe of her. I am so proud to call her my mum, and she has been far and away my best teacher, closely followed by my older sister. They have both shown me so much and given me so much gold to learn from, in so many different ways. Both of them are so different to me, it's been an incredible experience learning how to navigate those relationships. My dad and my stepdad were both more like me. They were more free-flowing and easy-going, so both of those relationships came with totally different kinds of reminders, and being honest with them was not difficult as they got it, and had very little judgement – as long as I was happy and safe, they were good.

Dis-Ease!

Time for an honesty checkpoint. Can any of you, from reading this, see a repetitive pattern that has been there throughout your life?

I was always distracting myself. If I think back to my first boyfriend, when that ended, I distracted myself with another man, then the next man, or the next shiny object. I allowed myself to get swept up in the matrix, and constantly fed by distraction. I was uncomfortable sitting in emotions and feelings. I had never observed anyone who was comfortable with it, so I felt this was the norm.

Anyone else, recognise sitting at home sobbing to themselves, when all they needed was a hug, like I did? Have you ever convinced yourself over the years that you were tough, when you really weren't? Like I did. I was here to show the girls what was possible, remember? I wasn't there to be weak.

Distractions, though, led to dis-ease in my body – and this is likely where a lot of you will start to feel slightly challenged in your belief system; so acknowledge it and go with it, if that's you.

Dis-ease is your bodies way of communicating with you. It's attempting to get your attention. It literally means your body is uneasy. I was riddled with dis-ease. Now looking back, it's so obvious to see; however, when I was in the middle of the hurricane of life, I felt it was 'normal'. Everyone else, including my 'safe guarders' were always experiencing dis-ease, so at no point did I ever consider that it was anything other than 'just one of those things'. 'You're run down; your immune is low; it's that time of year again...' These were some of the one-liners I heard each time I was struck down with tonsillitis, laryngitis, bronchitis, or chest infections. If you experience this even a couple of times a year, your body is attempting to talk to you. It's in trauma.

On top of that, there were issues with my hormones, thyroid and digestion. In all honesty, my body was attempting to shake me awake from the ripe old age of 20. Nothing like missing a memo. Each area I have discussed, when a physical issue arises, it relates to a different area of trauma.

As a really high level, as I can hear you all wondering what that all means? All of the 'itis' bugs and chest infections were related to my not speaking my truth. The thyroid issue was attempting to show me I had got misaligned from my life's purpose. And, both of these areas came from me wanting to please everyone else, rather than self — just to keep the peace.

The digestion problems were attempting to raise the awareness around unresolved anger, fear, jealousy, victimhood and self-sabotage. I feel even at this point of the book it's very clear all of those were prevalent.

The womb issues tied back to me holding onto the past. The perceived rejection of my dad leaving would have played a big part in this. On top of that, the lack of love I gave her — my womb — by constantly needing approval from others, and by being promiscuous.

When I think back at the conversations I had with the doctors, specialists, and those who I was in the medical care of over the years, at no point did anyone ever say to me, 'What foods do you eat? What stresses are in your life? What's going on with you? What are your relationships like? What traumas are you holding onto?' This is a key message from me now, the Lucy I am today, we must take responsibility for what is going on with our bodies. They are such incredible pieces of machinery. They require time, love and attention, and we need to remember to listen to our bodies; they communicate everything to us. They give us warning signs, just like the lights on our cars do; only there is no manual for our vessel. We must take ownership, take time to listen, and figure out what everything means, and then pass the wisdom forward. The answer to self-mastery is recognition of our trauma and dealing with it.

I know now that I created everything that went on in my body. I created it with my lifestyle choices, the relationships, the toxicity I *allowed in and around me, with my career, with me caring too much about what people thought of me. I valued other people and their beliefs and what they wanted for me, more than I did my own. There was all the hatred and anger from the circumstances and traumas I was still carrying from when I was young. I was pretending I had it all together, when really inside I was heartbroken and needing love. All those years of being tough, independent and not needing anyone. All of these things played a part in creating this manifestation of trauma in my womb.*

If you have read this section and you are in a place whereby you think you have not done any of these things, and yet you have had the dis-ease, I would suggest becoming super honest with yourself, which I know is bloody difficult to do. So many of the clients who come to see me now are delusional. They feel they have dealt with their stuff, they feel they should have moved on from it, but in all honesty, if you are experiencing what you now know to be called dis-ease, it might be time to recognise that honesty is required here.

34

I got to Heathrow airport and all of a sudden the nerves kicked in. It wasn't so much the idea of travelling, I had often hopped on planes to go meet friends that were away, but essentially, I was going away with a stranger. Also, I feel it was because the core of my being had started to soften. Where the shifts had started to occur, I was becoming – dare I say it – more sensitive, and vulnerable even. It felt like all of a sudden every step I took was leading to something much bigger than I could ever comprehend. I was going somewhere to experience something I had not yet experienced. It was like deep within my soul I knew I was about to embark on an adventure, but my human had not quite recognised it, yet. Thankfully, I had started to trust the intuitive pulls, which was a good start.

A couple of weeks before I left to meet Ricky, we had been chatting and he had sent me some information on something called ayahuasca. He asked me if I would be interested in going into the Amazon jungle to do it. It was so random, it came out of nowhere, he just said it to me, like I should know what he was talking about. I was so naïve back then. I had absolutely no clue what it was. I had never even heard about it. I knew so much about party drugs and felt I was totally street-wise in that regard, but this whole 'spiritual' thing, psychedelics, and plant medicine was all new to me.

"I'll be honest, I have got no idea what the heck you're talking about," I said to him. "Send me some information on it and I'll look into it." And that was my first introduction to plant medicine. When I investigated, it showed me that these plants could help you with a much greater connection to a different level of consciousness.

It still blows me away to this day how Ricky's soul knew on some level that he had to awaken mine. His intuition to be a smart arse to me as we passed on the path, all those months before in Thailand, had been spot on. And then him being honest and vulnerable enough to have some of the conversations he did with me, and then taking the lead in getting me to go and meet him in South America – magic. It was all divinely orchestrated. He had been the chosen one to kick-start my soul on her journey to awaken for the greatest good of humanity. It's just so bloody awe-inspiring when you actually stop and take a look at what is created for you to experience and live through, even if at the time it feels like the biggest shit show.

When he sent the information over about ayahuasca, I'll be honest with you, I got scared. I got really scared. Until this point, I had believed I was brave. I thought I could do everything. Then the mind games started — *How on earth am I going to go into the Amazon jungle?* First and foremost, there are snakes there, and that's enough to put me off on its own. Then, after reading all of the information I learned that this process helped people shift through their traumas and darkness. It had actually been shown to assist people with addiction. These, what they called 'ceremonies' were held in a group setting. People would have the opportunity to step through the darkness within them, and allow it to be remembered, acknowledged and stepped through. Just looking at this information made me weigh up all of my own darkness within — my parents have split up, my sister is a drug addict, I cheated on my boyfriend, I take drugs, I drink a lot. I reflected on this and was in no way ready to face all that. I convinced myself I didn't need to deal with that stuff again. I had my shit together after all! I was dealing with it, wasn't I? I had convinced myself — I'm good. I'm strong. I've got this. I've got my warrior on. On top of that, there was no way I was going to trudge through all that stuff with a complete stranger. There was such a thing as too much information. Knowing all my shit would have put him off for life!

Ric was great when I told him my feelings about the ayahuasca. He said, "Look, we'll just see what happens. You know you don't have to do anything you don't want to do. I've just thrown it out there as a possibility." It was so nice to be met with a confident, reassuring, kind manner. There was no judgement whatsoever. The thing was, once we had spoken about ayahuasca, it kept playing on my mind, the seed had been sewn. By this point, I was rarely doing recreational drugs. My fear was finding something new to replace the other drugs. I knew I had an addictive personality. I wasn't classified as an addict and I was definitely a functioning one, but whatever way you fluffed it up, taking drugs every weekend for many, many years, and drinking alcohol every weekend, was an addiction. I'm probably going to trigger the heck out of people by saying this, but it is an addiction. People generally are so unhappy, that they are addicted to feeling out of their body. I was starting to recognise that behaviour wasn't serving me, at last. It had been a long time coming. Finally, I was ready to get to know who I was, and who I was intended to be.

In the lead up to the trip, my fear of snakes became an unhealthy focus. The jungle was really going to test me. The Amazon jungle at that! They have bloody anacondas in the Amazon! My mind was going crazy. And that's when I heard the words again, "Lucy shine your light, you're here for better things." And as if by magic, those words bought me back from my head into my heart and to the love I felt for my grandad. It bought some much-needed focus on what really mattered, rather than the noise in my already extremely busy mind. It grounded me and gave me a huge kick up the butt that then drove me on. It did this many times over the years before I fully started to recognise it.

Finally, the day arrived when I was flying to Ecuador. I got to the airport in plenty of time. I checked in, handed my bags over, and then the check-in lady said to me, "Oh how wonderful, since checking you in, you have been given an upgrade. Sounds like you are in for a wonderful trip." I thought – *Thank you grandad. Thank you so much for looking after me.*

The airport was exciting, even more so than usual on this occasion. I felt particularly connected, wrapped in cotton wool, and protected somehow. I was allowed in the lounge, I had been upgraded. Quite frankly this trip was being set up to be perfection. I allowed my thoughts to run away with me. I truly believed this was a sign that this trip was going to be even more special than I had even allowed myself to believe. I really enjoyed being at the airport. It was a little bit of time to myself that I craved. It was rare that I ever gave myself any time back then. Sitting down, eating some food, having a glass of wine or two, felt great.

I had a lot going on in my head regarding Ric – *What is it going to be like when we meet? I wonder if it's going to be weird. I wonder if we're going to pick up where we left off?* I didn't know at this point if I was going to be a hook-up, or if it was going to lead somewhere. We never spoke about it. We didn't need to. He was travelling and I was just someone who he'd met on the road. We were both pretty easygoing with that stuff. We were in alignment with each other, despite knowing nothing about each other. We knew there was unfinished business. We knew that we wanted to spend more time with each other, and there were things that we wanted to explore. We both had a massive lust for life and for wandering.

My first flight was to Miami, then from Miami straight on to Guayaquil in Ecuador. The airline staff were beautiful and kind, and nothing was too much effort. I was properly looked after, which is what you want when you're flying on your own. I had a few glasses of champagne, watched some movies, and made sure I got a little bit of a lie-down. I made the most of this very precious time to myself.

When I got to Miami Airport, I could not help but notice how hectic it was. I had a few hours to wait before my next flight. I filled the time easily enough. I refuelled, walked around, bought myself a few magazines and then made my way to the next plane with about 45 minutes to spare.

When I sat in the pre-boarding area, I noticed that everyone waiting to board the plane was speaking in Spanish. They were all local to South America. I imagined Guayaquil must be an onward hub to get to other countries. As I boarded the plane, listening to the Spanish chat, fear kicked in again. My ego started having a field day with worry and anxiety. I had been so complacent with the fact I did not speak the language. How could I have been so lazy? And why on earth did I choose to spend a few days on my own before going to meet Ric? Was I making a big mistake going on this trip?

I eventually landed in Guayquil. When I got off the plane, I was like a deer caught in headlights. I was a complete standout foreigner. I couldn't understand a word anybody said, and they couldn't understand me. I was tired, having left my home almost 24 hours earlier. I was irritated lugging my baggage around, fed up with having to show papers and my passport, and embarrassed trying to figure out where to go without actually being able to communicate with someone. Fear kept surfacing. My head was all over the place.

I stepped outside and thankfully there were taxis ready and waiting for people. I got in one. It was such a blessing. I felt so grateful that it was so much easier than I had anticipated. Thankfully, he knew where he was going too. The hotel I was staying in was right in the city. I had picked it as it was the highest-star hotel I could find. Although I was on a travelling journey, I wasn't quite ready to give up all my luxuries just yet.

On the drive through the city, I could not help but feel vulnerable. It was dark. My mind was running riot as I sat in the back of the taxi clinging on to my mobile phone and passport, just in case something happened and I had to make a dash for it. There were groups of people gathered, congregating on corners and in parks. Of course, my mind ran away with itself believing they were up to something illegal. Back then, I had no idea how mind-controlled I was to fear – fear of travel, fear of freedom even.

We were about five minutes from the hotel and I heard a really loud bang. I totally freaked out. The taxi man just kept on driving as if nothing had happened. I quietly locked the door, in panic. We were driving right towards where I believed the bang had come from. I could not believe he was going to expect me to get out. *What on earth had I come to?*

As I got out of the taxi, I heard another loud bang, just like the previous one. It sounded like it was on the next road over from where I was. It sounded like gunshots. I was absolutely petrified. *I'm going to get killed tonight. No one knows where I am. No one will ever find me. What the fuck am I doing?* Two huge loud bangs within about two minutes of each other! I was really scared. With all I had heard about South America, it was proving to be true, and I had only just got there.

I grabbed my bags, paid the taxi man and ran like the clappers into the hotel. I had to navigate a ramp and a number of stairs with my huge bags. My life was in danger here, and so I found an inner strength that I didn't know I even had. It's amazing how focused you can be when you are fearful of your safety.

I walked in the hotel, and I didn't like it. The hotel reception was mainly dark mahogany wood, the lighting was dim and I could feel a really heavy energy in the place. It felt like there had been something that had gone on in there that was not pleasant. I felt scared and my mind did not do anything to appease that feeling. I was panicking that I was due to be there for the next couple of days, and I didn't want to be. I wanted to go home. I wanted to go to Ric. I wanted to do anything, other than what I was actually doing. I was angry with myself. Typical me! I always get myself in situations!

I was taken to my room by one of the porters who worked there. I said I was okay with my bags, but he absolutely insisted on escorting me. He was very sweet. He explained everything to me in Spanish and made it clear that if I needed anything, to call down and he would assist me. He handed me a card with reception's number on it.

Once in my room, I locked the doors, then attempted to sort my head out – *Lucy stop it, you can do this. You've got a couple of days. First thing tomorrow morning, you can get out and go and explore.* I decided that I wasn't unpacking. I wanted to be ready to go, so I took out what I required and left the rest neatly packed, ready for the next leg.

That night it took me about four hours to get to sleep. To start off there was a third bang, which sent me into a spin. I was like a nosey neighbour twitching at the curtains to see who was firing the gun. Then, there was the jet lag, the time zone differences and the serious lack of food and water I had during the travel day.

The next morning, I found out from someone at the hotel that the bangs I heard were firecrackers, they had been celebrating some festival when I arrived. I had created this entire drama from nothing. I also discovered that the hotel wasn't dark and heavy; it was me that was dark and heavy. I had been tired, dehydrated and hungry and in over-analysis mode. I never realised how programmed or judgmental I was. This story humbles me every time I share it. I called myself out on my stupid, paranoid behaviour and I felt much better. Something came over me, it was like the cobwebs had been cleared and I could see properly.

Two minutes from the hotel was the sea, exactly as the booking had suggested. It had something of a beach. There was a walkway that went all the way up the coast, and it was beautiful. Everywhere I looked there were beautiful, bright, colourful buildings. What really got my attention was a small mountain off in the distance with lovely houses on it, like you would see in Greece or Italy. I saw it and thought – *I'm going to go there. I'm going to climb to the top of it, to investigate the building at the top with a big cross on it.* I had nothing better to do that day. I didn't know how to speak the language, so it was not like I was going to go find someone to chat to. I made a decision that I would find something to eat along the way, and grab some water. It was time to go and enjoy myself. So, after my stern pep talk, that's exactly what I did.

I started walking in the direction of the houses in the distance. Randomly, a short way down the walkway, there were lots of iguanas. I was taken aback, I had never seen so many walking along, roaming free. I found it fascinating. It was a privilege to see them so up close. Had I done any research on the place, I would have known that I would meet these beautiful creatures on route, but of course, I did zero research. I was an ignorant traveller, or at least that is what I called it back then. I always trusted I'd see what I was meant to see. Clearly, I know this to be intuition now, but back then, I did not even begin to comprehend that it was even a thing. I carried on walking a little bit further and came across some beautiful, impressive birds. I'd never been this close to such beautiful, colourful nature. I was loving it, it was so inspiring. The colours. The way they allowed me to be so close. I felt so privileged to be living this experience.

I got to the bottom of the mountain, bought some water off a lady who had a little stall set up selling a few bits and bobs, and then I start climbing up. It was a pretty tough climb, but the views really did make up for it. The stairs were all uneven, so I really had to pay attention to what I was doing. I crossed paths with a few people, all smiles and 'Holas' as we passed. As I climbed a little further, there was a woman that was selling chocolates, sweets and water. I hadn't eaten anything, so I decided to buy something from her. This was back in the day when I didn't have a clue about what I was doing with food. I genuinely thought that the sugar would give me a little bit of energy to get to the top. I climbed up to the top that day, and when I reached it, the views took my breath away. They were stunning. It was in that moment I truly surrendered for the first time in my life to knowing and feeling that I was exactly where I need to be.

It was a glorious day, beautiful sunshine was beating down on me as I sat at the top of the mountain immersed in this feeling of euphoria. I closed my eyes and let the light flood my body. It was at this point I truly embodied the newfound energy that had started surfacing over the previous couple of weeks. I started allowing myself to think about things like – *What would I do if I could do anything in the World? What would I do if money was not a consideration? What would I do? Where are the places I would go if I never had to go back to work?* The floodgates opened. For the first time in my adult life, I allowed the juices to flow. I started to allow the 'Wanderess' that was inside of me, the one I had been suppressing for years – in favour of my career, money, and things – to start bubbling and become re-ignited. I sat there for quite a while allowing my mind to wander, allowing myself to slip into a world full of imagination and hope.

After a while, a man appeared who spoke English. It was really lovely to share some words with someone. We chatted about how beautiful the place was. He explained some of the sights we were looking at, and a little bit of the history. He was a really beautiful soul. I could tell he wanted to make sure I was okay. As a single woman, when you travel, you realise quite how protective some strangers are of you. It's actually a really wonderful quality.

On my walk back to the hotel, I started to get a little more confident, so I decided that rather than sticking to the normal path, the path I had taken on the way there, I would go off-piste and meander for a little while, to see if I could find some proper food, and see what I could stumble across. I roughly knew where the hotel was, so I figured I could easily get back there just by coming back to the beach and walking along until I recognised where I was. I gave myself a little pep talk – *Lucy you're never going to come back here, go ahead and explore, see where life takes you.* So that's what I did. I went completely off-piste and had an absolute blast. I saw some amazing buildings, incredible architecture, and lots of street stalls with food and items to buy. I went into some cool places, some museums, and spoke my best Spanglish wherever I possibly could. To make the day even more magical, I found somewhere nice to get some decent food. It had been a long time since I had that.

After my food, I carried on exploring. I stumbled across a really beautiful park. I was fascinated by it. It was in the middle of a really busy part of the city, yet it felt somehow like an escape, a sanctuary. It had some stunning trees in it and bundles of iguanas everywhere. They were hanging off the trees, moving around on the floor, it was like a little slice of their paradise. I gave myself another little pep talk – *Go in there, sit in the sun and let the world pass you by for an hour.* I made the decision, took a deep breath and started walking around the park, to see what was going on, and get my bearings. There was a small pond at one end of the park that was beautiful, surrounded by what looked like weeping willow trees. Everywhere you looked there were iguanas, of all sizes hanging around. As I walked, everyone I passed waved and said, "Hola." They were all so friendly.

All of a sudden, the world no longer felt quite as big as it had done.

After a good while of walking and taking photographs, I found a bench to sit on. I don't know what possessed me to sit at this bench.

I had an intuitive pull that I had to be there. I sat there for a few minutes before closing my eyes. I allowed my mind to wander and think about where I had come from and how I had gotten to this now moment. I thought about how brave I was being, and reminisced about my grandad. It was exactly 12 months earlier I had been sat on that sun-bed in Dubai, when I took that fateful call.

Exactly a year on. Wow!

A lot of reflection happened that day, in that park. I had been avoiding it for the previous 12 months. Not giving myself time to sit and be present with my feelings. I hadn't allowed myself to do it before this moment, even when I went to Thailand; I had the beautiful distraction of the people I met, my boxing training and then Ricky. This was the first time I had been on my own and I literally couldn't talk to anyone, which is obviously why I was divinely placed there. I was forced inward. I was forced not to speak. A total stranger had intuitively called me to the other side of the world, not knowing what a catastrophic journey he was putting me on. And that is the beauty of soul family. You do not need to know them this lifetime to trust them with your life. You remember them from many past incarnations, so when you meet again, it's just right. I didn't know any of this was going to happen, but my soul knew exactly what she was doing. She was starting the level-up process that was essential for me to step into the person I was always intended to be.

At some point in your life, you've got to learn to sit with yourself. If that means going to a country where no one speaks your language, do it! You need to learn how to be with yourself — which scarily I had never done in my life, up to that point, not since I was a child anyhow. I was a 35-year-old woman at this point, and I'd never sat on my own. I'd never sat in meditation. I'd never sat in peace. The only time I ever didn't speak or didn't communicate with people is when I was asleep or when I was under general anaesthetic. That's pretty heartbreaking when you stop and think about it. How many people do you think there are around the world in exactly the same position? I was never on my own, I never wanted to be. I couldn't get why people did it either. But here I was, sitting on this bench in this park, being on my own, having all these feelings come up, and for the first time ever, I'm loving every minute of it.

I still had my eyes closed but I could feel something near me, I thought it must have been one of the iguanas, so I opened my eyes. I was surprised to see an old man sitting at the other end of the bench. He must have been close to my grandad's age. He had such a beautiful, kind face. Really caring eyes. As soon as I smiled at him – the undisputed universal language – it was the green light for him to start chatting, so he did. He was chatting to me in Spanish, extremely passionately. I said, "Hello, how are you?" In Spanish – I can speak a little bit, but I connect more when people speak to me. He continued to chat away. As he spoke, I watched on in awe. This man could have been my grandad. And although at the time I didn't think this, every single time when I go back to reflect on this situation – that was my grandad sitting there, talking to me. He sent that man there to remind me that he would be guiding me.

I sat on that bench with that man for about 45 minutes speaking Spanglish, I would speak in English, he would speak in Spanish. Neither of us knew what the heck each other was talking about, but we sat and held space for each other. It was so beautiful. We really made a connection on that bench. He was so smart and so incredibly lovely. There was a beautiful warmth that came from him. I'll never, ever forget him. And clearly, that's the case because I'm here all these years down the line, and I haven't forgotten him yet. He left an everlasting imprint in my heart. Exactly when I needed a guardian angel, he appeared.

Eventually, he said he had to go somewhere, so he said goodbye and off he went. I sat there afterwards for a little while and reflected on that encounter. *Who does that? Who sits there and speaks to somebody that they can't even understand?* And this was the first of many, many shifts that happened inside of me. You don't need to be able to speak to people. They feel your energy. They feel your smile. They know your intention. I know I was divinely placed to experience that. I'm sure I'd had moments where I experienced that before but hadn't recognised the lesson, until this special moment with this beautiful gentleman, in this incredible park.

I truly believe that we will meet every person we are destined to connect with. I truly believe we all have contracts with each other and we will carry them out, no matter what. When the work is done, we move on. It doesn't mean we ever forget. Another point worth remembering is that the universal language of a smile is far more powerful than any word that can be spoken from person to person.

What was fascinating, after that man left me that day, everywhere I walked – no joke – everybody would stare. I know that sounds like a sweeping statement to make, but it was true. When I've got a suntan I can easily pass for Brazilian, or from somewhere in the Mediterranean, because I go quite brown. I've often been called Italian or Spanish, so I knew they weren't looking at me because I was different. They were looking at me because they could see something that I couldn't. All I knew was that they were looking, and I'd never had that level of consciousness on it before this moment.

I look back now and I realise it happened a lot, on trains, the tube, in bars, but back then I had such ego and attitude around it that I would say something like, "What the fuck are you looking at?" But, on this day, for the first time, I understood it. They're not looking at me because of anything bad, or because they fancy me, they're staring at me because they can see something that I can't. Admittedly, I did not know what that was then, but I trusted it was something I would figure out.

That evening I was brave and went out on my own. It was really lovely. I had a newfound confidence that I had discovered in less than a day. I had gone from someone who had told my mum that all I wanted to do was travel, and then the first place I go to where they can't speak my language, I hear some loud noises and I panicked and thought – *I can't do it* – to this confident world traveller who was willing and able to go and explore. What a difference a day makes.

That evening, I slept incredibly.

35

The next day I woke up early. I was travelling to the airport to fly down to meet Ric in Quito. I was up far earlier than I needed to be, so I went for a walk to stretch my legs and get some fresh air. It was never a thing that I did back then. It was a struggle to get me to go for a walk, but I felt intuitively guided to go. I had to get out for a walk, and get my body moving as I was going to be on an airplane for a couple of hours later on that day. I was sad to say goodbye when I left Quito, I had really bonded with the place. It was nice to meander through the city in the taxi on the way back to the airport and see it with fresh eyes.

I got to the airport about 45 minutes later. I was both excited and nervous. I had received a message from Ricky earlier on in the day, saying to let him know as soon as I got to the place I was staying, so he could come over and we could go for a drink and a catch-up. I couldn't wait to see him.

When I got to the hotel, I was blown away by how beautiful it was. Ricky had suggested staying in a hostel, but I decided to book somewhere nice for a couple of nights so we could ease into things gently. I'll be honest, I was earning a lot of money at this point, I was on holiday in my eyes, so I was happy to do it in style. You can take the girl out of London and put her in South America but you can't take London out of the girl.

The hotel was an apartment hotel. It was incredible. It had a beautiful lounge area, an amazing bedroom and a gorgeous bathroom with a massive roll-top bath in it. It was truly stunning.

Once I got settled, I freshened up and got connected to wifi. I popped Ric a message to let him know I was there. He messaged back almost immediately, my stomach dropped. It was time to go meet him.

I looked at myself in the mirror and thought – *It's now or never.* I didn't know if I looked the same as I did 6 months earlier. I didn't know if he would still feel like he did in Thailand. What if I had beer goggles on when I was there? What if this was different? I checked his picture again on Facebook, yep he was still smoking hot. *Pull yourself together Lucy, it's go time!*

I finished freshening my face up, but started to get really nervous – really, really nervous actually. So, in true Lucy fashion, I had a big glass of red wine – a big, big, big glass of red wine. We had arranged to meet in the hotel bar which was perfect because it meant I didn't have to get lost anywhere, especially now that I was a bit merry. I made sure I did not have red lips from my glass of wine, cleaned my teeth, put my heels on and off I went.

I looked at myself in the mirror in the lift and thought – *What the fuck am I doing?*

I got to the bar, sat down, and within a minute or two Ricky walked in. It was really interesting because in my head I had imagined there would be a level of awkwardness, but there was none at all.

He bowled over to me, gave me a massive hug, a double kiss on the cheek – because he's part Italian – and we instantly started having an amazing conversation, picking up exactly where we left off in Thailand. And again, for the second time in a 48-hour period, I felt totally at peace. It's a really weird thing to say about a stranger, but he made me feel like I was home.

We chatted for a few minutes, then Ric suggested red wine. I was not going to say no. Alcohol loosens you up, right? So I jumped in with both feet. I'm not sure he knew at this point that I had already had a rather large glass before coming down to meet him.

Oh boy, did we get drunk that night! We were putting the world to rights, all whilst guzzling the red wine, and then, all of a sudden, he leant in and kissed me.

All I could think at this point was – *Oh shit! I am in trouble!* Both of us knew we were going to be spending a few weeks together. So we both must have prepared for things happening between the two of us, but I didn't expect it. I certainly didn't expect anything on that first night, or I wouldn't have got so wasted! I actually wanted to remember this moment with a clear head. Oh well, when in Rome!

So we kissed, and we were both starting to get a little frisky with each other in the bar. The guy behind the bar was starting to giggle at us because he could see what was going on. We kept drinking for a while longer, and it's fair to say we'd both had a bit to drink, but, of course, I'm getting more drunk than him. Out of nowhere, I confidently said, "I really think we should take this glass of wine upstairs." We locked eyes. That fiery spark from Thailand came back in both of our eyes. He agreed, grabbed his wine, held my chair out of the way, and we went to my apartment.

On the way back upstairs to mine, in the lift, I was absolutely steaming. I was stumbling around. Ric was holding me up, plus the wine glasses, and he was laughing at me. I somehow found my way to the apartment and let us in. When we got into the apartment, things started to heat up sufficiently. We disregarded the wine pretty quickly and started to focus on each other. There was six months of pent-up frustration between the two of us. We had a good night, let's leave it at that.

After a while, I must have passed out. The alcohol had truly kicked my butt. I did not realise we were 3000m above sea level, so altitude was a real thing. Alcohol and altitude are really not a sensible idea.

When I woke up the next morning, he was gone. As I lay spread out on the bed, I thought — *Where the fuck is he? Where's he gone?* I checked my phone and I had a message from him. He'd left after I passed out drunk. So embarrassing.

I messaged him, and he replied immediately taking the piss out of me, "Yeah, I think you were a bit drunk, so I left you to it. Just give me a shout as soon as you're up and I'll come to you and we'll go out and do stuff for the day."

Cool. Things were okay. There's no awkwardness or anything. My kind of guy. I liked it. A previous wound of being rejected could have potentially kicked in there, but he mitigated it instantly. Good lad!

I messaged him back a bit later on and apologised again for being a drunken, dribbling wreck. I honestly hadn't realised we were at such a significant altitude at the time, and so every glass of wine I had was the equivalent of about three or four. Nobody told me that, and I didn't research anything. You would think I would have learned over the years, but I am still the same, I do very little research. But, I learnt a valuable lesson in Quito. The altitude was my excuse, and I'm sticking to it!

Ric messaged me back pretty quickly to say he had found somebody who could take us to a couple of key areas during the day if I was keen. He said he was coming to pick me up in a car and then we'd go off for the day.

The first place the driver drove us to was a cable car ride, Teleferico. It was unbelievable, the views were breathtaking and being with Ricky was amazing. We had so much fun. We didn't stop chatting the whole time. Just like me, he kept taking photos all day long. It's rare to meet someone who loves taking pictures the same way that I do. I just love it, there is something about looking back at snapshots, at those special moments in time. It takes you right back there, in the blink of an eye. And I knew this trip was going to be something I would choose to remember.

Everything between us felt very natural. Even with everything that had happened the night before, there wasn't any shame or awkwardness. He made me feel completely relaxed.

At the top of the mountain, it was bloody freezing and I wasn't dressed appropriately for it. In Quito, we were already high to begin with, the cable car took us to just shy of 13000 feet. It was amazing to see the views and the clouds below us. Despite the cold, it was such a wonderful experience. The altitude made us feel extremely wobbly, though, and I'm sure the previous day's alcohol didn't help the situation either. Regardless of the cold and the hangover, we had a blast.

Once we finally got back down from the Teleferico, the tour guide suggested we go to the town centre. He drove us over there, and it was actually really beautiful architecturally. We started off in an impressive square plaza in the middle of the town, but wherever we looked there were drug addicts. It was sad to see so many addicts littering the streets, laying on the floor, and leaning up against the walls. It really pulled on my heartstrings, and it was heartbreaking to witness.

There was a church and some other interesting buildings surrounding the plaza. We went into some of them. And even though the guide always kept a close eye on us, it felt dangerous to be there. I felt vulnerable. Everywhere we turned, the people were in a bad way. There was one woman, an older woman, and she was being quite abusive and shouting at the younger children. The guide explained to us that she was the drug dealer and the kids were her runners, and that's why she was shouting at them, bullying them, and bossing them around.

It took me back to my sister. I didn't realise it at that time, but it was all just slapping my healing right in my face. I had no idea about how the Universe or healing worked back then. I had no context of what healing was. All I knew was that I felt vulnerable here, something I was not used to feeling, so it was lovely that I was with someone I felt safe with. I felt scared that one of these people could lash out at us, or try and take our money. It felt aggressive, and the children were so erratic. It was almost like they'd done something like meth or a large amount of speed or crack or something that made them aggressive and violent. I felt safe with Ricky and the tour guide, though.

It was interesting meandering through the buildings and through the little side streets. Our guide was amazing. Ric did really well to find such a good guide. He always told us where we needed to be careful, and he really had our backs.

We finished our day by going to where the central line of gravity was. It was hilarious there, we had such a giggle. It's a cool place. They had made a little park there, making a big deal of the different energies. There were lots of different things set up to show you the centre of gravity. If you went one side of it the water moved one way, and on the other side of it the water went the other way. There was a line they told you to walk on and you physically could not walk straight along this line. Ricky was egging me on, "Go on, you do it." I thought I could, so I tried, but I couldn't, and he was roaring with laughter, then when he tried it himself he couldn't do it either. We had such a giggle. We were able to play around like kids, immersed in that really beautiful, innocent energy of each other. It was so refreshing to spend time with someone that I didn't need to speak to about work, or anything else serious for that matter. We were just two strangers, getting to know each other. It felt good.

Our first full day together was a really beautiful day. We had got to see some cool places. Ric had everything under control. I didn't really need to think about anything. I just allowed him to decide what to do and when. It was the first time in my life I had truly surrendered and handed the power over to a man. It was a huge milestone for me, but it somehow felt safe to do so.

In the taxi on the way back to our respective hotels, we started speaking about ayahuasca and when we were going to go to the Galapagos Islands. It was fun to be doing some planning. We decided that we would take a trip into the Amazon first, to see if we could find a ceremony to attend, then from there, we would go to the Galapagos Islands.

That was it, we had a plan.

Tomorrow morning, this guide was going to pick us up and take us on the 3 hour journey to Tena where we would look to see if we could find a shaman who would hold space for us to go on a journey.

Thankfully, my soul mirrored Ric's very quickly, we both surrendered to the intuitive pulls. We were winging it, but we stepped into our respective roles as The Wanderer and The Wanderess.

36

The next day we left the City of Quito. We got in the taxi with the guide from the previous day. We sat in the back listening to music, sharing a pair of headphones, and having a laugh. I kept wandering off in my thoughts, thinking about what we'd been up to over the last few days. We knew we would be in the taxi for a couple of hours, so we chatted for a little bit, listened to music for a while, and sometimes just drifted off, looking out the window and staring out at the world going by. We were so unbelievably at ease with each other.

The journey seemed to pass quickly. Time flies when you're having fun, apparently. We arrived in the most beautiful place called Tena, just on the outskirts of the Amazon. I looked around, and everything was wooden; it felt like we had arrived at some kind of a fishing village, with little cabins as shops. It was highly picturesque, and quaint. It had a high street setup, just an Amazonian version. We started looking around for somewhere to stay. We didn't know where we were going or what we were doing. Ric's entire focus was on finding ayahuasca. He didn't care about anything else. I liked the levels of determination he held. It reminded me of me. It's rare to find someone who, no matter what, will do what it takes to achieve what is required. The mission was to find a shaman. We needed to find someone who was going to hold space for us both to go through an ayahuasca journey. I wasn't too bothered by it. I just felt that if it were meant to be, it would be, and if it wasn't, then it wouldn't.

We walked around for a couple of minutes with our bags until we found a little touristy travel place that sold flights, hotel rooms and stuff like that. We went in and asked for somewhere really cheap to rent for the night, because all we wanted to do was dump our stuff and figure the place out, hoping we would go to the shaman that evening. We don't mess about; we're there for a good time, not a long time. Immediately, the woman began talking to us about this room that she had. It was cheap. Too frickin cheap. My monkey brain went off again – *Oh my goodness, this place is going to be a literal hell hole, this is going to be like something you've seen in a movie where people get murdered.* My mind started doing somersaults. Of course, when we walked into the place, it was exactly as I had imagined. It was awful. Ricky was wetting himself – *Oh the little princess is going to have to rough it for a night.* And he was right. I was thinking of ways to escape – *I don't want to be here, this is disgusting, someone has definitely been killed in here.* There were mosquitoes and creatures all around; you name it, it was all going on there. We dumped our bags and took a stroll down the high street. Suddenly, finding a shaman and going into the Amazon seemed like a preferred option over staying in that room. Well played, Ric!

It was time to find a shaman. We knew we just needed to speak to a few people, have the right conversations and we would end up with what we were looking for. Ric trusted this more than I did, at this time. We realised it wasn't going to be as easy as finding a sign up on a door saying, 'Shaman here, come on in, do you fancy ayahuasca?' We knew we would have to find the right people who would guide us to it. We decided that worst-case scenario, we would stay there for one night to try and find it, and if not, then we would leave.

That first day, we were walking along the road, I noticed that everybody was staring at me again, not at Ricky, at me. Now, bearing in mind, by this point, we've been in the hot weather for a few days, so my skin is starting to go even browner, and I don't look any different to the local women. I've got relatively olive skin, I've got dark brown hair, and I looked like all the other local women. I always get mixed up with the locals wherever I go. It's not like I had bright blonde hair or really pale skin and that was the reason why everybody was staring at me, but nevertheless, they were. I kept seeing them stare, and they wouldn't look away. I was so embarrassed. I thought — *Oh my God, what are they looking at? Is my boob hanging out? Is my bum hanging out?* I just didn't know. I got really uncomfortable with it. I said to Ricky, "You're going to have to do something because all these people are staring at me."

He looked back at me and said, "Oh stop being so bloody full of yourself. Who d'ya think you are? Everybody's staring at you!"

I said, "Dude, seriously, everyone is staring at me. Not just the young men, the older men, and not just the young women, but the older women. I need you to do something about it. Can you just walk behind me and watch?"

He sighed, but bless him he did it. He stepped behind me and walked like that for a while. He was shocked. He said, "Oh gosh, yeah, they're all looking at you, aren't they? I wonder what they're looking at?"

We had no idea, though.

We were on the cusp of the Amazon jungle, the energy there was so profound, something was going on. My body had tingles over it the whole time we were there. Now, looking back, I can see that it was almost like we had stepped into a vortex of powerful energy, that you can only really find somewhere so precious, like the Amazon.

At the time, it made me feel like I was in the book, The Celestine Prophecy – the part where the different levels of energy surround them, and they can experience things that put them into a certain state. The Celestine Prophecy was a book I read in 2000, and I loved it. I had become obsessed with it, but I didn't really get it all at that point in time. But now, looking back, being in the Amazon was just like that. It was everything The Celestine Prophecy had portrayed itself to be, and I was actually living in that energy.

We established that everybody was staring at me but we didn't yet know why, so Ricky just took me by the hand and assured me that everything was okay. We found a coffee shop and thought it would be a good place to meet people. It was a tiny little place, super cute. Ric and I ordered a drink, and we sat down. Over by the window, there was a lady and a man sat at a circular table, and they were huddled over and talking about something, intensely. I sat down near to them, and I could hear a bit of what they were talking about. I heard them say the word 'wizard', and then I heard them say something about a fire-walker, so I started elbowing Ricky and motioning for him to listen in to the conversation too, so he moved over to sit next to me so he could hear.

The girl and this guy, who were probably about our age, started talking about how dark the energy of this fire-walking man was, and how he was there to source the bright souls and put a spell on them. The conversation was dark and freaky, and I didn't like it. But Ricky's eyes lit up. I could see his mind working. He piped up and said, "Hey, guys, I'm really sorry. I couldn't help overhearing you. Would you know anywhere we could do ayahuasca?"

Now, one thing I love about Ricky is he's very passionate about anything he's dedicated himself to; he gives it his all. If he makes up his mind to do something, he won't rest until he's got it. I really admire that about him, and I respect that quality in myself as well because if I get the bit between my teeth on something, I deliver it. We are exactly the same in that way.

The guy sat with the girl said, "Actually, I'm a translator for a shaman. Would you like me to introduce you?"

"That would be great," Ricky replied.

Amazing! What are the chances? Clearly, the Universe wants this to happen.

The couple asked us to join them, so we got another drink and moved over to their table. We initially made small talk, but then Ric quickly navigated the conversation back to ayahuasca – where the shaman's retreat was and how it would all work. He was on a mission. I liked it. No bullshit or fluff. The translator was a guy originally from Chile. His native tongue was Spanish, but he could speak excellent English. He had started his own healing journey in Peru. He had somehow found the shaman he was now working with, and moved there to learn everything from him. I didn't know much about what they were talking about; it was all foreign to me at the time, but Ricky was holding the fort and asking good questions about the ayahuasca plants, about the set-up, and the way that the ceremony was going to work.

Whilst Ric was engaged with the translator, I began chatting to the girl, who was very 'quirky' – for want of a better word. She had a massive tattoo over her throat, which scared the fuck out of me. It gave me the heebie-jeebies. I didn't know why, but something about it felt very dark. I felt on edge just talking to her. I reigned myself in as I thought I was being judgmental. She seemed like a nice enough girl, although it was clear that she was traumatised. She had come from an addiction background, which I could resonate with because of my sister. My heart went out to her, but her tattoo scared me senseless.

Meanwhile, Ricky and the guy were exchanging details to organise the ayahuasca ceremony. The guy called the shaman and arranged for it all to take place the next day. We would be going for two days, doing two back-to-back ceremonies. It was agreed that the following day we would get a taxi to the retreat centre in the middle of nowhere, in the Amazon jungle no less. That evening we would do an ayahuasca journey with the shaman – my first ever plant ceremony.

We stayed there for a while longer, chatting to the guy and the girl. Ric and I were excited about how quickly we had arranged it, but we sensed in each other the need to get away from these people. Suddenly, they started to get edgy. They said they could see the fire-walker guy, the one that they had been talking about earlier when I was eavesdropping on their conversation. They pointed at him through the window and started freaking out. She said, "Oh my God, we need to go now. We'll see you tomorrow." And with that, they stood up and went.

"That was a bit weird," Ricky said. We both looked at each other and started laughing. How random was this trip so far? It was like being on a mission with one of your best friends who leads you astray at every opportunity – and just so you know, I am that person if you ever get to travel with me.

I took a look at what the translator had written down. Bless him, he had written down the name, address, the times, and a taxi number for someone who knew how to get us there. He was really helpful. I liked him. He seemed extremely kind. Ric was slightly less tolerant with both of them, but we had achieved what we set out to do, so we were both buzzing.

We decided to stay in the coffee shop for a bit longer to observe what was happening with the fire-walker guy they had been talking about. He had come into the cafe after they left. They had made such a big deal of who he was and what he was up to, that we decided to be nosey parkers and stick around to check it out. He actually seemed a nice enough guy. He had grey hair, and he did look a little bit like a wizard; he was definitely on the quirky side of normal – whatever that is. He gave off the impression that he had his shit together. We were naïve where energy was concerned at this point. Looking back on the conversations we had with him, I can see how he was blatantly trying to weave us into something. We told him we were passing through and didn't want to do the fire-walk. He was doing his best to convince us to get involved, but we both agreed it was not for us, so we made our excuses and went off to find some food.

Rick was excited about the ayahuasca journey the following day. On the other hand, I was a bit more – *'Oh shit, this is actually happening then. We're going into the proper jungle, and we're going to be doing this'*. Trust me, for a control freak, giving up all control, first and foremost to a jungle, and then secondly to a plant, was bloody challenging. I kept going around in circles of excuses about how I could get out of it. There was no way that was happening, though. Ric was on it. He was totally focused on the fact that this was something we had to do together, so after a little panic, I decided there was no option but to let go and trust that the Universe, and Ricky, had my back. I must have been really annoying in the lead up to it. I kept repeating to him, "You're a professional boxer, if anything happens to me, it's your job to protect me."

Her replied, "Yeah, yeah, don't worry about it. You'll be fine." So dismissive. He had done ayahuasca a number of times prior to this point, so he was comfortable with what he was doing. To me, though, it was like leading a lamb to slaughter. I had no idea what would happen, where we were going, or what I was likely to see. I had read about it on the internet, and it sounded terrifying, especially for someone who likes to be in control. I had also read many articles from people saying don't do it, due to shamans taking advantage of people or having your things stolen, and several attacks had taken place during ceremonies. As amazing as the internet is, my goodness, it corrupts people's minds with mistruths and disinformation. I had to trust this man that I was with. It was as simple as that. I had no choice but to go ahead with it – my ego and stubbornness wouldn't have allowed me to back out anyhow. Looking back, there was no one I'd rather have done it with. Somehow, I knew I was safe with him.

We wandered the streets for a while, looking at some of the shops; we found some food, and essentially tried to put off, for as long as we possibly could, the harsh reality of going back to that horrible room we were staying in. Honestly, I had gone from luxury to what looked like a brothel in less than 24 hours. It was a shock to the system.

We savoured our food that night. We were told that when you do a journey with plant medicine, you should not eat for several hours before doing it. We knew that evening would be the last time we would eat for a while, so we made a big deal of going out for dinner and loading up on the good stuff. We were both a little bit wary of the food we would get on the other side of the journey too. Thankfully, I was a meat-eater back then and so a little easier to cater for, although I was always a little scared about eating meat when travelling in case it wasn't cooked properly.

We returned to the room, and it was just as horrific as I remembered it. I was agitated, first and foremost, because I felt there was too much stuff that had happened in that room in the past, and secondly, I was very nervous about the mosquitoes. As a younger woman, I used to get bitten by them all the time, they would feed on me, literally, and I didn't like it. That night was horrible – it was too hot and then too cold, because of the air conditioning, which was intermittently going on and off. I could hear things running around the room, scratching. To top it off, I could hear mosquitoes buzzing around my ears. I did not get a good night's sleep at all. Ric, on the other hand, slept like a baby. Back then, I was so envious of people who could sleep well. It was very rare if I got a good night's rest. If it wasn't my digestion playing up, burning me as I was laid down, my mind was all over the place.

37

The next morning, when we woke up, Ricky was bouncing off the walls. He had done ayahuasca a few times before, and was so excited. He kept telling me that this was going to be an amazing experience and I was going to love it. I had to switch off to it in the end. I knew he meant well and was extremely excited, but every time he spoke about it, my head went off in a direction that I was not comfortable with. I am unsure if he had picked up on my fear and was attempting to get me to bring it to the surface, or if he was genuinely excited and just wanted me to be too. I was a bit quiet and distant on the outside. Inside, I was wishing the next two days away.

We got in the taxi, which we had arranged, and the driver tried to take us to the shaman's retreat, but got totally lost. He thought he knew where he was going, but he blatantly didn't. In all fairness, it wasn't exactly the easiest place to find. It was down a dirt track with no signposts and precisely the type of terrain you would imagine for a retreat in the middle of the Amazon jungle. You had to go down a bumpy, bouncy track for quite a while, then navigate through some trees, and then suddenly, out of nowhere, there were huts made out of wood in a ceremonial space. It was beautiful, in an extremely off-grid, rustic manner. I immediately thought there was no way I could live there for a week, but then countered that with – *It's just two nights, Lucy, you can do it!*

We were greeted by the translator and the girl with the tattoo. They welcomed us warmly, and the translator said, "The shaman's not here at the moment. Let's put your bags down and go for a walk, we can show you where you are, and what you've got available to yourself."

They took us to this beautiful area that had an amazing lookout, a really nice viewpoint where you could just sit and stare into the jungle. It was truly spectacular. Okay, the accommodation was not up to much, but those views! This is what we came for.

For the first time in my life, I felt genuinely connected to Mother Nature. It was almost like she acknowledged I had arrived by switching something on within me. We stayed there for a while, talking about the ayahuasca journey. Ricky said, "You know that normally when you go into ayahuasca, you will see a serpent or a snake. That's what basically greets you." Now I only have one fear and one fear only this lifetime, and that is snakes. So, of course, I went off on a rant! "I ain't seeing a fucking snake, no frickin way. If I see a snake, I'm going to run away!" Bearing in mind that I'm currently knee-deep in the Amazon, where there are real anacondas that can eat you, and all sorts of other different, poisonous snakes. I'm not freaking out about those ones, though, I'm totally losing it over the ones that I may potentially see in my mind's eye. I had a very unhealthy fear of snakes at that point in my life.

The translator took me by the hand and reassured me. He told me that once I had met the shaman, I should go back to my room and meditate on getting through this with ease and grace. That was the best advice anybody could have ever given me. I couldn't even meditate back then, but I thought that even if I just repeated it over and over to myself – repeat, repeat, repeat, repeat, repeat – I'm going to get it, surely? I was totally freaking out because as soon as Ric knew my fear, he started elaborating, "It's not just a normal snake, it's a massive snake and sometimes even shows up as a serpent." Either way it sounds like a snake to me. He was such a bloody smart-arse; he had me over a barrel at this point. I made my mind up I was not going to like it one bit. Nothing like a bit of positive thinking to get you ready. I said to Ricky that I didn't think I was going to be able to do it, it was just too much. He reassured me and told me I was stronger than this fear. He reminded me of the girl he'd met in Thailand, punching, kicking, and fighting. He reminded me of some of the stuff I'd done in my career. He knew that I was strong. He knew that I had that warrior inside of me. Thank goodness he was there for the pep talk. Had I been alone, I'd very likely have made an excuse and left. At this point in my life, although we had seen glimpses, the warrior hadn't quite come out in the way she needed to. Yes, sure, she came out in anger, pain, and things like that. Ultimately he said to me, "Look, what's the worst that's going to happen? You're going to see it, and you are going to be with the shaman and he is going to talk you through it." He was right. What was the point in avoiding it? I pulled myself together, brushed my ego down and started focusing on not seeing it. I trusted Ricky, and I really liked the translator too. I thought his energy was good; I liked his soul – despite him being kind of weird to me back then.

The shaman came back about an hour later. The translator took us to meet him. He introduced us, and the shaman asked, in Spanish, if we would like to go and pick the plants with him for that night's ceremony. We thought that would be a fantastic experience, so Ricky and I went off with him into the Amazon jungle in search of ayahuasca. We wandered down into the jungle until we found the plant – incidentally, at no point was I scared about the snakes. I was enjoying myself and really happy because the ayahuasca was literally a plant that we plucked from the ground. I don't know what I had been expecting, something more sinister, I guess. We picked the plant for ourselves, then we picked what I believe were cacao leaves. The shaman explained to Ricky, who was then explaining it to me, that they were going to make a brew from it; they would put it in hot water and brew it until it became like a tea, which we would then drink in the evening. I was fascinated by this because even at that point, I loved the thought that Mother Nature gave us everything that we needed to heal. I truly believed that, and here we were picking stuff from the ground; it wasn't pre-packed or pre-prepared, we literally picked it from the ground with the shaman, who would do his thing to it.

We walked back to the retreat, and the shaman explained that it would take about four or five hours to brew the tea. He went off to put the tea on, then he came back to us and showed us to our rooms. Ricky and I had both decided that we'd have our own rooms because of what we would go through. We didn't know if we would be purging, or too hot, or just need our own space, so we thought it best to stay separately. Ricky got shown to his room, and all was good and well. He wanted to check out my room to see if it was better than his because there was this really competitive thing we had going on between us. We walked into my room, and above my bed, caught in the mosquito nets which surrounded the whole bed, there was a black rat. I freaked out big time. I totally freaked out. Now, if I saw that today, I would look at it and think – *Hmm that's a beautiful sign, let me have a look and investigate that.* But back then, I was a proper girl. I screamed,

"Aaaaaaah, get that thing away from me." I had never seen a black rat before and this was a jet black rat. I screamed at Ricky, "Get me the fuck out of here. What on earth are you doing to me?" I went straight into victim mode. Thankfully, the shaman and the translator caught the rat and got it out of my room, but I was shaken up by it.

I thought it was a sign, but not a good one, saying – *Don't do it.*

Looking back on it now, I feel that it was ayahuasca saying to me, *"Okay, you don't like snakes or serpents, so I'm going to show you a black rat to let you know that I've got you, don't worry about it. You are far stronger than you have ever perceived yourself to be."* It's easy to see now with all these years of hindsight and wisdom, and the whole journey that I've been on, but back then, all I could think was that there was a bloody big black rat hanging above my bed. How on earth do you remove that image enough to be able to sleep?

I calmed down enough to sit there for the next couple of hours saying affirmations to myself – *I am ready to see the light, I want to be shown the beauty. Give me a beautiful journey. Everything light, love, happiness, and positive.* There was no mention of snakes. There was no mentions of serpents. There was no mention of any of that. I set the intention. I was not going to see it, not under any circumstance.

I was a total control freak back then, and the thought of seeing something that would make me lose control wasn't cool. Bearing in mind I was innocent about all of this, I had no idea what I was letting myself in for; I just trusted Ricky implicitly. I attempted to control the situation the best I could, but that was never going to happen. I later learnt that if you attempt to control the plant, she'll put you on your arse.

That afternoon, Ricky and I sat on a little table outside our rooms, and we started setting intentions for the journey ahead. I never asked anything about what was going to happen – what it tasted like, how long it lasted, why we had to do it so late at night. I didn't want to know. I thought that if I knew too much information, then I'd panic. I made the conscious decision on this occasion that less was definitely more.

When we talked about our intentions for the journey, though, I said to him, "You know, I'm ready to see where my future is going to take me. I don't feel aligned with my job anymore. I want to see what's next. That's my mission for today." And then I went and lay back down again and focused on my affirmations – love and light, unicorns and fairies. All of that kind of stuff because I didn't want to see anything dark.

The next thing I knew, it was time! The shaman arrived to come and get us. He mentioned the brew had been moved up to the retreat space, and it had been locked down, made sacred, there was a fire burning, and they were ready for us to join them. Ricky was so excited about this, he was like a kid in a sweet shop. The translator and the girl with the tattoo had all done it before, so they were also excited. I was freaking out! Totally nervous. My ego was piping! Walking down to the retreat felt like I was walking the Green Mile again. It was probably no more than a two-minute walk. I will never forget how dark and eerie it was, though. I wondered how I would find my way back later, once the ceremony was finished. My mind was all over the place.

When we got to the space where the ceremony was due to be held, it was all undercover, like a big tent or marquee. I was surprised at how big the space was. I was also a little perturbed that the sides were open. You can imagine what went on in my mind. It went from 0-60mph, questioning which animals from the jungle would be walking in on us. Did they not realise we were in the Amazon when they set this thing up?

There was an area in the middle of the ceremony space with lots of pillows and blankets. There was a fire pit set up too. At this point, I guessed this would be where people could go and sit and chat if they wanted to. I had absolutely no idea what was coming, clearly! There was another area close to the front when we walked into the ceremony space, where the shaman was. His area looked incredible. It was such a beautiful space. It felt very special and sacred.

We were all shown to a space where we would stay and lay down during the medicine journey. It was all so weird to me. I had never done anything like this before in my life. Usually, I couldn't even sleep in the same room as people I knew, let alone surrendering to be with someone I'd known for less than six months – and the rest of them there were complete strangers. I could have walked out so easily at that point, but something kept me there. Something about this intrigued me enough to let my soul take the reins. For the first time in my adult life, I properly surrendered to knowing absolutely nothing and trusting it was all going to work out okay.

I picked the space right at the front next to the shaman. I felt I could easily walk to the toilet, and disappear back to my room when the time was right. Ric went to the back of the space. I'll be honest with you, there was no way I was going back there; I imagined that if an animal came in, I'd be eaten before anyone even knew I was gone. At least where I was, I was closest to what the shaman had created as some form of civilised space.

After finding my spot and getting a little comfortable, the shaman beckoned me to go first. I was horrified. I had never done anything like this before. I really had it in my mind that I would watch someone first before actually having to do it myself. I just wanted to know what to expect, I guess. Looking back, I'm sure he picked me to go first because he could feel my inner control freak kicking in – wanting to watch someone else, and maybe even having the opportunity to run away. The translator explained to me that the shaman was going to give it to me first as I had never done it before. He wanted to make sure I was okay, so he would give me an amount he felt would be alright for me, then add more if I felt I wanted it. I'm not sure if it hits you for longer the first time you do this kind of thing, but maybe he wanted me to be coming around about the same time as the other people. Who knows? I should have asked more questions. I really did not ask anywhere near enough questions back then. Of course, being the first one called up, I was really nervous. I had absolutely no idea what to expect. My ego would have loved to have watched somebody else go through the experience first, but the shaman thought this was the best way.

I innocently walked over to the space where the shaman was. He smiled at me and gave me a beautiful, friendly, reassuring look, and then he stepped into his space to do what we had come there for. Suddenly, chants were coming out of this man that I was shocked he could even produce. He was confident, loud, and assertive. He started speaking to me in Spanish. I had no idea what he was saying, but I felt drawn to close my eyes and allow him to do what was required. He walked around me; I could feel him blowing the air, sweeping it with his hands. I feel this was to clear my energy field, but I'm no shaman, and I didn't ask after the event. Then he started moving around me whilst chanting. The next thing he did was blow smoke in my face. I believe it was tobacco. The smell was strong and potent. All of a sudden, I felt some sort of liquid being sprayed on my face. It felt like I had been spat on. It definitely came from his mouth. I remember thinking – *What the fuck is going on here? Is this absolutely necessary? What the fuck has Ricky bought me here to?* I didn't know what liquid it was either; best not ask. He was preparing me, getting everything ready, clearing my field, setting me up for what was about to happen. He continued to tap and blow smoke over me, for what felt like an eternity. I could feel my energy rising. I could feel my body doing something. There was a really intense few minutes towards the end of this part where he was drumming and building up the energy in and around me, in readiness to bring in Mother Ayahuasca. With that, he handed me a cup of liquid, and I heard the translator say, you must drink that. *Oh my God, I don't know what's in it. What am I going to do? Why did I have to go first?* I'd come this far, and it was time to surrender once and for all. With that, I thought fuck it and drank it down in one go. I remember feeling bloody chuffed with myself. I had done it! I had survived. I opened my eyes to look at the shaman under the candlelight. He smiled and beckoned his wife to come and get me.

The shaman's wife was a beautiful, kind soul. I could feel her loving energy. She smiled sweetly as she approached, took me by the hand, and then held me up as I walked back to my bed for the evening. As I got to the bed, I looked around, and one of the others had been called forward. They were about to go on their journey. The shaman's wife laid me on the bed and covered me with blankets. It was like going back to childhood and being tucked in by someone you love. The interesting thing was that even though I immediately went on a bit of a journey, I could hear him taking the next person through the process, and of course, that distracted me. I was fighting it.

I was not one to surrender to silence. I would never have been able to fall asleep in a roomful of people, so any noise around me kept me from allowing myself to go deep, at first. I feel that if I had gone last, by the time I drank the ayahuasca, I would have had to surrender my control and just go off without distractions.

I guess I will never know because that is not what happened.

38

The room went quiet. It felt so good. And that was when I really started to allow myself to surrender. I had no more distractions. I had to go inward. It was time to focus on me, myself and I. I did not see a snake or a serpent as I was told I would. I went straight into what looked like a kaleidoscope, seeing all of the colours and images merging into one to produce an incredible display. It was stunning. I will never forget it. Orange, red and bright golden yellow. I was in awe at how incredibly bright and vivid it was. I wanted to step into it and go through it. It felt like a window, a portal to somewhere that was beckoning me to explore and investigate what was going on. The more I focused on the colours and shape, they started to morph into a merry-go-round. I was on a horse, going round and round in circles. Music was playing loudly. I was laughing so much. The wind was blowing in my hair. I felt so free. I remember thinking – *I could happily stay here forever*. It was incredible. Everything was so light, bright and colourful. I remember feeling like there was some hidden message in this merry-go-round; something that this laughter and this sense of love was attempting to show me.

I carried on this merry-go-round for what seemed to be a long time; in reality it was probably only five minutes. I immersed in feeling such a powerful energy. I was truly, deeply there – with all of my heart and soul. I surrendered that little bit more; what came next was like something out of a movie. All of a sudden, it was like I had extra sharp sensory powers. It felt as if they had always been there, yet it felt like a switch had been flicked. It was like Mother Nature had opened up and said, *'Lucy – it's time to hear'*. I kid you not, I could hear animals. Yes, I was in the jungle, I appreciate that, and there were likely to be many animals around while I was off with Mother Ayahuasca, but I'm not talking about those kinds of creatures. I could hear little things crawling along the ground. It was like I could hear the ants making their moves, and hear what they were thinking and doing. I could hear the wings of insects moving. Not in the way we would hear or witness normally. It is so difficult to put into words. I had super-sonic senses. And rather than freaking out about it, I leaned into it. In my mind's eye, I asked a question –

Who are you? I had this beautiful, powerful, overwhelming surge of energy run through my body. It felt so strong; a strength and protection I had never felt before.

Suddenly, I felt I needed to take the trip down the dark path to the toilet. Surprisingly, when I opened my eyes I felt okay. The shaman came to check I was alright, as he saw I was moving about. I pointed to the toilet, and he smiled sweetly and held his hand out to show me the way. I smiled back. I felt he was proud of my efforts up to this point. I thought he was also possibly wondering if he should give me some more of the stuff. I had heard the others purging during the journey I had been on. I had not felt anything needed to be purged from me. I felt so full of love and hope. I could have run a marathon. In my mind, I felt so clear and connected at that point.

I started walking to the toilet, and that was when it happened. I had to walk past a tree; it was so big, the trunk was huge, I looked up, and it seemed to go on for miles. I smiled sweetly at the tree, then noticed Mother Nature. She smiled at me with an empathic knowing. I felt like she swept me up in her arms. I had to stop and hold the tree. Not because I felt weak, sick or wonky, it wasn't like that, it was like she wanted to feel me close to her. I found myself whispering, '*I've got you*'. I have no idea where it came from, it just felt like the right thing to say. I felt her breathe a sigh of relief, and then I got the feeling of her encapsulating me in her arms, reminding me I was safe. I had my eyes open at this point. I was not off in a dream, this was happening. I was being shown a world of magic and mysticism that I remembered from when I was a child. It was pitch black, yet it seemed to me as if there was a light on somewhere. There wasn't, though. It was my eyes, they were seeing so much stronger than ever before. I stayed close to the tree for a few moments longer to continue to benefit from the energy I was experiencing. That's when I clearly saw insects clambering up the tree. I could see them so clearly, even in the pitch black. *What was happening?* Even more interestingly, I could hear their footsteps working their way up the tree. I thought – *What on earth! This stuff is good!* Then the controlling side of me kicked in. *I'm losing it! I must be losing it! Who on earth will ever believe that I could speak to Mother Nature? Who would believe I saw insects in the dark and heard them walking up a tree? Lucy, you have finally lost it!* I could barely believe that this was happening myself. Not wishing to deal with what was going on anymore, I decided it was time to say goodbye to Gaia's energy, and finish the walk to the toilet.

I left the tree's grounding energy and continued to where the toilet was. I was a little bit wobbly after stepping out of that energy. It felt like I had been in a vortex or something, and I was attempting to balance myself on the other side of it. I have to add that at this point, I was feeling wired. The ground didn't look like the ground anymore. It appeared soft and almost fluffy. It looked like there was bright green moss all over the floor, and it was extremely bouncy too, weaved through with lots of colours. I could see lots of different animals, insects and plants. It was like Gaia had showed me how powerful her playground was. She had produced all of this, and I had to witness it, to remember it, to believe it all. Everything was super enhanced – bright, colourful, and pristine almost. It was magical. It took my breath away and made my heart feel like it was ten times bigger. I had so much love for nature, the earth, and animals. I had always been a fan of these things, but this was different.

After what seemed an eternity, I made it to the toilet. I cannot stress enough, it would only take a minute maximum to make that journey in normal daylight. Not this time, though. It was a magical mystery tour.

I sat down to go to the toilet, and actually managed to go for a wee with ease and grace. I remember back in my partying days, I could sit and attempt a wee for what felt like a week. Not this time. All was working exactly as it was required; thank you, Lord. Sitting there, I could hear people purging. I could hear them being sick. It didn't trouble me, though. I was just glad it was not me, and that I didn't have to see it. I allowed myself to wander off with my thoughts, and that was it, I started to go off again. Mother Ayahuascha had come in and was taking me on the next leg of the journey. I thought – *Wooah this is amazing.* I was looking around; I'm not sure at what. The toilet was just a tiny space – a toilet and a sink to wash your hands. Considering we were in the jungle, though, it was very clean. A fly flew past me, pretty close. It was bizarre; I could see every detail of its wings. I cannot emphasise enough to you, it was like I had supersonic hearing, and sight. There was a connection to myself I had never experienced. I sat there for a while, in awe of what was happening.

I then decided it was time to move. I thought I must have been gone for ages by this point. As I stood up, I looked at myself in the mirror. This was an old habit I used to have from back in the party days – I would always look to see how big my pupils were. As someone with very dark brown eyes, my irises would disappear on a night out, surrendered to my pupils. My pupils were huge. It was so weird to see them like this again. They were so dilated. This is one of the reasons you are required to use ayahuasca after dark, as your pupils dilate so significantly that you can cause some damage to your eyesight if you do it during the day – or at least that's what was explained to me. I was fascinated. A fair few minutes must have passed with me looking at my eyes and how different I looked. I looked more peaceful somehow, like I'd become one with nature. I had remembered who I was.

I decided I really should get back to the retreat. It felt like I'd been in the toilet for about a week, so I decided I should pull myself together and go back out. I could have stayed in that toilet all night. I was content in there, in my own little bubble. Not that I wasn't outside, because I was, but it was weird. I felt safe and in a little cocoon.

The walk back to the retreat was no different to the way in, only this time, as I walked from stepping stone to stepping stone, I felt like I was a fairy. I felt light on my toes like I had a newfound bounce. I felt playful, light, bright, and fun and to top it off, I could see lots of magic. I could see pixies, elves, imps, and bright coloured fruits and plants where all these magical beings were hanging out. In my mind, I could see badgers, deer and animals from back home in the UK. There was no way they were there in the middle of the Amazon, but I could see all of them.

When I got to the giant tree again, I was reminded of the answer to my question. It was Mother Nature. Gaia. This experience was the first true connection that I got to her energy, to how she would look after us if we looked after her – and to how protected we all are. I felt as if I was her. I stopped in awe again, hearing the ants walking and the insects buzzing. It was a very profound and extremely humbling experience.

I eventually made it to my space. I laid down and tucked myself back into my blankets, and instantly, in my mind's eye, I started witnessing lots of black and white photographs flashing up in front of me. It was fascinating; I love photography. Very few people know that about me, even to this day. Only those close to me would know that I love taking photographs, especially ones of scenery. All these photographs that appeared in front of me were images I had taken over the years when I'd been on holiday or exploring somewhere. It was truly stunning to watch. I asked in my mind's eye what this could mean. That's when an image of a plane going around the world started showing itself. They showed the world in a planet form; it wasn't like a flat Earth or anything like that. It was a ball, so I knew it was the world, and there was a plane circling around it continuously. I lay there thinking to myself – *Wow! This is amazing. I wonder what any of it means. Maybe I am just supposed to enjoy it. There is no meaning to it.*

Next up, they took me to a beach. The beach was stunning. It was like something out of a movie. Picturesque, bright blue sky, crystal clear water and the most wonderful white powder sand. I saw myself walking along the beach. I looked around and thought to myself – *I'm the only person here* – that's a bit weird with such an incredible beach like this. It was the most beautiful, magical beach I'd ever seen in my life. The water took my breath away. It was like the kind you see on the adverts for Bora Bora, or the Maldives. It was flat. It was calm. You could see fish swimming in it. It felt tropical. I felt that I just had to go there. All the colours and the feelings were overwhelming for my senses again. I could feel the sand between my toes. I could feel the tingle of the sunshine on my skin. I looked around and wondered where I was. I looked for something to show me a sign, so I would be able to locate it in the future. I noticed little brown boats in the distance and made a mental note of them. These little boats would be how I remembered it. Then words started flowing through me that made absolutely no sense for what I was doing – Trust. Surrender. Release. Cleanse. Today these words mean a lot to me, but back then, they didn't.

The next thing, I felt a tap on my shoulder, it was the shaman's wife with the translator. They beckoned me to go back to the shaman at his request. My intuition had been right. The shaman thought I was doing well and asked me to sit down whilst he reactivated me. With that, he started tapping and blowing tobacco on me again. The translator then asked me if I was comfortable doing some more. I have no idea how the translator could communicate as effectively as he was; he had done a big cup of ayahuasca just after I had taken mine. I looked at him. My soul really wanted to say, *'Yes, yes, yes'*.

My mind and my control were saying, *'You've had enough, Lucy'*. I had a fear I would want to take drugs again, even though psychedelics are nothing like recreational drugs. I pondered for another minute, then said, "I don't think I am. I think I'm quite happy where I am. I'm having a really nice experience." The translator told the shaman in Spanish what I had said and I felt he was a bit pissed off with me as he wanted me to go deeper. I now know this to be my own bullshit. Why on earth would the shaman be pissed off? I wanted to go deeper, but I was scared, hence my projection onto him. I recognise now that whatever we assume, whatever we judge, is how we really feel about ourselves.

Out of the blue, the girl with the tattoo on her neck started screaming and shouting out loud. Wow! I did not expect that. It was pretty traumatic in itself. Instantly it bought me out of where I was, that blissful place I had chosen to be. I thought – *Thank goodness I just declined it.* Do I regret that at all? Maybe. But, I trust that everything happened the way it needed to happen at that time. My decision proved to be the right one. I wasn't comfortable at all with this person screaming at the top of their voice. She was screaming that there was a dark energy in her throat that was trying to get her. She then started clawing at herself to get it out of her. I didn't like it. I didn't like that feeling. I didn't want to be around it. I would have run away if I could. What I was witnessing was not what I would call fun. Not in the slightest. I hoped Ricky would come round and grab me to take me back to my room. Being with the black rat would have been preferable at this point, trust me. I probably would have spoken to it, given half a chance.

As much as I would have liked to continue on the journey that day, I felt I had done what I needed. I said to the shaman thank you, but no thank you. He blew some more tobacco at me, which kind of brought me back up for a short time, and then I went back to my bed and laid back down. The translator came over and said that whenever I wanted to, I could go to my room and rest. As much as I wanted to be away from that woman, I had fallen in love with the world I had created around me. I lay there for a few minutes before surrendering myself back to my magical mystery world. It was very much a childlike place. It was somewhere an eight-year-old version of Lucy would be happy to be. There was no heaviness, no drama;

it was a magical world of mysticism. I had been reunited with that incredibly powerful energy.

There was no darkness at all during my journey with Mother Ayahuasca. There was no snake, no serpent. There was no dark night of the soul. There was no *'check your* ego' stuff, which should have happened, but it didn't. It was the most beautiful, connecting, and loving experience I had ever been through. I felt important. I felt as if I mattered. Would I have got to see all I did see if I was not important? I wondered what all of the images had meant. I wondered if it would all make sense at one point. Then I thought about Ricky. I wondered what he had been through, if he'd had such a kind experience as I had.

I believe that this experience set me up for the rest of the trip. To connect me back to Gaia. To connect me to the fact that love is a thing, that there is beauty in it and to it, that it wasn't all darkness and doom and gloom – which is what I had perceived up to that point in my life. It was like a cobweb had been removed from over my eyes, and all of a sudden, I could see clearly. It was like a fire had been reignited within my heart and my soul. Whatever this was, I was so grateful for Ricky at this point. I felt connected to my heart for the first time since I was eight years of age. You might find that weird, especially as I spoke about my first love not that long ago, but this was different to that. I loved myself. I loved what was around me. I felt content just being with myself, something that had been alien up to that point. I will always have so much gratitude for Ric, unknowingly pushing me to level up, and hard, I hasten to add. Without him, I would not be the person I am today.

39

At about five o'clock in the morning, I decided to trot myself to my room. I didn't know where Ricky was at this point, whether he was in his room or not, and to be perfectly honest I didn't really care. I was ready to rest and digest all that had gone on. I remember thinking I was excited about going for a decent shower in the next hotel we were in. I didn't get any sleep at all that first time with ayahuasca. I sat there thinking about the things that had happened. Wondering what those pictures had meant. What did the plane going around the world mean? What came next? There was gold, yellow, and there was red and orange. I wondered what it could all mean. Maybe there will be some meaning that I understand later in my life? What were all those photographs I saw of places where I had been travelling? What about that beach? What was the significance of the merry-go-round? I grabbed a book I had been writing key points of my journey in, and I started to piece the bits of the puzzle together. Was this telling me I had to be brave and go travelling?

I couldn't fully connect the dots at the time. Looking back, it was obvious, but when you're in it, it's never that easy to spot. It was only later when I took action that I started thinking – *Oh shit, Mother Ayahuasca actually told me I was going to do this. She showed me it all. Oh my god, this is magical. Thank God I did that experience.*

So many people need a dark night of the soul when doing plant medicine because of their circumstances. It was not my time to have that experience. Oh no, the Universe had much bigger plans for me. I was going to take myself to those levels on the next leg of the journey. If I had been given a choice, maybe I would have taken the plant journey to take me there, but I wasn't given a choice. I had to physically experience it, so that I knew how to heal properly and so that I could remind others.

I stepped outside my room at about seven o'clock in the morning without closing my eyes, since leaving the retreat space. I was wired; I felt as if I'd been up all night taking drugs, which essentially I had, but this was in a totally different way to the way I used to do them. I saw Ricky's room had the door open a bit, so I knocked. He was awake and looking in a reflective mood. I asked him, "How are you feeling?"

He looked at me and he said, "Can we have a chat?"

"Yeah, of course."

"How do you feel after yesterday?" he asked.

I said, "I feel really good. Wired. Probably should sleep, but can't." We both laughed, "I really hated it when she was screaming. I didn't like the fact that they were talking either. I just wanted to be immersed in what I was seeing."

He agreed, "Yeah, I'm a bit pissed off with it myself. Shall we go for a walk?" I nodded. We went for a little walk so we could talk in peace. He had something to say and didn't want anyone to hear. We both made a decision on that walk. We were supposed to stay on another night to do a second journey, but we decided that we just weren't with the right people to do it with. I loved how open and honest we could be with each other. We weren't happy, so why stay? It's rare you meet someone who is comfortable to walk away from something that doesn't feel right. We both agreed we were doing the right thing, so we decided to have some fun with it. We were like two little naughty kids. We planned to make our excuses and run, hoping that no one would see or question us. We had every intention to make it out unseen and unheard.

We had a lovely walk. It seemed to clear both of our heads. We both spoke about how we felt and the kind of magic that we'd seen on the journey. We then went back to our respective rooms and packed up what we had unpacked, which, I'll be honest, was nothing for me. I didn't unpack a single thing because I wasn't really interested in being there.

In the end, we made our exit public rather than sneaking off. We asked the translator to organise us a taxi to get out of there, and wished them success for their journey that evening. We settled the bill — we paid for the two nights, even though we weren't going to be there — and wished them every success for their next evening's ceremony.

While Ricky was packing up his stuff, I had a discussion with the shaman and the translator. Very proudly, I said, "I didn't see a snake. I'm really happy I didn't see a snake."

The shaman responded in Spanish, for the translator to repeat to me, "You obviously meditated very well on it. You are a powerful manifestor to have that power over the plant."

The shaman then gave me a piece of advice that I've never forgotten to this day. What he said to the translator was, "This girl doesn't realise it yet, but she's fully aware of all of her traumas. She just doesn't know how to deal with it. She didn't need to have it come to the surface through the medicine, which is why she got such a beautiful journey, because all she needed was the next steps of the path that will help her unravel this, and for her to go on to help humanity."

It was the most profound thing I had ever heard. I cried. I literally sobbed. All I could do was release the emotions that had been building over many, many years. *Was he really talking about me? Had my grandad been right all that time? There was something in me? How on earth did he know that? Were those feelings from when I was a child right? Was I really here to do something special? Something important?* Then my ego piped up and told me not to be so bloody stupid. Of course it wasn't. *Stop getting carried away, Lucy!*

Ricky and I were running away. We were following my usual pattern of disappearing rather than having to deal with things. I wondered if maybe Ricky had similar patterns to me. We were not running away from the shaman because he was lovely – as was the translator, who had a very sweet soul – rather we wanted to get away from the dark energy coming through this female with the neck tattoo. I had become extremely sensitive overnight, and I could no longer deal with being somewhere I did not wish to be, with someone that drained me.

That conversation with the shaman, as I was leaving, was a life-changing conversation. As much as I felt how profound it was, the full-body goosebumps made it clear this was a big deal. It still didn't mean much to me. It didn't yet make any sense. I thought – *What is he talking about? Trauma? I've not been raped or abused. What trauma?* I had absolutely no idea what he meant by trauma. Again, I could have asked, but I didn't feel ready to hear the answers. I must have instinctively known that at some point, when the time was right, I would be reunited again with this topic. It's fair to say that was the case.

40

The spontaneous decision to book the Galapagos trip was what would become the norm in this Lucy and Ricky relationship. We were like two peas in a pod. It was uncanny how similar both of us were. We were so spontaneous. We don't like to be tied down – or, more honestly – we were both scared to be tied down. We were free spirits. We both loved to say, "Screw it, let's do it!" And that's exactly how we were together. We would egg each other on, and push each other's buttons to do crazy shit.

It was beautiful because it was the first time I had been able to be a totally free spirit without judgement. You can't really be a free spirit working in Corporate because that's dangerous. They need you to sit your arse down at your desk and get on with your job. Likewise, in my family, my mum's number one value is security and safety, so to have a daughter whose number one value is freedom, is such a huge shift for somebody to accept. I honour my mum so much for this. It must have been a real challenge having me as a daughter. I know she loves me and I'm sure she's very proud of me, but I really do feel she would have preferred me to be someone who stayed in the corporate thing, settled down, had 2.4 children, and done that kind of thing. Sorry Mum, that was never my path for this lifetime. Maybe in the next one.

Our plan – if you could call it a plan – was that we were going to go and have a couple of days on the main island of the Galapagos, then do a week on a boat. The reason for the boat, for anybody that's never been to the Galapagos, is that the islands are so spread out that you cannot get to them unless you go on a boat. Ricky had been doing some research, and he had figured out that there were different islands with different animals on. We decided on the key animals that we really wanted to see and made a plan around that. We were both keen to do some snorkelling, maybe even some diving. The sea life in the Galapagos islands was truly remarkable. I have always had a pull toward water throughout my life. I was fascinated by it and head over heels in love with sea turtles and dolphins. We knew that winging it probably wasn't the most sensible way of going somewhere as beautiful and highly sought after as the Galapagos, but we continued to wing it all the same. You only live once, as they say!

To get to the Galapagos Islands, we had to make our way from Tena back to the Capital City of Quito. From Quito, we would fly to a tiny little island called Baltra. This was the access point in. It was a small island off of San Cristobal and Santa Cruz. We had laughed all the way back to Quito; every experience we had, so far had been absolutely magical. The interactions, the conversations, the connections. Everything had gone with such ease up until this point. We simply decided what we were doing, and we were supported through it all. We were shown how powerful our joint manifestation skills were – not that we acknowledged it to each other back then – we were too busy living it.

We had been warned that leaving it to book plane tickets would result in us having to wait a few days, but that just wasn't the case. We managed to get two seats with ease. We were clearly meant to be going there. We breezed through the airport and very quickly found ourselves boarding. The plane was lovely, much bigger than I had anticipated. I had been internally freaking out about going on a propeller plane, but again it was just my mind being overactive. It was a jet plane with three seats on either side of the aisle, so it was small, but perfectly formed. I had not had the privilege of flying anywhere with Ricky before, so I had no idea what to expect. I liked flying on my own as it meant I had no one to moan to if something went slightly off-piste.

We had a great laugh at the airport. It was so nice to have someone to be playful and banter with. Two out of the last three trips I had been on, I had been on my own. We listened to music, we were laughing and joking, and although I didn't sleep, I rested my head on him as we flew, taking time to be present, connected and peaceful with myself. Something that was slowly becoming more normalised in my crazy life.

We seemed to arrive quickly. It wasn't a long flight, just under an hour and thirty minutes. We got off at the other end extremely quickly too. At this point, our inner children were fully activated. We were like kids in a sweet shop. We had done it. We had arrived. We had brought the last few months of discussion into a reality.

As much as we had discussed the plan in the weeks leading up, I had moments of doubt that we would make it. Everyone back home had been telling me to book, not to risk it, but that was just not resonant to Ricky and I. I probably could have allowed my inner project manager and control freak to take over on several occasions during the lead up, but thankfully I had Ricky to guide me and ground me into much more of a divine feminine flow. Let's be real, I am a female this lifetime, so activating this beautiful energy was essential. I had been so heavily in my masculine energy before. Fight or flight mode. Survival. Keeping up with the men in my very male-dominated working environment. And let's not forget the toxicity I had created off the back of my interactions with men over the years. Someone had to remind me of the divine feminine energy I was here to embody, and thankfully it was Ricky. I had found him in the most bizarre of situations, our souls had recognised each other, and here we were starting our evolution. Not that either of us properly knew it at the time. To this day, Ricky probably still doesn't quite get the importance of this to me, and that's more than okay. He's on his own incredible path.

Lucy in the past would have booked hotels and got everything aligned in true project manager fashion, so this was a big deal. I would have known exactly where I was going, when I had to be somewhere and where it was. On this occasion, nothing was ever booked before we got there. It was such huge growth for me. I had become extremely controlling since becoming a project manager. I was controlling before, don't get me wrong – but that was more around the control in relationships and what people thought of me – the transition into project manager had amplified it to a whole new level, not that I could see it in myself. Anytime I would ask a question about the what or the how, Ric would respond with, "Oh, we'll just wing it." And although everyone had always said I was a free spirit throughout my life, he really taught me such a valuable lesson, that if you trust, then everything is going to work out exactly as it is meant to.

We got some transport from the airport to take us to the main area where there was a little more civilisation. When I call it civilisation, this was the Galapagos back in early 2014 – it was tiny and there was very little there. Nothing was very big, other than the sheer amount of wildlife that inhabited the place. We both had backpacks, so we couldn't do too much until we found somewhere to dump them.

We walked into a tiny little travel place and asked them if they could suggest somewhere that would be good for us to stay. The lady in the shop was most helpful. She made a few suggestions, and very quickly, we decided on a really cute, little place that was maybe five minutes walk from the restaurants and bars where we currently were. The lady showed us pictures and told us it was very quiet there. There was a swimming pool, and the rooms looked really beautiful. We agreed to stay there; she called ahead and we set off to find it. As we arrived, we both commented on the huge wooden gate at the front. It was enormous and really heavy. We were met by a friendly gentleman who, it turns out, had bought the place some years earlier and made some renovations. It was truly beautiful. As we got through the gate, the gardens and outside space were particularly stunning. The building itself looked like a castle. It was made of stunning grey stone. It looked extremely grand from the outside – it looked much more expensive than it actually was. I was excited to throw my stuff down in a room – rather than it being on my back – jump in the shower, change my clothes and immerse in the energy of this place.

The man took us to the room, let us in and showed us the essentials. Our room was in one of the turrets. We were only going to be there for a couple of days until we could book and join a cruise. The guy showed us the key to the main gate outside – the huge, fortress gate. He very clearly said to us, "I'm going to give you one key. If one of you doesn't come through the gates with the other one, the door will lock. There will be no way in." That all seemed very serious and sensible advice, but we quickly dismissed it. We were going to be going in and out together. If one of us was going out alone, we'd take the key, simple as that.

Once we had put our bags down and got changed into something more comfortable, we decided to go out for a little walk. Checking out a new place is always best on foot. People always ask me why I run wherever I go. It helps me get my bearings extremely quickly, which is why I do it. Ric suggested it would be a good time to pop to an internet café to check his emails, and do some research on cruises and a few other bits. We set off exploring, less than five minutes up the road and there were sea-lions everywhere. They were lolling around on the pathways close to the water, it was amazing. We walked past a kid's park and sea lions were on the slides, on the see-saws, they were everywhere. They were just so comfortable; chilling out and being a sea lion, I guess. I felt in awe, realising that on this island the animals were the number one priority over humans. It wasn't about humans. The humans were actually quite an inconvenience to the animals. The animals were what was important. It felt right that they had the same rights as us humans. It was unheard of anywhere else. The other thing we saw, was a lot of iguanas, again. I had recently experienced seeing them in Ecuador, and was absolutely fascinated by them. In the Galapagos, they were all different colours, camouflaging themselves against certain backgrounds, and interestingly, they were in extremely close proximity to the sea lions. It was a weird but beautiful place we had found ourselves in.

Ric checked his emails, and then we went to grab some food. Whilst eating, we spoke openly about our intentions for the cruise. We decided to look at what animals were on each island, then make sure we got as much variety in as possible. Once our bellies were full, and we had openly discussed what we were looking for, we went on a mission to start searching for this cruise. It turned out to be slightly more challenging than we had anticipated. We spoke to several different agents – everything was fully booked. What was left, the prices were sky high, as there were minimal spaces left. It didn't help that we were being extremely picky also. We knew what we wanted, which was to see several islands. We didn't want to be on a boat for seven days and just see two islands. It seemed pointless to go all that way to do half a job. That just wasn't Ric and I. Ideally, we wanted to see four or five islands. We were confident that we were going to find what we wanted; it just wasn't necessarily going to happen that day.

We talked to different people for hours and hours; we even went off on our own to speak to people, and then came back together to share our findings. It was fun, even though we weren't getting our way immediately. We knew it would happen eventually. That inner knowing drove us on, so we had fun manifesting it rather than getting upset about it.

It was time for dinner. All of this talking and organising was thirsty and hungry work. We continued to talk it through over dinner. We knew something would come up that would be exactly what we were looking for, and that in the next couple of days, we would be on the boat in bliss, surrounded by nothing but water and wildlife.

The next day, after a pretty passionate evening, we decided to go exploring again and lock in this cruise, once and for all. We knew we didn't have much time together, so we were desperate to get on a boat and experience the magic that was awaiting us. We didn't even really need to talk; something had happened to us since the ayahuasca. We had become much more connected to each other. We had both bared our souls and allowed our vulnerability, especially about having a shared wish to escape the place – and that had deeply bonded us. It was like we were tapping into each other's thoughts. Almost like our telepathy was coming online. We were finishing each other's sentences and laughing before the other had finished because we knew what was coming. In such a short time, we had experienced so much together – Ecuador, the people seeing my aura, the ayahuasca journey, running away, taxi rides, plane journeys, altitude, drug abuse. We had been through a huge evolution in a very short time – it felt like we were becoming one, rather than two separate entities.

Following more discussions with travel agents, we agreed to hire a private boat to sail around the main island – just the two of us.

We could have gone on a boat with other people, but he wanted to experience it alone. It was a nice touch. It meant we got to do what we wanted to do. We could sweet talk the captain into stopping where we chose. The captain of the boat we boarded was amazing. He was such a nice man. He made us feel completely at ease. He was fun, and playful and he kept encouraging me to drive the boat, which was great. It doesn't take much to encourage me to get involved with anything like that. Ric just rolled his eyes and smiled as I gave in to the man's flirting. I put his captain's hat on and fully immersed into the role as chief sailor.

A part of the journey was called 'The Love Channel' — of course! Where else would Little Miss Love end up? The boat owner drove us through the Love Channel and suggested we got off the boat in certain places, whilst he took photos of us. We were allowed to get out and explore. This is where I saw the sea turtles. I love sea turtles, always have done, so to be this up close and personal with them was absolutely magical. I never realised until this point in my life how fast they were. One minute they were there, then boom, gone like a shot. We dived in the water; the turtles and sea lions were so playful with us. I loved it so much. I was blissfully happy. The whole time I had such a huge smile on my face. We were experiencing this incredible magic together.

We got off at another place, and the floor was almost volcanic. There were oddly shaped rock structures and cacti. I was wandering around in my bikini, when I saw one of the rocks that looked like a penis, so of course, I had to play up to that. Ric was roaring. We were being silly and childlike. Exactly what both of our souls needed at that time. I think that's what was really important here. We were in our inner child. We were allowing them to come out and play because we felt so safe with each other.

When we got back to shore, we were both buzzing. Almost immediately, we decided we wanted to go out again, so we found another boat — a bigger boat this time. We got on board with about 20 other people and went snorkelling. Wow! It was unbelievable. We were out in the middle of the water, and suddenly the driver cut the engine. I'll be honest, my heart sank a little, thinking we had broken down, but the driver had done it on purpose. Out of nowhere, there were hundreds of manta ray flocking all around the boat. I had never seen anything like it. It was truly magical. Ric and I were sat at the back of the boat when it happened. We were lost in each other's energy, sitting with our heads together, listening to music sharing an earphone each. We were fully attentive and in total awe. What a trip! This was incredible. It was one of those moments that I wish I had captured on film, but at the same time, I was so grateful to be so present that my phone did not even enter my head.

Nothing could have made that boat trip any better. And although the boat was relatively full, we got lucky by getting a space in the sun at the back of the boat. Sitting there, next to Ric, watching these manta rays, I thought — *I wouldn't want to be doing this with anybody else. I am so happy right now. So grateful for all of this.* And remember, I didn't even know him from Adam. I had only spent a matter of days with him in Thailand, then reconnected months later. Yet here I am in the April, and I cannot imagine experiencing this with anybody else. This was a big change for me. Normally, that would be my cue to run a mile.

The boat owner asked if anybody wanted to jump in the water with the manta ray, and so, of course, without even thinking anything, I was straight off the boat. He motioned for me to put a life jacket on. I shouted back, *"I'm good, I'm all right. Don't worry about me."* Some of the other people jumped in with me. What an experience; it was incredible. The water was so clear. You could see all the fish and the stunning manta ray swarming all around us, it was such a beautiful environment. I had never been this close to creatures like that at any point before in my life. It felt so right. I felt like I had gone back to being a mermaid or something. I loved every second of what was happening. I was so confident. When I was younger, I was the girl that used to freak out about snorkelling because I always thought I'd swallow the seawater. I would put my head in a little bit and then lift it back up to ensure no water would get in. On this trip, though, I got my confidence back. I was diving down deep, and Ric and I were underwater, pointing things out to each other and having the most incredible time.

The connection between us was so special. Unique, in fact. I feel, looking back, that it was clear from the very start that he was obviously from a past life. I felt our paths crossed in Thailand because he needed to anchor some energy back into me this lifetime. Energy that reminded me that I could have this connection with myself and with the divine. It was like his soul had been chosen to reignite, activate and hand me back my power.

It's unbelievable really, just how much I surrendered my trust to him in so many different ways, in such a short space of time. At that period in my life, it was the first time I had actually surrendered to a man. Before that, don't forget – I've got the money, I've got the job, I've got it going on, I'm in control, I'm strong. But with Ricky, I decided – *I'm going to trust you more than I've ever trusted anybody in this physical lifetime.* I felt safe with a man, and that was the first time that I'd experienced that. Previously, I never trusted anybody, not even myself. Think mirror.

Before my human knew, my soul knew that he was somebody very special. He'd been placed in my life to reactivate me. He committed to coming into my life to plug me back in; to remind me where I'd come from and about the mission I had committed to. I had forgotten until now how to breathe underwater, but I was confident and free again. I felt like I was in Atlantis, with all these beautiful creatures surrounding me; witnessing it all. Everything felt like it had a whole new meaning.

I wondered how one person could deliver so many gifts in such a short time? And unknowingly, he was the chosen one. They had to send someone in who would get my attention. Someone confident enough to be cheeky, and to initiate my cheekiness back. Someone who would not take no for an answer, and even though he was not fully on his own path yet, he would trust his intuitive pulls enough to teach me.

After having much fun in the water with the wildlife, we got back on the boat; I was the last one back in. I wanted to stay there forever. I would have loved to gather up a sea turtle to take home with me, but I would never do that. And those sea lions! They were amazing, brushing right up against us because they wanted us to swim with them. They think humans are playful, we are there to play with them. They think humans are their toys, especially when you've got a snorkel mask on and you've got the bubbles coming out, they really love that, they just want to play with you.

Once we were back on the boat, we saw penguins, it was one thing after another. I'm not able to do it all true justice with my descriptions, but my jaw was literally open in awe the whole time. It was breathtaking. How on earth did I get here? How on earth did this happen?

I felt so grateful to be alive.

41

We got back to our room much later that day. It had been such an incredible one from start to finish. There were so many wow moments. We had a lot of sun and sea air and spent a lot of time in the water. We were very happy, exhausted, and content. We had that wonderful feeling you get after a hard day's graft on holiday; skin tingling, sun-kissed noses and a nagging need to go for a siesta. Despite all of those feelings of satisfaction, the only thing that could have made it better was food. We were more than ready to eat our weight in food. So rather than chill out and take our time to relax, we freshened up quickly and got ourselves ready to go out for dinner.

We walked from our hotel for a little while before stumbling across a quaint cobbled street we had not found previously. There were lots of restaurants laid out next to each other. There were menus at the front of each restaurant, and people were there to welcome us, without being pushy, though.

Ric and I were good eaters. We always got excited going out for food, especially when hungry. We would order options to share, so we could sample various choices from the menu. To start with, we ordered some drinks. We decided on alcohol, even though we were both exhausted. It was cause for a celebration. We had experienced the best day, and had survived over a week in each other's company. We also had finally managed to book the cruise, which we were starting the next afternoon.

We ate our starters, and then our main course came out – langoustines. They were the size of lobsters. I asked the waiter if he had got confused with the order because I had never seen anything like it. They were unbelievable to look at, and they tasted sensational. We had decided we were going all out that night. We had no idea what the food was going to be like on the boat, so we made a conscious effort to eat well and eat plenty. As the food flowed, so did the wine.

It was absolutely lovely, but I was starting to get a little bit cheeky. The wine was definitely kicking in, and I felt happy and playful.

At the end of the meal, we both felt full but comfortable. Although we had eaten how a king and queen would eat, the price tag did not match it. It was expensive compared to places we had eaten previously but not compared to restaurants back home in the UK. One of my favourite things ever is going out for dinner, enjoying good wine and good company.

It was strange to be sitting there sharing such a beautiful, intimate moment with a relative stranger. I knew nothing about Ric at this point. I knew he had Italian roots, and that he came from a beautiful big family. I learnt that he had left his home to get his head together after heartbreak. I knew firsthand that he was a phenomenal boxer, but I didn't know anything deeply personal about him. We had only met six months earlier, spoken for a few months, and spent a week together getting to know each other. That night, though — and I want to be honestly vulnerable and admit this — I made a judgement about him. As far as I was concerned, he was just some guy who was travelling with a backpack around the world, searching for something — he probably didn't even know what it was, even if it had bitten him on the butt. Our paths had mysteriously crossed in Thailand, we had then decided we wanted to go on an adventure together. I judged that the adventure he was on was probably too expensive for him, without asking if that was the case. I made an assumption about his situation. So I made the decision, under the influence of alcohol, that I would sneak off to the toilet and settle the bill. I made my excuses to disappear to the toilet with my bag. On the way back from the toilet, I grabbed the waiter and settled our bill, without consulting or sharing this with Ric.

When I went back to the table I touched Ric on the arm and said, "Okay, we can go now. All done."

He said, "Okay, let me just go and settle the bill for us."

"Ahh you don't need to worry about that," I smiled. "I've already sorted it." What came next I could never have anticipated. I had made a gesture — that I perceived to be kind and from a space of love — but it was not received in that way at all.

For the first time, Ric got angry with me. I saw a shift in him from the calm, assertive man that I had spent the last week with, to someone who was hurt. Actually, furious would be a better word to describe his reaction. He raised his voice and started to question what I had done, *"What the fuck are you doing paying for that? You didn't need to pay Lucy, what were you thinking?"*

I couldn't make sense of what I had done to upset him, and what was now unfolding in front of me. I was completely taken aback. And that's when the beast got released. I had never been good at being challenged, especially when someone shouted at me. Today I recognise that to be a trauma response, but back then, not so much. In seconds I went from 0 to 60. Angry Lucy surfaced for the first time with Ric, fuelled by the few glasses of wine I had during the meal. My armour, which I had been steadily dismantling over the previous weeks, very quickly resurrected itself, in readiness for an all-out war. *"Who the fuck do you think you are telling me that I can't pay? If I want to fucking pay for something, I'll pay!"* Boom! There she was, totally stepping back into the masculine energy. It came out of nowhere. I was so angry with him – yet only a few minutes earlier I had been in awe of just being in his presence. I quickly switched from my beautiful divine feminine energy, which had surrendered and was starting to become vulnerable and open – and someone I had become really proud of – to a full-on beast. I had trusted Ric so much, I had really let him in, and then in one decision, I collapsed all of that. My mentality was – *I must protect myself at all costs.*

I truly thought in my heart I was doing a decent thing. We had enjoyed a bit of alcohol, some good food and celebrated all that was and all that was going to be. I thought I was doing the right thing. I had money. I worked hard to do lovely things like this for people. Why could he not see this? Why was he not happy to accept the gift of me paying for something? I felt he had been paying for everything previous to this situation, so I guessed my return gesture would be met with thanks.

I had pre-judged Ricky. I had decided that he was somebody who was travelling the world and didn't need to be spending money on expensive meals, trips and cruises with some chick he met in Thailand just a few months earlier. I made a judgement that he needed me to pay for this – a total assumption – which I now know is really a sign of insecurity in myself. *If I pay for this, it will make him happy, he'll continue to like me.* He'd been so giving to me, he really had, he wouldn't let me pay for stuff the whole time we were together. I had felt guilty about that, and remember, at this time, my story was – *I'm an independent, successful woman. I don't need a man to survive.* The story that I had created and carried forward, off the back of my parents' marriage breakdown.

Knowing what I know now, and with the wisdom of hindsight, I would never have done it, and I would never do it again – not without a discussion first, anyhow.

What happened next was embarrassing. It erupted. To say it was a huge explosive scene was no overstatement. A face-off between two lost souls, staring at themselves in a mirror, seeing all they had to heal, but missing that point completely, and instead truly believing that their stance was the correct one to be taken. The red mist had descended over us, and neither of us was looking likely to back down. I got to the point where I told him to fuck off, and I walked off – there's that pattern again. That was what I did. If I was ever under attack, my natural response was to go. I couldn't, for the life of me, get where he was coming from. I just couldn't see it, no matter how I looked at it; I wasn't equipped with those tools back then. From my perspective, he was being a stubborn, pigheaded, selfish idiot. I couldn't remove myself from the fact that it was all his fault.

I stormed off in a mood, to which he responded by chasing me down. This is the reaction people generally want when they storm off, and I was no exception here. I wanted a reaction.

"Where are you going?" Ricky asked

"Fuck you, I'm going for another drink!" I huffed.

"You've got the key though and I need you so I can get in the room, remember if one of us gets locked out we're screwed? That's what the man said."

I didn't respond.

"Look Lucy, I appreciate you don't want to speak to me right now. Let's take a few minutes to calm down. I'll go and check my emails then come and get you when I'm done. Okay?"

In fairness to him, I think he handled me pretty well, yet again – not that I could see that at the time. I was furious with him; how fucking dare he! I pointed to a cafe bar and said, "I'll be over there." In all reality, going for a drink was the absolute worst idea that I could have had; it was another trauma response. I was not getting my own way, so I would lean on my crutch, and the only crutch I could get my hands on was alcohol. There was no reasoning when I was like this, though.

Honestly, it's embarrassing to be so vulnerable about this, but I know many of you may be reading this and recognising your own trauma responses. And as much as it's embarrassing, I know I was gifted this to assist humanity to ascend to much greater heights. It all starts with truth. Raw honesty and mastery of self.

I stormed over to the bar and the barman asked what I wanted. I feel he could sense I was a woman on a mission. "Glass of wine please, I'm on one," I confirmed to him. Yep, Lucy's angry and she's stormed off on a mission to get more alcohol because clearly alcohol will help resolve the situation. Talk about adding fuel to the flames. It was a stupid idea, especially as we had the seven-day cruise starting at lunchtime the next day. I drank the wine and started to talk myself down – *Right, Lucy, calm down. Just take some time.*

I finished my drink pretty quickly and the barman asked if I wanted another. Both sides of my ego were piping up massively at this point. The more prominent trauma side was saying – *Fuck it, what's the worst that can happen?* Thankfully, my more vulnerable side won over the pained inner child – *Another drink is going to lead to trouble. Go home.* I listened to that angelic guidance. Another drink was a very bad idea. I decided to breathe, let go of the hurt and anger, and went off to find Ric at the internet cafe. This was a huge quantum leap forward for me. I never backed down. I never listened to the calm inner voice. The angry version was so prominent, it was what I was used to hearing. It had kept me safe for all of these years, and stopped me from getting hurt. That armour had taken so many knocks in order to protect me, and I had to respect that, but I also realised there was another choice to listen to.

I sheepishly arrived back at the internet café and smiled. I hung by the door and asked if he was ready to go. He said he wasn't quite ready yet but he wouldn't be far behind me. Thankfully things appeared to be a bit more neutral after we took that little break from each other. I didn't like what had happened earlier. It felt horrible. All I really wanted was to be held, and to talk about it, without bringing all that stuff back up again. I knew that going over it all again would not serve either of us, although my inner control freak wanted to know what the fuck went on. How could we avoid it again, if we didn't know what triggered it? I smiled at him and let him know I was going to walk slowly back to the room. I told him I would prop the gate open with something so he could get in and I'd let him in if he called me.

I was tired and still a little upset by the night's events, so a little walk back, on my own, before bed, would do me the power of good.

On the ten-minute walk back, I started to feel better. I calmed myself down and was finally back in a fully peaceful state. Ric's suggestion of a little time out had been wise. He had done his thing; I had done my thing – drink alcohol. Regardless, we both had a bit of breathing space. Thankfully, everything seemed to be okay when I left the internet café, and I felt happier about that. As far as I was concerned, it was all done. That episode did not need to be revisited – unless he wanted to talk it through, in which case I would. *Thank God that is all over.*

When I got back to the hotel, I found a large stone to prop the gate open with and made sure no one else could see that the gate was propped open. I was happy with my work, so I carried on into the hotel.

I got back to the room and decided to have a shower to cleanse away the day, and set myself up for what was incoming tomorrow. In the shower, I let my imagination run away with thoughts of the coming cruise – the animals, the views, the sunsets. Once out of the shower, I decided to lay down on the bed and wait for Ric to call.

That ended up being a big mistake.

I lay down on the bed and fell asleep. It was so unlike me. I never slept until I knew the other person was safe, it didn't matter who it was, it was like a mothering instinct in me. And until this moment, it had never failed me. I had lost many nights' rest over the years, worrying about the whereabouts of people. I was also a very light sleeper; any movement would usually wake me. I'm still the same to this day. What I didn't know was that someone, probably the owner of the hotel, had removed the stone I had used to prop the gate open, so Ric couldn't get in at all. He was totally locked out. He pressed the buzzers of all the different rooms, and the reception, to try to get in. Then he started calling my phone, but I didn't hear a thing. He told me at a later time, that he had also tried to climb over the wall to get in. Massive fail on every level. Of course, because the gate was not propped open, and the fact I appeared to be ignoring his calls, he felt I was still in a mood with him, and that I was being a total bitch. I see now where he was coming from, but it actually couldn't have been further from the truth.

In the end, he had to go and find another place to stay for the night. I had passed out completely. I was comatose, likely because I'd had a couple of glasses of wine after a very busy day. The irony of it all was that I wasn't pissed off with him at that point, not in the slightest. What was done was done, as far as I was concerned. He didn't know that, though. To him, he was locked out of his hotel, late at night, after a huge argument with the person he was away with, and he had to find a room to sleep in – without his passport, or any stuff to check in with.

Oh boy!

The next morning when I woke up and he wasn't there, I thought – *Oh shit, where the fuck is he? Is he okay?* We were supposed to be going on the cruise soon. My mind went off on one.

I messaged him, "Where are you? Are you okay?"

He wrote back pretty quickly, "I was trying to get in that fucking room for two hours last night. I had to find a hostel to stay in."

My stomach sank. I felt sick. There was no way this needed to happen. I truly believed last night's argument was resolved and didn't need to spiral into another day, especially the day we were going on a cruise for a week. *Oh fuck! How did I let this happen?*

I fucked up massively. I really, really, really fucked up. I had no intention of doing it. There was absolutely no ill intent at all. It was an innocent mistake, he would see that surely when I explained – I had too much to drink, I was exhausted from the day and just passed out waiting for him to come back. The only light in this very dark tunnel was that he had been able to find a room to stay in that night. Just imagine if he'd been up all night or had to sleep outside.

He messaged to say he was coming back to grab his things. He was furious, I could tell. I could almost feel the venom coming through the phone. It was such a horrible feeling. I was really hoping I could sort things with him when he got back, but a big part of me felt like there was no chance of doing so before we got on the boat. I figured that being stuck with each other for a week on a boat, we'd have to sort it out and let it go eventually.

He came back to the room, and angry would be an understatement. He fucking lost it at me. I deserved it. I did. I really did. As far as he was concerned, I had locked him out purposefully. I had lied to him when I said I would leave the gate open, and the fact that I would answer my phone if he called. As much as I attempted to calm the situation and reason with him, there was just no way it was happening. He was so angry.

Looking back, it seems all of his wounds and his trauma had come to the surface to be faced and healed. Neither of us knew about any of that stuff back then, though, and even if I had done, this would not have been an appropriate time for me to start dissecting them.

I let him rant at me until he had said all he had to say. All I said back to him was, "I'm going to pack up my things, you pack up your things, let's just take some time and let's just get on the cruise and we'll sort it out when we are both ready." I had no idea how small the rooms were going to be on the cruise, I just knew by the size of the boat and the number of people on it, that they wouldn't be very big. Any animosity would have no place to hide, so we had to get it sorted, not only for us but for the sake of all the other people on the boat with us. Ric threw his stuff in a bag and said he was going to the internet cafe to check his emails. He was so pissed, I let him go. I wanted to stop him and talk things through, but I knew that in the mood he was in, he was going to erupt at me even for just breathing.

The interesting thing, when looking back on this situation is that both Ric and I had serious anger issues that we needed to deal with, all stemming from our emotional traumas, and our responses to them from a young age. We mirrored each other so much. We had to trigger the heck out of each other, in every way, in order to heal in the way that humanity and Gaia needed us to, for our future missions. I knew I had all this anger back then, but I did not know it was related to trauma. That concept was as alien as quantum physics to me at that point. Not knowing about it obviously meant I did not know how to work through the trauma and heal it. Ric was a great mirror. He mirrored everything back to me that I needed to deal with. I just didn't realise. I thought he was a fucking idiot, 'the biggest prick on the face of the planet' was a particular phrase that had actually left my mouth during one of our arguments. I projected everything out of me onto him. At no point did I consider he was mirroring me to activate my healing, nor did I accept the recognition and ownership of what I had to heal. I had absolutely no consciousness of that at that time.

42

Ric stormed out. I did not question it. He needed time to do his thing and hopefully calm down ahead of us getting to the port. I knew I would eventually find him somewhere, the place was too small to lose someone. While I continued to pack my stuff, Ric had made a decision to go and speak to the cruise people, and ask if there was any possibility of swapping rooms around. He was still absolutely furious with me. I turned up at the internet café, hoping that everything was going to be alright, and he told me he had moved me into a room with some random girl and that he had agreed to share with a man. The guy and girl were strangers, so it wasn't a problem for them to not be sharing – it was probably better for them to be in a room with the same sex as themselves. When Ric told me this, I went fucking ballistic – absolutely crazy. I lost it. I was ready to drown the arsehole in the ocean with rocks around his ankles. I left him in the internet café and started walking towards the port. I truly hated him at that moment. All of my abandonment issues flowed to the surface. *Fuck you, I am done. I'm not having anything more to do with you, you fucking arsehole.* It crossed my mind to find the captain and ask him if there was another boat I could join, so I never had to see this prick again.

Despite this awful animosity, the only choice we had was to suck it up and go on the cruise, or lose the money and not go at all. It was leaving imminently and I had to make a quick decision. For the first time in my life, I sucked it up, swallowed my pride, accepted not getting what I wanted, and decided to go on the cruise. This was another huge step for me, although I didn't fully recognise it at the time. My normal pattern was to run. I could easily have gone back to the hotel, left him to go on the cruise and organise myself a flight out of there. That was the 'normal' pattern, but something made me go on that cruise, knowing that it was probably going to be horrible. We had a massive black cloud hanging over the two of us, and an ugly amount of animosity. We could not even look at each other. I'll be honest with you, it was the most awkward thing I've ever done in my life. It was unbearably uncomfortable. The tension between us was palpable. Imagine how the others on the boat must have felt! Cringe!

The girl that I had been moved into a room with was absolutely magical, thank God. I really loved her and I was so grateful for her. I was actually really grateful Ric had behaved like he did because I got to spend special time with this sweetest of souls. There were some other girls on the boat as well, and they were just as amazing too. I am forever grateful to them all for helping me get through, and for distracting me from the fact that this person, who I had travelled halfway around the world for, was now ignoring me, like a child. They held space for me to be upset and allowed me to be frustrated, until one day I woke up and I just accepted it was the way it was. We would never talk about it. Never resolve it. He did not want to and I couldn't make him.

Ricky remained angry with me. He said some extremely hurtful things. He told me he could not even bear to look at me. That hurt me a lot. I needed to experience it, though. I needed to experience the level of anger that I had dished out to other people on many of occasions over the years. When, from my perspective, people had fucked up in the past, I cut them off and shut them down, never spoke to them again, without ever questioning it. As much as I hated it and I hated him for being the one to do this, he was mirroring every dark piece of my soul back to me, tenfold. He had been chosen as the one to slap me hard around the face with it, until I got it.

Of course, with hindsight and wisdom, I see this now, but I didn't know that was what was going on at the time. He didn't either, he just thought I was the most selfish bitch on the planet. We didn't realise that we were having a past life, karmic entanglement experience with each other, because the Universe needed us to be something very special this lifetime. I imagine the Divine was shaking her head at both of us wise, old souls having a meltdown with each other. This human experience sucks sometimes, hey?

So, rather than getting the memo, we continued in anger, blame and projection. It's all her fault; it's all his fault. She did this; he did that. And so it continued on, and on, and on. It was awful. Those poor people on the cruise. Mealtimes were hideous because we were supposed to sit around the same table, talking, and catching up on the day, but we both were not even making eye contact with each other anymore. It was so frickin awkward. If anyone who was on that boat reads this, please accept my sincere apologies.

One day, I woke up and thought – *Today, I'm going to be the bigger person. I'm going to speak to him, regardless of what he says back to me. I'm going to make the effort.* Rather than what a normal person may do, apologise sincerely, I took it upon myself to see if I could go down the banter route. He had been wearing pink that day – and so I thought I would show him a picture I had taken earlier that day in one of the caves, where I thought he looked pretty camp. For some reason, I felt it would crack a smile, remind him we could have banter, and if nothing else be friends. Big mistake again. He literally tore ten bales of shit off me for making that statement. And this had been my attempt to try to lighten the mood. He shot back at me with pure venom. I realised then that I was dealing with some serious heaviness. We both triggered the shit out of each other, and we couldn't see that what we were hating on each other was actually deep-rooted in ourselves – which is why this union had to take place.

We were two souls that were brought together for a very important purpose. Why else would we be so similar? There was a reason that we had to be connected. And it was all such divine timing, after my grandad had started waking me up. Ricky was divinely placed to help that awakening along. After the connection in Thailand, he had to take me to do the ayahuasca in the Amazon. We then had to go on this journey together and fall out. There was a divine reason that we had to have this massive eruption. We had to see in each other what was actually wrong with ourselves. Humanity could not have two powerful souls on the planet not doing their job. And this was the way that it happened, it kept banging us together, over and over at this period of time. It was absolutely bloody awful. I had never cried so much in my whole life over somebody who was essentially a stranger. Yes, we had been intimate and we were close, but he was still a stranger all the same.

Once again, looking back, because all souls have lived many, many lifetimes together, and done many, many things together, that's why my heart was really breaking, but I couldn't comprehend it. The divine plan was in full swing, but behind the curtain, so neither of us could see it.

Normally, I wasn't the kind of girl that would get upset at a guy. I closed it down and pushed them away if they broke my heart. Within a day or so, I would quickly put it back together and pretend it hadn't happened. I would shift to the next one, or start flirting, or maybe go out drinking with the girls to distract myself. This guy had really got under my skin, though. And because we were on the boat there was nowhere to run and no one to distract myself with. I had the whole seven days to sit with this feeling and figure out what was happening.

We did have certain moments where we were polite to each other towards the end of the week. He would show me a photo he had taken that I was in, and I would politely ask for him to send it to me when he got back to land. Things started to become a little bit more stable, but he had still closed down like a clam. He was not prepared to talk, and despite my best efforts, there was no way I was getting through to him.

On the morning of the last day, we were out snorkelling and he made an effort to point things out under the water. I was surprised but didn't make a big deal of it. I was hoping this would be a huge step forwards from where we had been over the last week. I hoped we could resolve this and be friends from afar, I mean there was no way our paths would cross after this anyway. He was from Australia and I was from England, it's not like we would bump into each other on a night out. It was such an interesting dynamic to navigate.

I became so aware of the decisions I was making and the words I was using. I'd never had to sit with myself for that long. I had nothing to distract myself with. I didn't have alcohol, well I did, but didn't dare drink it. I didn't have the food. I didn't have another man. I didn't have social media, because obviously there was no wifi in the middle of the ocean. For the first time in my life, I had to sit and recognise how angry I was. To top it all off, I had been so frustrated and sad, that I couldn't sleep, so I would just lie there and ruminate – *What would have happened if I hadn't paid that bill? What would have happened if I hadn't fallen asleep? What if I hadn't had that last glass of wine that night?*

All of this played on my mind. Ricky had actually said to me, "You drink too much wine. You know, this wouldn't have happened if you hadn't drunk that wine." My intentions were to pay for dinner even before we went out that night, before the wine. The storming off and falling asleep was one hundred percent about the alcohol. As for paying the bill, I still maintained I was doing a good thing. I thought I was doing something really beautiful for somebody I had started to care about. That was where I was at. I never comprehended at any point that he would feel like I had ripped his balls off, and taken on the masculine role to try to disrespect him. I did not see any of that. It was only through years of trauma work and being brutally honest with myself, that I started to connect the dots of how he had mirrored me. He had triggered the heck out of me, for me to realise what an arsehole I was, not him. Imagine a world where we all realised it was us, not those who we blame and project onto. That's a world I would like to live in.

I felt relieved and happy by the end of the cruise that we were starting to get on okay again – and when I say okay, I mean barely civil. We were never going to be mates at this rate. Our flights off the island weren't until the next day and so I suggested, "Why don't we get somewhere to stay tonight together, instead of staying in different places? We don't have to talk, we don't have to go out for dinner. But let's just not leave it like this." I was shocked when he agreed. I thought it was a massive step forward together.

Sharing the experience with the girls on the cruise was the right thing to do. I know that because if anything else would have been intended, that would have been what we lived out. Through all of the turmoil, I got to immerse myself more fully in the whole experience, without being distracted by him. It forced me to go inwards. That boat was the first time I ever picked up a book and started writing about how I was feeling, not realising that it was going to be a key part of my future.

We found a little hotel close to the port, nothing special. We went in, dumped our stuff and went off in different directions. I went for a swim and Ricky went to an internet café.

Later on in the evening, I met one of the girls from the cruise. We went for dinner and drinks. Whilst we were there we met a couple who were on holiday, so the four of us sat chatting over a few cheeky drinks. Ricky walked past the bar and he shot me a look as if I was a piece of shit. I had gotten over the crap that the two of us had been through. I was bored of it. I was on holiday and had endured a week of feeling like shit, so it was time to have some fun with people who wanted to be around me. I was not going to entertain the bullshit anymore.

I decided to get on with it and have as good a time as I could for the rest of it. No more drama, please! As far as Ricky was concerned, I just wanted to sit down with him and clear the air before we left because the next day I was going to be flying home, via Miami and Ecuador, and I didn't want to leave things the way that they were. Judging by the look on his face, he didn't have any desire to sort things out. I had to let it go. I had to be okay with never having my say, with not being heard. And then, never seeing this person again.

A little later, I got back to the room, and Ricky was not back yet. Out of courtesy, I dropped him a message to see where he was. We could not have a repeat performance of the other night. I went for a shower, then messed about on my phone for a bit, until eventually, I fell asleep, locking him out for a second time! Thankfully, this time it was only for a matter of minutes rather than for the whole night. I could hear him swearing and moaning. I opened the door, and he was raging, again. He walked in, grabbed his things and walked out. I get it, again. He must have been so pissed off, with the recurrence of something that had already happened, something that had already ruined our time together — and let's not forget I had been drinking again. I was absolutely heartbroken when he grabbed his stuff. I ran out of the room after him and asked him to stay, but he told me he wasn't prepared to do it, and he walked off. Him behaving like this, abandoning me, closing me down, not allowing me to speak — that was it, the final straw. I could not be around someone like this. I got back in the room and in a rage of anger removed him from Facebook and everything else. I deleted everything to do with him, even the photos we had taken with each other over the whole of our trip. I fucking hated his unreasonable arse, and was grateful I would never see him again. I didn't have time for that shit!

I called one of my girlfriends and sobbed down the phone to her. It had been a week of pent-up emotions. This was not the way it was supposed to pan out. This is not the way I had envisaged it. It was absolutely heartbreaking. Gut-wrenchingly heartbreaking. I just wanted to get back home and forget this had ever happened.

The next morning I woke up, got my stuff together and got a taxi to the airport. Thankfully our paths did not cross. I boarded the plane, and then sat there in my little bubble stewing on how much I hated him. From there, I had a connecting flight, straight on to

Miami. Getting out of there could not have come soon enough. I was done, I was over it!

On my way home, I stayed three nights in an exquisite apartment in Miami, looking out over South Beach. It was beautiful, and yet all I could do was keep processing the conversations we had. The same situations played over and over again – *What if I hadn't paid? What if I hadn't gone to that bar that night?* I met some amazing people in Miami and had lots of things to distract myself with, but the reality was that all I really wanted was to receive a message from him saying something. Anything.

During my downtime in Miami, I found myself contemplating. *What was that whole adventure about?* It speaks volumes about the person I was back then, but one of the things bothering me the most was worrying about how I was going to tell people what had happened, and what they would think of me. *How are people going to take the fact that I've spent a week with this guy having the best time of my life, and then a week where we argued and fell out and then ignored each other?* How do you explain to people that things got so bad between us that I removed him from Facebook? Which back then in 2014, was a big fuck you! That was the only way that we knew how to communicate. I wasn't on Instagram back then. I was a Facebook girl, especially as it enabled me to keep in touch with all the friends I had met from my travels, who were scattered around the globe.

After the hurt, came the anger. I thought all Australian men are arseholes, Italians are bastards – all the sweeping statements came out. I blamed him for everything. I wouldn't take any responsibility for myself, apart from processing what I possibly could have done differently. What I did focus on, though, was that my mouth was venomous, just like his. I was very cutting with the things I would say back then – which is now why I have to breathe and make sure that whatever comes out of my mouth is actually what I want to come out. We can be very mean with our words, and once spoken, it's very difficult to retract them. That Lucy hasn't disappeared completely, I have just learnt how to work with her and bring in beauty rather than anger.

I wanted to message him and say – *Sorry. Can we be friends?* But I didn't. I was too stubborn.

When I got back to the UK, it felt like the world and their dog was looking for an update on what had gone on. My best friend was desperate to hear what had happened. The last she had heard was me crying down the phone to her after epic fail number two. All my work colleagues were eagerly awaiting news because they had all decided there was something special in this relationship. I had my ex-partner, the one I had just finished with in January, messaging me and telling me he was missing me and still loved me, and could we please give things another go. The only thing that was obvious to me was that my life was a fucking mess, a total and utter disaster zone. In reality, the Universe had thrown a bomb into the middle of my life and said – *It's time to awaken. It's time to shift. It's time to make you so uncomfortable you've got no other option but to heal.*

Of course, I couldn't see it at the time.

My old programming went into overdrive, and I went on a mission of self-destruction. I went out drinking and partying at all hours. It was ridiculous – disastrous in fact. I threw myself wholeheartedly into destroying myself all over again.

Mirroring

Have you ever had a situation whereby someone has really annoyed you to the point it created a physical reaction within you? Maybe you got frustrated with someone for something they said, did, or the way they were being? That could have physically shown up as anger, your body temperature changing, your stomach going into knots, or many other uncomfortable physical reactions. I feel we can all nod our head at this one.

Normally we would point the 'finger of blame' and list off a whole array of reasons as to why whatever it is they are doing, is annoying us. Trust when I say, that was me too. That was until I remembered what mirroring was, this lifetime.

Mirroring is something I talk about a lot — I can almost feel the eye-rolling of my clients as they read this section. Mirroring is a principal I guide everyone to, especially when they are caught up in the past, in judgement, or blame. It is a very simple principal to understand; however, not such an easy one to put into practice when in the throes of a physical reaction taking control.

Before we look at mirroring, let's agree to work off the premise that everything we put out into the Universe we get right back. This may not happen instantly, but at some point, it will come back to you. A bit like how many people explain karma.

Mirroring is a wonderful principal whereby all of our healing is shown to us by the people we meet, the conversations and experiences we have day to day. Let's say you are in your car and you get irritated with a driver — who in your opinion is going to slow. Maybe you call them a few choice names before being able to overtake them, or they pull off in a different direction. At some point, the heat from that situation will come back to you. It may be as someone later cutting you up in the car, or it could be someone being rude to you in the supermarket for 'being in the way'. Every vibration we put out into the world is brought back to us for our healing.

Anyone and anything can be a mirror. The mirrors we mostly take notice of are those of our loved ones. Partners, children, siblings, and parents are always good mirrors, which is why we get so frustrated with them. A lot of my clients start my twelve-month course because they are at their wits end with their partner, or children. Very early on in the course, they are reminded about the effects of mirroring — and by the end of the course, they are much happier embodying new behaviours, which of course their loved then mirror back.

If you find yourself getting annoyed or upset with others, ask yourself what you are not doing to embody and experience what it is you are after. Take action and watch your life change. We basically vent our frustrations within ourselves by seeing it in others.

How cool is that for a principal to live by from here onwards? See how you go with turning the mirror on yourself with every situation and circumstance you find yourself in, and notice how much life can change for you.

A very simple practice in taking ownership can change you from being very reactive, to living more peacefully.

43

After I returned from the Galapagos, I was an absolute mess. There was no better way to describe me. I was not in a good place at all. In my mind, I had hoped that Ric was somebody who was going to be in my life in one capacity or another for a while, not just six months, which is all it had been. I had never imagined for one minute when I booked that holiday that we would end up in this position. As much as we had a magical time at first, I would have happily avoided all of the animosity. It all felt so dramatic and over the top in lots of different ways. *Why on earth was I feeling like this over a complete stranger? He wasn't in my life prior to that trip to Thailand, so why do I feel such loss now? Why was he acting like such a jerk, dragging it out and carrying it on? Why had he not bothered to reach out to see if I was okay?* I decided he mustn't really care, which made me care even less. That protective armour of mine kept getting stronger with each and every day.

I had met many people on holiday over the years and even embarked on holiday romances, and never once felt this way when we left each other or knew we wouldn't see each other again. This was a new one for me. How and why had I let this man get under my skin like this? I kept asking myself questions to try to comprehend what was going on within. I couldn't fathom it, though. What was it about him?

Going back into the office was a huge embarrassment. At first, I would talk about the magic, then stop before I got to the scenes of disaster, hoping that everyone would just leave it and let it go, but they didn't. They wanted to know the ins and outs of it all. Now, I have never been a good liar. I could withhold certain information without too much of a problem, but lying was not something I did – not since I was young and I realised how destructive it could be. I just could not bring myself to talk about the Ric situation. If I spoke about it, it would make it so much more real.

My body was hurting again. My digestive issues were playing up big time. Most of the time I felt like I had a hot poker in the chest area, where the hernia was. The reflux, which had stopped completely during the holiday, was back with a vengeance, and my womb issues had picked back up again on the boat in the Galapagos. Stress! What started out as a magical trip, ended up being so bloody painful, that it hurt everywhere. The fact I could not even shout at him or ask him to forgive me made it worse. I put on a brave face and internalised it all. After a while, I had convinced myself that he didn't exist.

Through all of this experience – good, bad, and very ugly – I did not realise that I was being humbled. I was being humbled to show vulnerability. I was being humbled by seeing myself in a mirror, via another person, and that really hurt.

I was also being shown gratitude. To be grateful for everything because things can very quickly switch from what we perceive to be good, to the perception of bad, and all in the blink of an eye. This situation was showing me how I was sabotaging myself, and to look at my coping mechanisms, and how I dealt with things. Or, how I grabbed the armour and got tooled up as quickly as possible when I felt challenged. It showed me how Ric had supported huge growth for me, allowing me to drop into the divine feminine energy, and allow myself to actually be vulnerable – until of course, the argument at the restaurant. All of those lessons were blatantly coming up for me to heal, and each time, I missed the memo. I was stuck in a place of – *It's everybody else's fault but mine.* Blame, project, and protect were my default.

I knew I had really fucked up, and my heart was so heavy because I knew I could not do anything about it. I knew it was going to take something pretty big and pretty special to ever be able to put it right, and I didn't know how. Let's face it, I had locked him out of the room, not once but twice. I can see why he bolted. I can see so much more clearly now through the wisdom I have gained. Even without wisdom and hindsight, most people would let you get away with locking them out once, but to do it again, was just frickin rude.

I had never connected the dots where alcohol was concerned. From a young age, we drank alcohol. It was what we did. So when Ric said it was the alcohol, I just felt like he was being controlling. I had not viewed the drinking as sabotaging myself. I was too scared to look at myself to recognise how unhappy I was. I wanted to feel needed. I wanted to feel wanted. And rather than ask for it, because that would be weak, I went about getting it in ways that were not resonant with my soul. That night I met him in Thailand, him being a smart arse and me responding, that was the way I got my needs met because that was how I saw things under the influence of alcohol.

The trip was a life-changing experience and I felt comfortable sharing that much information with my friends and colleagues. It was frickin amazing; I focused on the bits that really had been incredible. As I showed them photos of the places and animals I had seen, they were in awe. People could only dream of holidays like this, and there I was living it. Even to this day, some of the photos I look at give me goosebumps that I actually lived the experience. It was like a fairytale in so many ways, it's just that this one didn't have a happy ending. I was not prepared to admit that to people though. None of us want to admit it when we're wrong. Especially when we're living in our ego, and I was massively in my ego and materialism back then. I still could not comprehend, even after all these weeks, why he'd had such a reaction to me paying the bill. I didn't get it. None of it made sense to me. It was like I had committed a huge sin by just paying a restaurant bill.

In the end, I told one or two of my friends the full story. To everyone else, they got the version that it all went well and that was it. The issue with that was they carried on living in the fantasy world that Ric and I were going to see each other again one day, that we were going to embark on this beautiful relationship. "*What a wonderful love story it would be*", they would swoon. Even the men I knew loved our story. I was from the UK, he was from Australia, we had met in Thailand and travelled to South America together – they thought it was a modern-day fairytale. They were excited to see where this whirlwind, cross-continent, crazy journey was going to end. '*You must write a book on this one day*", many of them would say.

Indeed.

Gosh, it was so hard talking about it. It was harder still listening to them creating a wonderful story out of the handful of facts I had given them. They had it all mapped out for me, and yet inside all I wanted to do was cry. *Why did I tell anyone I had met him? It was crazy. Why on earth did I actually go to meet him? Who does that crazy shit? It's no surprise I'm hurting now, it was a disaster waiting to happen.* My insides were hurting too much because I had fucked up. I had royally fucked up. *Why could I not say sorry and allow myself to be vulnerable? Why did I have to act tough, like I didn't care, when I did? I cared so much. Clearly too much. How could I just pretend it wasn't happening? Pretend that everything was okay.*

Of course, it was far from okay.
And that's when it happened.
I got very sick.

44

Almost immediately after coming back from South America, I became much more lethargic. I'd lost my spark, if you like, and I put it down to the trauma of the holiday. It had not been the easy-going time away from the office I had required. I had to suppress my health issues whilst I was away, and then upon return, I had to suppress the truth to keep up appearances for those around me. I had got lost. I did not know who I was anymore, and my body had been communicating this for years, but I did not know how to read the signals.

I would go to work, and everybody there thought I was healthy, mainly because of my food choices and the fact I would go to the gym a few times a week. They knew about my drinking habits, and the after-work dinners loaded with fat and grease that would accompany the alcohol, but still, they thought of me as healthy.

It's amazing what we have normalised. It's amazing that at no point does anyone judge how healthy you are based on how much water you drink each day, how loving and open you are, what your relationships are like, and how much love you have for yourself. No, if you wore a mask well and ticked a couple of boxes, you were healthy. And trust me, I wore the corporate mask well. To them, I was a little piece of dynamite. I was a badass, successful Project Manager, who delivered everything that was asked of her. To everyone around me, I had my shit together. But in reality, I was falling apart on the inside.

Since returning from South America, even going to the gym became a real struggle. I didn't want to go to work. I didn't feel connected to it. I didn't have the energy. I just constantly wanted to lie down and sleep. It was an overwhelming sense of fatigue. On top of that my tonsils were always inflamed, there were always white spots on them. I would also regularly lose my voice or be coughing something up. My skin was also bad at this point in my life. The doctors would always blame hormonal issues as to why my skin was the way it was. They would offer a tablet or some sort of cream to mask the issue as an interim solution. If it got particularly bad, they would have the conversation about a new marina coil. The thing is, I felt in my gut that it was the coil that gave me these bloody horrible boils that I would get. I just felt really shitty about myself. I never understood why they could not get to the root cause of the issues – they were the doctors for goodness sake. If they didn't know, then who did? It was like everything was hurting from the inside out. At one point I could not even go to the toilet for two whole weeks. Two weeks for goodness sake! I am surprised I didn't explode with all those toxins inside me.

The irregular bleeding, picked up again big time. All of it was draining me. It seemed as if it was all coming in at once. I was being tested significantly. I was constantly in and out of the doctors or hospital. Constantly being touched, poked, and having tests done. I am not being rude when I say this, but hospitals are not the most uplifting of places. I know hospitals are essential, but gosh they are a negative environment; they can drain you and make you feel ill in themselves. You are surrounded by poorly people, people who are in their final days or dying around you. I get that it is a part of life, but when you are already low and feel like giving up, or like the world is caving in on you, they are definitely not the best places to boost your mental health.

I was really fortunate in the sense that when they got to a certain part of my treatment, I was able to go private, thanks to my work's private healthcare. Most of the procedures I had to endure during this period of time required sedation. I probably had 15 or more endoscopies in very close succession. Endoscopies are where they put the camera down your throat and into the top part of your stomach for exploration purposes. They're horrible, even with sedation you feel as if your throat has been violated. I would often get swollen tonsils, tonsillitis or laryngitis off the back of the procedures themselves. One of the times I had the procedure done, I woke up in the middle of it. My goodness did I panic. I was gagging and choking, and of course, I instantly reacted and attempted to pull the tube out of my mouth. Before I knew it, they had whacked a load more sedation through the tube to knock me out until the procedure was complete. You are not supposed to wake up, and if you do for any reason, you are not supposed to remember anything about it, but I remember it all. I remember how slimy the tube was. I remember it was black.

I remember the panic on their faces when they realised that I had come round and woken up. It was not supposed to happen like that.

If the tubes weren't going down my throat, they were going the other way, in the form of colonoscopies. There was something going on in my physical body that they couldn't get to grips with, and they were desperate to find out what it was, but no matter how much they searched, they would only find something minor and nothing to justify the intensity of the pain I was experiencing.

My lungs were also a mess. I was constantly coughing, and constantly on antibiotics. I could go on and on, the gist of it all was that I was an absolute mess. I don't think that there was one part of my body that was working effectively, apart from maybe my feet at this particular time. I felt swollen, I was inflamed. I have pictures of me from back at this time, and it's shocking the state of the inflammation that was riddling my body. It was everywhere. You could see it in my face. You could see it in my neck. There's a photo I've got where I have a bra and knickers on, the bra is folded down and you can see the whole body is in pain with how inflamed it is. You can see it clearly even just from a picture. It's so easy to spot when you know.

Of course, I had the hiatus hernia to consider too, which impacted the digestion process significantly. At a young age, part of my stomach had got trapped in my oesophagus, creating what they call a hiatus hernia. On top of that, I had been diagnosed with something called Helicobacter Pylori. I'd been diagnosed with it in my mid-twenties. The remnants of that bacteria lingered on. Helicobacter Pylori is a very intense bacteria that feeds off of the stomach acid, so very little kills it. When I was diagnosed, I had to be put on a huge cocktail of drugs to try to kill it. Unfortunately for me, it took three rounds of drugs in order to do it. Those drugs themselves then caused problems with my stomach, like ulcers. It took many months to get rid of the bacteria because it had survived so long in my body. I was constantly on drugs to attempt to neutralise the stomach acid, topped up with the medications for the other 'itis' bugs that were a constant for me back then. Then, just for good measure, throw in the tablets for my periods, irregularities with the bleeding, and the thyroid issues. That is some toxic cocktail – all prescribed by my doctors.

I had absolutely no idea what was happening to me, but I trusted the doctors and the specialists would fix me, so I kept going back.

I had to believe that they could do something. It was not until they suggested operating on my hernia, that I stood my ground and said enough is enough. I researched what that actually entailed and I scared myself shitless. It was not the operation itself so much, as much as what could happen if it went wrong. It was scary. *No, not happening* – I decided. I would do whatever it took. I just didn't know what that was, or where I would find the energy to sort it.

I was at breaking point. I couldn't take any more.

I was beating myself up over the situation that had gone on in South America. I was starting to get grief from my ex-boyfriend too. I was under so much pressure from my work. My mum was annoyed at me because I told her I needed to quit my job and I needed to focus on myself, and she couldn't get it. She was constantly asking me questions like – *What are you going to do? How are you going to support yourself? What if you can't ever get another job?* I know she meant well, but my goodness, I was about to break. Could no one see that?

It felt like the world was coming in on me from every angle possible, and I had nowhere to go. This was the downward spiral to burnout. I physically couldn't get out of bed, or speak to people without crying. I was completely and utterly broken from the inside out. Everybody knew me to be tough, and I was a tough cookie in all fairness, I was made of strong stuff. I was a boxer, I had been punched in the face on many occasions. I used to run. I used to go to the gym. I used to be able to hold conversations with CEOs of huge investment banks. I was the girl who was going to show all the girls how they could do it. I could stand on my own two feet. But here I was, a dribbling wreck. Allowing my world to cave in on me at last. I say at last because all of this was by design. This was the moment my grandad had prepped me for. Trust me! An awakening is anything but pretty.

I really couldn't take it anymore. I never had a moment of thinking about suicide, to stop it all, to get out of this life and the pain I was experiencing. But I just could not cope anymore. I couldn't do it. I didn't want to do it. I was broken. My body didn't work. My mind was playing games with me. I was no longer connected to anything. I felt lost. I had no idea which way to turn, who I could trust, or what I should do.

So, I quit my job.

45

I remember the day as if it was yesterday.

Things had been building for so long. I felt like I was losing it. In all honesty, I was. I was being stripped bare, to go through my dark night of the soul, but I didn't even know what that was at the time. I was changing and losing who I had always been. Nothing made sense anymore. My physical body was an absolute mess. My head could no longer retain information. I was an emotional wreck due to work pressures and all the physical issues, and also all of the trauma surfacing around the previous relationships. I wanted to run, but I had nowhere to go. I walked into the office on this particular day in May. As soon as I arrived, people were asking me for project plans and meetings, telling me information, and talking at me. I was there, but all of the busyness and the chatter were going over my head. I did not want to be around any of them. I sat at my desk and I wanted to scream. I was hurting so much, in so much pain and torment – physically, mentally, emotionally and spiritually. I just could not do this anymore. What on earth was all of this about? I felt like shit, and I looked like shit. Did any of these people actually care?

The decision was made.

I had been wanting to quit since my trip in October and the only thing that had kept me there was fear, but this was a different kind of fear I was feeling now. That day, I knew if I stayed on for another year, I would probably be dead. I was spiralling out of control. I could barely keep my head above water. Something drastic was required. With that, I logged into my PC, ignoring all of the noise around me and started typing out my letter of resignation. I was doing it. Today was the day. I wrote the letter very quickly at my desk. Thankfully my mum had sent me on a touch-typing course, much against my will when I was younger, but at times like this, when things were required immediately, I always thought about her and thanked her for giving me the opportunity to be able to get away with sneaky shit at work. I drafted it, read it, and printed it off, signed it, then popped it in an envelope, ready to go. Everything I used to do this was the bank's property – the paper, the envelopes, and even my time, the bank paid for it all that day as I was on the clock. *Fuck it* – I thought – *it's done.*

Once the letter was safely in the envelope, I stood up, walked upstairs to my boss's office, and knocked tentatively on the door. He told me to come in, so I walked in, said hello, slid the envelope across the desk to him, and then turned to walk out. As I was walking away I said, "I'll speak to you in a bit." He instantly stopped what he was doing and said, "Hang on a minute Lucy, what's this about? Before you go anywhere, let me just open this letter."

He opened the letter, and I burst into tears. "Oh Lucy, I had no idea. Let me get you some help. Let me get you some sort of support. You don't need to quit your job. There are other options on the table here. Let me get you a sabbatical. Let me get you an extended holiday. Let me do something to help you. Quitting is so final, you don't really want to do that."

I pulled myself together enough to say to him, "Thank you, but there is nothing you can do to help me, other than accept my resignation and let me go as soon as possible." He did not accept that, though. I was one of his superstars – and those were his words. I was a Director. I was climbing the ranks. He wanted me to be there as part of his team. He was happy for me to take a three-month sabbatical or whatever I needed at that point, to come back to my full-time, very well-paid job. I knew I could not do that, though. There was something inside of me saying – *Don't put a timescale on this. You've got to go. You've got to figure out who the heck you are because if you continue to work in this environment, you're probably going to end up dead.* It was almost like I had somehow gained an insight into the future. This life was not serving me. If I did not do something about it, it would take me down.

I went back to my desk, and bless him, he ran around the office like a headless chicken that day, speaking to people that he thought would be able to get me back in alignment and agree to a sabbatical. He spoke with the H.R. department, asking about the potential of a sabbatical. He was on a mission all day to attempt to sort me out. Later that day, he called me back into his office and said, "Lucy, I'm worried about you. Do you think you are having a breakdown?"

"I don't believe I am having a breakdown," I said. "I feel for the first time in my life I am waking up." Let's be honest, at this point, he probably felt his suspicions were being confirmed. I mean who says stuff like that? The irony of it all was that I didn't know what it meant. It just felt right to me. It felt like it was the truth. I realised that I had become suppressed, that I had become a version of myself that I fucking hated. I was stuck in a cycle of sabotage and I just could not see the light at the end of the tunnel, or the way to actually navigate myself out of there.

Almost a year to the day from my grandad's passing, I got that final kick – probably from him too. I got that big boot up the backside, that shoved me into making that major decision, and that would be one of the first stepping stones to freedom from these low vibrational feelings that I had normalised.

That initial feeling of freedom was pretty short-lived. I knew as a Director I had to give three months' notice. I prayed that out of the goodness of their hearts that they would let me go early – bearing in mind what I had been through in the previous 12 months. It had been such an intense year. Losing my grandad, the significant health issues I had – the womb, the breast cancer scare, digestion problems, the hiatus hernia, and the operations. The list seemed to go on and on. In the end, work came back to me and they wanted me to work and ride it out until the bitter end. Three months is a heck of a long time when you are at rock bottom, and then you are told you have to be somewhere that you don't want to be and that is already making you physically, mentally and emotionally ill.

Despite the emotional rollercoaster, I was proud of myself. I'd done it. I'd been brave and made the big decision, going against everything that I had been conditioned to believe. Everything that my friends and family believed in. I went against everything that was normal, and I trusted – just like I had trusted myself going to South America – that this was going to be the best decision of my life. It was brave that I trusted myself at all, so soon after such a letdown with Ricky. But, this version of me was becoming so brave. She was someone I was just starting to like.

People were absolutely shocked when I eventually told them. My big boss, the one who had convinced me to go over to that company in the first place, poaching me from the previous place, was really shocked. He tried to coach me and talk me out of it. He tried to do everything in his power to get me to stay because I was a superstar from JPMorgan. I was the strong woman who was going to make a ripple. They offered me all sorts of different things to stay – trips, bonuses, and they actually offered to almost double my salary again.

I knew that was a final test. I was already on ridiculous amounts of money, doubling it would have set me up for life. I could have retired super young – if I could curb the spending and the lifestyle that would likely accompany such a salary increase, of course. You know what it's like living in this consumer world? Increase the salary, the expectations increase. Change of house, car, acquiring more shiny, new objects to match the new salary. They threw it all at me. I don't know where the strength came from, but each time I was offered something, I would respond with, "No, thank you." It was the first time in my life I used 'NO' as a full sentence and I truly meant it.

I could safely say, for the very first time – *When you know, you know*. It's really interesting because people would often say that about finding their forever partner – *when you know you know* – but I had never experienced that, until now. I finally got it. I absolutely knew that if I didn't take that action there and then I was going to die. It sounds so dramatic, but everything had taken its toll. The trauma over the years had built up so much that I was ready to explode. My body was doing its best to take me out, or at least to warn me. It felt like all of the suffering was down to working in an environment I hated, and being around people who no longer resonated with me. However, that newfound strength to walk away felt totally right, and it sparked a renewed energy within me. It was almost like my brave decisions had lit a fire inside, and somebody up above had recognised it – O*kay, she's made a decision, let's light that fire back up within her. Let's give her a little bit of her power back.*

In all honesty, the next three months were awful. That little spark of fire was the only thing that kept me going. One day I would be feeling – *Yes, I'm getting out of here, it's so amazing* – and the next day I'd be in a mess, questioning my decision – *Oh, what if I can't ever get another job? What if nobody ever wants me?* It was a complete battle between the ego-mind and the heart. On the one hand, I was at the top of my game; I was a phenomenal Project Manager, and they wanted to double my salary to keep me, but then here I was also thinking who the heck is going to employ me? It made no logical sense, but this battle continued for three whole months. Ultimate highs and ultimate lows. And let's be clear, I had no plan. I had absolutely no plan at all.

There was actually only thing that I had planned as soon as I left work in late August; my best friend and I were going to get on a plane and go to Vegas. We were going to enjoy an extended holiday, party, watch a boxing match and go on a road trip. Many years prior to this, I had fallen in love with boxing. I felt it really sorted my head out. I went to watch my sister and other people fight for many years and at any opportunity I got, I would go and watch it live. There was just something about boxing, I loved it. The fight we had tickets for in Vegas was Mayweather vs Maidana. It was a pretty cool thing for us two girls to be doing. We knew Vegas was going to be messy, so we decided to start there, and then take a road trip to San Francisco afterwards.

That was the only plan I had for my life post-corporate. I had spoken about travelling. I thought about flying to South America from San Francisco, but I was scared. Although I had been there just a month or so earlier, I was really frightened. My ego was piping up constantly, doing its best to keep me safe. During the three months of my notice period, there were many times I looked on job sites and thought – *Fuck it, I'll just get another job*. I was petrified. I had been earning a huge amount of money each month. I had the ability to save a few grand a month because I physically couldn't spend it fast enough. I was paying off my car, and the mortgage. I was going out for expensive dinners, drinking a bottle of wine a night, and buying anything I needed or wanted, and I was still saving plenty of money because I couldn't spend what I was earning.

Interestingly enough, though, no amount of money I spent made a difference to my health. During my whole three-month period of notice, nothing really changed with my health at all. I didn't get any better, put it like that. I was still going in for tests all the time. I was constantly on the phone with the doctors and constantly in surgery, or having exploratory tests being done.

My hair started falling out as well during this period of time because my body was in such bad shape and I was stressed to the max. My physical vessel was broken. The only thing keeping me going was that small flame that had been reignited again. It was almost like psychologically I had to hold on for those three months, like we had an unwritten agreement that we only had a few months to get through, and then we could take a rest. Maybe we could even become friends again. I had hoped that handing my notice would shift a few things, and release some of the pressures and burdens, but through June and July, things got a whole lot worse.

My digestion was awful, it deteriorated really badly during the summer. The acid reflux, which I had since my mid-twenties worsened terribly. I was in agony more often than I was comfortable. I had to sleep sitting up because it was so painful. Every time I would lie down, it felt like something was burning in my chest. Almost like a bunsen burner being held there until it burnt me. It was the hiatus hernia – everything would congregate in that space because it had nowhere else to go. Just imagine the wine, the crap foods, lack of sleep, stress and all of my emotional trauma in a tiny little space in the stomach, churning away to get your attention. Not nice. The crazy thing was, despite all this pain, I still didn't stop drinking. I just carried on doing what I was doing. I would go out drinking. I would go out partying. I would eat all the rich foods. And all of that stuff would cause pain and suffering.

I know now that any physical ailment is a sign that there is emotional trauma caught up somewhere in your vessel. Your body is only designed to go 'wrong' when it is out of alignment. But, I wasn't ready to connect the dots. I wasn't ready to change my life or take ownership of what I had created. I wasn't ready to stop drinking. I literally had to drink to get through the crazy shit show that I had going on, and yet all the time, I knew the drinking was worsening everything. I didn't have any other coping mechanism at that time. Every single day I would plod forwards. I just had to keep my head high enough above water, and keep putting one foot in front of the other, and that's the only way that I managed to get through it.

46

A few weeks later, about a month before I was due to leave work, I decided to get really brave, and I made the brave decision to travel the world after the trip with my best friend to America. When I say I was brave, I was absolutely petrified at this point. I was thirty-five years of age, and what most people would call 'washed up'. At that age, for a woman to not be married and have children, or be secure and settled down, was really considered to be wrong. And I was about to break that mould completely to go off and travel the world with zero plan. I did not plan anything. All I did was book my first plane ticket from London Heathrow to Phuket, Thailand. I would fly in for one day after getting back from San Francisco, swap my bags out and get back on the road, so to speak.

Once I had made the decision, it felt like another little spark had been ignited. I was so sad to be leaving my best friend. My goodness, she had deserved a medal these last few months for what she had done for me; I was so grateful to that woman for so much. Her support, her love, accommodating me into her home. I had bent her ears on many an occasion and lent on her shoulder for me to cry on more times than I could remember. She really did look after and protect me, and that was all I wanted and needed.

I was scared of so many things in my final weeks before leaving. I was scared that people were going to judge me. I was scared that I was too old to travel. Scared that I wouldn't mix with people, because I assumed everybody travelling would probably be in their early 20s. This goes to show the power of the mind, I have always mixed well with people. Not once have I ever not found people on my wavelength or people that resonated with me in one shape or form. I was a shadow of my former self, though. I had been poked and pulled, used and abused too much for any one person to deal with, and all in the space of about a year. I knew this trip was the only way out.

My leaving do was an affair and a half, to say the very least. It was absolutely humongous. In truly Lucy fashion – or what it was back in those days – it started in a strip bar. Nice and classy, Lucy! We got absolutely annihilated that night. There were so many people there, probably 50 or 60 people, maybe even more, and that was just from my current work. I had aligned the evening to be split over Canary Wharf, where I was just finishing up working, and then a little jaunt over to the city to make sure I could catch up with all of the wonderful souls I had worked with at JPMorgan and BNP Paribas. Oh my goodness, did we get on it. The first bar was extremely messy. We went completely overboard. Wine, bubbles, vodkas, cocktails and shots – lots and lots of shots. The hours were flying past. Things were moving very quickly. I looked at my watch and I was already late for the city bar. My friends from over there had been calling and messaging asking where we were, so I rounded up the troops, and we headed to the DLR and went into the city. In the city, we went to Henry's bar. We had an area booked downstairs and when I arrived loads of my friends were there already lining up the shots for my arrival. It was so emotional saying goodbye to work colleagues, some of whom had been in my life for over ten years. I really did question if I was doing the right thing at this point, but there was nothing I could do to change it, even if I wanted to. It was just fear trying to keep me safe once again.

I've got an incredible photo from that night, all my old 'big bosses' from JPMorgan and the current company from over the years stood around me as we celebrated our goodbyes. It's a photo that I'm never going to delete, it's a memory I will always cherish. Every single one of those people really saw something in me that I didn't see in myself. I am so grateful to them all. They gave me hope, they gave me opportunities. They actually helped me to become the best Project Manager in the business that I would later grow on my own, because now I see things in people that they don't see in themselves. And actually, it's a massive part of my Self Love Club. I make sure that people have my love until they get it themselves. I share with people what I see in them until they see it, and they can hold their own with it. And that's what these guys taught me, in a roundabout way. They would cringe if they read this – too macho to admit that they showed me love. That's what they did, though, in their own special way. A phenomenal bunch of men. Overachievers, and incredible souls.

That night got so messy. I got so drunk, I was a complete handful. I was doing shots at the bar, dancing on the tables, it was a bit like the night of my birthday, but this time it was me having all the fun, rather than watching it unfold. I was the thing that was unfolding, though, I ended up an absolute mess. Thankfully, as always, my best friend, my earth angel, had been there to look after me. We had decided way before the evening that we were going to stay in a hotel that night. We knew that I wouldn't get home safely on a train, so we just did not risk it. I got to a certain point in the night and I told her I really had to go, I was too drunk to carry on. She guided us to a taxi to head back to the hotel and that's when the emotions kicked in. All I did was cry – *I've made the wrong decision, I shouldn't be leaving. What if something happens to me? What if we end up not being friends anymore? What if I never got another job back?* The poor girl had to deal with this blubbering mess. There was no other word for it. At this point, I'm sure she was ready to hand-deliver me to the airport with a one-way ticket.

We had our fair share of these situations over the years. More often than not it was her who did some crazy shit on our nights out and I would have to deal with it, but these last few months made up for everything I had ever had to support her through. I guess that's what friends are for, right?

My best friend decided that to keep me sober and from falling asleep, she would call a good male friend of mine to chat to, so I was distracted. I was pouring my heart out to him on the phone, and I kept banging on about eating pizza to sober me up. So bless him, he drove all the way from Southeast London into Central London to buy me a pizza and delivered it to my best friend, who fed me because I wasn't capable of doing it myself. Oh my, I had such a good bunch around me. What amazing people, willing to do these things for a drunken little mess like me.

I partied hard that night. I made sure I went out with the biggest bang you could possibly imagine – not to be forgotten. I woke up the next day with the biggest hangover I've ever had too – I mean let's not forget my body was already broken and hurting, and my digestion was all out of whack – and here I was fuelled up on booze and pizza, just to remind myself of how shitty I can feel.

My mum was very worried about my health, she'd been really worried about it for a long time. I went through so much in my early twenties with regard to hormones and digestion. My mum would always be there with me at the appointments, listening to the doctors, and what they had to say about my operations and my prognosis. Many of these issues were a trauma line that had run right through the whole of my mum's side of the family for many generations. My mum, my nan, and my great nan had all experienced things like I had been going through, so it was really hard for her to watch her daughter going through it. It must have been pretty horrific because she understood how bad things were. She knew I was constantly in hospital. She knew I was on a daily concoction of lots of different medications. This is not me judging my mum when I say this, but my mum had been on so many medications since her early 30s, it was pretty normal to her. It never sat right with me, though, even though I kept doing it. It wasn't right that my thyroid was playing up. It wasn't right that my weight was all over the place. It wasn't right that I was having intermittent bleeding after my periods. It wasn't right that I couldn't go to the toilet for two weeks at a time. However, because my mum had a number of similar issues, that she took medication for, she would often say, "You just have to take the pills and get on with it. It's just one of those things."

But, something in that statement didn't quite resonate with me, even though I didn't know what to do with that feeling yet. I was just trusting these experts because I didn't know any better. And the fact that my mum — one of my teachers and my safe space — trusted them, I just followed in her footsteps. Something kept niggling me that it wasn't actually right.

Thank God, I eventually listened to the calls.

47

That was it! I was officially a bum — as my mum kept reminding me in the days following my leaving bash. I had not been out of work even a day when she asked me, "What are you going to do with yourself? What are you going to do with your life?" The pressure was real. She knew I was intending to go travelling. I had made absolutely no secret of that since February when I initially broke the news to her. I think she had hoped that over the passing months I would have changed my mind. Her questioning me was her last-ditch attempt to get me to rethink my course of proposed action. Of course, that was never going to happen. I had not thrown a literal bomb into my life just for a bit of attention. The Universe made it very clear there was no other option but to go.

The holiday to America, with my best friend, was booked and paid for, so everyone knew that was happening. I was in a bit of a quandary, though. I wanted to go straight off travelling afterwards, but I was travelling to America with a huge suitcase, due to the nature of the holiday we were going on. We needed heels, cute dresses, and swimsuits to wear to pool clubs, all of which I would not require whilst travelling. I had absolutely no intention to wear any type of footwear for the year I was travelling, let alone heels. I'm sure this is where my love for Australia stems, no one judges you as you walk down the road barefoot, even in the middle of their winter.

We had this dream trip to look forward to, just a couple of days after I left work. We had been to lots of boxing matches together over the years, but Mayweather v Maidana was a big deal. It was the biggest fight we had been to together, and it was in Vegas. We were both absolutely ecstatic about it.

I had gone home to my mum's house in Bournemouth after my leaving do. In the weeks prior to that, I had moved all of my things out of the apartment I had been living in – the one where we had the big party – as there was no point in me keeping it on. I didn't know how long I would be away. The way I was feeling I was hoping I would never return. I had donated most of my things to a woman's refuge charity. I had moved my bed to a friend's house as he had just bought a new place and had nothing for his spare room. I even dumped my television at my mum's house for safe keeping. My clothes were boxed up and put in her loft. I officially had nothing, other than the things I was initially taking in my suitcase, and the stuff that was loaded in my backpack, ready for when I got home from America. It was really happening. I had no trace of a plan at that specific moment in time, I just knew I was leaving and heading off in one direction or the other.

The day before I flew to America, I booked some accommodation in Thailand. At last, I had a destination. Still no plan. However, I knew the first stop. I was going to be home for just over 24 hours before I disappeared off again.

It was quite fascinating, I had only been out of work a matter of hours and I was already rebelling, being repelled completely by the thought of a plan. My life, for the prior 13 years or so, had been one big, long planning session, and I was now well and truly ready to remove myself from it. I thought – *If I never saw a project plan again in my life it won't be a day too soon.* I was so ready to be footloose and fancy-free for as long as possible. I learned some amazing skills during my time. Really amazing things I never thought I would be able to do when I started, but I became an expert at them. However, now in the big wide world, they wouldn't any longer serve me. Or would they?

I was so excited about the trip, but also extremely terrified. I had never done something like this, with no plan. When I was 21, and had gone away for a short time, I had a plan and a group of friends I was going with. This was different. And I was older. Would people even accept me into their circles? So many thoughts, patterns, trauma and sabotaging responses were spinning through my mind. I was about to leave my friends, my family, my security, and everything I knew, to head off on my own merry way. My Thailand trip in October 2013, was the first time I had ever flown on my own with no one to meet me at the airport upon arrival. I knew I was going boxing and that I would meet people, plus that trip was only for ten days — worst case scenario I would have just talked to myself for ten days and then gone home. This was different. This was going to be saying goodbye to people and not knowing if, or when, I was coming back. I had an inner knowing that life was not supposed to be what I had settled for up until this moment.

It scared me that I knew in my heart this would be the end of my amazing relationships back home. We would all grow so significantly in the period of time I intended to be away. It is such a weird feeling throwing a bomb into every area of your life, when some of the people you really love, and would not choose to change. However, unless you do make that change for yourself, you cannot change those you are discontent with. I knew that if I could do this, life would never be the same again. I just knew it. I had to keep reminding myself that I had made the decision to quit my job because I truly felt it was killing me. It was slowly suffocating the true essence of who I was really destined to be. Now I know that sounds very dramatic, but it's the truth.

My health was in a really bad way and although I carried on drinking, partying and pretending I was okay, I wasn't. I had totally lost myself. Every situation I had found myself in for months was toxic. Relationships, work, even going out drinking. It was as if the Universe was conspiring to make it so bloody painful for me to ignore.

A little while before I quit my job, I actually got spiked at a bar in London. It was a relatively cool evening, we had been at work until late and then agreed to go to a bar, one where we could stand outside and chat. My best friend had come to meet us, as she regularly did. I went into the bar to ask where the toilet was, and the guy behind the bar directed me there, with a flirtatious smile. When I came back up, I ordered some drinks for the group, and then took a couple outside. I went back in to collect the other drinks from the bar, and we all carried on drinking. My glass of wine didn't taste funny or anything like that, it tasted normal, but then a couple of sips into that glass I started to not feel normal at all. I grabbed my best friend and asked her to take my wine from me and take me to the toilet. She looked immediately concerned. As we walked, I could feel all of my muscles starting to go limp. I started walking as if I was going to fall over, so my best friend grabbed me, to support my walk. I was all over the place. I felt completely off it – a little bit like I had done on the ketamine many years earlier. She got me to the toilet where I collapsed in a heap. I had been spiked. I was a mess. A few sips of wine did not make me feel like this. She formulated a plan to get me out of there. Again, my best friend came to the rescue. Once she got me in a taxi and to safety, I spent the rest of the evening throwing up. I should have gone to the police the next day and got tested to see what it was. I should have reported it to the bar, but I didn't. I felt awful for a few days afterwards. It was only then that I thought about reporting it but apparently, it would have gone from my body at that point. There were things like that happening all the time. The signs were there, I was being shown every which way that I had to do something drastic. I had missed the memo for such a long time. At last, I was starting to pay attention.

The day came for Catherine and I to head off on our trip together. We were like children at Christmas. We were so filled with excitement. It did not feel like I had quit my job at this point. It just felt as if I was going on a holiday. I love Las Vegas. I have always said that when I get married, I'm going to Vegas with the girls on my hen do because it's just amazing. Everything is bigger and better, everywhere stays open later, and is completely and utterly over the top. It's so weird because I can't say I'm a fan of super busy places, I don't even like gambling, and I certainly don't align to massively bold things, but I always love Vegas; in all of its contradiction.

Vegas has always had a very special place in my heart and always will. I have had many memories there, very special moments, both before, during, and after the awakening that I lived through. Back in the day, Vegas was about raw, boozy fun. Then, it became about conferences and running down the strip at the start of the day – when most people were wandering home from the night before. Then, it ultimately became about shifting consciousness.

The whole setup with Vegas, from landing at the airport to the time that you leave, is all about money. It's about getting you to spend as much as possible under the guise of fun. It is very much about gambling. The hotels are created in such a way that the casinos have no windows, no daylight, and no clocks anywhere. The whole point of that is so that people lose themselves in gambling, and parting with their money, with no idea what day it is or what time it is. You can get free drinks if you are gambling, so you part with more money. There is food available round the clock because they want you there round the clock. You could smoke anywhere. And on top of that, the rooms were pumped full of oxygen, to make sure you rarely felt tired. Vegas was a place to be wide awake and indoors, despite most of the year having the most incredible weather.

Catherine and I were flying with Virgin Atlantic, from Heathrow Airport. We met inside the terminal, and were so excited and giddy with anticipation. We were probably most excited to be going to the boxing because we had been talking about doing a huge fight in Vegas for such a long time. And now, here we were, speaking it into existence.

Boxing had been a huge part of my life for some time. I had started training in boxing when I lived in Wimbledon. It felt good to punch things and let off steam after a hard day's graft in the office. I never thought that it would be one of the catalysts to changing my whole existence. The sport had taken me all over the world. It was in my blood. When Thailand called me in October 2013 with the promise of doing boxing, it was always going to happen. Little did I know, I would fall head over heels in love with Thai boxing whilst I was there.

Back at the airport, the two of us had our massive suitcases to navigate through the airport. We had so much unnecessary stuff with us, it was ridiculous. However, on this trip, we were going to the boxing and we really wanted to look pretty and make an effort. We had planned to go on a few other glamorous nights out as well whilst we were there. This was going to be the last time for a while that we went out together, so we had to make the most of it. Not only did we need glam outfits, but we also needed to make sure we had enough clothes to travel up the coast on our Thelma and Louise road trip. We had booked a Ford Mustang convertible to drive from Vegas to Los Angeles, then up to San Francisco. We were buzzing for that part of the journey too.

We got through customs relatively hassle-free and then headed to the first bar that we could clap our eyes on. Catherine and I were boozy birds when we got together. Especially when we were in any kind of airport, or on any form of transport. So despite it being about 10 am, we got straight on the wine. There's no sense, rhyme or reason, but in airports, anything goes. Wine for breakfast it was.

A few glasses of wine later and we boarded the plane, feeling good. We were off to Vegas, so the celebrations started now as far as we were concerned.

I'd had a few previous visits to Vegas that I was keen to forget and this trip was my way of attempting to do that.

The first time I had visited Vegas was in 2009 with an ex-partner. It was not really the introduction to Vegas that I had wanted or expected. We had stayed in a beautiful suite at the MGM Grand Hotel that had a jacuzzi on the balcony. It was incredible. We could sit in there, having cheeky champagne, looking out over the strip, whilst no one could see us. We were there to watch boxing on that occasion too. This time it was Manny Pacquiao and Ricky Hatton who were going head to head.

We were only due to be there for a few days and so we didn't have time to adjust to the timezones properly. We were there for the boxing and that was it. We had been out enjoying the jacuzzi and champagne a little too much, so we decided to have an afternoon nap, to liven us up in time for the boxing. Unfortunately, we woke up late just as the fights were starting, which set us off on a really uneven footing for the evening. We had a major panic to get showered and ready. Neither of us had eaten anything, and as the tensions started rising, we ended up having some strong words. We were walking through the boxing to get to our seats, and a man grabbed me and started speaking to me. As always, I like to stop and chat with people who want to chat with me, but this was not on my boyfriend's radar. He was in a rush and I was slowing him down, so he made a short comment directed at me, and well that was it. It erupted. Feisty Lucy kicked in. I was not disciplined at all back then. If someone launched at me, my protective layer would kick in and I would launch back, loaded with extra venom. I did not like being spoken to like that. I did not feel it was necessary. It triggered the absolute heck out of me. Now I know that it's their shit and not my own, but back then I was like, "Fuck you, you're not going to speak to me like that. How dare you!" And then, more often than not, I would not let it go, for a very, very long time.

As a result of this argument we never really got to experience Vegas properly. I never had the chance to fully immerse myself in the place. The argument left a bitter taste in my mouth for many years, so I was absolutely determined to re-write that old story and have a great experience this time around.

Catherine and I landed in Vegas after almost eleven hours of being on the plane. There is nothing that can quite prepare you for landing in Vegas. Each time I go, I forget what it's like. You step off the plane, into the air-conditioned, oxygenated airport, and then you get hit with the fruit machines, the gold, the lights, and all the noise. It hits you like a thunderbolt. There is just no way you can afford to be tired in Vegas, there's no time for jet lag, so they make sure you are buzzing from the minute you get off the plane, until the minute you leave. It's so weird seeing all the people who have just got off a plane transfixed on the fruit machines. It really is a wonderfully weird place.

We were so excited to get going. However, we had to wait at the carousel to pick up our humongous luggage first. The two of us had a competition every time we travelled as to whose luggage would come through first. One of us would notoriously always have the last case off the plane, and the other one would more often than not be one of the first. On this occasion Catherine's case came off very quickly, so she was smug, ready to go, and pretending to be impatiently waiting for me. Mine was nowhere to be seen. I was thinking – *Fuck, please do not do this to me. Not this time.*

Eventually, we grabbed our bags, jumped into a taxi and headed off to the Aria hotel. It was one of the newer hotels on the strip at that time and it was in a really good location in the middle of the strip.

We got to the hotel and I was blown away by quite how incredible it was. It was beyond anything I had experienced before. I had completely forgotten how big everything was in Vegas. And this hotel was grand. From the outside, it looked like a huge mirrored building that reflected the sun. At night, it looked truly stunning.

We got to our rooms and we both decided to have a quick shower to freshen up after that long flight. We had decided we were going to put our bikinis on and get out by the pool for a little while. I was desperate to relax for a bit, and get some much-needed vitamin D on my skin and get in the pool.

After, we had been for a swim, we were exploring the hotel, and decided it would be rude to not stop and have some wine. While we were sitting there sipping on our wine, my best friend came up with a bloody genius idea, "Why don't we go out tonight? Why don't we go clubbing?" She said with a huge grin on her face.

"Seriously babe? I'm going to be hanging out my arse by tonight if we carry on like this!" I said to her.

"Lucy Davis. There's only one way, and that's to plough on through."

Welcome to the world of Lucy and Catherine. So, typical me, I said, "Fuck it, let's do it."

We both agreed that with the jet lag, it would be best to have a little nanny nap before we headed out. We figured out how to use the iPad in the room to close the posh, electric, blackout blinds and we dozed off.

An hour later, when the alarm went off, it was awful. Both of us were like bears with sore heads. We were wandering around saying things like, "Why are we doing this?" "Why on earth did we have a sleep?" "I feel worse now." We opened the blinds, and it was still daylight. Vegas felt like it was just starting to get its heart pumping in readiness for the evening ahead. It was September and the peak of summer in Vegas. I just couldn't get my head around it. I was grumpy. I wanted to go back to sleep. I would happily have stayed in the UK time zone at that moment. My eyes were stinging really badly because I was so tired. It's fair to say, we both felt rough. However, we knew what we had to do – get out of the room and move. Showering at that point would have resulted in us sitting back down or even laying down, and well that was going to be dangerous, so out we went on the search for food, which let's be real is not a challenge in Vegas.

We threw on the clothes we had been wearing during the day and decided to go and find some food in the hotel for ease before heading out for the night. We agreed that if we could make it until about one o'clock in the morning, we would easily slot into the time zones the next day. The mission had been set and we were ready to embrace it.

That night we got spruced up in tiny little dresses and killer heels. We had absolutely no sense in our choice of shoes considering the size of the hotels in Vegas. To walk through a casino is bigger than most clubs, so we were going to do some serious steps that night.

The first stop was our hotel lounge bar, which was close by. We took a seat and within seconds of sitting down, we had a waiter come and take our order. That's Vegas service for you. Even before our drinks had arrived a guy made his way over to us to kick start a conversation. This gentleman was lovely. Really attentive, funny, cheeky and very attractive. He and his friend were doing their best to get us to join them at their table. He kept attempting to win us over by saying, "Let us buy you girls drinks." He was in awe of our English accents. Every now and again when I was talking he would just stop me and say, "Oh my God, that English accent is amazing. Please just talk to me all night. We won't even speak. You guys just talk to us with your sexy accents." Welcome to Vegas baby!

These guys kept flirting with us, which was fun. It made Catherine and I feel good before we went out to the club. The guy who had initially come over, I actually exchanged details with before we left that night. They had asked us to go out with them that night, but we kindly declined as it was our first night. We said we were keen to go out just us two and see where the night took us.

By the time we eventually left the hotel bar, we were already very drunk. We got in a taxi, and as always, Catherine and I were chatting away to the taxi driver. We got him to crank up the tunes, and we had a party in the cab with him.

After drunkenly clopping along like two ponies on our high heels, we arrived at the club and there was a massive queue. As I always do in any situation, I observe deeply. I spotted a security guy parading up and down the queue, picking people at random to go to the front. Me being me, I thought it might be time to be a little cheeky and use the British accent. I caught the guy's attention, smiled and I said, in my best English accent, "Hey, can I just ask a few questions about the way this works, please?" Of course, the English accent got him instantly. He was beaming from ear to ear with a beautiful smile. Within a minute or so, the girl he was working with came over, heard our accents, and asked "Where are you from?" I said, "London, England. My friend and I are writing an article on what Vegas is like." The girl very quickly whipped us out of the queue, took us to the front, got us into the club, and, most importantly, gave us a table to sit at – which was really quite amazing.

We met some incredible people that night, mainly because we had a table. People came over wanting to sit down and rest their feet, so they started chatting, I guess they were just being polite before they joined us. The music was amazing. Surprisingly, we were having a really good time, knocking back the drinks. It got to about 11:30 pm, we had only been in there an hour or so, and the time difference suddenly hit us, hard. We were starting to struggle. It was about 7.30 am back in the UK and all we wanted to do was go to bed. My dear best friend was a real warrior though, so Catherine being Catherine said, "No we made a promise. We made a commitment to each other. We're going to stick it out until one o'clock." Good on her, she was disciplined when it came to staying out. Off the back of that decision, we thought it best to have a dance, get our bodies moving and try to get involved a bit more, throw ourselves into it rather than just clock watching and sitting in the shadows of the dance floor.

Once we did that, we really got into it. We ended up having such an amazing night and massively overshot our target of 1 am. We rolled in at about 2:30 am. We were so proud of ourselves and utterly convinced we would sleep right through until about 9 am.

However, it was just not meant to be. We managed a couple of hours sleep at best, and then we were wide awake again; I don't care what anybody says, alcohol and jet lag do not mix well.

That day, we decided to chill by the pool and allow ourselves to recuperate and restore our energy. Vegas in September is boiling. It's one of my favourite times to go. It's still hitting the high 30s and into the low 40s, but cools down a little in the later evening. The hotel had a really good vibe. It was very busy, but we didn't mind that. There was a lot to see. Lots to watch. Plenty of nice people to meet in the pool, and by the bars. We had a great day – we swam, sunbathed, slept and enjoyed a couple of cocktails by the pool. Super chilled.

We had done a little exploration of our hotel the previous day, so whilst out by the pool, we decided that we would go for a wander around some of the other hotels that evening. No drinking, just walking, checking it out, getting some food and saving ourselves for the boxing the next night. We knew we were going to walk a long way, miles in fact, so we decided to go super chilled in our shorts and pumps for ultimate comfort. We also made the decision that if we went out in shorts and pumps, there was no way either of us would lead each other astray. It was time for a chilled night in preparation for the boxing. There was no way I was going to mess it up this time. We had to be fresh to be able to appreciate it at its best.

We showered, stuck on some casual, comfortable clothes, and some flat shoes and headed off to explore the strip. At this point, I had only been to the Venetian, MGM and the Aria, so I was excited to see what the big deal was. Next door to the Aria was the Cosmopolitan, so we walked through there, checking out how beautiful it was. There were massive chandeliers hanging down from the ceilings. Everything looked very pristine and modern. We both mentioned how we would love to go to their club, Marquee. It looked and sounded amazing. We made a conscious note that would be on our to-do list. If not this time, then next time for sure. Next on our list was the Bellagio. The Bellagio, to walk through, is extremely over the top. We wandered through huge indoor gardens. It was absolutely spectacular, loaded with Halloween decorations which both Catherine and I loved. They were everywhere. Although It was only September, the Americans were getting right into the spirit of it. Outside of the Bellagio, it was pretty special. Every thirty minutes – on the hour, and half past – there was an incredible display of fountains outside. They would go off in time to the music. It was very incredible, especially the first time you watched it. It drew a huge crowd, every night. We stopped and watched in awe, before carrying on to our next stop, the one I had been most excited about – Caesar's Palace.

I had always had a bit of a thing about Caesar's Palace, because of the mythology, how grand it was, and also because it used to be the place where they did most of the original boxing matches. We walked into the hotel and I was in awe. It was so big, and so incredibly well done. The architecture had been captured magnificently. I loved it. I felt like I was there, back in ancient times. I also recognised it all from the movie 'The Hangover'. It was a real pleasure to be there, walking through where so many movies had been filmed. The straight path from the Aria to Caesar's Palace is just shy of a mile. We had meandered through the shops, casinos, and whatever else they had on offer. We had walked a long way by this point, so we decided to stop for 'just one drink' – famous last words. We were tired and fancied a refreshment stop, and well 'when in Vegas' and all that. We wandered through the casino and found a cute lounge bar that sold champagne. Without even questioning it, we ordered a couple of glasses. 'We will only have one' – we both nodded to each other as we clinked glasses.

Within seconds of us ordering and taking a seat, we had a couple of guys, a white guy and a black guy, ask to come and join us. Catherine rolled her eyes as she always did when this happened. Somehow it was always my fault. They had overheard us ordering the drinks and having a giggle at the bar, so the opening line from the white guy was, "Oh, that's a sexy accent." I just smiled and carried on chatting to Catherine without actually speaking to him. He carried on chatting, the black guy with him looked embarrassed, which actually made me want to speak to him. He did not want to be annoying or attention-seeking, I liked that. His friend persisted, and continued to chat and ask questions, so eventually, we gave in and spoke back. Oh my god, if ever we made a collective bad decision, it was talking to these two. It was the worst and best decision we could have made that evening, depending on which way you want to look at it. Bloody good story, though.

We ended up sitting down at a table with them, and they took it in turns to buy rounds. We found out that the white guy owned a limousine company there in Vegas. I decided to be cheeky, "Brilliant, you can give us a lift home later on then, as our feet are hurting big time." They gladly agreed. What we did not know was that my pure cheek of getting us a lift home was about to take us on our own personal version of 'The Hangover' tour.

48

It started with champagne, and then very quickly moved on to vodka. The white guy said, "Why don't we go to the club here in Caesar's Palace? We know people who can get us in VIP." Before we knew it we were at the front of the queue, heading up to Omnia, the club at Caesar's Palace, and because we were with these guys, we didn't have to pay anything. Not entry, not drinks, not a thing. All we could do was laugh at each other at this point. We had such good intentions; this was going to be a failure of epic proportions.

We were placed at a table, and on the table were vodka and champagne. We both kept looking at each other like – *Oh my God, what's happening here?* And from that point onwards it became the movie 'The Hangover' – featuring Catherine and Lucy. We got fucking smashed that night. Bearing in mind, we were in shorts and pumps, we had no make-up on, and we were dressed like we had just come off the beach. The boys didn't give a shit. They were enjoying being in our company. They were egging us on. I was dancing on the tables and on the chairs. We had an absolute ball.

At some point, someone decided it was time to move on to another club. The boys drove us around in a limousine. The black guy wasn't drinking, so he was driving. He was such an amazing guy. We actually became very good friends later, and although his friend was on my case all night, I wasn't interested in him whatsoever. I actually said to Catherine that I needed to stay away from him, there was something about his vibe I didn't like. We left another club, then the guys told us we had to go to a hotel to pick up a rapper and his friends to go on to yet another club. They asked us if we wanted to join them, so of course, we agreed. We were past the point of no return at this point.

When, earlier in the day, we had committed to going on a tour of Vegas, neither of us had imagined it would end up the way it did. We were on the craziest tour of Vegas that anyone could ever imagine. What a night it was. We moved around bars and clubs, getting drinks everywhere we went. After we picked up the rapper and his friends, we ended up in a dingy place; absolutely no idea where we were. It was probably about four o'clock in the morning by this point. This weird little place was full of pop stars, rap stars and all kinds of people like that. We were thrown onto a table with all these people, blatantly off their heads, and ignorantly, we had no idea who they were.

It was a seedy little joint, I didn't like it. It felt like a really dark underground kind of place. My gut instincts were telling me to leave; I wanted to go back to the Aria. We were having fun, but sensible Lucy kicked in and it was time to go. I said to Catherine, "I'm heading home. Do you want to come with me?" I'm embarrassed to say that we were a bit like that, if one of us wanted to leave and the other didn't, we would just leave them. Actually, on this occasion, Catherine agreed to leave with me, which surprised me as she was having such a great time. We told the boys we were going to go and they kindly offered to take us back to the hotel, to make sure we got home safely.

As if enough wasn't already enough, once back at the hotel we went into one of the hotel bars. We did not realise at the time the boys were following us. This was turning into a bit of a nightmare. There was no way they were coming to our room. Catherine shot me 'the look' as if to say she didn't think we would get rid of the boys. It was about 7 am at this point. We had boxing that afternoon. I had done everything I said I would not do. So then I pulled up my brutal honesty pants and told the boys straight up that they had to go. They were actually cool with it. They said their goodbyes, we exchanged numbers and then headed off. Catherine and I could not stop laughing, as we navigated our way back all the way through the casino and back to the lifts. We always got ourselves in so many interesting situations. Every time we left home together it was an adventure.

As we walked back through the hotel to the lift, the staff who had already got to know us were shaking their heads and laughing. We totally encouraged it too. Pulling the innocent 'who us' card. As we got closer to the lift, I ran into the guy who I'd met earlier on, the previous evening, before we'd gone out. "Oh hey," I slurred and started roaring with laughter. He took one look at me and said, "What the fuck has happened to you?" All I could do was laugh, I looked like a total disgrace. What a sweet guy, though, he helped us get into the lift as we were too drunk to figure it out.

Somehow we got back to the room, and very quickly got unchanged, took off our make-up, closed the black-out blinds – to shut the start of the day's sunshine out of our room – and passed out. I don't know how I ever got over it, or how my liver has ever recovered from that night. It was a messy evening. Bloody good memories, although I'm not sure I would ever do it again.

49

We woke up the next morning, feeling shocking. All we could do was laugh at each other. We always ended up in these predicaments, no matter where we went.

We realised we did not have too many hours before we would have to get ready for the boxing. The first stop had to be food. We decided to keep it super simple and easy on our feet, after the mileage from the previous day, and so we headed to the hotel buffet. We needed to soak up last night's alcohol and get us in a position to be going out again in just a few hours' time.

At about three o'clock in the afternoon, we decided we needed to start getting ready for the boxing. We wanted to be at the boxing early so we could enjoy the atmosphere and watch some of the undercard fights. After my last experience of boxing in Vegas, this time I really wished to change the story. I wanted to fully immerse in the occasion, as did Cat.

Now I'm not a girly girl. It does not take me long to get ready at all. I'm not one of these girls who paint their nails before a night out, puts on fake eyelashes, or anything like that. I normally just have a shower, put some makeup on, brush my hair and put some clothes on. This afternoon, though, we made an occasion of getting ready – we had wine because it had been such a long time since we had some, put some music on, danced, and sang our hearts out until it was time to go.

We got in a taxi from the Aria in the direction of the MGM, which wasn't far. We got out onto the main part of the strip and it was rammed. We sat in the taxi for a while not really moving too far, so we decided to jump out of the car and walk the rest of the way there. At least the night before we had flats on, but here we were parading up the strip in tiny little dresses, huge heels, and in the late afternoon sun, which was probably the hottest time of the day in the desert. We were trotting along, laughing at how our makeup was rolling off our faces with the beads of sweat gathering there. Such a good look girls.

Eventually, sweating like pigs, we arrived at the MGM hotel, but even then it was still an enormous walk to get to the stadium. Thankfully we had the air conditioning and carpet under our feet. First stop was to go and check out the lions. At this point, the MGM still had lions roaming around in part of the hotel. Looking back it was bloody cruel, and today I would likely set them free; however, back then it was not in my consciousness to consider how cruel it was what they were doing.

We eventually got to the boxing arena and it was absolutely heaving. It was buzzing. There were so many people there, so many famous faces too, which was really nice as they were intermingling with the normal people. It was such an incredible feeling to be there, being part of something of that size is pretty special.

My eyes were feeling sore, though, and getting worse and worse every minute. I put it down to a mixture of the heat, tiredness – having hardly slept for two days – plus the smoke and the oxygen that was being pumped into the room to create the atmosphere.

We sat down in our allocated seats and next to us was Amir Khan. Cat very quickly decided that she wanted a photo with him and was going to do whatever it took to get one, even if from afar. That was not good enough for me, though. I bowled over and asked him if we could have a photo. Of course, he obliged, and was really nice and friendly as he chatted with us. We stood and spoke with him for a short time before his commentating duties were due to start. The arena started to fill up very quickly. The fights were getting a little bit better, the atmosphere was starting to build. We were leading up to the main fight and you could tell. Everything started to get a little louder, until the main event, Mayweather vs Maidana started. The room was so alive during their walk-ins and the actual fight itself. It was a really great experience. We both loved it. This was also probably one of our most sedate evenings that trip. We barely drank that night as we were so engrossed in the fights, and it felt good to be clear.

50

After the fight, we were shuffling our way out of the crowded arena. People were chatting about their thoughts from the fights, giving their opinions to total strangers who were all united in their conversations. All of a sudden, out of nowhere somebody just shouted, "He's got a gun." And then there was a gunshot. Everybody either ran or dropped to the floor. There was so much panic. I grabbed Catherine and shielded her by putting my arms around her. I've no idea what I thought I was going to do but I just thought – *Fuck it, if we're going to go then we're going together*. It was pandemonium, people were panicking. There was only one gunshot, but it was enough to scare the shit out of all of us walking through that area – and it really did. I grabbed Catherine by the hand, and we ran. We were running through people, elbowing people out the way. Absolutely no thought given about our feet that had been hurting earlier. *Fuck this, we're not ready to die yet.*

We asked someone who worked there the quickest way out, and they guided us out of one of the side doors. We got away from the perceived danger, stepped outside and all of a sudden felt safe.

We stood there for a few minutes, just staring at each other. "What the fuck just happened there?" I said. We couldn't believe it. We thought about what the most sensible thing to do was and we decided to call the guy who we had met last night, the one who had driven us around in the limousine. We told him what had happened and that we didn't know anyone else in Vegas. He told us to get back to the hotel and that he would come and see us the next day to check that we were alright.

We navigated our way back to the hotel on foot, completely shocked about what had just unfolded. When we got back to the hotel it was all over the news that there had been a gunshot at the fight. People were talking about it everywhere we went. We were in total shock that we had been so close to a situation like that. That is something you hear about on the news, it's not something that actually happens. It's a hair-raising experience having something happen like that, so close to you. We could have been shot or caught in the crossfire. To take the edge off our fear we did what we did best, we went to the hotel bar. We only had one, maybe two that night, just to help us wind down.

The next night, though, was a different story. We met up with the black guy, the one I had spoken to the night before after the gunshot. He was actually off work and so decided to come to see us at the hotel. He had arranged with a friend of his to go to the Marquee club with him in the Cosmopolitan hotel. We had earmarked that club as being the one we would really like to go to out of all of them. We had an absolute blast. He arranged a VIP table for us with free vodka, champagne, and wine; plus, David Guetta was guest DJing. What an incredible, super random, off-the-cuff night.

The next morning we were supposed to be picking up our car, a Ford Mustang, to start our road trip to San Francisco. As the night went on, that early road trip start looked less and less likely to happen. We were in the zone, completely caught up in the holds of Vegas nightlife. We had drunk a lot of alcohol, and we were dancing the night away to some phenomenal music. It got to around two o'clock in the morning, and I thankfully put my sensible pants on again. I said to them, "I've got to go, I'm driving in the morning. Are you coming with me?" Catherine won't drive abroad, so I was going to be doing the driving over the coming week. She was having such a good time that she said she would stay with the guy. In all fairness, she looked so happy dancing around, so I checked he would get her home safely, which I knew he would, and I left.

I got back to the room and passed out immediately. I did not even manage to take my make-up and clothes off. I must have laid down on my bed to think about what an amazing evening we had and just drifted off. We had a skinful of alcohol that night.

Catherine came staggering back into the room at about six in the morning. She was absolutely wasted, bouncing off the walls, turning all the lights on, and causing absolute carnage. Then if that wasn't enough, she started puking. It was absolutely ridiculous. When you wake up after a skinful, just a couple of hours later, somehow you feel worse than when you went to bed. That was definitely how I felt. I got her to bed and then managed to get back off for a couple of hours of sleep before I was due to go and pick the car up. I wasn't in the mood to do anything, let alone act sober enough to take possession of a Ford Mustang. I suggested to Catherine we postpone for a day. We agreed that it may be a sensible option, but decided we would discuss it further after a shower. I got in the shower to freshen up, wash my hair, and do my best to wash the hangover and lack of sleep away, but it didn't work. When I got out of the shower I just slumped on the floor in my underwear, with my towel around my head crying, "I can't do this, I just can't do this Catherine." Catherine thought it was hilarious. She was still drunk at this point. She didn't have to drive a car for six hours, on the wrong side of the road, hungover. I suggested again we postpone until tomorrow, but we couldn't keep our room at the Aria, there would be charges involved, so we decided to suck it up. If you're out, you're in – was the old motto from work.

What an absolute mess we were queuing for check out. It was bloody embarrassing. We checked out and then had to go for a lay down on the couches in the reception area. We could not compose ourselves. It would have been funny if we had been watching other people feeling that rough, but no, it had to be us two. We felt sorry for ourselves for a little while longer, then I made the move. "Right, let's do this! We gotta do this now, or we will never move!" There was a little cheer from some of the people who we had met during our stay. They had been laughing so hard at the state of us both. Yes, it was a low point. However, there's only one way to go from low, right?

51

When we got to the car rental place the queues were humongous. Catherine had a total meltdown when she saw what we had to navigate, and ended up lying on the floor resting on her suitcase. We were in there for a good two hours, which was torture considering we were already feeling rough. I guess that's God's way of rolling his eyes and shaking the finger at us. When would we get the memo about sabotaging ourselves?

Eventually, we got to the desk, I was talking to the guy with my face turned away from him subtly, so he didn't pass out from the alcohol on my breath. He gave us the keys and told us to go find the car in the car park. No delivery to your door service here, it seems. We were doing our best to navigate our monstrous suitcases, with the scorching heat, hungover, looking to find a car we had no idea where it was, other than we had the key for it. It was a scene, let me tell you.

We finally found the car. It was beautiful. I felt a little guilty for being too hungover to appreciate it in all its glory. It was a gunmetal grey Ford Mustang with a black hood. What we hadn't planned for, though, was how small the boot space was. We really had not even considered that when we were ordering the car. We had enormous suitcases and loads of other much smaller shopping bags, as we had picked up loads of unnecessary stuff, as you do when you are in America. Catherine was huffing and puffing, both of us totally challenged by the puzzle of having so much big stuff to fit into a small space. The car was plenty big enough, we just wanted to embrace the roof down without worrying about something flying out of the car as we drove along.

We got in the car, and I said to Catherine, "I'm not sure I can do this. I can't drive far, I am way too tired to keep us safe today. Can you find a hotel for us, somewhere close, where we can go relax, eat and sleep this off? We can get up tomorrow and start afresh." Catherine looked relieved that we were going somewhere to rest, imminently. She went online and found us a room at the Luxor hotel – the one with the big black pyramid – not quite the standard of the Aria, but perfect to rest and get an early night.

We drove all of fifteen minutes from the car rental place to the front of the hotel, handed the keys over to the valet, sighed a huge sigh of relief and went to get checked into our new room. As soon as we got to the room, we both collapsed on our beds in a heap. We had made it! We had totally messed up the start of our road trip, but we laughed hard about it. We knew that one day it would make a good story, and we would not have missed the previous night for anything in the world.

We had such a magical time in Vegas. Much heavier than it ever needed to be, but this was the last dance. I had no idea when I would be seeing my bestie again.

The next morning, we quickly got our stuff together, as we had not unpacked anything other than our toothbrush. We had breakfast, as we knew we had a long drive ahead, then hopped straight in the car and got on our merry way. We felt fresh. We looked good. We looked human. We were back at it and ready to hit the road, immersed in the glorious sunshine of the desert as we went on our way. Thelma and Louise, out on the open road, at last.

We had decided the night before that rather than going straight to Los Angeles and up to San Francisco, as the original plan, we were actually going to drive further down, to San Diego, then make our way up north to San Francisco. I had always wanted to visit San Diego and despite the number of times I had travelled to America, I had never quite made it that far. It was almost always just slightly out of the way; however, this time, we were the rule makers, so we could do anything we chose to do. We could stop anywhere we liked. This part of the journey was about winging it. Or as I refer to it these days – intuitive travel.

The initial part of the journey through the desert was amazing. It was scorching and so many people we drove by were looking at us as if we were crazy for having the roof down. We were having the time of our life. What a difference a day makes! We were singing at the top of our voices. Music was blaring, we were beeping our horns and waving at anyone that was drawn to look at us. We were setting the tone for the rest of the way this trip was going to go. This was about fun, about connection. As much as we did not speak it, this was a goodbye. We both knew life would never be the same again.

52

The initial journey to San Diego was a long one. It was about five hours. As much as we had a lot of giggles, there were moments where we felt totally bored of the scenery. For many miles, it was just desert as far as the eye could see. We had to stop at one point, as we were approaching the midday sun and it was just too hot. We had to put the roof up to stop ourselves from getting burnt. We were slightly pink and crispy, but not burnt, not yet anyway. We were also having to guzzle as much water as we possibly could; the challenge was finding a toilet, though. Trust me when I say there were not many opportunities. As soon as one appeared along the roadside, we pulled in and ran against each other to see who could get in there first.

About five hours later we arrived in San Diego. We had absolutely no plan and had not booked where we were going to stay, so we decided initially to go and check out the area, then make some simple decisions.

As always, whenever I get to a new place, my intuition guides me to the water. This was no different. Within minutes of arriving, we found the beach and parked the car up to take a closer look. It was stunning. Typical American beach. Vast, wide, and sandy. It felt so good to be by the water's edge, after being tucked away in the desert.

We wandered along the beach and then got back in the car to see if we could find somewhere to stay. We liked this place and wanted to stay close by. We noticed the sky looked a bit grey, and a little bit temperamental, but we kept the roof down. We agreed if we got a bit wet, it wouldn't be the end of the world. As we started to drive, we noticed lots of cars on the road. It had not been like this a little earlier. Everyone had their lights on and seemed in a bit of a hurry. The further we went, we noticed a lot of leaves flying around, then big branches lying in the middle of the roads, and debris scattered around everywhere. We thought it was a bit odd, but carried on regardless. We had never been here before, so who were we to argue about what was normal or not. Then came the rain. It started gently, then as we drove a little further, it started to get extremely heavy. We had to pull the car over at the next safest spot and put the roof up. We were roaring our heads off. In all the years I had my convertible mini back home in the UK, we never got wet. I would never have had the roof down with clouds like that, but we chanced our luck being on the West coast of America and all.

The rain became relentless. Sideways rain. I turned to Cat, "What the heck is going on here?" She shrugged and laughed. We drove a little further and had to slow down to crawl along the road as I could barely see where I was going. It got really bad very quickly, I had to put the hazard lights on so the other cars could see me easily. With that, the car started shaking and the windscreen wipers could not go fast enough to deal with what was going on. People on the streets were running to get away from the weather. It was so weird, it had come out of nowhere. I had never seen anything like it. It was like a scene out of a movie. Minutes before we had the roof down, singing songs and basking in the sunshine, then a short drive down the road and the weather was so traumatic we couldn't see.

Whilst I had been driving and navigating the torrential rain, Catherine found us a hotel that was relatively close by. We headed in the direction of the hotel, in the hope we would find some safety.

We stumbled upon the hotel, dumped the car outside, and ran into the hotel, leaving all the bags in the car as we did not want to navigate that whilst this weather was persisting. As we entered the reception, in typical British fashion, we asked, "Hey, what's with this weather going on here?"

The lady looked at us in disbelief, "We have just had a massive typhoon rip right through here. You girls are lucky to have been able to get here safely. Is your car okay? Any damage?"

What the actual fuck? Catherine and I looked at each other in shock, then burst out laughing, as the lady looked on totally bewildered. This could only happen to us two – gunshots in Vegas, Typhoons in San Diego. Two near death experiences in just a few days. What the heck is going to happen next? This was only day six of our trip!

We checked in to the hotel and decided it was probably a good idea to just chill and relax until we had a better insight as to what the weather was going to be doing. We had made it there safely, we were not keen to keep testing how much lady luck was on our side. We used the time efficiently, to put a loose plan together as to the route we would take to San Francisco. We identified some key spots along the route that we would like to go to; we also wanted to see some whales and go into the forests.

The next morning, we woke up excited to start the next leg of our journey. We had the most magical mystery tour loosely planned. We were open to change and going wherever we were taken, all we knew was that we had to arrive in San Francisco to do what we were going to do there. We found some of the most incredible places along the route. Breathtaking scenery, places that no photograph could ever do justice to. The images were etched in our memories forever, though. We had a really wonderful time chatting, giggling and being present with ourselves in the car. It was amazing how simple it was, yet how eternally rewarding it felt. We were often distracted by work, our phones, or any number of other things when we were together. This gave us such a lovely amount of time and space to remember why we were such good friends, and why we had chosen to do this section of life together.

After a couple of days of exploring the route, we arrived safely in Santa Monica to meet up with a lady we had met on the cruise at Christmas; she lived in Santa Monica and so we had arranged to catch up with her. I had zero expectations of Santa Monica, and, in all honesty, if we had not been stopping to see this lady, we may well have just driven past it. I'm pleased we did stop, though, because Santa Monica was beautiful.

We parked the car and went to explore, as we always did. We found the beach and went for a beautiful walk along the pier, and then meandered around the shops and around the central area before we met up with our friend for dinner. Over dinner, she asked me how my trip to the Amazon was. She had seen some of my recent pictures on Facebook. She was talking about my time with Ricky. Why would she bring that up? She mentioned that she felt really happy for me when she saw how happy I appeared to be with him. She joked that the Canadian guy must have been heartbroken to witness it. Catherine agreed, whilst I played it down, "It wasn't like that," I blushed. It was so beautiful that the Universe had divinely placed us to meet this lady in the first place, and then to stay in contact with her, and to meet up with her on our latest adventure. When you stop and look, you may notice that every person is, or was, a messenger. She was such a sweet soul, and her son, interestingly enough, was qualifying to be a barrister at the time we met him. It is very interesting now, looking back – the introductions that took place would be extremely poignant for the future work I would do.

I really liked Santa Monica, but Santa Barbara was my favourite town along the coast. There was something special about it. The energy was beautiful. It felt as if we had stepped back in time there. It was picturesque and very obviously an area where there was an abundance of wealth. People were very friendly, they would go out of their way to engage with you, which I actually really like when I am away from home. I remember a man being so helpful, he assisted us in crossing a road to get us to a restaurant we had found. We were able to spend some time on the beach in Santa Barbara, burying our feet in the sand, as we lay chatting about what was going to come next and where we were excited to be going.

We carried on driving over the next few days and several hundred miles – exploring, and only stopping for somewhere to eat or rest. The memories from that trip will be etched in my mind forever. It was the last dance with my bestie. It was solidifying our bond and cementing our friendship before I packed up and left.

53

Eventually, we arrived in San Francisco. I really didn't enjoy it there. It was not my place. It was a bit of a downer to end the trip there, to be honest. It was cold, grey and wet. I felt I had just landed back in the UK. The man at the car rental was rude, it was busy, and it just did not feel like a holiday anymore. We both said had we known we would have started in San Francisco and ended up in Vegas on a high. San Francisco just wasn't the place that I expected it to be. We were staying in a beautiful hotel, that we'd spent a lot of money on, but it felt dark. The whole city felt dark, to be honest. There was a lot of poverty, homelessness, and a lot of begging. Now I appreciate that is the reality for some in this paradigm; however, it was not resonant with where we were at that time. Of course, we had to have that bump down to earth. We had been living in paradise, in a higher vibration, a higher level of consciousness for days, but this was such a huge shock to the system. It rained most of the time we were there, which probably didn't help. For those who know me, you know the rain is not my thing. I appreciate it so much for watering the plants and allowing things to grow, but being out in it is not my preferred choice. The day that we went on an open-top bus, it pissed it down. We both sat there freezing cold in the rain and wind, grumpy, without jackets – as we didn't feel we would need one on for the trip.

There was one saving grace after our miserable open-top bus tour. That evening we found the most amazing Indian restaurant ever. It was a strange-looking place – Catherine didn't even want to go in there, she said it looked like the kind of place we could end up getting murdered in – but I insisted we try it because it was convenient to our hotel and I had read a couple of reviews that said it was good. I normally do quite well picking food places and this was no different. We went in there and had the most amazing meal. The food was stunning. The restaurant itself was nothing special, but the food was fabulous. It was my little, tiny pocket of hope for San Francisco.

On reflection, I may have been feeling low because I knew this bubble with my bestie was going to be the last stop before I had to disappear off on my own. We were flying back to the UK the following day and then I was switching over my backpack to go off again this time solo. I didn't know when I would see Catherine again. So it's pretty reasonable I was panicking about going travelling and my ego was kicking in somewhat, to keep me safe. I was scared to leave my best friend and go on my own. She probably never knew it, but she had become my safety blanket.

Cat suggested a couple of glasses of wine in our hotel bar before we ended the evening. It was only early, we were flying back to reality tomorrow, I had no more driving to do, so I was all in. It had been about ten days since my last alcoholic drink, which was unheard of back then, so after our amazing curry, we headed to the busy bar in our hotel. It was so lively when we got in there. Music was playing and seeing people having fun livened us up a bit. We walked over to the bar and found a couple of empty bar stools, so decided to pitch up there for the evening. It saved us from moving too far, and the plus side of sitting at the bar is, you always meet really interesting people whilst waiting for a drink. It's always amazing the messages you get from strangers; they're always exactly what you need to hear. We ordered a couple of glasses of wine and took our time with them, appreciating the taste – there are some phenomenal wines in California.

We laughed so much that night, we met some incredible people, got some amazing insights from the barman and had some really quality conversations between my bestie and me. I was so grateful to have her in my life. I'm not sure I ever told her how important she was to me. She really was someone I trusted with my life. We went through everything together.

At some point during the first few glasses of wine, feeling slightly under the influence, Ricky surfaced in my mind. I went back to that dinner in Santa Monica, and how the lady had brought him up. I know she was on my Facebook, but why of all the things she'd seen over the last nine months did she mention that? Then, all of a sudden I felt as if he was near me. I could feel his energy. There was a feeling in my body that I just had to know where he was. I had to say sorry to him. Now, this freaked me out. I was so stubborn back then and very rarely apologised; however, I felt this overwhelming urge to do it now.

I mentioned it to Catherine who was shocked to even hear his name. I had banned us from speaking about him after the trip back in April. I had wanted to forget about him and move on, and yet here I was, a few glasses of wine in, on the last day of our trip and I had mentioned his name. She told me it was best to leave it. I knew she was right, but alcohol thought otherwise. I couldn't help myself. Thankfully he's not got the most common name in the world – unlike Lucy Davis – so I went to my Facebook account, put his name in and boom, it was there. My stomach flipped. Did I really want to do this? Was this really the right thing to do? Then the alcohol kicked in even further. The little devil on my shoulder was screaming 'DO IT!' at the top of his lungs, whilst the angel was saying – *See how you feel tomorrow when you're sober.* Catherine firmly believed I should leave it alone, so when she went to the toilet, I seized the moment. I messaged him. I did not add him as a friend, I just messaged him, which gave him the huge opportunity to ignore me without offending me. I told him I could feel him around me and that I was really sorry for what had gone on between us, and then I put my phone back down and ordered another drink.

What on earth had I done? What possessed me to do that? What was I thinking? I immediately panicked – *Oh God I really wish I could delete it.* Catherine returned from the ladies and asked why I looked so guilty. I burst out laughing. She knew me too well and never once did she judge me for it.

"I messaged him," I shyly said.

"Lucy Davis – I can't leave you alone for a minute," she giggled. "What's he said?"

"Babe I feel sick, I can't even look at my phone. I cannot bring myself to ever look at it again," I explained, very dramatically. With that, she turned over my phone and I had a notification from him! I was shocked. I never expected him to respond, and he had, immediately. Cat was desperate for me to open my phone and check it, but I needed a moment. I felt sick. *Had I really meant to apologise? Was I really sorry? Did I want to connect in with this person again after the way he spoke to me? What if he's still angry with me? Did I really want to re-live this? What the heck was I thinking?*

After a few more swigs of wine, I took a deep breath and opened the message. I was shocked to read, "Lucy, good to hear from you, how are you? Where in the world are you? I'm so sorry about what happened too." I showed Catherine and she smiled in a way that only a best friend would. The previous six months, I had held onto so much baggage about this person, I had convinced myself he was a total arsehole – and yet all it took was one olive branch. Maybe it was the amount of time that had gone by, water under the bridge. Maybe we had both realised we had been bloody idiots dragging it on this long. Maybe we were both intrigued to see what had been going on, away from each other. Who knows why I messaged? Or why he responded. And why our souls had decided it was time to reunite. We chatted for a while that night. It was so good to hear how he had been. He was so excited I was just about to embark on my travels. So much had changed for both of us. However, somehow, we remembered that we were supposed to be a part of each other's lives this lifetime.

Before I went to bed that night, he said he would be back in Thailand from around November to January time. He was not quite sure when, but it would be around that time. He was ready to get fit again and get his boxing training back on track. We agreed to meet up there and have a good chat about everything. I went to bed really happy that night. I felt so much lighter, by allowing myself a level of vulnerability I had never experienced in my life. I had allowed myself to be wrong, whether I felt it or not, and to get back aligned with someone who I truly felt connected to.

The next day, we flew back to the UK. It wasn't a particularly memorable flight, we were both absolutely exhausted. It had been a really weird end to the holiday. Despite putting on a brave face, and not really looking after myself, my health was really struggling. I had been suffering with my stomach and acid reflux due to my hiatus hernia. At times it had felt as if someone was holding a blow torch into the upper part of my stomach. The alcohol had really taken its toll on my body. On top of that, the sizes of the food portions had not helped with my digestion issues. There was not a salad in sight that trip; rather deep-fried everything, loads of bread and lots of starchy foods.

The trip had been predominantly plagued by digestive issues. Usually, digestive issues are trapped emotions in your system, mainly anger. Of course, that's what was causing my body to hurt, to get my attention. I was suppressing angry, hurt, guilty, and frustrated emotions. I was pushing them even further down with alcohol and food. They were doing their best to get my attention – the health issues, the gunshot, the tornado. It's fascinating that the signs from the Universe were there, clear as day, but I had my head up my arse and I didn't realise it.

I didn't know it at the time, but this trip and the Vegas experience were truly symbolic of the last dance. It was my last dance with my old self. The one I was clinging on to for dear life. I was panicking. I had planned to go travelling on my own, I was starting to open up and feel into the things my grandad had said to me, but I was desperately holding on to the old me, the party girl, and the familiarity of it all. *What if I lost my best friend because I'm not going to party anymore? What if I don't have the fun times anymore because I don't drink as much as people would like me to? What if I'm not fun anymore and people do not wish to hang out with me?*

I think I knew intuitively, and on a soul level at that time, this was the start of something, I just didn't know how it would play out. My soul took over that night and made me message Ricky. My stubbornness would never have allowed that in the past. I was changing. I was healing. On some level, I knew this was going to be the next part of my story.

And with the last dance, came saying goodbye. Saying goodbye to a piece of myself that had been my identity for all these years. I was saying goodbye to the identity that I, Lucy Davis, had created. There was this person, this ego, driving the Lucy Davis vessel, but it wasn't the soul. The soul was saying – *I'm about to wake up, get it out of your system because once we go from here, there is no turning back.*

Straddling Two Worlds

There is a really odd period of time during a journey like this one I am taking you on, whereby everything is collapsing around you. Your friends who you have known your whole life start to step away, your health, career, and anything that you would relate to as being 'normality' all of a sudden starts to change. It doesn't feel as if it is yours anymore, it no longer aligns to you. You start to question it all. You wonder why people are leaving you, or not including you anymore, and why you no longer feel like you belong. It's almost like you are forced into isolation and it feels horrid, it's not something you asked for, so why is it happening?

Welcome to your spirit awakening! Some would call this the dark night of the soul. At this point, your soul has given your physical vessel lots of opportunities to remember what it came down here to do, and you are starting to feel it; however, fear holds you back from fully immersing in it.

It's at this point you are what I call 'straddling two worlds'. Things don't feel right anymore in the life you've had up to that point. The fear of the unknown is such a real thing, and in desperation you cling onto anything you can.

My grandad passing created a ripple within me. His words of wisdom on his death bed, the inspiration that he handed me, created a physical, emotional and spiritual shift within my energy field that led to all of the events up to this point. No one else around me was going through what I was. No one else understood what was happening behind closed doors, as it felt too weird to talk about it, but there was no denying that I was changing. I felt totally alone in a world where I had hundreds of friends and worked in an environment with thousands of people, but nevertheless, I felt totally alone.

As much as I was desperate to evolve and to move forward and experience all that I was starting to believe was possible, losing my old world of security, popularity and the certainty that came with it; well it scared the absolute shit out of me. Of course, I was nowhere near ready to admit that I was scared either. Vulnerability — what even was that?

I was in a vicious cycle of being scared of the unknown, and so sabotaging with the known — alcohol. Every time I would take a step forward, alcohol would be my nemesis to keep being the good-time, fun girl that everyone knew and loved about me from over the years. I was shedding an identity that had been with me since I was 16, and it was bloody scary.

When you find yourself in the position whereby you realise changing means you are about to lose everything in your world, know this is the ultimate test of whether you are in fact willing to evolve and step into your role as one of God's servants. I am not going to pretend it's easy, what I will say, though, is once you do it, you'll never look back and say you wished you stayed where you were.

You've got this!

54

It was September 2014 when I arrived back in the UK from America. There was a brief moment of excitement, but very quickly the reality kicked in. My stomach flipped. Oh shit, I've got no home, no job, and I had even sold my car. So, I had nothing, literally. I had said a sad goodbye to my best friend, we would to keep in constant touch whilst I was away, and she had promised to come to see me wherever I was in the world on my birthday. That was four whole months away at the time, though, but something to hold on to.

It was true, I was officially a bum. I had to navigate getting the coach back from Heathrow to Bournemouth, where my mum was storing my stuff for me, but it all seemed like such a mission. I messaged my mum, and she agreed to come and pick me up from the coach station in Ringwood. It would be lovely to see my mum, although it was just one night. I had to be back at the airport the next afternoon, and then who knows when I would be seeing her, or any of my friends and family again. It felt eerie in a way, but it needed to be done. I knew this would change my life on one level or another.

I was feeling extremely vulnerable. I was excited to go off on my own, but also really scared. I was having doubts, feeling as if I should just stay in the UK, get a job, find a new home, and get back to what normality was. I was also scared because of the 'what ifs'. *What if something happened to me whilst I was away? What if something happened back home whilst I was gone? What if everyone forgot me? What if....?*

I had to have a pep talk with myself, but my mum was on my case to stay and sort my life out, so she was unknowingly feeding those doubts and feelings of fear. Those fears had held me back for so much of my life. Even my successful career had been forged out of fear. I had been fearful that I would not make anything of myself as my schoolteachers had threatened. I had created my whole life based on a determination to be successful. I thought that was the answer to happiness. Those same fears had stopped me from stepping forwards and travelling in the past and also from allowing myself to love and be loved. The fear I was feeling at that moment was real, though. I was about to step on a plane to Thailand, with absolutely no idea when I would see any of these people again. I did not have a return ticket, a plan or anything.

Most people found it weird. I had been so meticulously planned in every area of my life, and it was time to truly let go and hold on for the ride. Some of my friends – my best friends at that – were placing bets on when they thought I would return. Some of them reckoned a month, and some said six months. Some of them thought I would end up married, living in some off-grid community and never coming home. In my heart, I felt I would be gone eight to twelve months, maybe a bit longer. I had plenty of money to play with. It was not going to be money that brought me home, though, it would be missing people. On the one hand, I wondered if there was such a thing as too much travelling. On the other hand, I figured I could go forever if I wanted to because I could easily get another job somewhere in the world. I could create a life wherever I wanted. I was open to it on some level, which is why it scared the shit out of me. For the first time I had ever allowed in my life, the world was literally my oyster. I could choose where I would like to be and who I would like to be with. If I wanted to be around people I could be, if I didn't, then there was no forcing it.

As much as it excited my soul, it scared my human. *What if there was no one to talk to? What if I don't make friends?* There are those 'what if's' again.

I made it back to my mum's without too much hassle and packed my backpack, ready for the next phase of my life. Once you have travelled, you have a really beautiful connection to your backpack. I had chosen a red one. I felt it would be easy to spot coming off the airplane each time. I did not realise how that colour would end up being so important in the coming years. Our intuition always knows. My beautiful red backpack got loaded with so much shit that night. I had no idea what I was doing. I packed as if I was going on holiday. I packed as if really weird random things were going to happen. I had no idea at the time that packing into a backpack was a definite art. Almost the second you arrive at your first destination, you very quickly realise none of that stuff you packed serves you. So you end up donating it to charity or binning it all, and then filling it with stuff that you're actually going to need for your journey. Life skills like these have been seriously missed from the school curriculum.

I had decided my first stop in Thailand would be to go and do some training for a little while; back to the place I'd been to in October 2013, where I'd met Ricky. I decided that I was going to go there because it was safe. I knew where I was going. I knew what I was doing. It was familiar. I had been to Thailand a couple of times over the years before 2013, with friends and an ex-boyfriend. We had travelled to Koh Samui, Koh Lanta, Koh Phi Phi and Krabi. We had never done it justice, though, especially when I went with the girls. It was more of a beach day thing, to recover from the night before, and then get blind drunk again in the evening. There had been no depth to my experiences until that point; however, this time I was looking to step out of the old Lucy and start dipping my toe into this new vision of me – the one that was excited to experience life. The ayahuasca journey had bought all of this into consciousness for me. I had connected with something special. It had been validation of the pulls I had been feeling – and ignoring – for years. It had given me a clear vision that this was what I had to do. The signs had been there throughout the whole of that journey, and here I was about to embark on it. I could have ignored them. It would have been so easy to ignore them.

I was scared, really fucking scared.

After a great night's rest, I got up knowing that today was going to be the first day of the rest of my life. My mum said, "You've not changed your mind then?" as I was preparing my backpack for the next leg of my journey. I smiled sweetly at her. I adored my mum so much. She was so kind, and caring and wanted everyone close so she could nurture them. I cannot imagine how it must have felt for her. In her eyes, I was running away. She didn't realise why this was important to me. I'll be honest, I wasn't totally sure myself, at the time. I just knew there was something inside of me that I had to go and investigate. There was something that had been telling me for years that there was more to life than what was going on, and what my reality had been like. I could not explain it, it was something deep down, wisdom I could not quite touch yet.

I was lucky enough to get a lift to the airport. It was lovely, and a welcome distraction, to have people to chat to on the way. It helped pass the time when I would have been mulling things over and convincing myself not to go. When we got to Heathrow, Terminal 2, my stomach flipped. It was time!

I got out of the car, grabbed my bag, threw it on my back, hugged them, and walked quickly away before the tears started to flow.

I banished them from coming into the airport because I knew damn well it was going to be emotional enough, without a send-off party. I felt like I had to be tough. I was doing this on my own and I knew I had to get used to it. I walked into the airport, it was so hectic that it made me forget that I was going off on my own. It was utter pandemonium. After a couple of hours in the airport, I actually started panicking I would miss my flight due to the carnage taking place.

My flight route was London Heathrow to Bangkok, then down to Phuket. Other than the bedlam checking my bags in at Heathrow, everything went really smoothly – getting my connecting flight and picking my bags up safely in Phuket. It was a dream.

The moment I touched down, I had an inner knowing rise within me again. It felt like home. Everything was exactly as I had described when I landed here previously, nothing had changed. The overwhelming noise, the speed at which people were speaking, the scents from the orchids, the smell of the food.

I giggled to myself as I passed through customs and saw people bartering their way through more quickly by paying 500 baht. I just loved how this place worked. I truly loved how it was such organised chaos.

I got picked up by a taxi, like last time, and driven to the hotel, where I also stayed on the previous visit. Familiarity was all I had to hold on to at this point, so I went with it. The only difference this time was that I knew exactly where I was going. I didn't have any fear around getting lost, or not being able to communicate effectively. As much as I had only done it once before, it was enough. I wasn't scared that they didn't understand me. I wasn't scared to go into the supermarket to get supplies. I was just so happy to be back here – in the land of smiles. It felt special. I had a feeling of excitement in my gut. I felt as if this was going to be the start of something magical. I was open to experiencing anything that I needed to, to help myself become the person I knew was hidden inside of me.

I got to Coco Ville, where I had decided to stay for my first month. I felt that this would give me the time to meet some friends, and get my bearings, then it would likely be time to move on and travel, or something like that. When I checked in, they remembered me. It was really lovely to see everyone again. The first time I had been in room 222, this time it was room 144 – no surprises there. Interestingly, 144 was the room that Ricky had been staying in back in October when he had told me to swing by his room on my way back from being out for the night in Patong. The Universe works in such mysterious ways.

I woke up really early the next morning, but that was fine. I felt remarkably settled, considering this was only day number one of my travelling experience. The first thing I did was make a loose plan. I had to grab some essentials for my room, such as water and nibbles. I also had to organise my gym membership. I had decided to sign up for a month's training – even if I decided not to stay for a full month, at least I had the option to use it if I chose.

Later that same day I started training. I was not going to sit around and ponder, I wanted to get straight at it. It was so weird to think that not even a year prior, I had arrived in this exact location looking to get my head together and do a little bit of boxing, and I ended up falling head over heels in love with their national sport, Muay Thai. I had been passionate about boxing before that trip to Thailand, but now Muay Thai was my drug. Since that first visit in October 2013, I had been training consistently back home in the UK. I was lucky because about 20 minutes from my house, my sister's fiancée, at the time, had a mixed martial arts gym, so I used to go there. I had actually become quite good. I had toughened up a lot, and become extremely strong, and the most important thing was that I was focused in a way I had never known myself to be before. I was not fit like you have to be in Thailand to train, but I had come on a lot since I left in October, so I was pushed through the ranks of the classes very quickly.

The Thai trainers were really quite surprised with how much I had improved in such a short period of time. They would hold pads for me in the class remembering what we had done previously and then they realised I was serious, I had become strong. So they then became serious and started correcting me, pushing me harder. I mentioned to them that I would like to fight one day. The words came out of my mouth before my brain engaged. It was an interesting situation. I had not processed what I was saying. The Thai trainers asked if I had a Thai boyfriend back home. I looked at them oddly, not knowing what they were talking about, and then they laughed and said it was because I had improved so much in such a short space of time. They would then ask if I wanted a Thai boyfriend whilst I was there. We had good banter. We really did laugh a lot, it was a lot of fun. I was truly saddened to find out that my first ever Thai trainer, from the previous October, had recently passed away from cancer. Just a short time earlier we had been training together. I will always remember him, he was the one who lit the match for my flame to burn with Muay Thai. From that moment forward, I decided to cherish his memory and do him proud.

As much as I loved being back and being immersed in the energy of this place, I missed Ricky. I would be training and hear something, turn round and it was not him. I had such huge memories from that short visit in the previous October. It made me think back to our trip to South America. I felt sad about the unnecessary stuff that went on there. Things could have been so different. I was happy we had spoken whilst I was in San Francisco, though. I never knew why I wanted to be friends with him so much, and why it bothered me about us staying in touch. It's weird. Why did I care? Why did he bother to respond? It was highly likely that we would never have crossed paths again. However, I had messaged him, and he had responded. We obviously had not quite finished our journey together, and it was weird for him not to be there and to not hear his cheeky, smart-arse comments. I smiled at the thought of him. I knew one day we would be friends again.

I tend to make friends wherever I go, though, and very quickly too. This trip was no different. It was silly me having that story running through my mind that I might not make friends. I have never been in a position where I do not find people to hang out with. I'm pretty social and I like a chat, so I tend to make an effort with people, even if it is just saying hello, or being nosey about the food they are served in a restaurant.

I quickly became friends with an Australian girl. She was over there wanting to get the confidence to fight. She was so passionate about learning about boxing, it was amazing to watch her. She wanted to experience everything. She had a passion for really immersing and learning from the best, so she put herself in front of people to get her needs met. Where we were training, there were some of the best trainers in the world. This girl would place herself in front of them, ask questions and force herself to do things that maybe she didn't want to do, just to get recognised and in their vision. Initially, I thought – *Wow, she's full-on*. It must drive people crazy with someone doing that, around the clock. Nevertheless, it was inspirational. She knew what she wanted and she was going to get it, no matter what. I judged her as it was so uncomfortable for me to put my hand up and ask. I did not want to seem like a pain or too full-on, so I let people come to me, I did the hard graft on my own, for fear of being rejected. I had a level of envy that someone could be so vulnerable, and get everything they asked for, rather than sitting back and waiting for someone to notice them, which had been a thread throughout my life up until that moment.

Over the coming days and weeks, we ended up becoming really good friends. She took me under her wing and started introducing me to some other people. Likewise, when I met new people, I would introduce them to her. We became besties for the period we were together. She was really confident and had a little moped that she would come and pick me up on. I would jump on the back of the bike and we'd go off to the beach, go training together, or maybe head off to the night markets. She gave me confidence, and I know that's why she was placed in my life. I had to be shown the strength in vulnerability, not shirking from the traumas we were all carrying – and she taught me how to ride a moped.

Within a couple of weeks of me being on the back of her moped, she decided it was time for me to grow my wings. She was heading home in another couple of weeks and she knew I had to get on a moped by myself, so I could travel around and experience life in its fullest form. Oh my goodness, it was hilarious. I hadn't ridden anything like that in such a long time. I got on it the first time and floored it too quickly. The bike went from under me, straight through my legs and sped off without me. We were crying with laughter, it was so funny. How no one got hurt is beyond me. After that, I was really not keen to go again. However, she had so much confidence in me that she encouraged me to get straight back on. She had confidence in me that I could not see for myself at that time. I was really confident speaking to people and training, but she gave me the confidence to do other things, like riding a moped, and really experiencing what Thailand was about. There was a much bigger picture, and thankfully, she held space for me to see it. I had to be honest with myself, I was travelling, so I had to be willing to learn new things. That was the whole point of being here. There was no point me sitting in this comfortable cocoon that I'd been sat in for the previous 35 years.

55

One afternoon, towards the end of my first week, I was coming home from training, absolutely shattered, dripping in sweat after a heavy session in the afternoon sun. I walked past the gym that was near to my hotel and could not help but notice the extremely attractive man training there. He was gorgeous. Now it had been a while since I had looked at a man like that. Don't get me wrong I appreciated good looking men and there were plenty around this area, but this man really caught my attention. Not wanting to be too shallow, but just to set the scene – tall, dark, handsome, six-pack, nice muscly arms, sweaty – you get my drift. He had a very kind face too. He really caught my attention, and his Thai trainer noticed and was not going to let me get away with it. In true Thai fashion, the trainer called me over, "Come here, come here. Come and train with us, join us," he said. The Thai trainers are always doing their best to get your attention, and this one knew he had a hook with me with this guy. He persisted, but I carried on walking, ignoring him. I was dripping in sweat, my hair was all over the place, I had mascara all around my face too, because not only had I just done a two-hour training session, but I'd walked down the road in 40 degrees heat. His persistence paid off. I reluctantly wandered over to the trainer, and the gorgeous guy said, "Hey, you alright?" I was so embarrassed. I was totally off men at this point. I had perceived that Ricky had been a twat in the Galapagos Islands, and my ex-partner had ended up being crazy. I had made the commitment to myself when I was being chatted up in Vegas, by all these different people, that I was going to travel the world single and get my head together. I said to Catherine, "I'm not ready. I don't want to meet someone. I'm not ready to do it. I want to travel the world on my own."

I said hello and goodbye, almost in the same breath, to the guy and his trainer, and headed back to the hotel. I was so hot that I dumped my stuff outside my room and went and threw myself into the swimming pool, fully clothed. After a little dip, I went back to my room and got changed into my bikini. I had some time to relax before my next training session, so I thought I would sit by the pool and see what was going on. I loved the sunshine, it made me happy, so vitamin D on my skin was what was needed. My mission for the trip was to be the brownest I'd ever been. It was going to be an interesting challenge as I tanned pretty well, even just on a week's trip. I continued to sit there minding my own business, pottering about between my room and the pool, grabbing some water when it was required. The next thing, I looked up and the gorgeous guy I had just seen earlier, arrived back from training and went back to his room, which coincidentally was just one room away from mine. *Uh oh* – I immediately thought. *Oh shit, this is going to be dangerous.* I started having a conversation with the Universe and pointing to the sky and saying, *"No, no, no, no, no, I'm not ready. Do not do this to me!"*

The guy appeared again, a few minutes later, he'd changed into his swimming shorts, and he threw himself into the pool, exactly as I had done minutes earlier. He got out of the pool, which was a vision in itself, I tell you. I looked at him and thought – *This man is absolute perfection.* He wandered over to me, "Is that sunbed taken next to you?" All I could think was – *Oh Shit!*

I was trying to display some dignity, but failing miserably, "Err no, feel free to lie down if you wish." If you wish!!! What the fuck! Lucy! Of course he wishes otherwise he wouldn't have asked! Inside I was thinking – *Fuck, fuck, fuck! Oh well, here goes!*

Within a minute or two, he started talking to me. It transpires he was from St Albans in Hertfordshire. It was really nice to hear an English accent and to be able to chat about things from home. He was a really nice guy. Quite shy, hardworking and super dedicated to his training. He had taken ten days off work to train in Thailand because he had a fight coming up back home. What was so interesting, was the more he talked, everything he was doing reminded me of the trip to Thailand that I had taken the year before. He needed to get away, he needed to get his head straight. It was uncanny the similarities in our journeys and the connections we both had off this short conversation. He mentioned that whilst he was having a great time training, not many people were up for doing things outside of training. I guess he was kind of hinting. I was chatting with the Universe inside – *No frickin way, not today, I'm not doing it.*

I was polite, but I quickly made my excuses, "I've got to go now, really nice to meet you," and I walked off. As I walked off, he shouted, "What's your name?"

"Lucy. Yours?"

"Kyle."

I got back to my room, shut the door, and cursed the Universe big time – *Fuck, fuck, fuck, fuck, fuck.* Why is this happening right now? This was not part of the plan. I was not ready to meet anyone or even flirt with anyone. I needed time to be me. This time was meant to be all about me.

My head was muddled, in week one and I'm already in a pickle. I messaged my Aussie girlfriend to come and get me, so we could go out for dinner and talk things through. We were both in a similar spot. We had run away from home, relationships, life, in search of something. Whilst we were out that night, she introduced me to loads of other people; really, nice people too. Everybody was there to train, they all had the same kind of mindset which made it really easy to keep focused. We all decided to organise a dinner for that coming Saturday night. We decided we would go to a lovely Mexican restaurant that some of them knew. A number of people were leaving the following week, so it was an excuse to have a good get together. The Thai gyms are closed on a Sunday, unless you are training for a fight, so Saturday was the perfect night to go out and not have to worry about training the next day.

Later that night, I went back to the hotel and sat in the reception area, where people would usually relax and have a few drinks. I ended up meeting a few other people – as I do – and I mentioned to them about the dinner on Saturday night. I was gathering up all of the lost souls for a reunion, if you like. It was looking good, we had a really good crew; it was looking like about 30 of us would be going out on Saturday. Suddenly, Kyle, the gorgeous guy from the pool, came over and he asked what I was organising. I told him, and then he looked at me, waiting for me to ask him to come with us. I reluctantly asked, "Would you like to join us?" I wasn't reluctant because I didn't like him, I was reluctant because I knew there was bound to be alcohol being drunk, and I wasn't sure I was ready for the repercussions of being in close proximity to this person whilst intoxicated.

A couple of days later, we all gathered at the restaurant. I purposefully sat away from Kyle at the start, but as the night progressed, we started gravitating toward each other. At the end of the meal, everyone wanted to go to a bar. Ideally, I wanted to stay away from bars, but so far on my trip I hadn't been out or doing much socialising at all, so I agreed to go. At the bar, another friend I had met, from the Gold Coast in Australia, could sense my resistance to drinking. He shouted over at the top of his voice, "Davis! Another drink! What do you want?" He was not taking no for an answer. He got me a glass of wine, and as I said thanks I could feel things were about to take a slightly different direction from what they had been so far on this trip.

We were in a dancing bar, there were people all over the place drinking, sitting on stools at the bars, and girls were serving drinks and dancing round poles on the bars. It wasn't a strip bar, this is just what most of the bars were like over there. In this particular bar, there was also a pool table. Now I love playing pool, so my girlfriend and I decided we would play on opposite teams, to keep it interesting and play with the boys. My Aussie girlfriend went with my Aussie guy pal, and of course, Kyle appeared and said he would pair up with me. It was on! Australia versus England. We started playing, and we were having cheeky banter from the get-go. I thought to myself – *Lucy, stop it! You don't need to be cheeky and get involved.* It was on the cards, though. The more time went by, the more flirting occurred. The Aussies were laughing at us. Everyone could see there was some serious sexual tension between the two of us. As the night wore on, the more pool we played, the more alcohol we drank. Then suddenly, the shots started arriving. It all started getting really, really, messy. Then the flirting moved on to touching; not groping or anything like that, at first it was just gentle brush pasts, then hand touches as we exchanged the cue. I could see exactly what was happening and as much as I really fancied this guy, I could not get involved. Kyle hadn't had a drink for months because he'd been in a fight camp, and I hadn't drank since San Francisco, so we were both totally out of practice. It was all starting to get a bit naughty by this point. My girlfriend was falling all over the place. Some of the others were totally wasted as well. We were doing our best to continue playing pool, and pretend we had it together, but we weren't doing a very good job of that – but we were having fun, and it felt good.

I got to a point where I knew I needed to go home. I was getting too drunk and I knew I did not want to feel rough the next day, even though I had the day off. I said, "Guys, I'm going to go." I have always had a tendency to do that, actually. Most people carry on until they are totally obliterated; however, I knew when it was time to go — most of the time. Everyone was keen to stay on that night, or else they were heading in different directions to me; that's when it happened. Kyle said he was ready to go home too, and as we were going to the same place he would get in a taxi with me. Inside I was thinking — *Fuck, fuck, fuck, fuck, fuck*! On the outside, I said, "Okay, yeah fine." You know, playing it cool. I had no idea how I was going to navigate this situation because I knew myself and I could see what was going to happen. This was going to be a test of my willpower, and even though neither of us had actually indicated we liked each other, it was obvious.

In the taxi, I had a moment of clarity and decided to try and throw him off a bit. I said to him, "I think I might go and see my friend in his bar."

Kyle responded, "Okay, I'll come with you."

This wasn't going to be easy. I had made my excuse now, so I needed to follow through and go to my friend's bar. I had met this guy, my friend, on a big night out, through one of the Australian girls I was friendly with when I was last here in October 2013. He owned a few places around where I was training. We had become good friends. He had a cool little reggae bar, and I always felt safe with him, so I knew he'd talk sense into me. There was a connection between the two of us. It was like a brotherly sisterly love, we had a beautiful respect for each other, and we could talk about anything. We had spent many days and nights putting the world to rights. I figured that he would look after me if I went there.

I walked in and he was so happy to see me. Then he clocked the guy I was with and gave me a cheeky knowing smile. He offered us drinks, but I didn't really want one, I had only gone there to try and get away from the awkwardness of having to say no to Kyle. I had not mastered the art of 'no' being a full-sentence back in those days. Neither of us wanted drinks, he knew I was distracting from going home. He must have wanted to witness me squirming. We were now trapped in this bar making small talk, knowing each of us did not want to be there. I had actually made things so much more awkward because we were now going to have to do the walk of shame from the bar, back to the hotel together. Everything I had tried to avoid, I just bought in ten times worse. Well done, Lucy.

I got to the point where I thought I would try it once more, "I've got to go, you can stay here if you want?"

He looked at me strangely, "Why would I do that?"

It was a very valid question. I tried to answer and then surrendered to the fact that I could not avoid it any longer. I had to go home. I wanted my bed. (I said 'my bed' – not his!) It was time to surrender to whatever the Universe had intended for us, and let this situation unfold.

We started walking back and we were chatting. Of course, we're both a bit drunk so we kept colliding into each other, not on purpose – or at least it wasn't on purpose from my side. We were laughing. We had such a good night together, which is what we were mainly reflecting on. There had been some absolute characters out with us that night, so we were wondering where they were and what they were up to. We turned down the road of the hotel and I was thinking – *Yes! We've almost made it home safe.* We were passing the gym where he had been doing his training. The hotel was just within eyeshot, 50 yards away, maximum. We were almost there, and that's when he pulled me in and kissed me. He kissed me in a way that I had wanted to be kissed since Ricky. It was magical. Everything I had wanted to avoid was happening and as much as I wanted to stop, I couldn't. It felt so right. I knew that this situation was really frickin dangerous. I was so far from healing from the trauma of the previous year. He was only there for a few more days, and I thought – *This has just got a lot more complicated.* Let's face it, my whole story has been complicated, but where men are concerned it seemed to be more so. They were definitely my kryptonite, back in the day. At that moment in time, all I wanted to do was travel. I wanted to go and experience life without complications. Without a man. And then this guy comes along out of nowhere and sweeps me off my feet.

We were kissing, passionately, and then he picked me up to carry me the rest of the way. You can imagine what's going on in my head. There is something really sexy about a man who can effortlessly pick you up and carry you. I was so caught up in the moment, it felt so good to be that connected to someone, especially someone who was as gorgeous as he was. We stumbled back into the hotel reception. The people working there were laughing at us. They knew exactly what was about to go down, most likely they saw this kind of thing regularly. We were giggling like schoolchildren. I was telling Kyle to be quiet because most normal people were fast asleep; this was a place focused on fitness, so most people were looking after themselves, and only let their hair down once in a while. However, as much as I shushed him, we would end up laughing out loud at the mischief of what we were getting up to. We got to his room and he said, "Are you coming in?"

"No, no, no, no, no. I can't do that. Can't do that at all." We had another kiss and then I ran back to my room. I walked in, closed the door, looked at myself in the mirror and smiled a massive smile. It had not been on my radar, but I liked how I was feeling. I sat there revisiting everything that had gone on. Was I doing the right thing by saying no? How would things be tomorrow?

The next thing, there was a knock at my door.

Oh shit – he's at my door. What do I do now?

Well, the good intentions very quickly left the building. We had a crazy night that night, let's put it that way. There wasn't much sleeping taking place, for us – or our neighbours, I hasten to add. We had the most intense, crazy night ever. And from that moment onwards, we were pretty much inseparable. We'd go training together, then come back and go to the pool. We would go off and explore. We went to see the elephants and the tigers. One time we drove, in the middle of the night, up to this place called Big Buddha, where you could see the whole of Phuket. We had the most amazing time together. Everything that I never thought I would have, had found me when I least expected it. He had thrown a curveball into my life, in a really beautiful way. He had been divinely placed to assist my healing journey, that is for certain.

He scared the shit out of me, though. Not in a bad way, but because he was so vulnerable. He was so open, and I had never met a man like that. He wasn't damaged, or at least on the surface, he didn't appear to be. Obviously, like anyone, he had his baggage, but he wasn't damaged at all. He was not scared to be vulnerable in the slightest. He would ask questions without giving a damn if anyone judged him. It was like he knew assumptions were the mother of all fuck ups, so he wasn't afraid to ask questions.

I knew when we connected, that he only had a number of days of his trip left. I also knew it was going to pass very quickly. We had a beautiful friendship group around us, and they watched this relationship bloom out of nothing, and grow into something very quickly. There were even nicknames for us. We didn't care. We were happy in our little bubble.

Each day, we would do our own training, but we also trained together. We would go on runs and do stair and hill sprints together. It was a different kind of bond to any that I had ever experienced before. At no point did it scare me that he was going to leave in a few days, although I didn't want him to. I was more fearful about what the future was going to hold for me where relationships were concerned. So much had happened in the previous 12 months, before I left the UK, to make me feel that I had to stay away from men for a long while. This man had swooped in and reminded me of the absolute beauty there could be in the divine union between a man and a woman. I was desperate to be vulnerable enough to talk about what was happening between us, but I really did not want to ruin what we had, or mess up my future travels. It was a predicament. It could have been so easy to get caught up and swept away. I did to a point. We made some plans to see each other again. Well, when I say plans, we spoke about it. I did not necessarily believe they would happen. At this stage of my life, vulnerability was not a thing. Since my early years, I had learned to be tough. I had learned to suppress what was going on within me. I had also learned over the years that whenever I wanted to know what was going on between myself and someone else, as soon as I knew it either put me off them or things changed. I didn't want that to happen here. We were in a beautiful bubble of healing energy. He had kindly and unknowingly taken on the role to heal the hurt in me, to put my heart back together and lead me further down the path of enlightenment and love.

During this time, there was a real struggle taking place between my head and my heart. My head was telling me to remain single as I travelled the world. I had no idea who I would meet on the journey. I thought I might miss out on other opportunities because of Kyle. I also knew Ricky was coming to meet me at some point too. My heart, on the other hand, was telling me in no uncertain terms that this man had to be a part of the journey for a while. I didn't know how that would work out, though. No matter how much I attempted to pull away from him, my heart knew that this guy was the one to assist my healing.

What were the chances that I would travel to the other side of the world, then be in my first week of a trip of a lifetime, and meet someone from back home? How come I did not meet someone from Brazil or somewhere exotic that I hadn't travelled to before? God works in mysterious ways, that's for sure. He was a curveball; a lovely one at that, setting me on my path to love. Not all curveballs are there to lead you astray. It is worth remembering, we will receive all of the lessons we have chosen, whether we like it or not, when the time is aligned.

There was something about this guy, at this time. He was chosen.

56

The day before he was due to leave I stepped into mother mode. I asked him, "Have you checked your flight details? Got your passport? Checked in for your flight? Are you sure you've got everything sorted?" That was the project manager in me and the female motherly instincts all surfacing at once. He told me not to worry, he had it all sorted. So of course, I trusted it. The old Lucy would have said something along the lines of, "Show me your paperwork. I'll check it for you." And maybe I should have been more like that and saved him a whole heap of shit because he ended up missing his flight. Hilarious! The funny thing about it was, for days leading up to it he was talking about extending his trip and staying on a bit longer, and how he didn't want to go home yet. We were so caught up in our own little bubble that he completely missed his flight. We experience all we ask for, sometimes it takes a while, sometimes it is imminent. The Universe truly wanted to keep us together. That's the way we read it anyway. He didn't get to stay for long, though. The airline ended up putting him on a flight that seemed to take him all around the world, on his journey back to London. My goodness, that gave me so much fun over the years. I took the absolute piss out of him about that for a long time afterwards.

Once he had gone, I felt a bit lost. I had a lot of really beautiful friends that I had made, but for the last ten days, I had been immersed in a little bubble of love. I felt as if I had lost my right arm. I allowed myself to feel sad about missing him. For the first time, I did not distract from it. I allowed myself to recognise that this was actually a beautiful feeling I was experiencing. It meant I had feelings for this person and had not run away from them, despite everything that had gone on before my great escape from the UK.

Once Kyle got home, and I had stopped taking the piss out of him for screwing up his journey, we talked regularly – once a day, sometimes more. We never spoke about 'us' and what was going on, though. We were building a really beautiful friendship, and a connection. Each time we spoke, as much as I missed him physically being there, we grew a little deeper in friendship, which was something I had never really experienced before in a union. This was such huge, and necessary growth. How had I had such a distorted view on what a relationship could be? Especially as I had been in them for a huge part of my life so far.

I had it in my head that at some point I would like to do a fight in Thailand. I had watched my sister fight for many years, doing her mixed martial arts, and I'd been her chief cheerleader. I felt it was time to see if I had the discipline to focus on something like this. Up until this point in my life, I had not been the most consistent person in anything other than my career. I wondered if I had the guts to get in the ring and actually do it. I wanted to know if I had the strength and the dedication because to actually fight and be fit enough to go five rounds – which is what it is in Thailand – you've got to be at a whole new level of fitness. There is a mental strength required to get into a ring, knowing it's just you and your opponent. You've got to have something in you that will get you through those rounds because the first time you get kicked or punched, you are going to have your mind tell you to get the heck out of that ring. To keep going for another four or five rounds, you have to dig deep. It takes a lot of willpower, a lot of mental strength, and a flawless mindset. And I didn't have any of that at this point. I couldn't even turn a guy down! Now admittedly, he was a very attractive man, but that's not the point. The point was I was far away from a place of great discipline.

I started making stronger decisions, so the fight could become a reality. I decided I was going to stick around Thailand and train for a few more weeks, then do a visa run somewhere close and convenient, and then hop back. I thought about Malaysia or Laos as they were on my to-do list. Most tourists are allowed to stay in Thailand for up to 30 days, I had an extended visa, so I was ok for 60, then I had to leave, and I could re-enter again for another 60 days. My visa run conveniently coincided with a fight night that was taking place in Malaysia. There were a number of fighters from my gym on the bill, and my Aussie girlfriend was going, so I thought I would go over and support, and I could have a good explore around while I was there. I could get my new visa on return. The next trip after that would be to go off to Australia for a month over Christmas and New Year.

For now, though, I was going to focus on my training here in Thailand. My Aussie friend had introduced me to one of her good friends from Ireland. She was a beautiful, psychic soul who had settled over there with her business for some years. As she had been there for some time, she knew a lot of the Thai trainers. When she found out I was keen to do a fight, she introduced me to a trainer that was really good, and who would support me in my lead-up to a fight. I jumped at the chance. At that time I was in the intermediate class, and this trainer taught the fighters, so it was the perfect introduction to where I was focused on going. It was difficult to get in the eyesight of these trainers at the time. I wanted to be around somebody that was shit hot, super disciplined and, in all honesty, would not take my bullshit when I did not want to do something. I got away with quite a lot with some trainers. I could flutter my eyelashes or be super playful to distract from doing something I didn't want to do. It was an ego trick that I had mastered over the years. If there was an easy route, I would take it. However, there was no more easy route for me. I was choosing to level up and I knew it had to start with my physical. I was looking for somebody to get me ready, fight fit and mentally prepared to step into the ring. She introduced me to a phenomenal Thai trainer called Sanong. You only had to take one look at him to know that he would not put up with my nonsense. He scared the shit out of me. He was very tall for a Thai trainer, maybe six feet or more, relatively attractive, and extremely confident in his teachings. He took no nonsense from anyone, and pushed even the toughest of fighters to the point of them almost wanting to quit; however, he got results. His English was not very good, but that didn't matter. In fact, it made it much easier for me to focus and tap into the energies of the sport, rather than relying on the words. It was always interesting when I did something wrong, though, attempting to figure out what on earth he was talking about.

Looking back, I didn't realise it at the time, but what he had was true divine masculine oozing out of him. He was soft but extremely tough. You wouldn't mess with him or he would put you on your arse. He was extremely protective, yet he had won hundreds of belts from thousands of fights where he had caused serious amounts of damage. He was very well known around the world, and well sought after to train with. I was flattered, excited and a little scared when he agreed to train me. He held pads for a few minutes, and asked me to show him my technique. He said, "Strong, very strong for a woman." Yes, there were improvements that needed to be made, but my right hand was a bomb and they knew it. Every time I connected with a cross, you could see a little light ignite within him. A woman who could punch, and punch hard.

As much as I was scared about what I knew was coming from a training regime, I knew that this was it. I knew that this was going to be the opportunity that I had asked for. I said to him, via someone who could translate for me, "I'm here for a couple of weeks. I would like to train with you every day for a couple of weeks, and even Sundays if you will do it. I've got to go on a visa run to Malaysia, so I'll be gone for a little while and then I will be back." I promised him that I would still run and keep fit whilst I was in Malaysia, so that when I got back I was ready to start training again for a fight. "Will you organise a fight for me if I can improve my fitness?"

He touched my abs, laughed and said in Thai, to which my friend translated, "There is some work to do. I will train you and we will aim for a fight next year." *Perfect* – I thought! It's officially on. I have daily one-on-one training with this awesome guy, who I knew I could learn so much from, and I would also still do the classes and go running. Welcome to the world of training martial arts.

The training regime he put me through was rigorous and brutal. You were expected to run 5k before training in the morning. Then you would do a one and a half to a two-hour group training session which would involve more running, rounds on the pads and sparring. You were expected to focus on strength and conditioning, which I did around lunchtime. After lunch, you would be expected to run another 5k, followed by another two-hour training session in the evening, which was then followed by another run. It was about seven hours of training, every single day to toughen you up, lose the fat, and make you lean enough. When I say 'toughen you up', at the end of the session your trainer would more often than not punch you in the stomach, throw heavy medicine balls at your abs, just to prepare you for when somebody knees you or punches you in the fight. Your muscles are required to protect yourself. It was tough. It was not for the faint-hearted.

I had felt already, after just a month, that I was becoming fit. The runs were becoming easier, the training was becoming more pleasurable, and I was handling the punches to the face better. It was like a total rewiring was taking place in my brain.

During this period of time, I completely stopped drinking alcohol. It actually gave me the excuse to stop I had been looking for, since I was 16. I no longer had to do that to fit in. I had this new community that involved health and fitness instead. There was no way I could drink during this time as it would completely mitigate what I was doing. I was going through a massive transformation from this crazy, party girl. And even though I did get wasted on that night with Kyle, and I dipped back into the old world for one night, I did not like the person I'd been the next day. I felt resentful. I felt shame, I felt guilt.

I'd been training and I'd been really working on myself, and honestly, for the first time in my life, I started to fall in love with my body. I took photos of what my body looked like on my first day of arrival in Thailand because I knew that I was going to go on a transformational journey. She was broken. She was so poorly. She was so sick. And I've still got those photos, I look at them every day to give me the inspiration to remind me of where I came from. I started to embrace who I was, and the direction in which I was heading. Something really beautiful happens the moment you decide to be your body's friend. When you decide to make the commitment to look after her, honour her, even become friends. You may be reading this thinking how on earth can all that training and being punched in the face mean you want to be friends with your body? The truth is, I had not given her any attention for years. Here I was, focusing daily on what was best for her. What she required. What felt good from a food perspective. I became extremely conscious of her communicating with me, I was yet to find out what it all meant, though.

So even just a month in, my body was starting to physically change. I was starting to get a little bit more muscle, starting to feel like my lung capacity was much better, but the most important transition, from my perspective, was the shift in strength in my mind.

I asked my trainer if I could enter something called the 'Beatdown'. It was a once-a-month event at the gym I was training in. It gave people the opportunity to have an amateur fight if they so wished. He looked at me, without speaking, and shook his head. I accepted, I had been told, but I wanted to know why. I asked one of the other Thai trainers who could speak English to ask him his reasoning. The guy came back to me and said, "You are too strong, you will hurt someone." I felt a little flattered, actually, but at the same time, I was a bit concerned that he thought I needed something tougher. Some of the fights I had seen were pretty tough, and he was saying no to me being in them. What did he have planned for me?

After that conversation and a subsequent sparring session in the group, they stopped me sparring with women at all. I had been in a class sparring with a girl and she had been throwing bombs all over. We were supposed to spar quite lightly in the classes, but after a few occasions where she lost control and hit me full pelt a number of times, I hit her back, properly. That was the end of my sparring with women. I still needed practice, though, so they started throwing me in the ring to spar with the Thai young men, those who were around 15 to 17 – who I hasten to add had well over a few hundred fights each. They start young in Thailand. They were throwing me in the ring with people that were incredible fighters because I was very strong. They felt as if I could handle myself and it was good discipline for me. I was not technically gifted, I was still very much learning, and nowhere near as nimble as they were, but it was great practice for me.

I felt like I had a new lease of life, I was more focused on this than I had ever been on anything in my life. I really didn't want to go to Malaysia, it was an inconvenience. I wanted to continue training. I was becoming addicted to the feeling I got from being that fit and healthy. I would have stayed there forever if I could have done at that point. I really was in a truly healthy bubble for the first time in my life. Something that I had been craving for years. I was eating clean. I had more energy. I was connecting with people who genuinely saw something in me and wanted to help me, and more importantly, I was open to being helped and being guided. I was training with the most incredible guy, and his English was becoming better by the day as I had started teaching him. I had become very good friends with the mixed martial arts team, a well-known team of trainers who supported many UFC fighters around the world. They were phenomenal. I felt part of the family. They welcomed me into their community with open arms. A lot of the team were American, so of course, they loved the English accent, which helped. They would take the mickey out of my accent when I was training, to make me laugh. In their best British accent they would say, "Pass the cup of tea madam." Once again, I became one of the boys, even though they really honoured me as a female. They were very supportive of my dream to fight and would often cheer me on from the sidelines as I was training, and provide advice as to how I could navigate things better. I was loving being a student again. I trusted these people to help me. Very quickly, they were becoming my family. It was amazing how quickly it all happened.

57

It came to the time to fly off to Malaysia. I had finally accepted that I had no option but to leave for a while, so I started to get excited by the idea of waking up in a different place and a time when my body needed to, rather than at the crack of dawn to run 5k. It was going to be nice to have the freedom to eat when I needed to, rather than having to squeeze it in when I could, and that would also ensure my hernia wouldn't give me any discomfort whilst training. I always had to leave two hours between eating and exercising, or my hiatus hernia would cause issues. With the rigorous training schedule I had, it often felt like I was skipping meals, which was not the case, I was just having to eat smaller portions, and much more quickly. This was time to refuel and rest my body, to return stronger. I left all my stuff in Thailand and took a little backpack with me.

It is an extremely short flight from Phuket to Kuala Lumpur, about an hour, so as soon as we were up in the air, it was time to start our descent. Once we got there, the boys went to start weight cutting, running, and getting their bodies ready to fight. Us girls started exploring. It was extremely hot and humid. Much more so than in Thailand. It felt much busier than Phuket too. It was interesting to walk around, immerse in the culture, experience the food, and explore the key sights in all their glory.

A few days later, it was the weigh-ins for the fights. It is quite normal for people to fight at a much lighter weight than what they walk around at. The process leading up to the fight can be extremely rigorous on the body, so it must be done carefully. To put it in to context, Connor McGregor would walk around at eighty kilograms and cut to just under sixty-six kilograms for his fights. That's a significant weight loss to gain an advantage over smaller fighters. In later years, when I fought, I would drop five to seven kilograms to hit the weight I chose to fight at. In Thailand, they were slightly more lenient for the lower level fights, you could get away with missing weight by a little bit. In the UK, that was not the case; you had to hit the weight, or not fight, simple as that.

We were staying in a beautiful hotel in Malaysia, which felt very grand compared to where I had been staying. It was the hotel the fighters had been put in, so we chose to stay with them. It worked out well. Whilst the guys were doing their thing, getting weighed in and doing all of the promotional stuff that is involved in the fight scene, my friend and I were able to go off and do our own thing – swimming, running, training and exploring. We were able to go to the gym and train with the guys, but running in those temperatures is not fun, so we pretty much left them to it, until they were through the toughest bit of the weigh in.

The fights later that night were amazing. It was so great to be there and be immersed in it. I had been around this kind of environment for years by this point, so I was used to it, but being so closely involved in it in Malaysia was a cool addition to the memory books. A couple of the guys won that night, which was amazing, so we all agreed after a good refuelling that we would go and celebrate at the after-party that was being thrown for them.

Now, after a fight night, no matter the standard of the show, there is always an afterparty. Always. I had made the decision that I wasn't going to be drinking. I was so focused on my fight, even though I didn't know if there would ever even be a fight, but nevertheless, I wanted to prove I was serious. For the first time in my life, I felt disciplined enough to go out and not be involved in any of the shenanigans. I thought about Kyle over in England too. He would have loved the night we had just been to. Despite not knowing what was going on between us, I did not want to jeopardise anything. I was happy. I didn't feel drawn to join in the drinking activities at all. I knew I could celebrate in style with these people without drinking. I grabbed my bottle of water, and off I went. I was processing a lot that evening, in a good way. I was observing things that I would never have seen, had I been drinking.

The afterparty, as they always do, got a little bit crazy. Everyone was drinking, to celebrate their wins. And as much as there was a lot of alcohol being consumed, there was a really beautiful vibe about the place. There was no trouble. Now bear in mind, it was a roomful of fighters, and their supporters, plus lots of alcohol, so there was the potential for it to be feisty; however, everyone got on really well and had a good laugh. It was lovely to chat to lots of different people, and hear about how they got into fighting. It always fascinated me that most people I spoke to, found boxing or Thai boxing through feeling lost. They had come from challenging backgrounds and situations that they had needed to run from. Whether that be family, friends, gangs, or drugs. There was a thread that joined all of the fighters together. It was their escape. They had used the sport as an escape route, to get their discipline and life back on track. I was no different. As much as I had come from a high paid job, an abundant, some would say, privileged life, I had been lost in the murky waters, and had been unknowingly looking for something; and thankfully, found it. Deep down, as much as fighting is an individual sport when you are in the ring, we were all searching for our soul family; the ones who truly got us.

As we were leaving the party in the early hours of the morning, one of the guys who had been fighting that night asked us all to get into a selfie shot. There were about 15 of us in the lift in total, although only 11 of us actually made it into the shot. It's a great image and one I'll keep forever. It captures how happy and content we all were. All from different areas of the globe, with one commonality that joined us all, which was our passion for martial arts. That picture is one of my favourite travel pictures. Unknowingly, it was the calm before the storm.

58

We rolled out into the street, laughing and playful. We had such a blast that night. I was the only one who was completely sober, although no one was particularly wasted. One of the trainers that was with us – an ex UFC fighter, who I hasten to add was very attractive – put his arm around my shoulders. We were only friends, but it just felt right. We were walking along, laughing, deep in conversation with his arm around my neck. We were following the others to get taxis back to the hotel. As we were walking, we passed other people walking the other way. Out of nowhere, two men approached us, one of them made a beeline for me, knocking into me and shoving me out the way. As he did that, my earring went flying out of my ear. I was sober, but there was no way I was going to let someone do that to me. I shouted after him, "What the fuck are you doing? Who do you think you are?" I was pissed off with the way he had run into me and did not even apologise for doing it. The guy who had his arm around me asked the guys what they were doing. The guy who knocked into us was being extremely derogatory. As this standoff was taking place, a beautiful Asian lady came over to me and handed me my earring back. I thanked her so much. She said if I needed any witnesses, to let her know. It was very sweet of her, but I felt it would be over as quickly as it started.

I was wrong.

The coach who had his arm around me, stood in front to protect me. I remained quiet and let him deal with it. I have absolutely no idea what got said after that, but one of the other lads, who had won his fight and had been drinking, must have seen something that I did not. He launched a running superman punch straight at the guy who barged into me. I thought – *Oh shit! This is not going to end well.* The guy who had barged into me did not realise he was starting on a whole group when he picked on the smallest person to bully. He must have thought we were a couple and we would be an easy target.

It kicked off big time in the streets of Malaysia. The local guy then attacked one of our guys, so he defended himself, and then it all went off. There were people coming from all angles to join in. It was like some sort of crazy fight scene from a movie. People who were not part of the fight team – I can only assume they were friends of the two guys who started the fight – started getting involved. It was the most bizarre situation ever. I had never seen anything like it, and I'll be honest, I'd happily avoid anything like it again in the future. The two instigators were obviously looking for a fight, and unfortunately for them, they picked on the wrong people. The fight team were shouting at us girls to get in a taxi and get out of there. Unfortunately, we didn't listen, we were pecking away like mother hens, protecting the men – which we really didn't have to do. They did not ask us to, and quite frankly, if anyone had it covered, it was them.

We heard the sirens coming. We were worried about the guys being arrested. That would not have been good, at all. We somehow managed to gather the guys and bundle them into taxis, but there were only enough spaces for them, so we told them we would get the next one. They did not want to leave us, but they couldn't afford to get into trouble. They didn't fancy spending a night or three in a Malaysian cell. We assured them we would see them back at the hotel shortly. As they were pulling off in their taxis, the two guys who had started the trouble spotted us being left behind and started running towards us. It was so dramatic. Thankfully, our guys spotted this happening so they stopped the taxis, piled out and went after the two guys again. What a mess! It was crazy, it was mayhem.

Eventually, the two troublemakers got away, and we got most of the boys out of there before the police arrived. One of the guys stayed with my friend and me to get a taxi home with us, and to make sure we were safe. What was really interesting was, as soon as I got in the taxi my girlfriend started having a go at me, saying that everything that happened was all my fault. I thought – *Wow!* But, I didn't say anything at all. I hadn't asked for somebody to rip my earring out, I certainly didn't ask for him to start on the guy who stood up for me. I didn't ask for any of that to happen, but she clearly thought I did. She projected all of her shit onto me that night, and I allowed it at the time. I hadn't had anything to drink so I was more rational about it, thankfully. The old Lucy would have lost her shit, especially if I had been drinking. In this instance, I kept my cool. I sat there quietly and just thought about what had gone on that night. The highs and the lows.

Looking back on it, there were so many lessons to be learned from that situation. I was proud of myself for not feeling that I needed to defend myself to my friend. It was her shit, not mine.

We eventually got back to the hotel, and everything was a mess. One of the coach's hands had swollen big-time, where he had hurt it in the street fight. He was okay, but there was definitely a little bone broken in there, you could tell by the way it had swollen. Other people in our group were buzzing around, chatting about what had gone on, revelling in the adrenaline of the situation. There were lots of cuts and bruises, from both their professional fights and the street fight. It was a shit show. And all I kept doing when I got back, because of what she had said, was apologising. I had stepped into emotional trauma response mode. "I'm so sorry. I didn't mean to create that situation," I kept repeating that to anyone that attempted to talk to me. Everybody, without exception, told me it wasn't my fault, and that I had done nothing wrong. They all believed that those guys wanted a fight with the person that I was walking with. They thought that they could humiliate him and bully him, not realising he was part of a team, and part of a family that had each other's backs, through thick and thin.

I decided the best thing to do was leave the situation with my girlfriend until the next day. I had said sorry as many times as I could, and tomorrow we could do whatever it took to make sure that everything was good again. She passed out very quickly anyhow ,thank goodness. It saved any more uncomfortable discussions. She had been drinking through the evening, so I sat there for quite some time processing what had gone on because I felt bad. She had made me feel bad. She had made me feel as if it was all my fault, and I took it on board. I know now that we get to choose how we respond and I clearly wanted to be the victim right then.

The next day, we were flying back to Thailand. We had been there a few days, and besides the incident the night before, we had had an amazing time. We had done what we needed to do in Malaysia, which is such a beautiful place. I will always have a lot of love for it. I ended up visiting there a number of times during my time away, and it was only this once that I had any sort of issue.

As we were getting ready to go back to the airport, my friend was really hungover and really quiet. I apologised once again to the guys. They were adamant that I had done nothing wrong and that I should stop feeling bad about it.

On the journey back to Thailand, there was a massive crew of us at the airport. We had a lot of fun. Everyone kept calling me Scrappy

Do, mainly because my friend had accused me of starting the fight, so they decided to keep the banter going. They were playing with me because they knew she had got under my skin. One of the guys said, "Oh my God, we're all going to come to your fight because it's going to be an absolute brawl." I loved it to be honest because from my perspective the whole experience had been an eye-opening opportunity to experience that world. They had opened up their hearts to allow me to be part of their team, which was really amazing. The protection I had felt from these people, who just a few months before had been total strangers, felt good. For many years I hadn't felt like I'd been part of anything, I hadn't felt like I really belonged anywhere. And here I was being myself, not the alcohol, drugged-up version of Lucy. This was me being me. This was me with a raw honesty that was accepted and appreciated.

59

We arrived back in Thailand, after a fun journey. I spoke to Kyle, who was back in the UK, and told him what had happened. He was absolutely roaring with laughter, "You're a fucking nightmare. What are you like?" He wasn't wrong. Then he said to me, "Why don't we meet up somewhere soon? I can get a week off work in November if that works for you?" Wow! I was not expecting that. What a nice surprise. So we banded around a few ideas and then agreed to meet up in Dubai. Now, this was something to look forward to.

It was still really weird, though, because neither of us knew what was going on between us. We got on really well. We spoke all the time. It was like we were in a relationship, but we'd never actually spoken about it. As much as I wanted to know for my ego's sake, and to feel safe, I also didn't want to know because I was travelling and I did not want the responsibility – even though it was clearly already there. I guess I still wanted to do what I wanted to do. By that, I do not mean sleeping around or anything like that. I never looked at anybody else, even though I didn't know if we were a thing or not. It just was not resonant to me to be intimate with many people. I was becoming more myself. It wasn't the true essence of my soul to hurt or cheat on somebody, and although I had done it when I was younger, that was because I was hurting myself back then. At this stage of my life, I didn't want to be sleeping with lots of different people. I was starting to value myself. I really just wanted to be loved. I wasn't going to damage this situation with Kyle because I actually really liked him. I felt as if we were going to go on an adventure together.

Over the course of the next few weeks, I upped my game significantly because I had the full support of the fight team. They were keeping a close eye on how things were going, in readiness for this fight I was hoping to have. They would offer up helpful advice and guidance on how I could improve and be stronger than any opponent. They would hold the pads for me, pull me up on my stance, encourage me to do more, and just push me harder and harder. I was open to receiving all of their wisdom. This was all brand new to me, so I surrendered. I remembered my friend and how I had admired her ability to learn from the trainers and so I did the same. I was willing to put in the work to achieve it all. It was a really beautiful experience. It really helped me to get aligned and disciplined. It was the catalyst to start feeling into this sense of who I was always meant to be.

I didn't quite realise it at the time because I was training, and then after the intense training, I would have to rest because I was exhausted, but essentially, I was being forced to go inwards. I didn't want to watch anything on TV – Thai television is not the best anyway. The stuff I used to like made me feel drained, so I just stopped doing it. My intuition was working overtime. I did not feel drawn to sit on social media. I did not want to sit on my phone at all, so instead, I would go to sit by the pool or walk on the beach, go in the ocean, and immerse in nature. I felt really drawn to stuff that I had never invested in before. If I only had a couple of hours in between training sessions, I would get my bikini on and go down to the beach – which was only about 20 minutes away on my moped. I would get there and throw myself in the sea, then on the way back I would grab some food and get ready to go to training again. It was so beautiful. It was such a simple life. I didn't need anything. I didn't want for anything. As long as I had food, the beach, the sun, and training I was more content than I had ever been.

Now, towards the end of October, my trainer told me he thought I was doing really well, I was getting stronger by the day, and he thought I was ready for a fight. Not the best timing, though, because I had to tell him I was buggering off to Dubai for a week. With hindsight, it was a silly move because I had worked so hard to get fight-ready, but I guess that's what happens when you have emotions and feelings running through you, you do crazy shit. It was Kyle or the fight. I felt that I could fight anytime. Who knew if Kyle would still be there in the new year when I was maybe ready to see him?

I was due to be going to meet Kyle at the beginning of the second week of November. We were really excited to see each other. Neither of us knew what to expect. He wasn't particularly good at flying, as you've heard, so I wondered if he'd even show up at all, or end up in a different country. We had a lot of banter about that leading up to our reunion. And then, before long, it was time for our trip.

I trained hard leading up to going away. I was determined not to lose that level of fitness in a week in Dubai. On the plane on the way over, my mind was working overtime again. I was thinking – *Is he going to show up? Is he going to be there on time? How is this whole thing going to work?* I arrived in Dubai first and went straight to the hotel to check in. It was stunning. We had made such a good choice. I had received a message from him whilst I had been in the air to confirm he had boarded and would see me at the airport when he landed. I had a couple of hours before he arrived, so I went to the room, got freshened up, and then headed back to the airport where I grabbed a tea and waited.

The next thing I knew, he was standing there in front of me. It was so weird seeing him again. A good kind of weird, I hasten to add. Reunited after a couple of months of only seeing each other on a screen. I had changed a lot in this time. I was a lot fitter. I was a lot browner. Aesthetically, there was so much that had shifted, but there was also a catastrophic shift that had taken place inside of me. I had found a level of peace, something that I had actually admired in him. I had found a level of honesty too, something else I had admired in him. When he found me at the airport, it was like we'd never been away from each other. He scooped me up and gave me a massive hug and a kiss – which, let's be honest, is really inappropriate in Dubai Airport. Getting arrested wouldn't have been the best start to our trip, but we made it out of there safely.

The trip was incredible. We did some really cool things. We got on just as well as we had done in Thailand, if not better. We went to loads of water parks, beaches, shopping malls, deserts, skiing, and loads of different places to eat. We had the most incredible time together. We were so comfortable in each other's worlds.

One night, I suggested that we went to the hotel that I had stayed in when I took that fateful call from my mum about my grandad being sick. They had a good bar with a pool table, and we both loved playing pool, so we headed there for a couple of games. We were having a couple of drinks, playing pool, and being cheeky and flirty with each other. It was getting towards the end of our time together, so we were doing whatever we could to create nice memories. It had been such a lovely trip. We decided that we would have a couple of drinks as a bit of a sendoff, but nothing too much. I noticed there was a guy, dressed all in white, sat in one of the booths near the pool table. He was on his own, although clearly waiting for someone. He engaged in conversation with me. I was fascinated by him. He seemed a very kind man, genuinely interested, and clearly oozing wealth. Although I had been to Dubai a few times before this trip, I had never bothered to find out what the different colours meant on the outfits that the men would wear. So I seized the opportunity to ask him all about it. As I've mentioned previously, I'm not a fan of research, I prefer to talk to people. That is how I like to learn. I was always a bit of a social butterfly, so Kyle would roll his eyes at me. He joked that he thought the guy had a soft spot for me, even though he was old enough to be my dad, if not older. Whilst we were talking, another guy came into the bar to meet him, a much younger American man. The guy in the white excused himself from our conversation and told me he had some business to attend to, but that we should join him afterwards if we felt drawn. Kyle wasn't best pleased with the thought of it. He tried to coax me out of the bar before their business was complete, but I was oblivious. I chatted to anyone and had a good time doing it. I was nosey, I wanted to know everything about everyone and everything. I wanted to love everybody. I loved getting to know people. Kyle just wasn't like that. It was good, in a way, because we were opposites. We balanced each other out in so many ways.

We continued to play pool, and we got more drunk – unintentionally. The two men invited us over to their table, as they had finished their meeting. We obliged and said we would join them for a short time. We went over and immediately they asked us what we were drinking.

I said wine for me, so they ordered me a bottle of expensive wine. They asked Kyle what he wanted, he said Jack Daniels and coke and so they ordered him a bottle of JD. Kyle and I were already slightly well-oiled at this point. We shot each other a look of surrender. We had not even formally introduced ourselves at that point, so we did. Once we were acquainted, the guy in the white said to me, "So Lucy, tell me all about yourself." I found it a bit weird, to be honest, but the alcohol kicked in, and so I told him what I thought he might want to know. I said, "Well to cut a long story short, I'm currently on a break from work after working in the investment banking world as a project manager for over twelve years. I suffered burnout a short time ago, and now I'm travelling the world."

He said, "Oh my gosh, that sounds amazing. Not so good about the burnout. Are you okay now? I am actually looking for a project manager for a big music project I've got. Would you be interested?"

The old Lucy programming kicked in briefly. It did not help that I was under the influence of alcohol, and probably wanting to show off a little bit in front of Kyle. For the first time in months, I was back thinking of the money. I was sat in the company of someone clearly very wealthy. Both Kyle and I had mentioned his watch within seconds of noticing it. It was stunning, it had diamonds all over it – but at the same time, it somehow didn't look ostentatious.

I had said to him, 'Your watch is beautiful." Kyle nodded his head in agreement. There was no denying it, it was stunning.

He replied, pointing at Kyle, "When you marry this man, I will give this to him as a gift."

I jumped in, "Wait a minute, what about me?" and started giggling.

"Only joking," he said. "I'll buy you a matching one too."

This was where Kyle joined in, "Well we better get married then," and he winked at me.

"Excuse me, can we stop pimping me out here, please?" I joked. We were having a laugh with these strangers. It was funny how we connected so quickly.

After a little while of joking around, he navigated the conversation back to the project. Basically, what he was doing was creating a project whereby people could buy music online. Back in 2014 in Dubai and the United Arab Emirates, this wasn't a thing really. We have normalised it now through Apple Music, Spotify and companies like that, but back then it wasn't so prevalent, people were still using iPods and devices to listen to their music – so this guy was well and truly on it. I was interested too in one sense. I trusted this man, but Kyle kept rolling his eyes at me, to keep me grounded. He reminded me that I was travelling and should really stop getting distracted. He was very good like that. I thought about things for a moment. What a random, incredible opportunity that had fallen in my lap. Divine alignment I had believed. I thought that there must be a sign in this. I said, "If I were here on holiday, I would take you up on the offer. However, I'm travelling, so I'm going to have to say no. I have worked so hard to get here, to where I am now, with freedom, travel and living out my heart's desires. Thank you for the offer, and thank you for recognising something in me. But, I have to say no."

The guy was a bit shocked and taken aback. Clearly he was not used to being turned down, which of course made him even more keen. "When are you flying home?" he asked. "Let me take you to meet my whole family. You can meet my wife. You can meet my children."

"I don't know what that's going to achieve," I replied.

"I want you to know I'm a family man. Come and see where I live. I live in a very lovely house, you will like it."

"I bet you bloody do," I said cheekily. "It is still no, though"

The guy went to the toilet at that point. The American guy that was with him leaned in and said, "His house is not a house. It's like a fucking castle, it's like a palace."

Oh gosh, what am I doing? How have I ended up in this situation? Thank goodness for Kyle. Mind you I would never have been in Dubai, being put in this situation, if it had not been for Kyle. When he returned from the toilet he persisted, "Just come and meet my family and check it out. If not tomorrow, the next day. If you have to extend your trip, I will fly you, first class, back to Thailand."

At that point, my ego really piped up, because flying first class on Emirates had always been on my bucket list. My ego was screaming, *"Do it, do it, do it, just imagine the experience."*

He kept going, "I'll put you up in my hotel in your own private suite. You can both stay"

He had a hotel for fucks sake!

"I'll put you up in the best suite in my hotel. I will make you so comfortable."

He was trying to buy me. And as much as I wanted to say, "Heck, yes" and name my price, all whilst living the dream, flying back to Thailand from Dubai first class! I was buzzing with the whole idea of it, but something inside of me, the real essence of Lucy, had to say, "I'm sorry, I can't do it."

At that point in my life, bearing in mind the world I had just come from, I was really proud of myself, I was teetering on the edge. It was like the gymnasts that walk on beams; they have to have incredible balance, and sometimes they wobble over on one side and they have to correct themselves. That's what I was doing. I was navigating this new voice. I was navigating this new person. And, most impressively, I was doing it under the influence of alcohol at this point. The old Lucy would have said, *"Heck yes. Thanks Kyle, now jog on."*

But I didn't.

Instead, I said, "Thank you so much, I really appreciate your offer, and in another lifetime I would have said yes." He had really massaged my ego. I felt really important that somebody like that would want me. Looking back, I had dodged a huge curveball. It was a blatant test from the Universe. As a last-ditch attempt, in the typical fashion of someone who doesn't take no for an answer, he gave me his card and he said, "Lucy if you ever change your mind, call me. Keep in touch with me, and if you ever come back to Dubai I'd like to catch up with you." I looked at his card, and of course, he was a Sheikh. All of a sudden, it made sense.

I actually kept in touch with him a little bit after I left Dubai. Every now and again, we would drop each other a message. I did see him one other time when I was back in Dubai, which was really nice. I made a friend for a short period of time, but I lost touch with him eventually when I changed my phone.

The next morning, we didn't feel so great. We had drunk a lot of alcohol the night before, completely unexpectedly, so we just chilled around the pool. We were both flying back to our respective countries that night. Kyle was going back to the UK, and I was going back to Thailand, so we enjoyed some special time together, being present and connected before we had to say our goodbyes once again.

We had the conversation, though. That conversation. He actually started it, because I was not going to do it, let's be real. He vulnerably asked, "What's going on with us? What are we going to do?

When am I next going to see you?" As much as I had wanted that question. I really did not know what to say. I was emotionally stunted when it came to situations like this, and I had so many conflicting thoughts running through my head. The problem was I was going back to Thailand to do a bit of travelling. I was going to carry on with my Muay Thai training whilst on the road, so I did not know how much time I would be able to free up to connect with him. I was going to different areas to explore and finish Thailand in its entirety. Then I was going to go to Australia for Christmas for about a month, which was even more of a time zone difference to what we were already on. It wasn't going to be easy. I had my own plans and they weren't really involving this beautiful soul that was looking back at me.

I looked at Kyle and I just didn't know what to say to him because I didn't want him waiting for me, but I also didn't want him to find somebody else. I really liked him. We had a very special connection. He was making me evolve in ways I never knew possible, even though I wasn't fully recognising it. He was really helping me step into my truth. He was starting to help me get connected back to my true heart and what felt good to me. He was holding space for me to heal and to remember who I was destined to be. There was no way I wanted to let that go. I also had a little niggle in the back of my mind about Ricky. He was going to be in Thailand sometime soon. I felt guilty thinking about Ricky because I truly liked Kyle, but I couldn't help feeling that there was something unfinished there too.

There was a lot going on at this particular time. I didn't want to lose Kyle, so I reasoned with him, and said, "I have a wedding to go to in Cyprus in March. We will keep in touch regularly. We'll video chat and talk all the time, but wherever I am in the world, on the way to the wedding, I will fly back to the UK. I will come and see you for a few days so we can spend time together, just us. Then I will fly to Cyprus. How does that sit with you?" He was happy. He picked me up off the floor and gave me a huge kiss. When he put me down, I said, "Please do not tell anyone that I'm in the UK otherwise people will expect to see me." He was cool with that. And so, that was the plan we made. Six months later, we were going to see each other again.

Six months seemed like two minutes away. It sounded so easy, but in reality, I was asking a lot for someone to wait around for me, whilst I was off doing my own thing.

That night, I flew back to Thailand. I was gutted to be leaving him. A massive part of me thought about going back to the UK. It was so strange, I had travelled to the other side of the world and finally found someone from back home. I thought – *Fuck it, just go home and enjoy it!* But then there was another part of me that also thought – *You've waited all your life to travel like this. Don't fuck it up now. You know you'll resent him one day, if it goes wrong.* So I stuck to the plan.

On the plane back to Thailand, I was all over the place mentally and emotionally. I reflected on the plane about the offer that the Sheikh had proposed. I felt as if I'd made the right choice, even though the money was still playing on my mind a little bit. The programming runs so deep. It's actually quite scary when you realise quite how deep it does go.

I thought about Kyle a lot on the journey home. One moment I was really ecstatic because we'd had such an amazing week together. The next moment I was heartbroken that it was going to be six whole months before we saw each other again. We had talked about the possibility of him coming out to join me and travel. He had itchy feet too and had openly talked about the possibility of quitting his job to join me travelling. That was playing on my mind as an option too. I thought that would be the best solution all round.

I landed back in Thailand and realised I had not even given the place a second thought whilst I'd been away. As soon as I landed, though, I remembered why I loved coming back here as much as I did. I was greeted with all the incredible sights and smells again. The smells of the orchids, the food, and also the heat. There's no suitable description for the smell of the heat when you get off the plane. It hits you out of nowhere and it's such a familiar sensation. The colours were so bright also. Now that I was back in Thailand I realised what a sterile environment I'd just come from. Everything in Dubai was super clean. It was white, it was glistening. Don't get me wrong it was beautiful too, but it lacked the heart and soul that Thailand had.

I went through Thai customs very quickly. I knew what I had to do, having flown in and out as many times as I had done recently. I knew how to navigate it with ease and grace. I was becoming a local. I knew who I needed to smile at to get to the front, and how to speak a little Thai, which always went down well. Being there was really starting to feel like home.

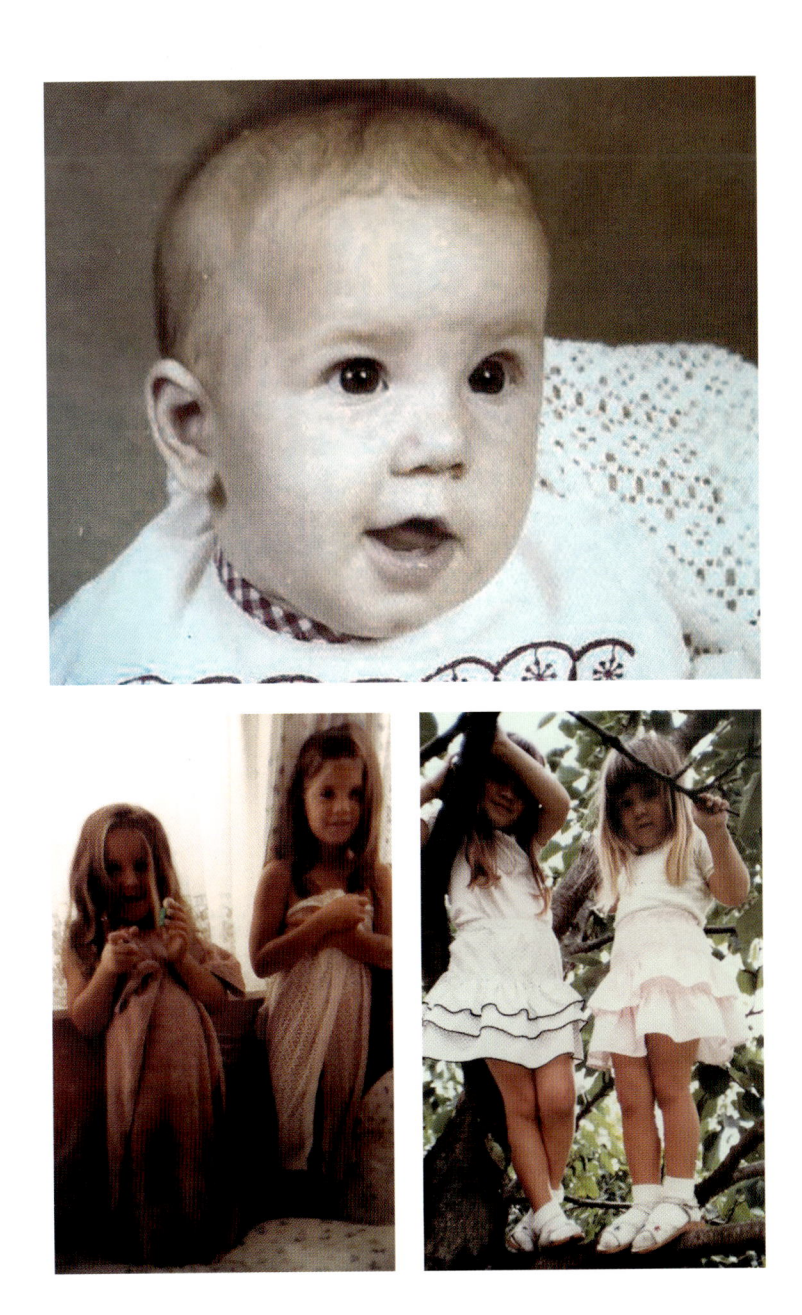

Top: Me as a baby, around 9 months. Bottom left: Kirsty (5 years old) looking like butter would not melt and me (3 years old) being cheeky. Bottom right: Kirsty (6 years old) and me (4 years old) up a tree hiding out.

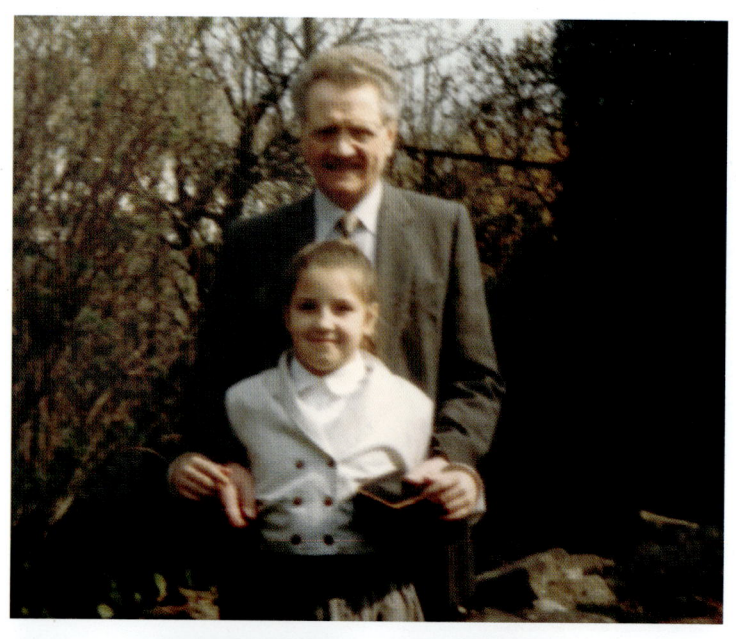

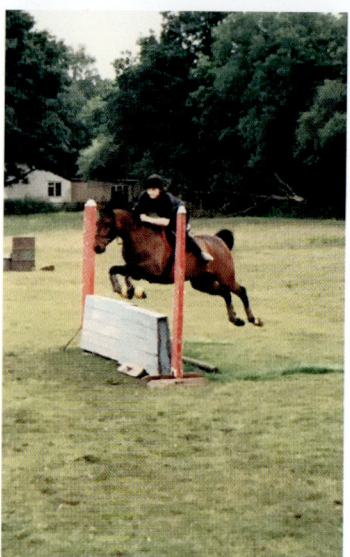

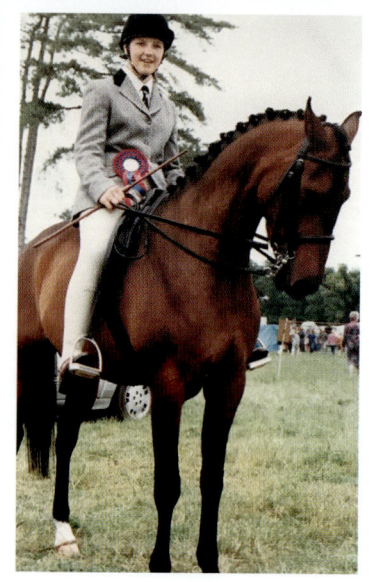

Top: My late grandad and I when I was about 9 years old. Bottom left: Harry and I flying round a cross country course. Bottom right: Harry and I after winning Working Hunter Pony Championship.

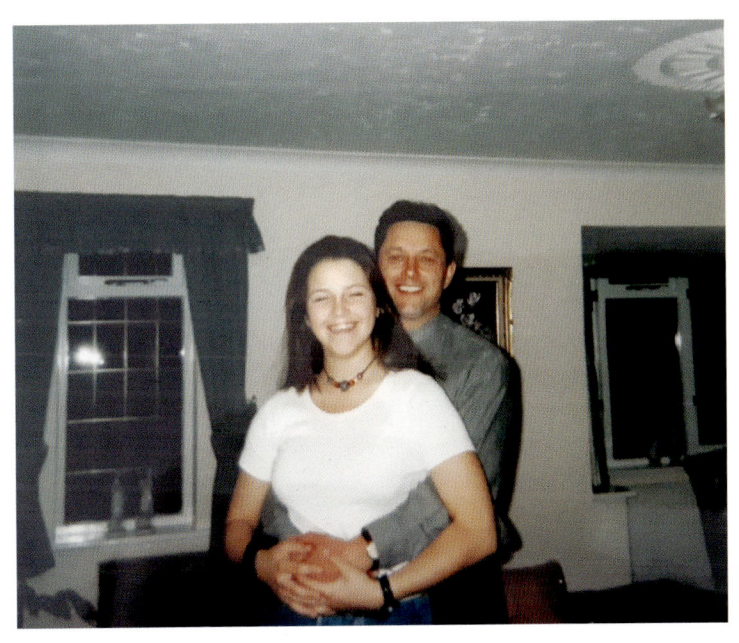

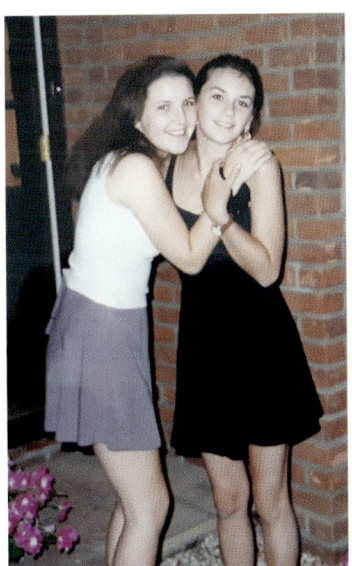

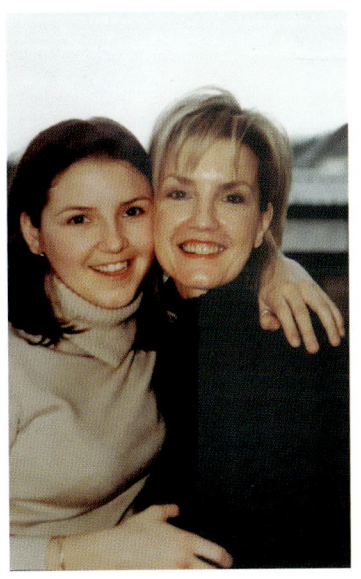

Top: My stepdad Mark and I. Bottom left: My sister Kirsty and I in the doorway of the bungalow where all the revelations took place.
Bottom right: My beautiful mum and I.

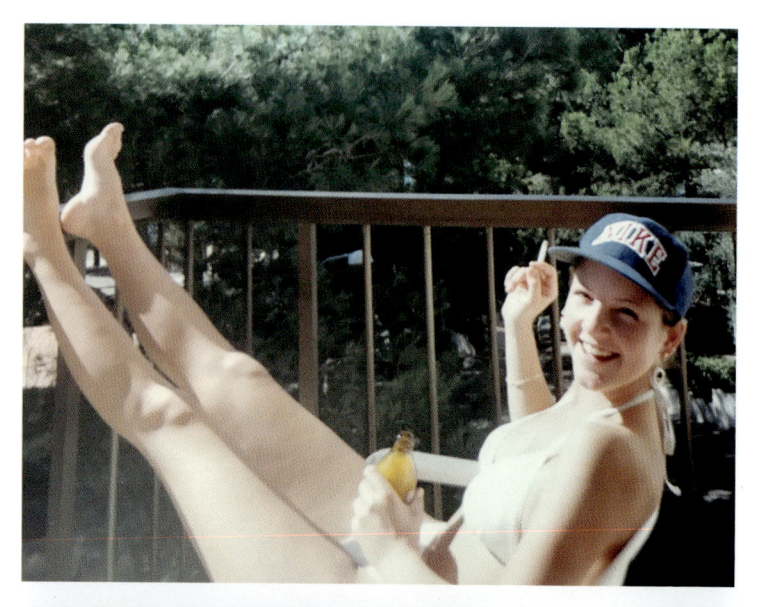

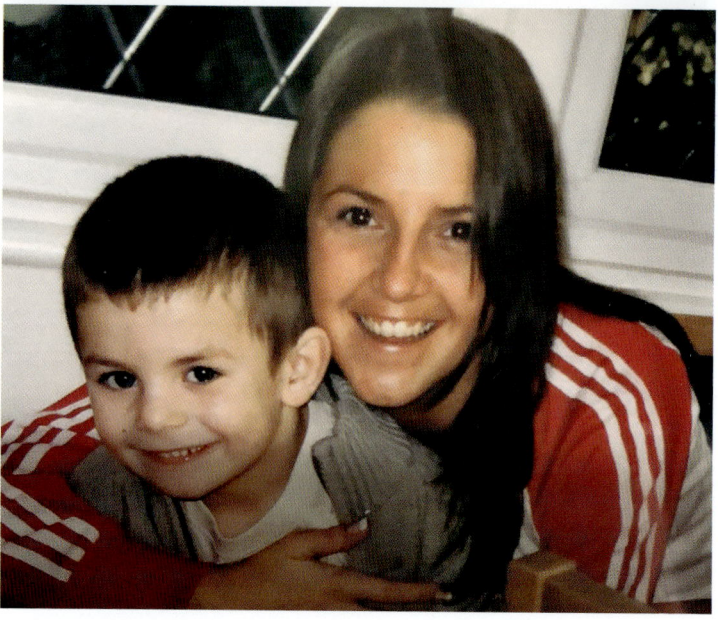

Top: At 20, in Magaluf smoking! Bottom: My gorgeous nephew Josh and I.

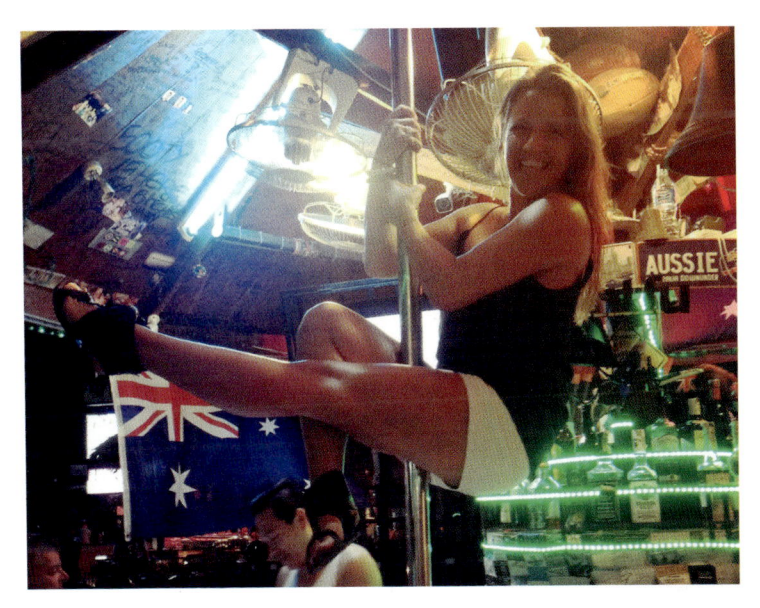

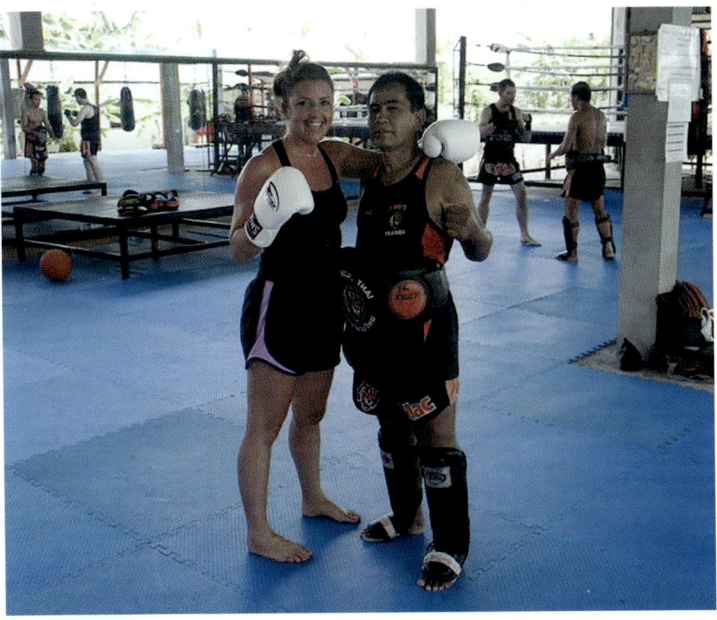

Top: Pole dancing in a bar in Thailand in 2013. Bottom: My first ever Muay Thai trainer in Thailand who passed from lung cancer between visits.

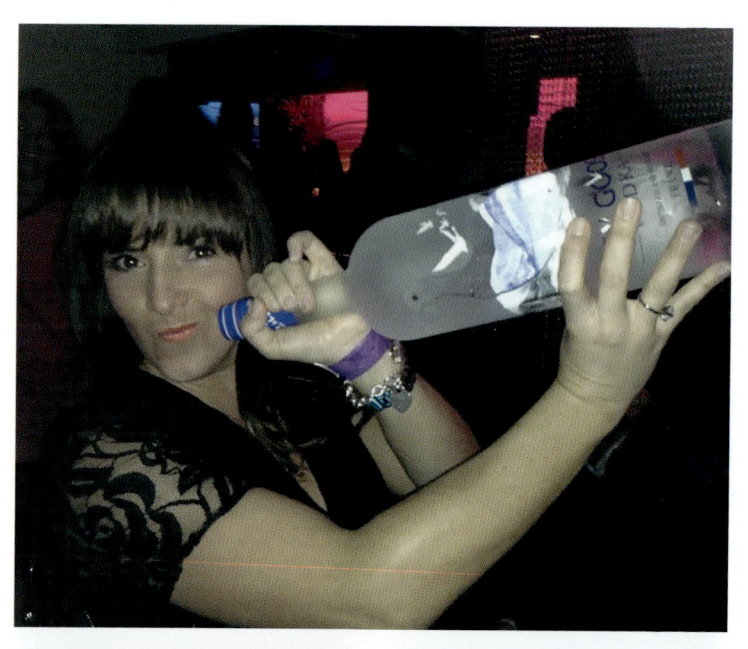

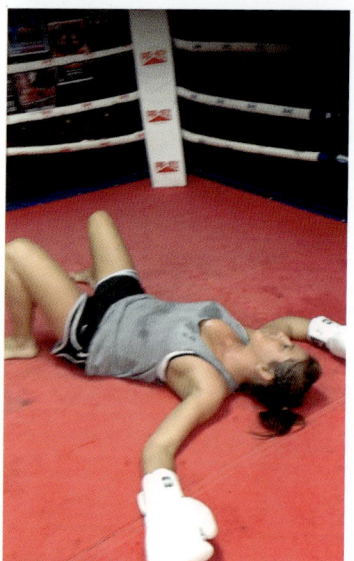

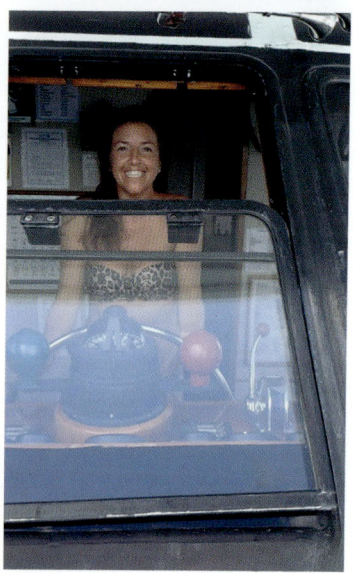

Top: Birthday antics in February 2014. Bottom left: KO'd during training at my sister's ex-partner's gym in Kent. Bottom right: Driving the boat in the Galapagos Islands.

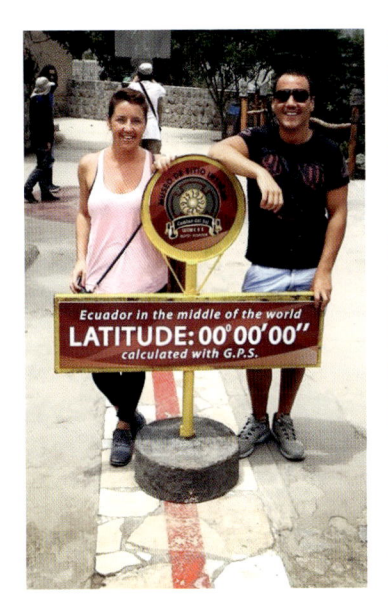

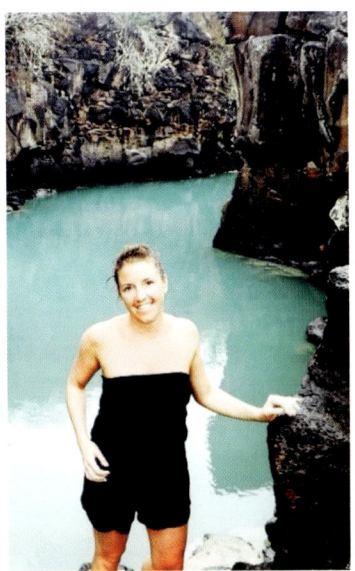

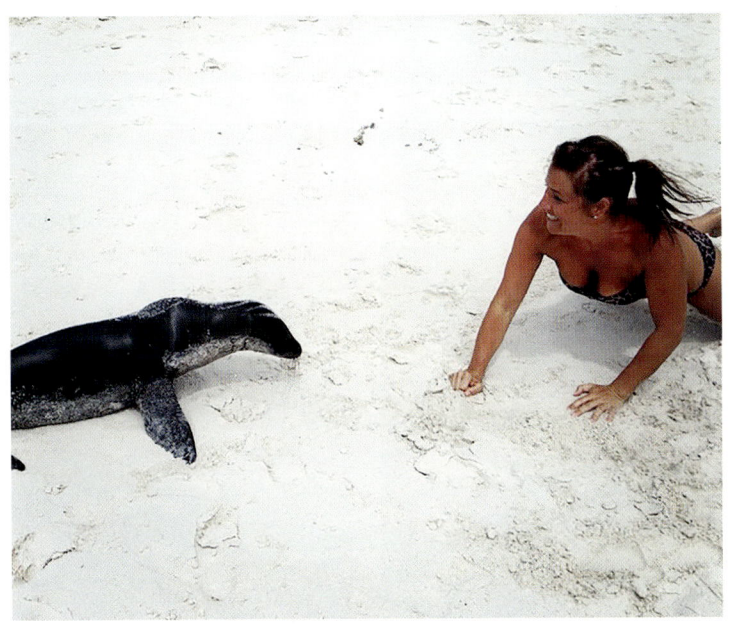

Top left: On the equator line with Ricky in Ecuador. Top right: The Love Channel, Galapagos Islands. Bottom: Fun with the sea lions in the Galapagos Islands.

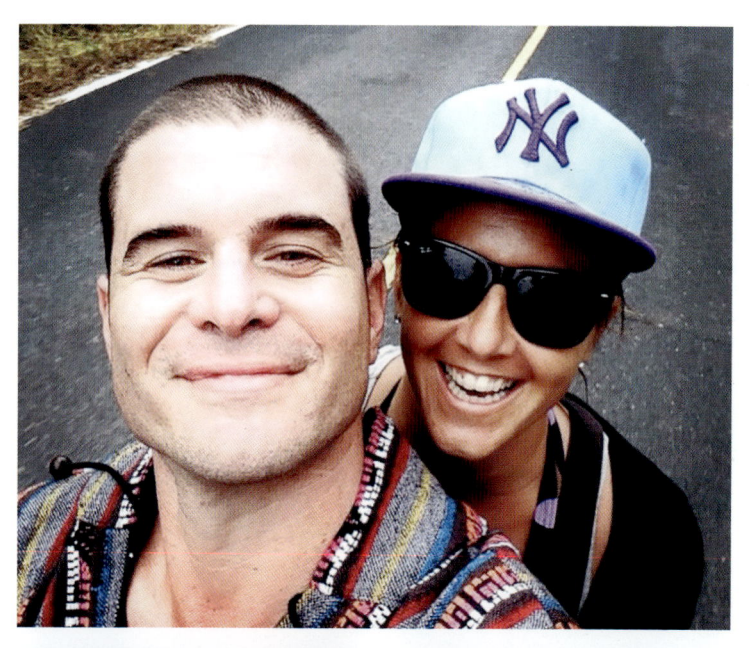

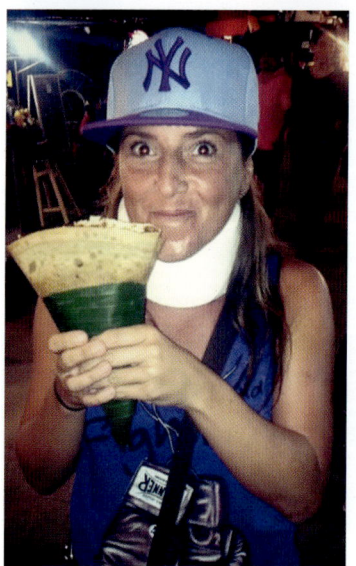

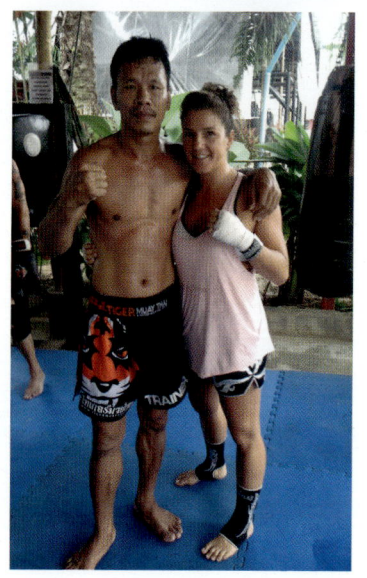

Top: Jared and I (Bert and Ernie) cruising round North Thailand on a moped. Bottom left: Post fall neck brace with the biggest Nutella and banana pancake possible. Bottom right: My Thai trainer for my first fight, Sanong, and I.

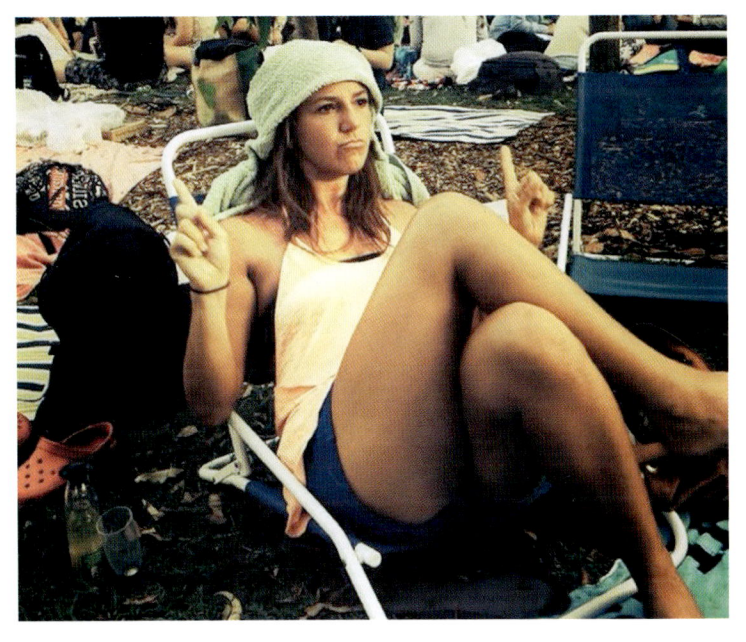

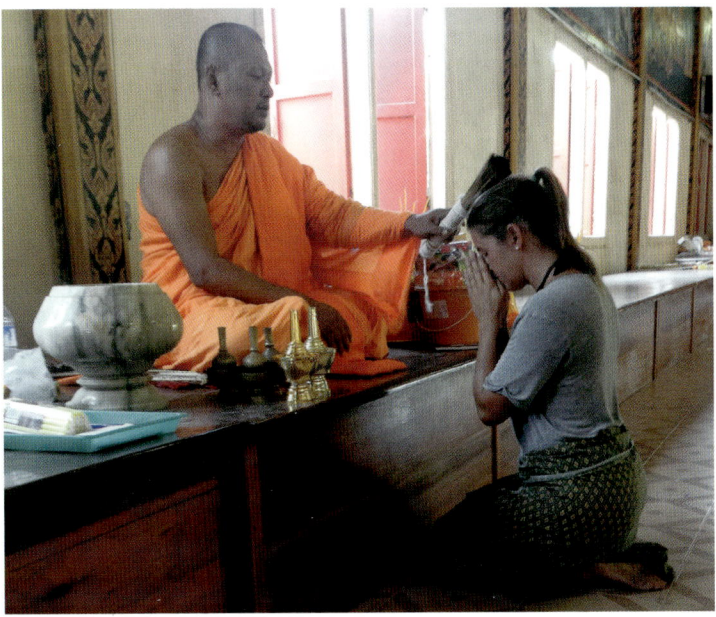

Top: New Year's Eve in Sydney. Bottom: Being blessed by a monk for the second time in one day prior to my first fight.

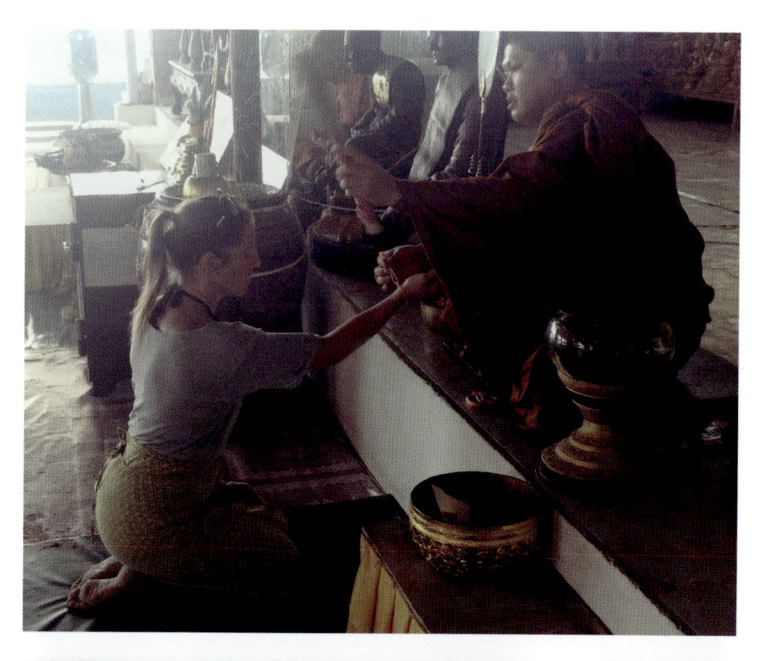

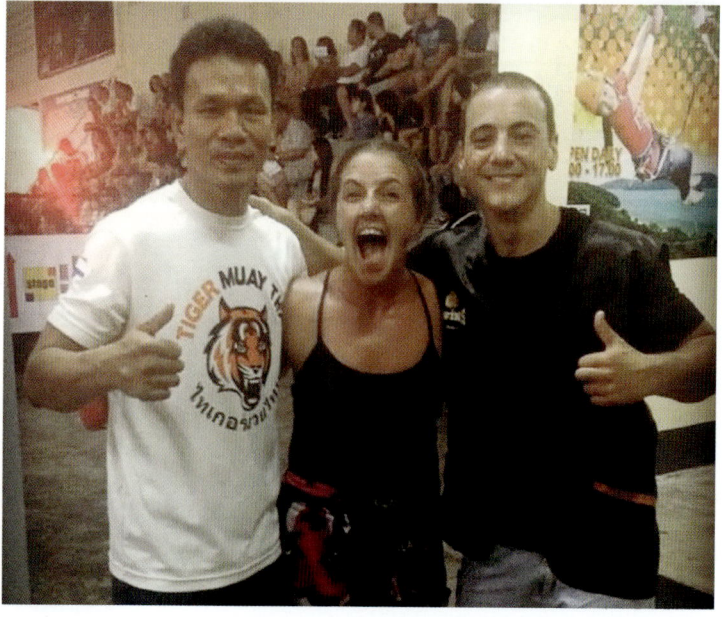

Top: Monks started to become a big thing in my life at this time.
Bottom: The Dream Team! Sanong, Ricky and I happy with the result.

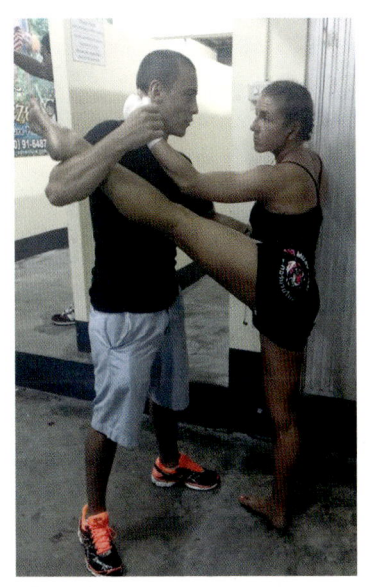

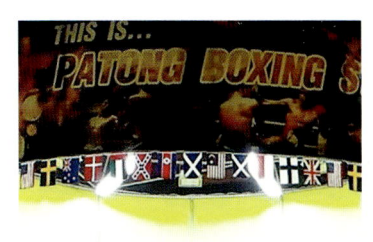

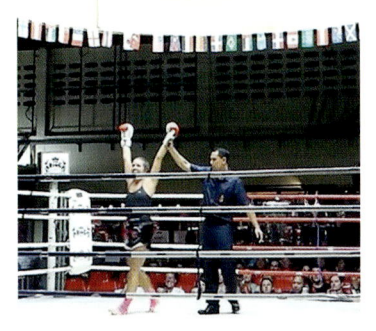

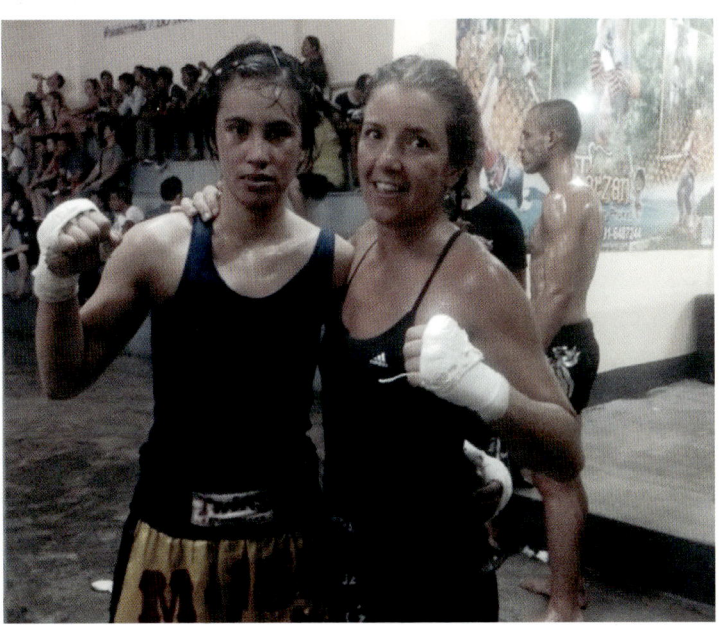

Top left: Ricky stretching me out whilst giving me a firm pep talk before my fight. Top right: That winning feeling! Bottom: Second fight, losing against a girl who had 220 fights.

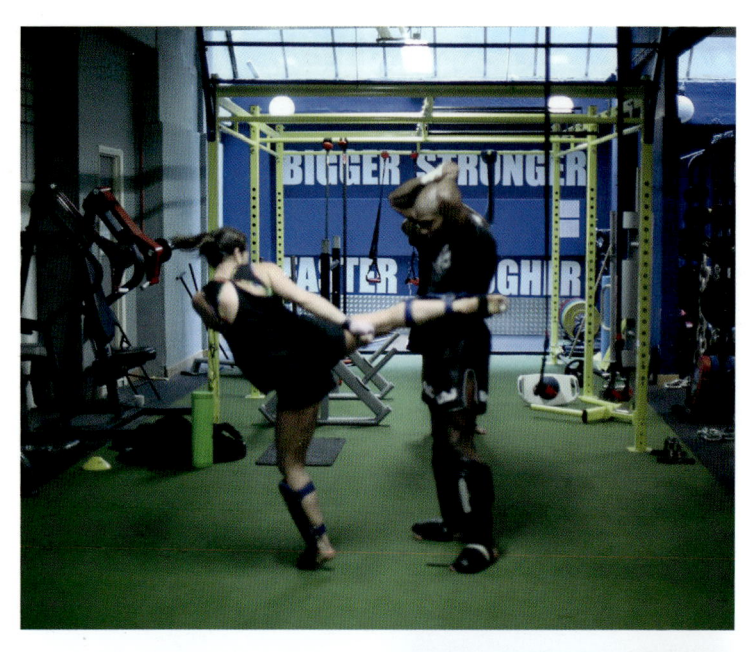

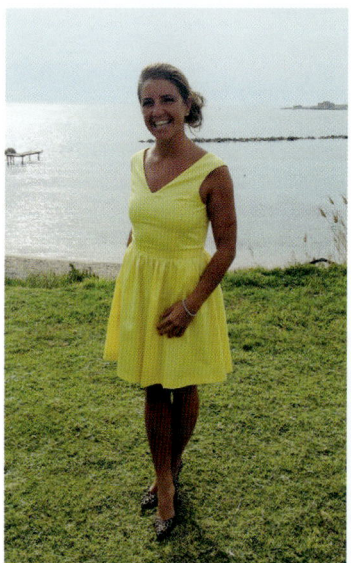

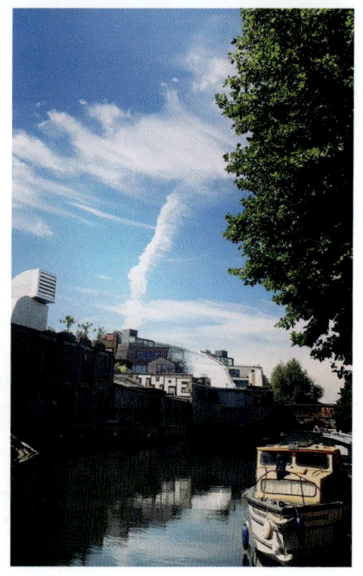

Top: Lunchtime training in the city during my UBS days.
Bottom left: Laura's wedding in Cyprus. Bottom right: The most powerful image of the sky to date. Angels, dragons….what do you see?

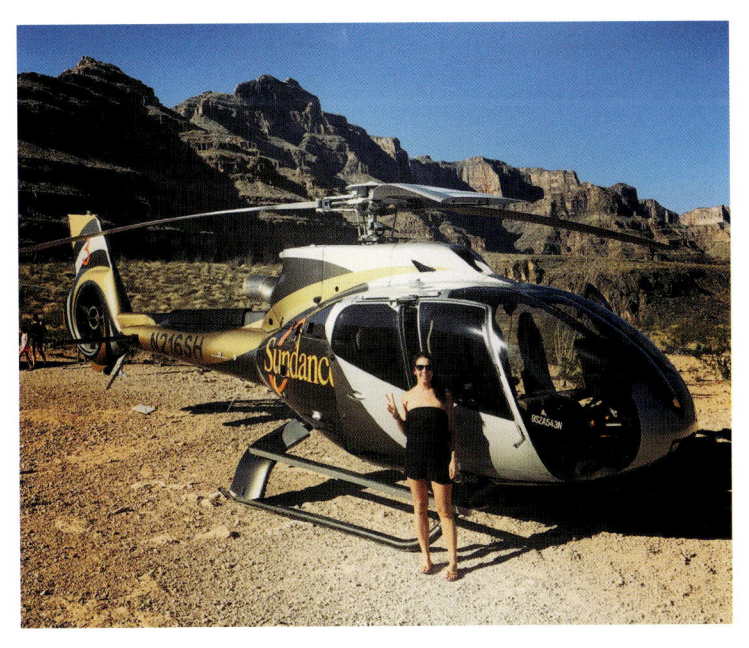

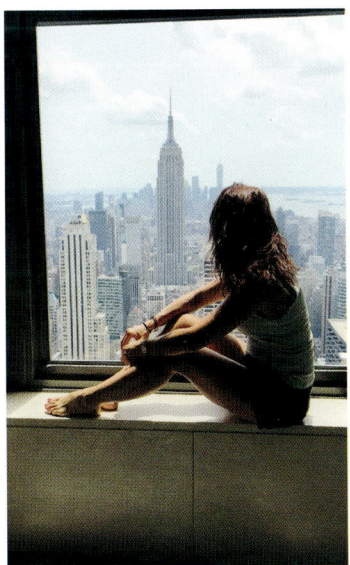

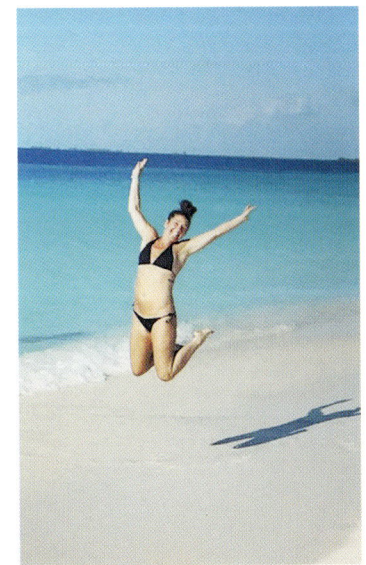

Top: Helicopter into the Grand Canyon whilst in Vegas for a friend's 40th birthday. Bottom left: After leaving Vegas, heading on to explore New York. Bottom right: Cuba baby! Happy times – Christmas 2017.

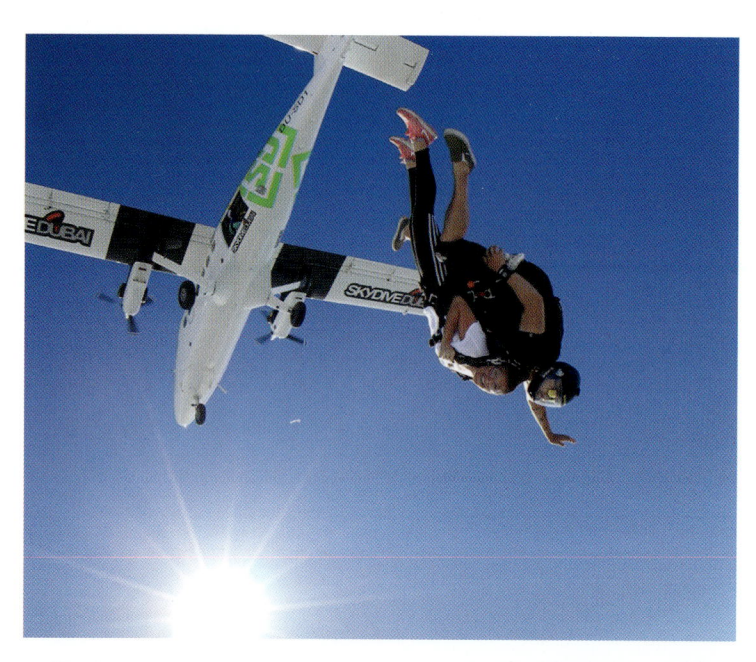

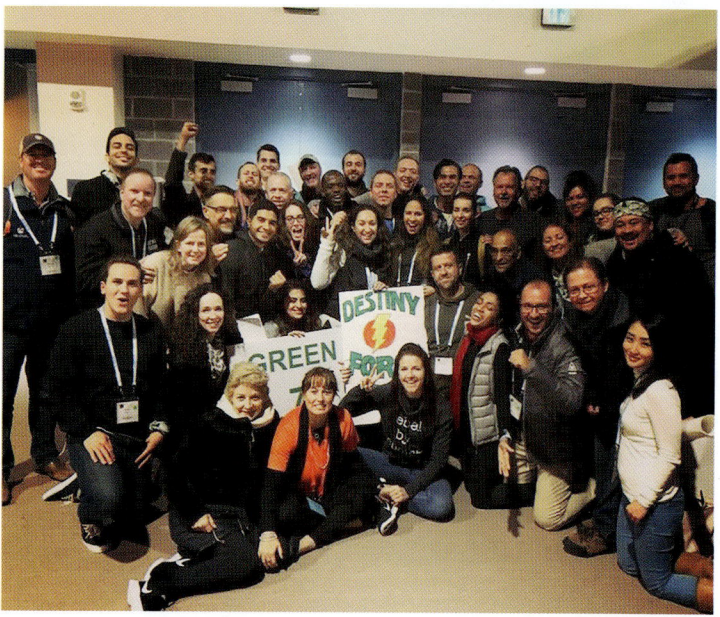

Top: Sky dive in Dubai. Bottom: The Date with Destiny team – Katrina and I at the front.

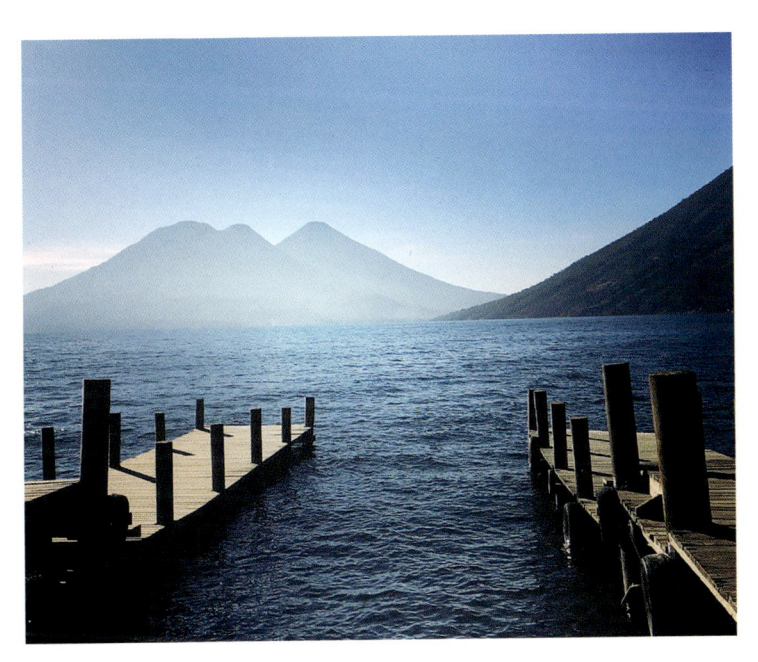

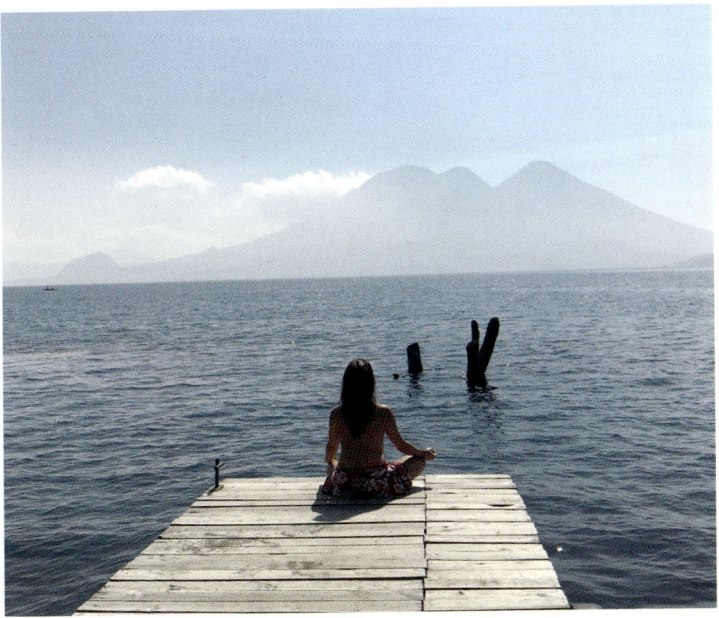

Top: The port in San Marcos, Guatemala. Bottom: Daily meditation and connection looking out over the lake.

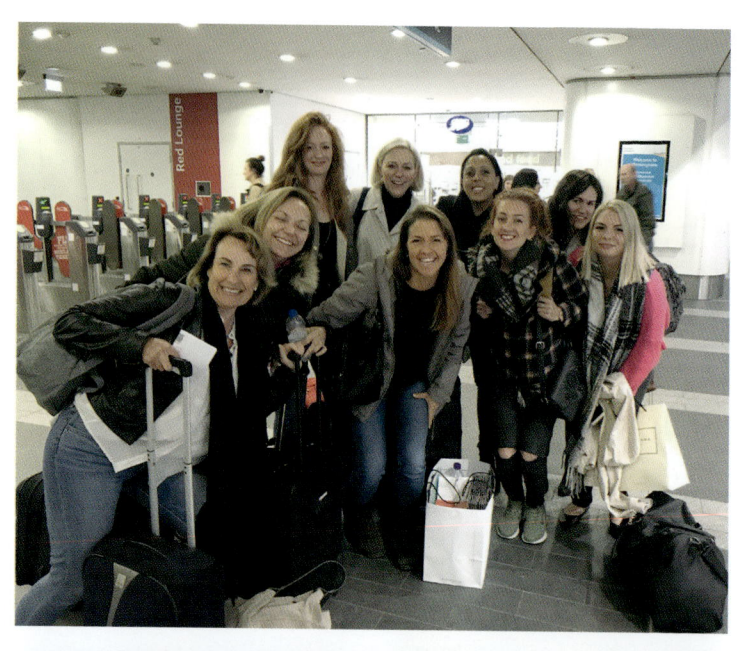

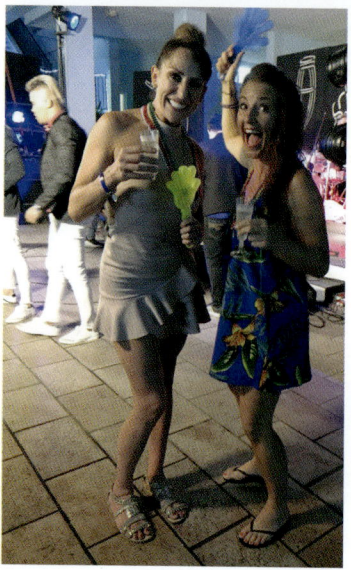

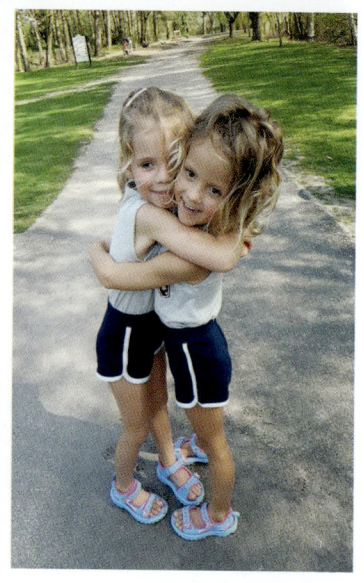

Top: My team and I arriving in Birmingham New Street station, ready for my outing on the big stage. Bottom left: New Year's eve in Cuba. Bottom right: Everything I do, is to make the world a better place for these two. The Little Beans.

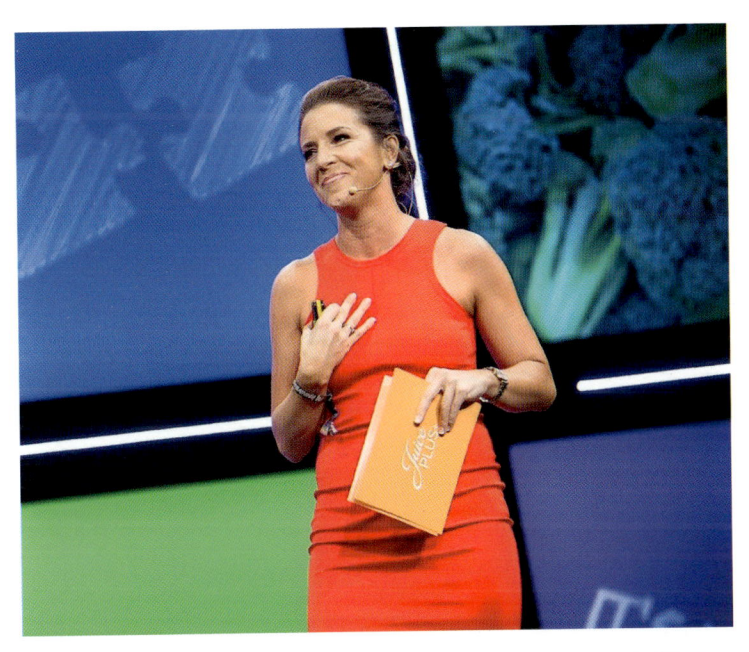

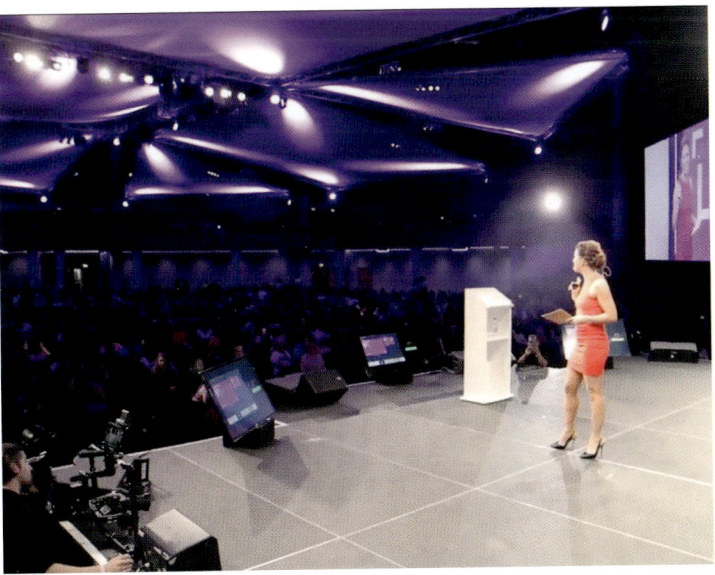

Top: On stage in Birmingham in 'that' red dress. The first of many talks given around the world that activated the souls of thousands.

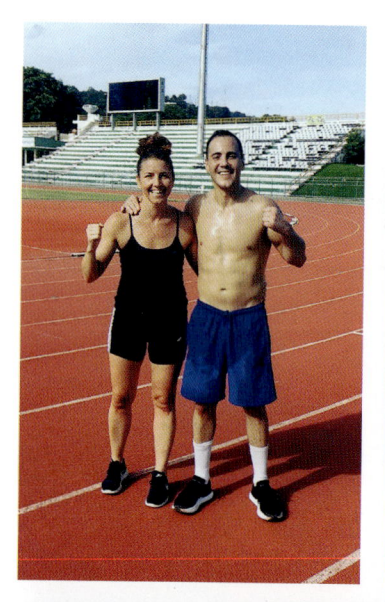

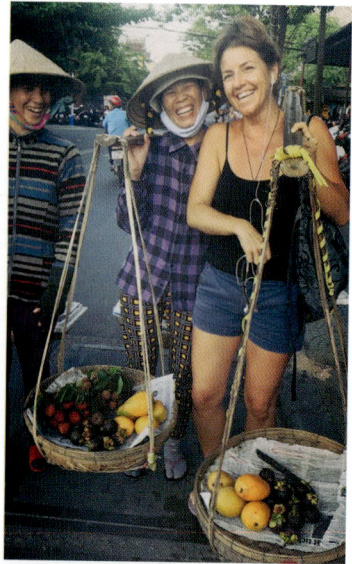

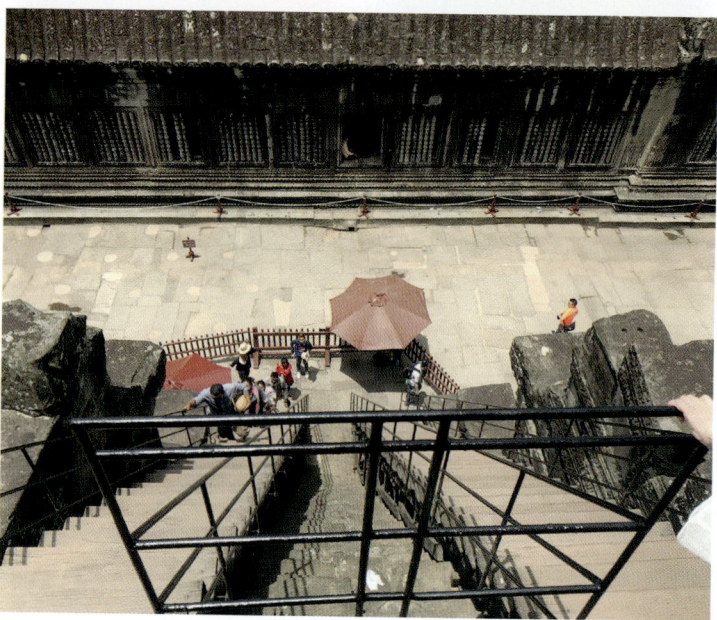

Top left: Ricky and I training after the epiphanies I received in Thailand, June 2018. Top right: Activating Vietnam! Bottom: The view from the Nirvana point at Ankor Watt, where the storm raged.

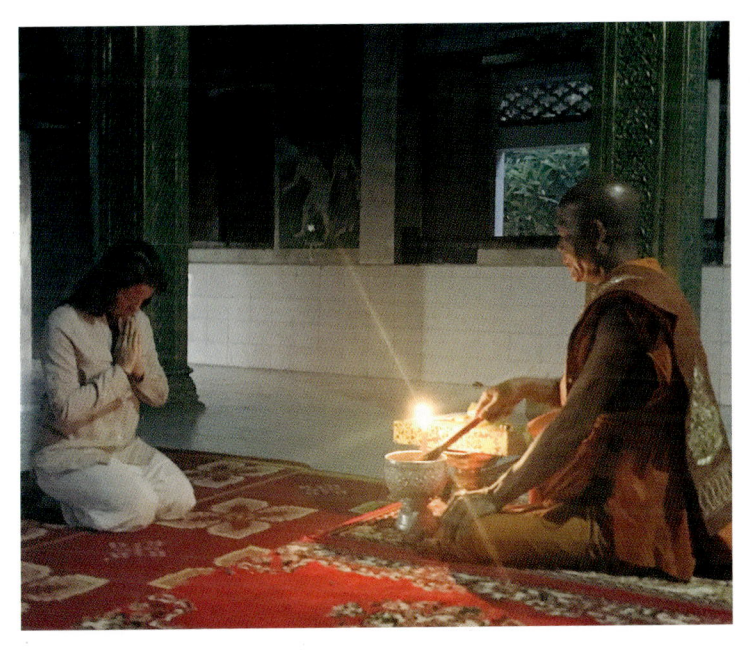

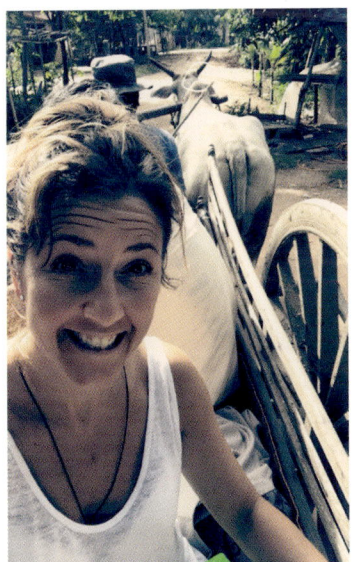

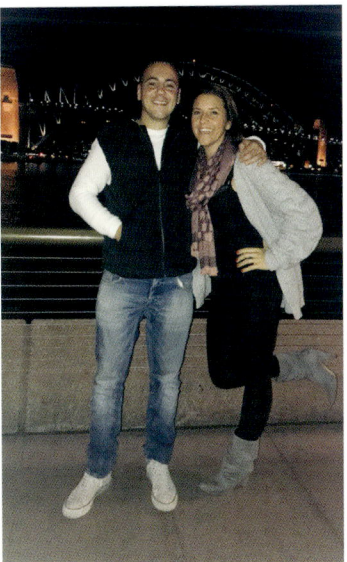

Top: Meditation and blessing with the monks in Cambodia. Bottom left: Riding the water buffalo after a random day. Bottom right: Ricky and I out for dinner in July 2018 when I found myself back in Sydney, unexpectedly.

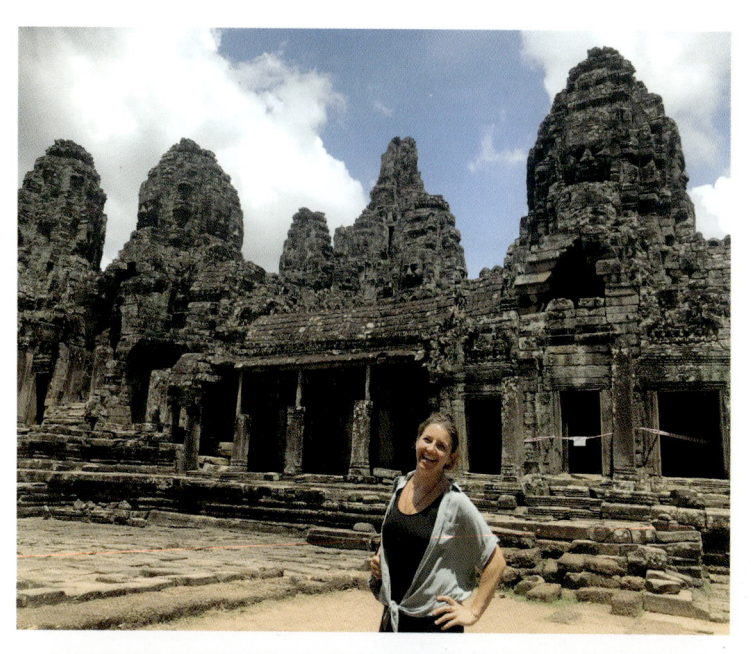

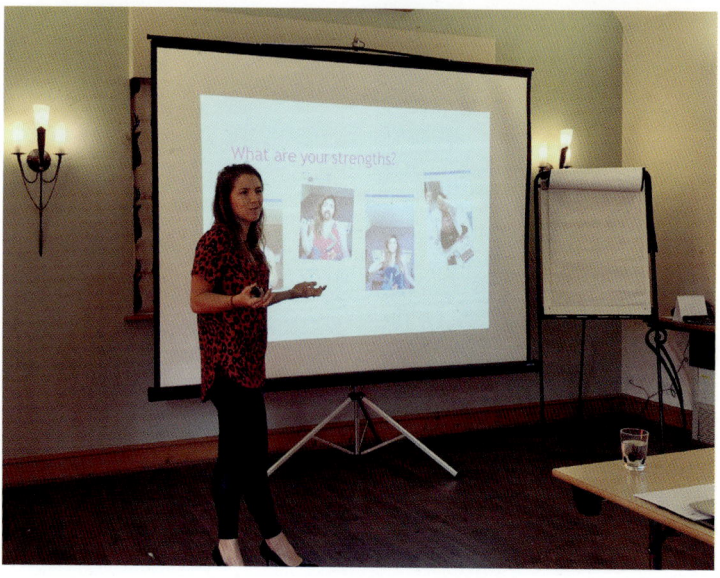

Top: In Angkor Wat June 2018. Bottom: Speaking at the Social Media summit in Windsor. This was the day I lost my voice, two days before I ended up in hospital.

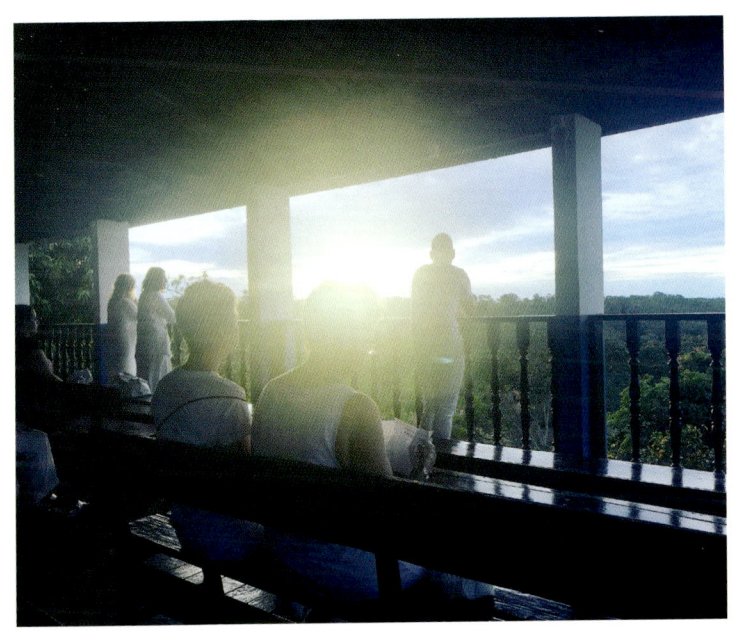

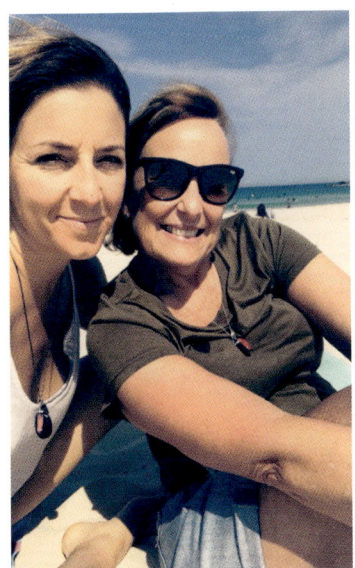

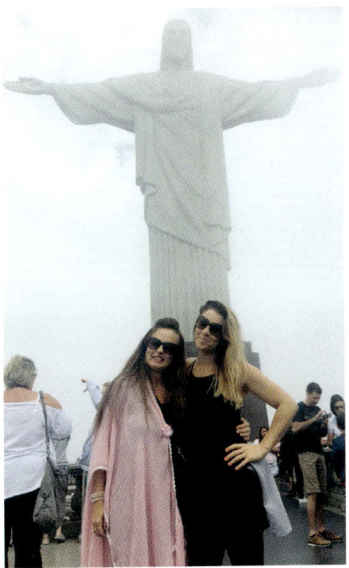

Top: The view from the Casa in Brazil. Bottom left: Donna and I on Bondi Beach, breathing a sigh of relief after landing in Sydney. Bottom right: Katrina and I in Rio de Janeiro at the Christ the Redeemer statue.

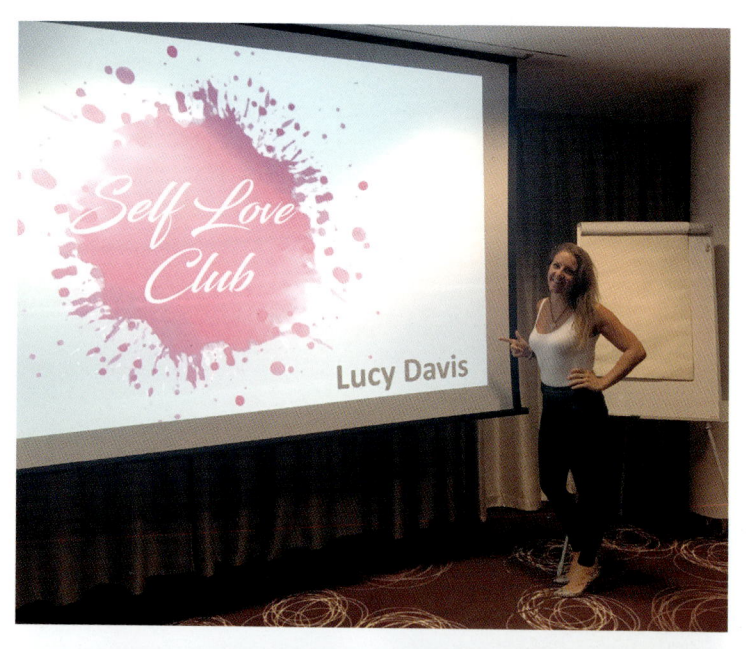

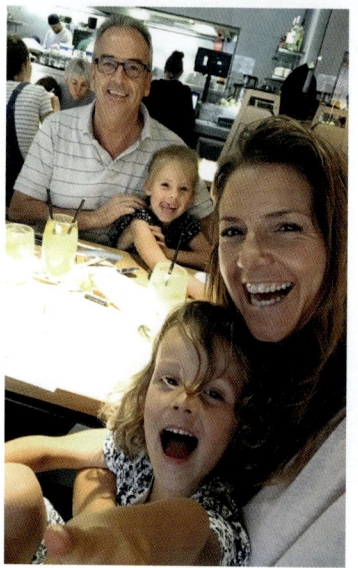

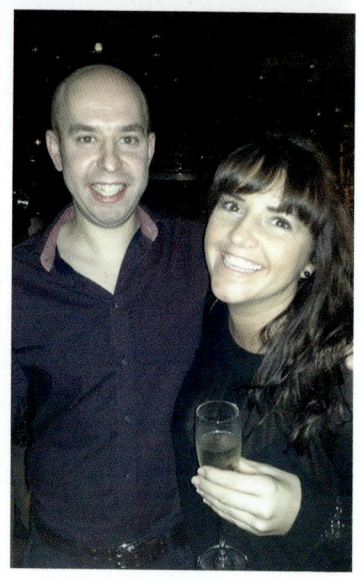

Top: The Self Love Club Launch event in London. Bottom left: My Dad, Gabi, Bela and I out for a late lunch. Bottom right: My best friend Jimbo and I from back in our party days.

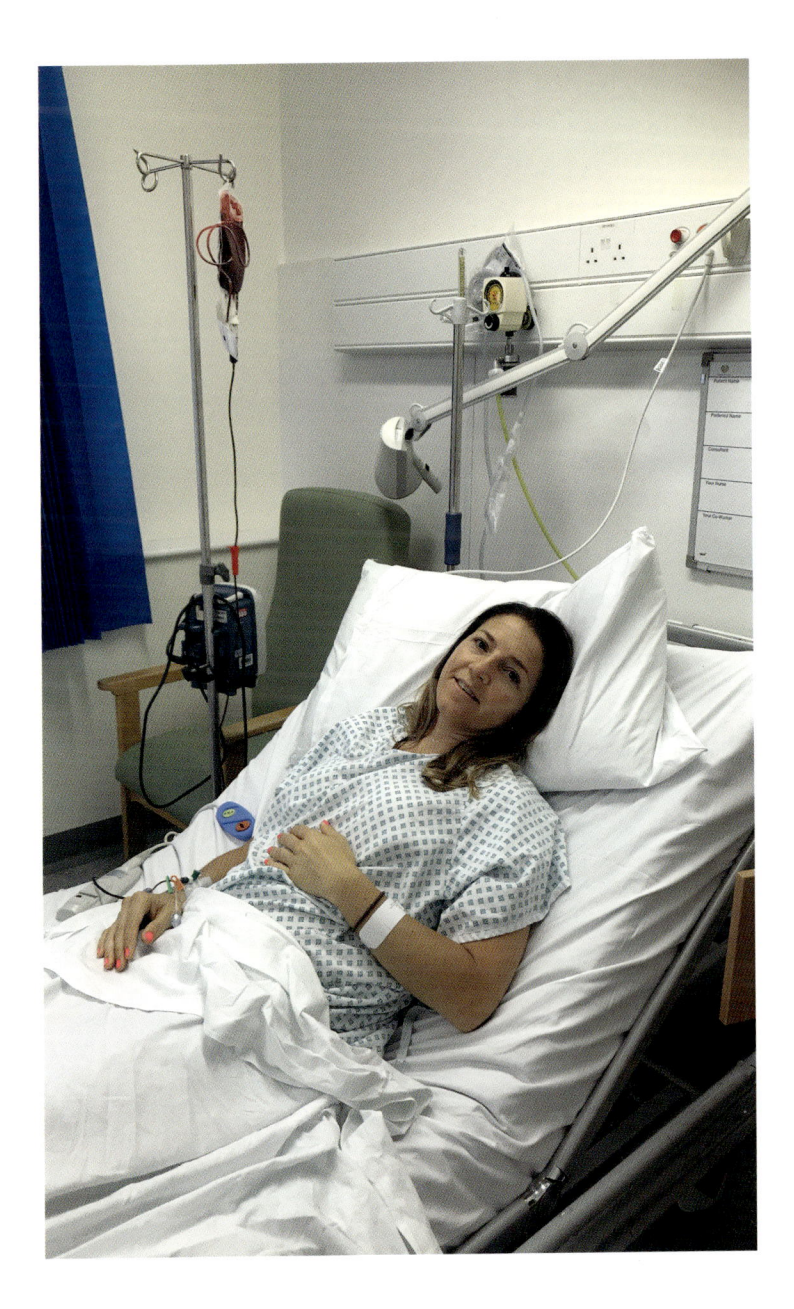

Above: The day I nearly died. The blood transfusion that I desperately didn't want but that saved my life.

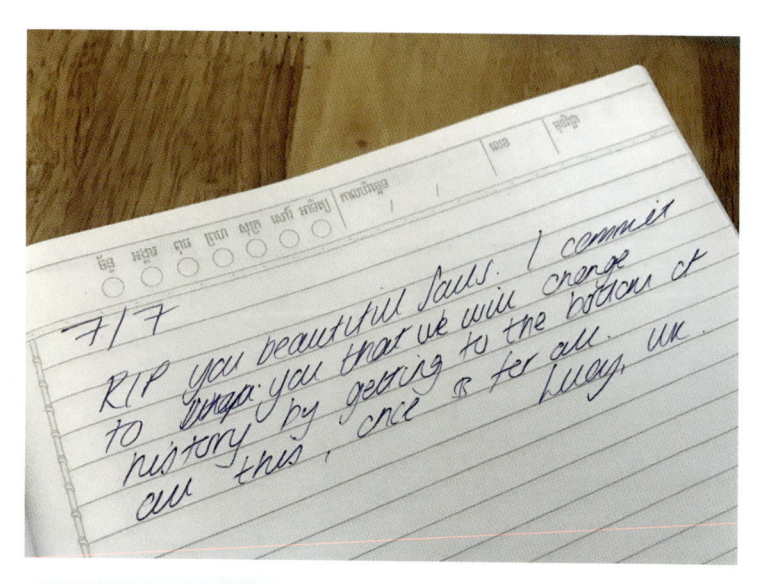

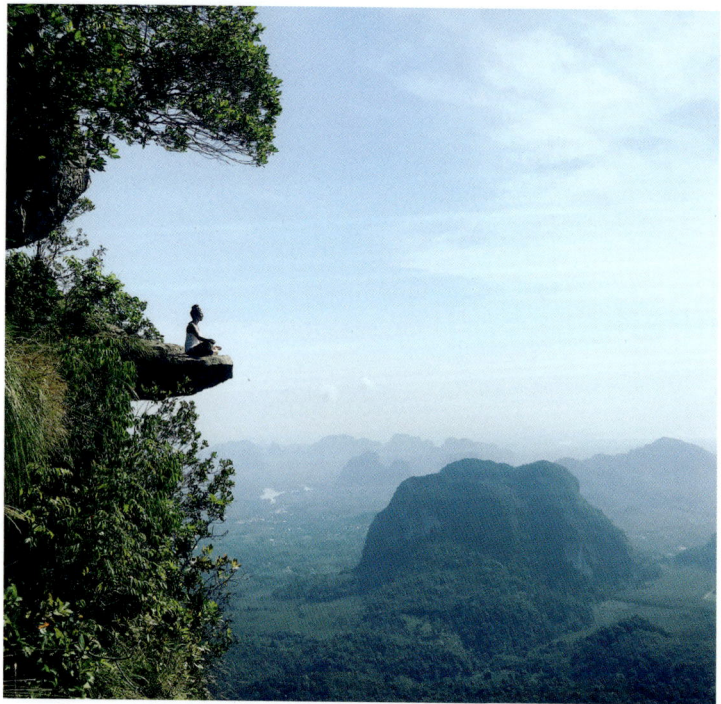

Top: The note I wrote in the guest book at Tuol Sleng Genocide Museum on the 7th of the 7th 2018. Bottom: A brief glimpse into the future.

As soon as I got back to Thailand, though, I switched to being more present. I stepped right back into training mode and to being disciplined and thinking about my fight. I also had a few weeks of travelling around Thailand and Australia to look forward to. Very quickly, I thought of the Dubai experience as something that was in the past. That little adventure was done, it was time for me to recommit to myself.

60

Although I was back in Thailand and had hoped to move on from my experiences with Kyle, it wasn't that easy. We had such a great time together. I knew in my heart there was unfinished business. It all felt a bit weird. Why I had to meet someone from back home, just when I had been brave enough to leave, was beyond me. Curve balls come in all different shapes and sizes, and I liked the shape and size of this one. At least we knew in six months, when I had to attend my friend's wedding in Cyprus, we could see each other again. Six months seemed such a long time away, though.

This was the first time I had stuck strongly to my own vision. When I look back, there were so many times I changed plans for other people. I own that it was always my choice, but I was usually influenced by how I felt about them. There was a time with my first serious boyfriend when I wanted to travel for a year; he suggested that if I went, we would have had to finish. I get it now, but back then, because I loved him, I stayed. Hindsight is such a wonderful gift. This time, with Kyle, I had to follow my heart, I just hoped he would stay around while I did.

I got my head down and focused on my training to keep me from dwelling on Kyle. I was back out running, doing my 5km run before our group session. I was then in the gym doing my two-hour class. I decided to skip my strength conditioning for a few days because I had just had a week of eating lots of food and having a few drinks and stuff, so I was sensible to ease myself back in – how funny that sounds now – that training 5 hours a day was 'easing myself back in'.

Nothing stopped me from badgering my trainer, though, poor guy, "When can I do a fight? Surely there must be something for me soon?"

I have seen so many westerners thrown in the ring with Thai fighters and had their asses handed to them on a plate, but with me, I feel my trainer was teaching me a valuable lesson that helped create the person I am today. He demanded consistency. I think he wanted proof I was going to show up regularly. He knew 100 per cent that when I was there, I was the most committed person in the ring, but the Wanderess within me often won the battle and led me to places that took me away from training. He was teaching me patience, discipline and consistency in a way nothing else could or would have taught me. As much as I could usually get him wrapped around my little finger, he was not taking any of my nonsense. He was making sure I was fully ready for every eventuality that may unfold in the ring. It would have been easy to throw me in the ring to teach me a lesson in patience, thankfully, though, he taught it to me before I got in the ring.

During that first week back, I really missed Kyle. I missed our connection and started feeling as if I was missing out on things by staying in this one place. Was I having the best experience I could have by focusing all of my time on a fight? What was it about it that I could not let go of?

Over the previous months, I had become excellent friends with a guy called Jared, from New Zealand. Kyle had met him too when he was over. We had done some cool exploring trips, the three of us. We often shared our desires to travel, go on adventures and explore the lands around us – Laos, Cambodia, the rest of Thailand, and Vietnam. As much as I wanted that fight, I also had a burning desire to explore, and I mean really explore.

One night, we went out for dinner, and that was it; we planned it all out. We can fly to here, then get a bus to there, and stay there for a few days. Nothing deeper than that. We just mapped out our journey. I knew my trainer would be pissed off, but I also knew that this was something I had to do. Training could continue whilst I was on the road, and I was certain that working with different trainers would make me a better fighter and more adaptable. I was not so sure he would see it that way. I guess I was distracting. I was running away again. Although I wasn't running away from Kyle this time, I was running away to distract myself from the fact that I missed him, especially where I trained because we had made such magical memories together. That was our place.

I was ready to explore and figure out more about this country that I had fallen in love with. I had heard that Thailand was very different down South to up North. I was told the North was very mountainous and plush, whereas the South, where I had spent a lot of time exploring, was much more about the beaches and the glorious sea. Of course, due to it being such a pretty tourist trap, the South was also much busier. I loved the beaches, and quite frankly, every time I returned there, I attempted to figure out a plan to move there, so I was intrigued to see how well I took to the North.

I justified it to myself that I had nothing to lose. I spoke with my trainer about my plans, and like every previous time I had announced I was off for a while, he rolled his eyes and tutted at me. I had only just got back, and I was telling him I wanted to fight, but then I was disappearing again. My actions and words did not marry up. I could see why he was saying no to putting me in the ring. Where was my dedication? He told me that as long as I trained as much as possible when I was away, he would evaluate where I was up to when I got back, and then we would start looking at when I could do my fight. I was pulled in several directions because I wanted to fight and maintain the incredible fitness I had established; however, I had also reached a point where I needed to take a bit of time for myself, to focus on having more fun for a while. It had all become so serious in such a short space of time. It was time to immerse in the beauty of the place and continue my journey of going inwards and connecting to the beautiful heart space I had ignored for so many years until now.

We booked a flight from Phuket to Bangkok, just an internal flight, super easy. Like flying anywhere domestic, you don't need to go through any of the international processes. It was a breeze, ten minutes, and we were through, ready to go on the next adventure.

61

We arrived in Bangkok quickly and easily, then boarded a bus and travelled through the night from Bangkok up to Chiang Mai. We had such a laugh as we travelled together. It was weird because although I had become friends with him over three months since we met, I had never considered if he would be easy to travel with, whether he snored or anything like that. We laughed a lot, though, and created absolute mayhem – quite often leading each other astray, in a good way. He started calling us Bert and Ernie from Sesame Street, and it stuck, and we still call each other that to this day.

Up in Chiang Mai, we explored the city for a little while. I didn't like it. I had heard so many beautiful things about it, one of my ex-partners had spent a lot of time there and spoke so highly of it, but it just didn't feel resonant to me. It felt pretty drab. It seemed grey and almost reminded me of a very hot, sweaty England.

We spent two days exploring the city. We had written a list of things we wanted to check off whilst there. Thankfully, Bert did not feel much about the place either, so he was keen to check things off and move on to the next place. We went into a small café-type place to grab a drink and some food and make our next plans. We decided that we would be heading out the next day, on a bus again, to a place called Chiang Rai. Chang Rai was slightly further North again. We had researched the best temples in Thailand, and Wat Rong Khun came up as a very impressive place to visit. It was stunning. A bit like how you might imagine a castle or palace made out of ice to look like. It was entrenched in the Buddhist religion that was prevalent all over Thailand, and there was also a stunning art side to it. We were both sold on this. It transpired that Bert and I were able to travel together easily. We got each other and were able to make quick decisions and go with the flow. It was great. I would never have guessed we would travel so well together.

Bert was a fantastic guy, but up until this point, whilst we had been down South, he had been a boozer. He was hilarious. He would do a few days of training and then disappear for a few days, getting wasted, or because he had fallen for a new woman. He was one of those kinds of guys. I absolutely love him dearly, and we're still excellent friends to this day, so he won't mind me saying this, but that's what his pattern was – training then disappearing. Whenever he would come back he'd say, "Oh, I'm not going to be doing that again." And then he would just repeat it again a few days later. It was so funny. You could tell that he was desperate to break the cycle, but he was also so desperate to fit in and be loved. This is one of the main reasons why he said he wanted to go away with me. He knew how disciplined I had become. He knew I had Kyle back home, so there would be no leading me astray or getting into too much mischief. He felt safe with me, and the beautiful thing about this friendship was that I felt safe with him too.

Whilst we were on this magical trip, he started to get the fact that you did not need to be out and about boozing all the time to fit in. The epiphany hit him that there was more to life than that. I was not really a big drinker at this point – if at all, and because we weren't drinking in the evenings, we needed to find stuff to do, so I would badger him to go for a massage. He kept saying, "No, we're not going for a massage. I don't want a 'happy ending'. That would be embarrassing." We were just winding each other up. We made a deal, though, on the way back from the palace that day we would get a massage – as that was what I wanted, and then we would go for dessert because he was obsessed with getting dessert.

The temple was stunning. It was incredible. It was hectic, being a tourist trap, but it was incredible all the same. Any of the temples you visit, or the kind of places that have monks and religious connotations, you must cover yourself up. If you are a woman, you must cover your shoulders and your legs. If you're a man, you can get away with wearing shorts as long as they're not short shorts, but you've got to cover your shoulders as well. It's respect. A huge part of their culture. I personally am very respectful when in other countries. I've been to countries where you literally can't show any skin, and I respect that. I'm not one of these travellers that just thinks – *Fuck it I'm on holiday, I'm going to wear a bikini.* I believe if you are in somebody's country, you should respect them and respect their rules. That's my personal belief system.

I had to get wrapped up in a sarong around my shoulders, and another to cover my shorts. Bert – in true Bert style – was taking the piss out of me because I was looking like a pretty girlie for the first time ever. We walked around this place, and the energy was beautiful. It was something else. I was starting to feel the energies at this part of the journey, and at certain times I would become extremely sensitive to them. It did not make sense to me at the time, but looking back, this was the point when it all started to come online.

We spent a good few hours in the temple, looking at the orchids and all the beautiful flowers, especially the lotus flowers. I had become slightly obsessed with them during my travels. They often grabbed my attention. They really appealed to me, and I never quite knew why. I just knew that the lotus flower was somehow going to end up being a big deal for me – and later on in the journey, when I got to Vietnam and Cambodia, that would make absolute sense. What I learnt and love about the lotus flower is that no matter how murky the water is, it would still shine, and shine brightly too. That was a really important message for me at that time in my life. I had come from the darkest depths of hell. There's no other way to describe it, and I was just starting to navigate my way back through the murky waters to find the surface so I could bloom again. The lotus flowers reminded me of how you could choose to transform.

After we spent several hours at the temple – walking, observing, investigating and admiring all of the incredible artwork – we decided we were starving and couldn't wait until later for dinner. I was always either starving or stuffed, there was no middle ground with me back then.

We hopped on the back of a tuk tuk to take us to the town closest to where we were staying, so we could get something to eat. Now I don't make any secret of it – I love to eat. I can eat lots of food. I am good at eating. I enjoy it. I appreciate it, especially in places like Thailand. Thankfully Bert was no different. We found a little traditional Thai restaurant and ordered pretty much everything on the menu. Lots of different tasters and small plates are my favourite way to eat. I love to share food, and I have always admired the way people ate in the Mediterranean and places like Thailand. The table was filled with plates of beautifully coloured and delicious-smelling foods. It was sensory overload. The food looked, smelt and tasted stunning. We ate as if our lives depended on it. It was like we had not been fed since the previous day, which was pretty much true. We had eaten early the previous night, then went off early exploring, so here we were about three in the afternoon, starving and getting our first feed in. And my goodness, it was a good one.

Once we were fully satisfied, we decided to explore some more, and plan the next leg of our journey. As we meandered through the pretty town, we chatted about where we were drawn to go next. Bert and I never stopped talking. Looking back, we had a really beautiful connection. We were so at ease with each other, and I took it for granted at the time. It's only now, sitting here writing this I feel in awe of how comfortable we were with each other. We spoke about everything and did everything together for those few weeks, and never once had cross words.

As we were exploring more and more, we met people who were sharing their travels and ideas of places we should visit. On more than one occasion, Pai had come up in conversation. It was a place I had suggested we go to when we initially left Phuket, as so many people had mentioned what a truly wonderful place it was, and nothing like you would find anywhere else in Thailand. I was intrigued. It was meant to be really beautiful and plush in that area, but we had also heard the journey there was a bit of an experience. The more people mentioned it, the more Bert and I decided it was on our to-do list. That afternoon, we decided we would go there the next day, so we hunted down a little travel agent and spoke to the lady there about our onward travel. Typically, we had done no research. We were winging it completely, deciding on the spur of the moment, there and then, that it was going to happen tomorrow. Thankfully, the lady was really helpful, and she sorted everything out for us. We would have to travel back to Chang Mai on a bus and get connected to a minibus that would take us on to Pai. She organised a beautiful place for us to stay, one with a swimming pool, I hasten to add. Bert and Ernie were back on their adventures again.

So many people who have travelled with me since this experience cannot appreciate how I like to travel. I went from being an over-the-top planner to feeling into things and trusting it would all work out as intended. Bert helped me relinquish all my travel control and go with the flow. I quite often, even to this day, book a flight and have no idea where I am going when I land.

We were excited to be going back on another adventure tomorrow. Yes, it was a pain in the butt to go back to Chang Mai, but if it all went to plan, we would only be there about 20 minutes before setting off again. We had a newfound spring in our step as we continued exploring before leaving the next day.

62

Later that evening, I took Bert for his first-ever Thai massage. He was so nervous that he made sure we were in a double room. He told them I was his girlfriend, so no funny business took place. It was hilarious. It's so funny when you go for a massage with people in Thailand,

and they don't know what to expect. An authentic Thai massage can be brutal. They contort you into some positions that you never knew you could get into. You get folded like a pretzel. And then they dig their elbows in so deep it feels like all of your bones are going to pop out. I could not stop laughing as Bert was screaming like a little girl. There was him focused on the 'happy ending' – if he had experienced it before, he would have realised there is nothing happy about a Thai massage, unless you're used to them. Don't get me wrong, afterwards, you feel incredible, but during it, you want to punch them in the face and run! We had such a giggle. I've got some fantastic photos of us sitting in the outfits they put us in, right before our massage. I will never forget that night for many reasons, starting with the yelps from the big, strong Kiwi lad.

Oh, how karma has an amusing way of working!

After the massage, we decided we would return to our hotel for a little bit. We were laughing at what had gone on, although both of us were feeling pretty amazing by this point. We had only been back in the room maybe an hour, just starting to pack up again for the next leg of our journey, when Bert decided he wanted to go out and get some snacks. This was a frequent thing in Thailand. It would get to a certain time, and you would need a little bit of something. So, off we went, on the hunt for a shop. We were walking down a relatively busy road; there were no street lights, just the lights from the cars that were highlighting the way for us. It was dark by this time, and as there were no pavements we were trundling along the side of the road, just having a chat and typically putting the world to rights about one thing and another. The next thing I knew, I fell down a massive hole in the road.

I heard Bert say, "Where the fuck are you?" He couldn't see me. It was like I had disappeared – because I had! I had fallen straight into a massive hole. There had been no barrier around it, nothing saying that there was a big fucking hole here, or a sign saying 'watch your step' – as you would have in the UK. There was nothing. And, of course, it had to be me that fell in and slammed myself to the floor.

When he found me, I was wetting myself laughing because as much as I had dropped a decent amount, down to my waist – which is a pretty decent drop when you are not expecting it – I just laughed at how random this was. Thankfully, I seemed alright, I couldn't feel any damage. It could have been so much worse.

Bert was laughing hysterically; he was literally on the floor rolling around, so he didn't help me get out the frickin hole for ages. "Look at the fucking state of you. Look what you've got us into this time, Ernie." All we could do was laugh. The laughter I had enjoyed whilst he was being whipped into shape in the massage parlour was now gifted to him in the form of me stuck in a big bloody hole in the middle of a road. We were like a comedy double-act. "This is going to be a great story for the books; Bert and Ernie's Magical Adventures," he declared.

"Just help me out of the hole," I shouted back at him. I had to laugh because there's nobody else that this would have ever happened to, except me. He lifted me out, and I was able to walk perfectly. "If it wasn't for you needing your bloody snacks, then I would have been okay," I was winding him up to a point, but there was a level of truth in what I was saying. Yep, I was looking to point that finger of blame. It could not have been my fault. Oh no no no! It must be someone else's fault when things go wrong.

We grabbed the snacks and headed back to where we were staying. After all of the excitement, I was so tired and fell asleep straight away, ready for our trip to Pai the next day.

The following day, I woke up early, at about five o clock. Before I even opened up my eyes, I was in absolute agony. I was screaming. I woke Bert up through my discomfort. He was shocked, "Oh my God, what's happened to you?"

"I can't move, I feel as if my whole body is in a brace." It was excruciating; I didn't know what to do. I tried to move but I couldn't. I couldn't even sit up, or turn my head at this point.

"Shit, what are we going to do? We're travelling on coaches to Chiang Mai and then on to Pai today, Lucy."

"I'll be fine. I'll get through it." Tough old Lucy – can't possibly show weakness. *Must keep going* – is all I kept thinking that day. It was a poor decision to get on that coach.

The first part of the journey to Chang Mai was okay, they had recliner seats, so I could lie flat and let the world drift past without too much hassle. It took us about an hour and a half to get there. Bert carried my bag for me, so that helped navigate that piece of the puzzle okay. It was a bit painful but manageable. When I got to Chang Mai, I decided to go to the chemist and buy some of their most potent painkillers – something that I wouldn't do today, but back then, it was a case of 'when in Rome!' Popping a pill to fix a problem was common back then. And what made things much more interesting is that in Thailand you can go to a shop and pretty much buy morphine or any other drug over the counter, without a note from the doctor, unlike back home. I walked into the chemist and asked for their strongest painkiller.

We got on the minibus to Pai, and it was a disaster. The first half an hour was fine, we were on proper roads, and it was relatively smooth, but then all of a sudden, we hit the mountains, and it turned into the bumpiest ride you could imagine. It was like a bucking bronco. We were sitting at the back of the minibus too, so we were bouncing even more than anybody else. I was in agony. I drove Bert mad, telling him I was in pain every five minutes without fail. Even the super-strong painkillers weren't touching the sides during this journey. We were told that loads of people often have to stop the minibus to be sick because it was such a bouncy, hairy journey. I could not have chosen a worse time to damage my neck.

We eventually arrived in Pai, and despite my agony, I could see why everybody had told us to go there. It was breathtaking. It was just so incredibly beautiful. It felt almost like a beautiful, quaint village in the UK on a summer's day, only in the sweaty heat of Thailand. It was a real contradiction.

I gingerly stepped out of the minibus, I was so thankful to get off that damn bus. I felt as if I had done some serious damage on that journey. It had felt painful before, but all of the bouncing and bobbing around made me feel like something was broken. I started to panic a little bit, but without letting on to Bert. He grabbed both of our bags because I was next to useless at this point. He had one on his back, one on his front and both of our hand luggage bags in either hand. What a hero! Thank goodness I wasn't on my own. We beckoned a tuk tuk to take us to the hotel, where we would also be able to get our moped. That journey was also excruciating. Typically, we had picked somewhere out in the fields, in contrast to where we were in Phuket so that we could enjoy the best of the mountain area. We had decided to immerse in nature and then dip into the town when required, rather than the other way around, which is what we had been doing.

PART TWO – TO THE HEART

When we got to the hotel, it was incredible. It was almost like a honeymoon suite for the two of us, although we did have separate beds. It was beautiful. There was such a fantastic amount of space. The bathroom was amazing, like a tropical paradise. It had this massive outdoor, grassy area and a swimming pool. We were both in awe and gratitude for where we had found ourselves. Despite the pain I was experiencing, I felt so glad we were finally here. In the end, the journey had been worth it!

I told Bert I needed to take some time out and relax before doing anything else. I needed to get my body back in alignment. We agreed to lay out by the pool for a bit and relax. He thought that I needed to go and see a doctor, and he made it very clear that I should be going to the hospital to get checked out – 'given the once over' as he put it. I was having none of it. I was hoping the painkillers would do the trick. I figured if I went to a doctor, they would only prescribe them to me anyway.

I lay out by the pool, doing my best to get comfortable. Bert was being a typical boy, annoying me on purpose by jumping in and out of the swimming pool and splashing me, knowing I could not run away. After an hour or so, my neck was getting no better; it was actually getting a lot worse. I eventually succumbed and told Bert, "You're going to have to take me to a hospital, or a doctor, or find something to help ease this." He was such a gent. He could see the pain in my eyes. He could see how serious I was, so he marched off to ask the owners what to do. The owners of the place we were staying said there was a hospital in the town centre of Pai; they said it was a very busy hospital, but it was a hospital nevertheless, and it did take accidents and emergencies. They asked us if we had insurance, and they told us that it would cost us if we didn't. And to be clear, this was not a private hospital, it was a standard, local Thai hospital.

Thankfully on this part of the journey, we had already decided to get just one moped. We had decided I would sit on the back and let Bert drive me around, like driving Miss Daisy, so I could capture the beautiful scenery in photographs as we went. Bert was cool with it. I think he quite liked being allowed to be the man, and my goodness, I needed him to be at that time.

When we arrived at the hospital, I took one look at it and said to Jared, "Please don't make me go in there. I'll catch something horrible." It looked awful, but I had no choice. I figured it was only a bad neck, I needed to stop making such a drama of it all. They would probably send me straight away with a new prescription. The trouble was, I had this in-built thing in me, from being a child around a lot of hypochondriacs and it really made me feel weak. So rather than showing pain, hurt or letting people know something was wrong, I had made myself tough, and strong to withstand whatever pain was thrown at me. That story has definitely served me in so many ways over the years — I've had fillings done at the dentist without having any anaesthetic; that's how good my pain threshold is. In this scenario, though, when it was my neck and potentially my back, it possibly wasn't the most sensible approach.

I staggered into the hospital, and they didn't understand a word I was saying. There was one English-speaking doctor in the whole hospital. They had to go and hunt him down and extract him from whatever he was doing to be able to come and speak to me. Thankfully he was lovely and so kind. He examined me and sent the fear of God into me when he said he felt I had potentially fractured or broken a bone in my spine. Bert took my hand and gave me a knowing, calm smile. *What the fuck will I do if it's something serious like that?* I told myself to keep calm. The hospital organised an x-ray as a first step to ensure I was okay and that any future treatment would not cause too many issues.

As stupid as this sounds, it was only when the doctor asked us if anything had happened to cause it, that we even connected it to me falling in the hole the night before. I had come out of the hole absolutely fine, so I thought this injury was just because I had slept funny, or maybe the massage had created some trauma.

They put me on a bed and told me not to move, at all. For some, that may have been an easy thing to do, but little Miss Ants-In-Her-Pants had hardly ever sat still in her whole life up to this point. It probably would have been easier if they had actually pinned me down to the bed. I tried my best, but Bert wasn't helping. If he wasn't making me giggle at the mess I'd managed to get myself into, he was walking around saying, "Can you fucking believe it? We're in a Thai hospital. Only you would have put us here."

Of course, the Project Manager in me surfaced, "Go and ask them what they're doing."

"None of them understands me, Lucy. What's the fucking point?"

Eventually, the doctor returned and confirmed they would take me for an x-ray. They took me to a room; it was the creepiest room I had ever seen. I mean, x-ray rooms are a bit strange anyway, but this was like going back in time, and probably to a time when x-rays were first invented. It's judgemental of me to say it, but it felt like a real spit and sawdust kind of place. Let's just say it was rustic. They did what they had to do and then took me back to the bed, after placing a brace around my neck. *Oh my goodness, it must be serious if they are putting a brace on me. What on earth have I done?* My hypochondria officially kicked in – my mind was off on one. I was creating scenarios about how I would get left in this hospital, trapped for months, with no one knowing where I was. My family having to fly me home to be treated 'properly'. I could really create a drama back then!

After a while, the doctor came by and told me that I had severe whiplash. They had checked the x-ray, and everything seemed okay structurally, so they put it down to whiplash. I was relieved! Thank goodness, I was going to be okay. I needed to man up! Then they dropped a little bombshell about needing to have an injection to take the pain away. I looked at Bert, and said, "No way! Whiplash isn't too bad, so what's the injection about?"

Bert said, "If it means you're going to be okay quicker, then take it for the team Davis. Remember, you've got your fight."

I was thinking I couldn't box my way out of a paper bag at that moment in time, let alone actually consider a fight. I had found a gym that I really wanted to train at whilst here in Pai; apparently, the trainers were excellent, but there was just no way I was in any fit state even to be walking, let alone running, punching and kicking. One punch and I would have been on my butt! I was really pissed off with this whole scenario and probably would have taken anything to get me fixed more quickly.

I agreed to go with the injection. The nurse indicated that she needed me to spin around to inject it into my bum. I told Bert to leave immediately, but he said he was not leaving under any circumstances; he was laughing and joking about wanting to see my butt. The nurse did her best to chase him out of the room, but he was being a total pest. Fair play to him, he'd been patient with me and likely worried about me too, so now he knew I was safe, he was going to misbehave. She eventually drew a curtain around me, so I was in some privacy. I was laid down, butt hanging out of my shorts, which were down around my knees, about to have this injection, and all I could hear was the woman shouting in Thai. I looked up, and Bert was peering over the curtain with his camera, snapping pictures of me with my butt out. He was roaring, "Oh my God, this is a fucking comedy sketch, and I am absolutely 100% going to post this on social media." With that, the woman jabbed my butt! Ouch! I wanted to punch both her and Bert! My butt on social media, I don't fucking think so. Thank god the nurse was a professional and jabbed me in the right place. She easily could have gotten distracted with all the commotion he was creating.

I pulled my shorts back up, and they handed me a massive wad of paperwork and told me I would have to take this with me wherever I went, just in case anything happened on the rest of my journey. I had to keep the massive brace around my neck to support it. Under no circumstances was it to come off before I was ready. I wasn't sure how I would know when I was ready but didn't bother to ask. My head was tilted awkwardly backwards as the brace was so large that it didn't fit me in the slightest. What a picture!

We left the hospital, and I was completely off it. Whatever was in that injection – and to this day, I do not know – but my goodness, it was fast working. I was slurring my words and all sorts. God knows how I was going to hang on to the back of the moped.

We decided after the day we had, we deserved some treats, so we went to this beautiful, quaint little tearoom. It was just like being back home in England in a proper tea shop, all the tables were set up beautifully, and they had tea, teacups and proper teapots. It was fascinating. Nothing I ever imagined seeing in a little Thai village.

We sat there with our cups of tea and planned the next part of our journey. With my neck the way it was, we realised we had some limitations now, but we only had a few days left, so we decided to go exploring and make the most of it. We had found some natural thermal baths in the mountains that we could go to, and we both wanted to see the poppy fields too – where heroin was made. So we thought we would just see what was on offer in the mountains.

And that's what we did. We explored.

63

My neck started to improve. It felt instantly much better after the injection. I felt like I could have gone dancing. To be honest with you, I felt completely off my head; like the good old days! I genuinely believe I could have gone training, but no doubt I would have done more damage. The effects did start to wear off during the later parts of the day, but for most of the day, I was completely off it. It was also unbelievable the things that were coming out of my mouth! I feel now, looking back, that I was being channelled. I don't remember any of the things I said, but, according to Bert, the stuff coming out of my mouth was profound. At the time, we both thought I was going crazy. I was high on drugs, only these ones had been prescribed to me not bought in a nightclub.

We had a lot of fun exploring during those two days. We ended up in strawberry fields, poppy fields, lakes, thermal baths, and did endless hours of driving around the picturesque scenery. We made a good team Bert and I. We laughed non-stop, chatted all day, every day and allowed each other the space we needed – other than when I was getting pricked in my butt!

We decided to do a little bit more in central Thailand before heading back down South. Thankfully, by the time we had to do that bloody awful minibus journey back to Chiang Mai, my neck was all but recovered. I could actually have a bit of banter and enjoy it on the way back. We had decided that from Pai, we would get the minibus back to Chang Mai, then fly to Bangkok to save time and have some comfort, before hopping on another minibus for four hours to get to a place called Koh Chang. Koh Chang was a beautiful, idyllic little slice of heaven. It was just a tranquil island where there were excellent restaurants and beaches, and they had a Muay Thai gym, of course. We decided to stay there for a couple of days and relax before going back South. I was keen to start doing a little bit of training again, and Bert was eager to get back to doing some weights. So, we decided to do that – take it easy and get a moped to get us around so we could explore a bit and find some beautiful, idyllic places to hang out. It was so freeing being there. We would go off on the moped and stop at places with incredible viewpoints and take photos. We found some of the most stunning beaches, and there were magical swings and fallen-down trees that lent themselves perfectly for some amazing pictures. We also stumbled across the gym that was there, and it looked nice. It looked really clean and extremely quiet. We asked if they did any training, and they said the classes were at eight in the morning and four in the afternoon. Perfect, we thought. Tomorrow, we will do just that!

The next day, after we had finished at the beach, I told Bert that I fancied going to training. I hadn't been able to train for a while because of my neck, so now it was feeling much better, I wanted to get back to it. Bert wasn't in the mood for it, so I asked him if I could take the moped and go. He looked concerned, not only about my neck, but the fact that I was going to ride the bike without him. He replied, "Just put on a helmet because you're a fucking liability." What a friend!

When I got there, it was empty. Nobody was there. I must have got my information wrong, or maybe it's cancelled, and Bert's intuition was correct; I should not be training. I was about to hop back on my bike when the guy appeared. I looked around, and he nodded, "Yep, it's just you this afternoon." I thought – *Shit, he's going to kill me.* Bearing in mind, this is my first session back training since way before I fell down the hole.

We started training, and it felt great. It was super smoking hot, but it was really good to be back. At four in the afternoon, it's so humid in Thailand. It would have been much better in the morning when it's cooler, but I had wanted to go to the beach then. Tanning and training were a constant internal battle. I loved both so much; they made me feel alive. I had a great session, and the guy loved training me. He was encouraging me to stay on and train with him. He said, "Let me train you and put you in a fight." Now my ego was getting a real rub from this. I had not trained for a couple of weeks, this was the first session back, and here I am smashing it. I'm strong, and he now wants me to fight for him. It would have been easy to say yes and meet my needs immediately. Then loyalty struck. I owed my trainer back in Phuket. He had invested so much time, love and energy into me, and I knew he had my best interests at heart. Loyalty was, and still is, a massive thing for me. I'm very loyal to people, and this guy had invested months in me. He worked so hard, even when I wasn't paying him and wasn't in the class, he'd show me certain tips and tricks to keep me safe. If he saw me training on the bag, he would come over and show me different moves and spins, correcting my stance and technique. So as much as I enjoyed this first session and the little ego rub, I decided to say no to him. I did continue to train with him for the next few days until we left to head back.

Bert and I had a really good time on our little exploration. I felt that in another life, maybe something would have progressed between us. We became so close, and nothing happened because of Kyle – and a girl Bert had met in Phuket – but there was a special bond between the two of us. Looking back, we were an amazing team. Probably how a relationship should be, but we definitely missed that memo this lifetime.

During these days in Koh Chang, he started getting hassled by the girl he had been seeing back in Phuket. She wanted him to get back there. She kept accusing him of being up to no good. Her insecurities were clearly kicking in. He was a perfect travel companion, and I can 100 per cent vouch for the fact he did nothing whilst we were away. Not even drink. He was somebody that kept me very grounded, and I obviously did him the world of good because there wasn't any boozing at all. We didn't go out drinking or looking for ways to block things out; we experienced life together. We found waterfalls, discovered beautiful scenery, and found amazing bugs and creatures and things that people wouldn't usually see. We would go off into the middle of the jungle and just ride and see where we ended up. It was a beautiful experience, and it felt so good to be doing it with somebody, rather than on my own. I don't think I would have been confident enough at that point to just go off on a moped and see where I ended up. He had given me the confidence to realise that I was actually in a position to be able to do that – something that over the coming months would become the norm.

On the way back to Phuket, I got a message from Ricky telling me when he was going to be arriving there. This was a bit weird. Since I had last seen him, and we had made up, I had fallen head over heels for another guy. Kyle and I had spoken on Facetime almost daily since we'd left each other in Dubai; even Bert had been joining in on the calls. I was enjoying talking with him, and I was excited about seeing him again. However, I also had this other situation running through my head regarding Ricky. He did something to me, ignited something in me, and I couldn't explain it. We had been on a magical journey in the Amazon jungle, and nobody could ever replace those memories. Yes, Kyle and I had made our own memories here in Thailand, but there was something about Ricky. He had come into my life to shake me up, turn me upside down, and spin me around so that I had to see everything that was in me. With Kyle around now, I had this feeling of loyalty towards him. I wondered how I was going to be able to spend time with Ricky as a friend. I really wanted to be his friend, but how could I be a friend with somebody when I had this other man? There was this weird triangle dynamic going on. It was almost like I was being given these different choices to see which one I was going to take, to see if I picked the right one, or if I chose the forbidden fruit. When Ricky messaged to say that he was coming back, my stomach flipped. *Oh God, I'm not sure I'm ready to see him.* The last time I had seen him was in the Galapagos Islands when he had stormed off with all his stuff. This was going to bring up a whole heap of shit for healing.

I was nervous and apprehensive about seeing him, but excited simultaneously. I wanted to see him because I knew what we had was special, but I was not sure how it would go. I wanted to know. Like anything in life, I wanted to know the outcome, so I could avoid any discomfort. You would have thought by this point I would have realised that was not an option, but that inner control freak was still attempting to do her best work.

It had been over a year since we had first met each other. A lot had happened in that year. From two total strangers who had bumped into each other one day, the magical journeys we had been on, the massive bust up and now we were reconnecting.

When I got back to Thailand, I saw Ricky within the first day. We were training at the same gym, so there was no way that we wouldn't see each other. When we did see each other, it was amazing. It wasn't awkward at all. All my worries about being a bit weird with each other were wrong. We gave each other a massive hug, caught up a little bit, and did a little bit of training together, just like the old times. It was like that awful situation in South America hadn't happened. We were back together in the place where we had met, and nothing had changed. Absolutely nothing had changed. It was just bizarre. We didn't even speak about what happened in the Galapagos Islands or anything like that. We spent a little time together, just going out to dinners and stuff like that. It was nice. I didn't speak about Kyle, we didn't bring up anything of the past, but I felt he had a few things to say on a couple of occasions, but he never did. I was keen for us to start over and actually be mates, in the hope that one day we could forget the Galapagos situation. Kyle had completely turned my head, and although Ricky was still a really good-looking guy, I was nervous around him. He had really hurt me. Okay, in reality, I know now that I hurt myself, but at the time, I felt he had hurt me, massively, and I no longer felt safe with him in the way I had before South America. It didn't mean that we couldn't train together and be friends, or maybe even become close again, but at that particular time, I was grateful that Kyle had come along and distracted me because I would have had to deal with my wounds a lot sooner. And who wants to do that? Distractions, avoidance, and running away were my tools to avoid dealing with the traumas.

Now that I was back in Phuket, and had seen Ricky, I decided to stay in a place that was quite close to where I was training, so that I could be there early and train as much as possible because I only had a little bit of time before The Wanderess was flying off to Australia. Christmas in Australia wasn't going to be a time for training, it was going to be spending time with friends and family, and we were going to eat a lot of food, drink alcohol and generally enjoy life. I knew I wasn't going to be living in the cleanest way, so whilst I was here, I was committed to being focused.

I threw myself into my training again for the next week or so; my trainer was impressed. He said, "Lucy, we can get you a fight in December. You're good, and you're looking strong. I'm putting you with strong people, and you are beating them. You are winning." He tried to convince me to put my Australia trip off. The Thai trainers earnt money off you fighting, so it was in their interest to ensure you were good to go. Their reputation was on the line. Some don't care, but luckily mine did. He wouldn't throw me in the ring knowing that I would get obliterated, as he valued his reputation. This guy had won hundreds of fights, he had some of the best fighters in Thailand fighting under him. And so he didn't want to throw me into a ring for me to get battered, as it would look shameful for him. We had an open, honest conversation, and once again, he was a bit pissed off with me because I was disappearing, for the fifth or sixth time since he committed to training me. During the conversation, he asked me if I was scared to get in the ring. And I said, "Well if I said that I wasn't scared at all, that would be weird. But it's not something that I'm really fearing. It's something that I know I've got to do." Of course, I was a bit worried about it, I was fearful of breaking my nose or something like that, but there was something inside of me telling me that I had to do this. It was not about the fight; it was about more than that. It was about seeing what I was capable of doing. I didn't honestly know why I had to do it, I just knew that my life would never be the same again if I did. It's so difficult to explain. It was intuition. Something was guiding me and telling me that this was my path and I needed to do it.

When the time came to go to Australia, I was upset because I was in the best shape of my life. I looked good. I had shed so much weight. The inflammation was going down. I felt strong. I felt energised and healthy. I felt happy, driven, and more motivated than I had ever been. I had become consistent and was loving every second of it. I could see the light at the end of the tunnel. I knew that the fight I was going to do was going to be my moment and that I was going to win. I knew so much was going to happen off the back of it. When it came down to me getting on that flight to go to Australia, as much as I was looking forward to seeing people, I really did want to stay in Thailand. I knew I was going to undo some of the amazing work that I had done up until that point.

The friend who I was staying with in Australia was a boozer. He was a friend from the UK, but he left after his relationship broke down and his ex-partner had taken his son away from him. He had run away to Australia years earlier, and I had only seen him once in that period of time, and that was when he came home because his mum had passed. The friends I was going out with on the new year were big drinkers too. New Year's Eve is a big deal in Australia, they have an incredible firework display going off from Sydney Harbour Bridge, that is admired by people all over the world, and I was going to be there in person enjoying it with some of my besties. On New Year's Day, my friend, who was a deejay, was playing for a massive production over there, so we were going to be going out partying on that day too. This was going to be a real test of my discipline, to see how I would behave.

64

In the middle of December, I was heading in the direction of my beloved Australia. I had been very much in love with the country from the age of 21, when I had first touched down on Aussie soil. At the time, the strong feeling I felt didn't make much sense, but something about being there just felt right. Looking back now, it felt familiar, like home. There was a longing and a knowing in my soul that felt extremely comfortable being there.

I was so excited to be going back. When I first went, I met up with one of my good friends who was travelling there at the time. I had another friend out there too, they had very recently gone through a relationship breakup, and so we had agreed to meet up and travel up the East Coast of Australia together for a few weeks. It was the first time I had flown on my own, and the first time I had gone away anywhere for over two weeks.

After several incredible months of being there, seeing such beauty, and beginning to step into my 'wanderess' shoes for the first time, I sat on the plane and sobbed as I left. I felt I was leaving something behind; leaving the place where I should be.

I visited again a number of years later whilst working for JPMorgan. I was in a fortunate position to do so because I was working very closely with a team in Sydney. As a sweetener to keep me there – because it was another time in my life that I let them know I was thinking of leaving – they sent me to Sydney to work for a few months. I was based in an apartment in the city, and I walked every day to an office that overlooked the Sydney Harbour Bridge. I was in heaven. Every cell in my body wanted to move there, so I applied for an internal transfer, and I got it; then the fear kicked in. My grandad was getting older, my mum had got very sick with skin cancer, and the fixer within me felt I was the only one keeping everything together, so I pulled out from going. I put everyone else above my own needs. It was my choice. A choice I regretted for many years, until I eventually connected why things had to happen the way they did.

So, all these years later, here I was going back to Australia for Christmas and New Year – something I had dreamed of doing ever since I first saw the Sydney New Year fireworks celebrations on TV.

And this year, I was going to actually be there. From the minute I knew I was going to travel, it was always going to be Sydney for New Year. I knew in my soul it was going to be such a magical trip.

A moment of vulnerable honesty here; I always believed I would meet my husband in Australia. The connection that I had with the place had to make sense at some point. My logic always went in the direction that it was because I would meet someone from there. Of course, this was only a story I had convinced myself of. I was making up the end of the story to suit my needs. Welcome to the world of Ego. How many of you have wanted to know the way your story ends? In doing so we display zero patience for the path we are walking; we want to know the end result with as little effort as possible. When you look at it with such brutal honesty, it becomes very obvious why so many of us go for tarot readings, visit mediums and do things like that.

I'd had the most magical time in Asia. I loved becoming part of the team with my new fight family. I never realised that I had been longing to be part of a community until I had been in Thailand for a prolonged period of time. I never realised I wanted something to get involved in, a community of like-minded souls that were aligned to the person I was transforming into; people who supported my future mission, with similar ideals, values and principles. Travelling with Jared, and exploring Thailand had been the most magical start to my journey.

It had been four months since I had left home, though, and it was time for a new chapter. It was time for me to live out some experiences outside of the fight world and training bubble I had encased myself in. I knew I would have to come back to Thailand and revisit the previous chapter at some point, but I also knew that I had to go on and do this. I was open to being guided as to when that time would be to return, and I knew in my heart that it would all work out exactly as it needed to; if I surrendered. Letting go, though, was not so easy. I desperately wanted to fight before I left Thailand for Christmas, and I wondered if knowing I had to return to Thailand to fight would stop me from enjoying myself fully in Australia, and if it would affect my decision of how long to stay there for.

On this trip, I had planned to cover bits of Australia I had never seen before. Initially, I was flying from Thailand to Perth to see a girlfriend – the girl I had been in Malaysia with when the street fight kicked off. She was originally from Perth and was back home at this point. I was going to stay with her for a few days and do a bit of exploring together; she was keen to show me how beautiful Perth was. I had never been to Perth before and so was totally open to being shown another area of Australia, which would no doubt make me fall even more in love with the country than I already was.

I also had a plan to fly over to the Gold Coast to stay with a really good friend from back home in Bournemouth. He had moved over there when his relationship ended and when he wasn't able to have access to his child. I knew it was going to be interesting spending time with him. He had been one of my party associates back in the day. We always ended up partying the small hours away. This time around, though, I was a very different version of myself to the one he knew. It would be a test of my willpower to say no to the boozing because I did still enjoy a little drink from time to time.

My favourite part of my plan was to head to Sydney – my favourite place in Australia; you've got the city, the beach, and for me, the combination and contradiction of both peace and hectic, is central to my life. Let's be honest, it pretty much sums me up as a person – a total contradiction.

I was going to finish the Aussie leg of the trip off at Ayers Rock, with another of my girlfriends, who was flying in to meet me on the Gold Coast. Remember the girlfriend I was in Portsmouth with, having dinner when I decided to go on that magical trip in 2013 after my grandad passed? That's her. She was coming over to Australia with a couple of her friends and we were going to spend some time together.

I'd never been to Western Australia before, so when I landed there, it was the start of a magical mystery tour. It was exciting discovering a brand-new aspect of Australia. This is the reason behind the love I feel for travel. The new experiences, the connections, the foods you get introduced to – all of that excites me so much.

My friend, Kim, picked me up from the airport and, bearing in mind we had only seen each other a few weeks earlier, we were so excited to see each other again. It was a whole new experience being here together, rather than being in Thailand. Over there we were driving around on mopeds and living life without a care in the world. Here, though, she was picking me up in her car and I was experiencing her home. We were acting like kids at Christmas.

And why not? It was the festive season, after all. Her partner ran a successful fight gym in Australia, so we had every intention to train and continue what we had been doing in Thailand. I was shocked and a little excited when as soon as we had stopped squealing at each other in excitement, after landing, she said "You'll come to the gym's Christmas party today, hey?"

And I thought – *Well yeah, why not? If I'm going to be here, I may as well throw myself into the swing of things.*

Now Christmas in Australia is hot, so when I say a party, I don't mean a party like back home in the UK. It was an outdoor party, a 'throwing a shrimp on the barbie' kind of party – please tell me you said that with an Aussie accent as you read it? The party was starting in the afternoon and the intention was to wind it up later in the evening, but Kim did suggest that we may well end up going 'out out' after it had finished. I was open to whatever we were doing. I had no intention of getting boozy. I was keen to spend some quality time with Kim, get to know her fella, and meet anyone else who was destined to cross my path. I was much more accustomed to travelling by this point. I settled into places very quickly. It's quite a fun skill to have picked up, actually. Now I have this innate ability to be able to pack and unpack very quickly, knowing where everything is so I can just grab and run.

I sat out in the garden at the party later that day, enjoying being around like-minded people. Most of the people there were fighters, boxers and people on a mission to look after themselves physically. It felt like a home from home. I stepped into another community that welcomed me with open arms. There were some really lovely people at the party; the couple that Kim lived with were very friendly, and made me feel very welcome. There was one girl there who I clicked with instantly. We hit it off, and as we conversed, the synchronicities we shared made it clear we were always destined to meet. She was a nurse based out of Perth and had just quit her job when we met. She was going to take some time out before going into a new role. As we sat chatting and getting to know each other, she asked me about my time in Thailand. She knew that was where I had met Kim and that I was intending to do a fight. She asked me where I was training, and her jaw dropped when I told her. It transpired that she had booked to go to Thailand in the New Year and to the exact place I was training at. What a small world! This was true confirmation that we were destined to meet. She was excited and relieved knowing she knew someone who was going to be there with her. She had recently been on quite a journey with her career and her relationship and had booked the trip on a whim, and then, like most of us, she had started panicking once she had booked it. Getting connected that day at the party was perfect timing. We exchanged details and promised to keep in touch with each other, in the event that something changed. We both knew it was the start of a beautiful, magical friendship, and I knew in my heart that we were destined to connect again – unlike the countless other people you exchange numbers with but never see ever again. I had found a soul sister. That night we talked, we laughed, and we resonated so deeply with each other; we both knew in our hearts we were about to embark on a journey.

After a few fun days in Perth, I flew right over to the other side of Australia, which is just mad. I thought that a typical flight from one side of a country to another would probably only be an hour or two. Oh no! In Australia, it's 5 hours plus. I had to fly down to Melbourne, which is about 5 hours on its own, then up to the Gold Coast, another decent flight.

After a day of travelling, I eventually got to the Gold Coast and met up with my guy friend from Bournemouth. He remembered the 'party girl' and the 'crazy' Lucy. He remembered the version that I was desperately working hard at trying to forget. I had changed a lot by the time I arrived at his house on the East Coast. I looked different. I felt different. I even spoke differently. Although, I hadn't entirely stepped away from drinking at this point – let's just say I was in a 'transformational stage'. He couldn't get his head around it. He kept trying to hold me back into that older space.

He kept on saying, "Come on, Lucy, let's go out drinking. Let's go out tonight and get off it, like the good old days."

For the first time in my life, I had the discipline to say, "No." I was navigating things in a new way. I was figuring out the language that felt comfortable to me, and it all was a whole new experience. I was in a place where I could happily go out and have fun, but would step aside from the 'other' antics. I was more interested in going on road trips, exploring places, and being more childlike and innocent.

Thankfully, he embraced this new me, although it was a little weird for him, and so we went on lots of road trips whilst I was with him.

We drove all over the East Coast. We went to Byron Bay, which is one of my favourite places in Australia. I feel very at home there, I love it so much. We went to Noosa, which was somewhere I had not been before; what an amazing and intriguing experience that was. It felt so good to go on road trips with my friend and to truly get to know him. Despite us spending many years in each other's company, we didn't know each other properly. It's funny, with party friends you spend hours chatting to each other on a night out, but you don't ever get to know them on a deep level.

We had a barbecue on Christmas Day – a very Aussie thing to do. It was weird. I could not get my head around the fact that there was no roast dinner.

On Boxing Day, the two girls arrived from Portsmouth. It was so lovely to see them. They had been such a pivotal part of my decision to head off to Thailand, after my grandad had passed. That decision had led to this magical experience that was still unfolding with each new day. My guy friend and I picked them up from the airport and we went out for a few drinks, so everyone could get to know each other. It was interesting to see the different friends I had connected with at different times in my life all coming together. I sat and observed, in awe of how lucky I was. It was so random. I had met my guy friend on a night out in Bournemouth. The girls I had met at V-Festival in 2012. All of these connections were made through having fun times and partying. And here we all were coming together on the other side of the world.

When it came time to leave the Gold Coast, though, I was ready to leave and head to Sydney. It had been amazing, but straddling the two worlds was becoming draining. I was caught between the new version of me – transforming and growing – and the old version of me that my friends remembered. I wasn't really in one camp or the other. I was straddling the two. This experience, though, would serve me well.

When we got to Sydney, we were all splitting up. One of the girls was staying with me, and the other girl was heading off to stay with some friends who lived out there. We would still see each other, and meet up for New Year's Eve and New Year's day, but we were going to be based out of two different houses for a short time. Me and the girl who was staying with me had become really close in the months before I left to go travelling. She had been an amazing friend. I would often be in Portsmouth at IBM, so I would stay with her and we would hang out. She was a rock when my grandad died too. She was very reliable, and a friend I always thought I would have. We had such fun in each other's company, and being in Sydney together was no different. We would go running in the morning, we discovered beautiful places to eat, spent time with my friends, and totally immersed in the beauty of Sydney. We had arranged to go to Ayers Rock together after the New Year, just the two of us, to explore this magical site. We had invited the other girls, but they had not wanted to go.

On New Year's Eve, we went out at about 11 am – apparently, that's what you have to do to get a decent spot for the fireworks in Australia. We intended to have some beers and food throughout the day, so we headed to the park carrying a lot of stuff – wine, beer, food, and everything else that goes along with being out all day long. We had a great time. We sat out in the sun all day with music playing, we danced and played games, and joined in with the thousands of other people who were doing exactly the same thing as we were. The only real downside to the day was the toilet situation; you had to fight your way through the crowds, queue up and then remember where your friends were on the way back – this was fine in the daylight, but the minute it got dark, it took on a whole new level of complexity.

Regardless, I had an amazing day surrounded by some amazing people. However, I started to feel a slight undertone with one of the girls. I'm not sure if she had been feeling left out or if she was feeling insecure, but there was something going on. Admittedly, back then, I did not know how sensitive I was and that I could read energy, but I felt something was up. One of my favourite lines in a movie is 'assumptions are the mother of all fuck-ups'. That line stuck with me ever since and it taught me not to assume anything; I asked good questions to extract the right information. That night, in Sydney, there was a strange dynamic going on between the two girl 'best friends', and it was making everybody feel uncomfortable, not just me. It really started bugging me, but I didn't want to get involved in it and ruin the night, so I carried on regardless.

We stayed for the full day. The fireworks were breathtaking, an absolute extravaganza. We all wished each other Happy New Year and watched in awe as the sky lit up with colour and beauty. I had never experienced anything like it. This was a massive tick off the bucket list for me.

I went back to my friend's house shortly after the New Year celebrations had finished, for a little decompress and debrief. We were not having a crazy night that night, as the next day he was deejaying at a daytime party, and we knew we had another day of dancing and being 'out out' to come. We ended up heading to bed at about 3am on New Year's Day, and we had to be at the party in just a few hours' time.

On little sleep, we made it to the party by midday. My friend was DJing towards the middle of the set; his fiancée and I spent the whole time dancing to the tunes he was dropping. It was amazing. He was an amazing DJ. I had fallen back in love with dancing. Dancing around on a terrace, in Sydney, on New Year's Day, with the sun beaming down on us. Could life get any more precious than this?

I had some guy friends who had flown over to Sydney for Christmas, and they came to meet us for the day. They had managed to secure some 'goodies' to get them in the party mood. The two girls, the ones who were giving off the bad vibes the day before, decided to get involved in the 'goodies' too. The animosity from the day before seemed to have disappeared, which was a step in the right direction.

At some point in the early evening, I reminded the girl who was due to be flying to Ayres Rock with me, that we had an early flight the next day. It was just a reminder – call it intuition, or maybe my inner control freak – but I thought it best to let her know. After that, I carried on dancing and having fun. I'm a real fan of letting your body flow, whether that be Thai boxing, dancing, sex, or whatever your jam is. Allowing your body to do whatever it needs to do is important.

It got to just after midnight and my friend had finished his sets, so we decided to head back to his. I told the two girls that I was going, but they were happy to stay on. I reminded my friend once more, that we had the flight the next day, and then I left.

We got back to my friend's house, chilled out and chatted for a bit, and then went to bed.

The following day, I woke up and I had received a text message from the girl that I was supposed to be going to Ayers Rock with; she messaged me to say she wasn't coming to the rock with me.

Hmm, pretty interesting. I fell straight into victim mode – *Oh shit! I'm going to have to go there on my own. Why has she done this to me?* I was pissed off. There had been this weird vibe on New Year's Eve, and then they had got off their heads at the party yesterday. I had asked her a few questions, but she wasn't very forthcoming. I even thought that they were probably still out partying – not that it was any of my business. My guy friend, the DJ, got wind of what was going on, and he said that his fiancé should take her flight and come to Ayers Rock with me. I got on really well with her, so I was well up for that, and so was she. We both got excited by the idea of a cheeky road trip, to a place where neither of us had been before. We switched the names on the flight ticket and headed off later that same day in search of the red rock.

65

We landed in Ayers Rock, and nothing could have prepared me for the feeling I got as my feet connected with this special earth, known as one of the chakras of the world. It's worth remembering, at that time I was still very three-dimensional, and so was my friend's fiancé. She was in recruitment for banking technology – similar to the kind of roles I was in, and I was still only recently distanced from my old trading floor paradigm. We got there and the place blew us away, though. I wasn't aware, at this point, that I could feel energies or anything like that. All I knew was that there was something very special about this place.

We were staying in one of the closest hotels to the rock. I got to our hotel room and told my friend that I had to lie down for a bit, before we headed out. The heat was overwhelming. It had an intensity that seemed to come from nowhere. Obviously, it's in the desert, so naturally there was heat there, but there was a warmth running through us, through our veins, and in our cells that is difficult to explain unless you have been there. Interestingly, it was the first time, since being a child that I remember feeling drawn to have a nap in the afternoon. Looking back on it now, with the knowledge I have gathered from my journey since then, I was starting to get upgrades. I was starting to get the communications, and the activations from the light codes. That's why our bodies need to nap sometimes. Not through laziness; to allow the integration of very important DNA shifts that enable us to embody the energy coming in. I didn't know at the time that this precious site was the Solar Plexus chakra of the world. I do now, though, and I can appreciate exactly what was happening, and my reason for being called there.

Whichever way you look at Ayres Rock, it is red. The whole landscape is red. Our trainers were changing colour as we walked because the sand is such a profound colour. We had a beautiful connecting experience as we trotted slowly through the cactus plants and wildlife. It was so hot – early 40s that day – with absolutely zero moisture in the sky. I have no idea how people survive out there without water and shelter.

That night we both had the craziest, vivid dreams. My friend's fiancé woke up, and she was freaked out by how intense her dreams were. It was almost like we were caught up in a vortex of energy – which we essentially were – but neither of us knew that at the time. We both just thought it was a bit weird. She was dreaming about all these bizarre scenarios, and I was getting insights into what had happened with lots of different people. It was like all of a sudden my psychic abilities had come online. I didn't know how I knew stuff, I just knew. It was fascinating. I was a bit weirded out, and I didn't really want to talk about it. I wasn't quite ready to be sharing what was going on in my head.

The next evening, we arranged to go back to the rock and get as close to it as possible. On some evenings, aborigines play their local music. You can buy their stunning artwork and artefacts. We really wanted to embrace that experience. It was so incredible too, we were so glad we went. It was probably my first experience of truly, deeply feeling how magical a place is, where it is nothing more than mother nature in all her glory. To your eyes, there's nothing really there in front of you other than a big red rock, albeit one that you're told is very special. However, on an energetic level, there was a level of peace that was running through our veins and into our cells. We found ourselves sitting there in total silence, reflecting. Not because we had nothing to say but because there was nothing that needed to be said. It was like a special energy was working through us, bringing us back online. I felt deeply rooted in nature and attached to something exceptionally sacred and ancient. Interestingly, something else I did not know at this point in my journey, was that the solar plexus was where I personally held my trauma. Anger, resentment, guilt, and shame were all building up in this area of my physical vessel, without my awareness.

When we eventually started speaking, we had some interesting conscious conversations that were totally out of character for us both. We had become good friends, but I wouldn't say we held a particularly deep relationship up until this point. There, though, we spoke about lots of different off-the-wall things. And some of the messages coming out of her mouth were profound. I'm pretty sure she won't remember much of it, but I know now that she was channelling. It took me back to my grandad in his dying weeks. I was absolutely certain that my nan was channelling him to get the messages to me, so I would awaken and go on my path of enlightenment.

We had such a magical night with the aboriginals, listening to their music. There was something in that music that was captivating and activating. It was the activation point, I'm sure; everything changed for me after that. I completely let go of any animosity I may have felt towards the other girl for letting me down and not going on the journey with me as I had expected. I accepted that she was not part of this chapter and that was okay. I totally let go. I relinquished everything that I needed to. It was almost like I had listened to the tones and the frequencies and become plugged back in to get my vibration going up again. I sat there that evening, in the balmy temperatures of Ayres Rock, and sent her so much love for her onward journey, with tears rolling down my face.

The next day, after that magical experience, we left Ayers Rock and flew back down to Sydney. I stayed there for a few days with my friend and his fiancé, and then I got myself ready to make my way back to Thailand.

Unfortunate Accidents

It might be a good time at this point to say buckle up – trigger warning incoming!

It's my personal belief system, since going on this magical journey, that everything we experience and all the circumstances that arise in our lives, show up to remind us of what we need to heal and why we this lifetime. All accidents, arguments, illnesses and even insect bites. They are all brought to us to bring to the surface all the hidden emotional traumas that we have buried deep within us and have pretended to have dealt with.

When I look back on that bizarre accident with the hole, it's really interesting. The healing journey I went on off the back of all these experiences, led me to revisit every injury, every unfortunate accident, and every freak situation that I ever found myself in over the years. I looked at what I call the 'energetics' that created the situation and why it needed to show up. My personal belief system is that what we experience as a physical sign, is to get our attention to whatever trapped trauma is in our body.

The accident with the hole is a perfect example. Walking along a road and falling down a hole would, to most people, appear as an unfortunate accident. Nothing more, nothing less. The way I view things now, was that I was missing something, not paying attention properly and so I had to be stopped in my tracks. I had to be pushed. I clearly needed to be jolted, to have a little bit of a shakeup in my body, so that I would take some time out and actually sit and reflect. When I think about what I was doing, I was totally distracting myself – with boxing, with men. I had not been prepared to sit with my feelings. I was not prepared to sit there and realise I was falling for Kyle, and so what did I do? I distracted myself with travel.

I was not ready to sit and feel all of the emotional pain I was carrying around, and the reasons why I had become so sick and burnt out. From the minute I left Corporate, I went on a whirlwind tour with Catherine, then on to Thailand, and straight into training and boxing mode. From there I went to Malaysia to the fights, and ended up in a street brawl. I even looked into the reason why the guy ripped my earring out. Now, the right ear relates to being angry or annoyed. And this was true, I was constantly replaying things in my mind around childhood, and getting angry about it, stepping through the old traumas. At that particular time, I felt like I'd had an earful of it all, hence I ran away.

After the Malaysia fight, I went back to training, and then ran off to see Kyle in Dubai. It was one distraction after another. I was not sitting with myself, so the Universe kicked me up the backside and made me fall down that hole and hurt my neck, so I could realise the weight of the world was on my shoulders, in the shape of emotional trauma. Everything needed to be looked at and faced head on. There was no more running away. I was going to keep being hit with more and more scenarios, until I actually sat with it.

This was just the starting point where it appeared in my consciousness. Don't get me wrong, I was not fully there yet, but I was coming online and starting to recognise a few things. It's like I could see the memo, but the words were blurry. Now though, when I look back, this was the actual start of it. This was the start of me recognising that I had been missing something very important for all this time, and that I had to deliver it to the human race.

There is no such thing as a simple common cold in my world anymore! It's all showing us something.

Trust me, it becomes easier the more you lean in.

66

I arrived back in Thailand at the end of January 2015. I was excited to be back. I was ready to get on with my training and that discipline again. I'd had almost a month off proper training and let my hair down somewhat. I did train whilst I was in Australia because I had access to my friend's gym, but it wasn't like Thailand. Nothing can prepare you for the training in Thailand, I'm not sure anything compares actually; having no air-conditioning in those temperatures is a whole new level. Even having the heating on in summer doesn't come close – and yes, I have trained at a gym in England where they did that to prep us hard. Honestly, the things fighters have to endure!

Even though I had been away a month, my sights were still very firmly set on doing a fight. I was going to do whatever it took to get there. I was absolutely focused – no distractions; it was head down, bum up time!

My first training session back was hell. My trainer was shaking his head at me, winding me up, "What's wrong with you? What's happened to you?" I was in so much pain from kicking the pads because my shins had five weeks off it. Before I went away, my shins were tough, they were hardened from all the sparring, bag kicks and pad kicks. I had lost something whilst I was away, and I was bruising like a peach again. I had a long way to go. It completely humbled me. If you stop whatever it is you are looking to do – diet, get fit, write a book – you can lose it all in a click of a finger. It's okay to take a short break, but keeping going is how we achieve things. I was laughing at myself. I did like to make life harder for myself than was necessary. I had the old paradigm running through my mind- no pain, no gain. I knew it would likely take me a week to get back into shape and get used to dealing with the humidity again, so I tried to be gentle with myself while I adjusted.

It did only take me a week too. My muscle memory was returning quickly. In my second week, I was beginning to get more confident, and so I started up again, "When am I going to fight? Come on, when are you going to put me in?"

My trainer laughed at me and said, "You're strong, you're so strong, we need to get you out there." He wouldn't commit to a fight though. I actually felt by this point he loved our training sessions as much as I did. We had such a laugh, although he was tough as old boots and took absolutely not one ounce of shit from me; we loved each other. We had a beautiful relationship, built on respect and fun. He would often see me doing my own training in the gym, and call me over so he could throw medicine balls at my abs. I know it sounds like hell to most people, but it was what was required. He wanted me to win. He needed me to be in the best shape of my life; and I was getting there.

I got tired of waiting for him, though, so one day towards the end of January, I proposed to him again that I did my first fight at the monthly event called 'BBQ Beatdown'. To give you a little more insight, on the last Saturday of the month there was a barbecue for all of the trainers, staff, clients and some of the locals from in and around the gym. Everyone was welcome. They would have alcohol, food, and amateur fights, and then a big party to close the night out. These events were massive. More often than not, there would be a hundred people there. They were good fun and really good exposure to what a fight would be like. I would be able to fight with all of my friends around me, supporting me, and getting in my corner. I thought it was a win-win situation; it would meet my needs to practice for a real fight, and my trainer would gain confidence by seeing I was ready. He cut it dead immediately again, though. He said, "No, you're too strong for that. No, I'm not going to put you into that. You'll hurt somebody." I was furious. I was not getting my own way with this man at all, and I wasn't happy about it. *Why is he doing this? What's his problem?*

My ego was roaring like a lion. I went into full-blown victim mode, blaming everything and everyone. In my head, I accused him of just wanting to make money from me. I knew that the trainers got paid when they put you in a professional fight, not an amateur fight. People also gamble quite heavily in and around the fight scene in Thailand – they say gambling's illegal, but that's nonsense. Anyone who has been to a fight there would have seen it all unfolding, and maybe even got involved. I also thought that maybe he didn't trust I could do it, and he had no faith in me. In my heart, I knew all of this was nonsense, but my ego was raging. I believed I knew better. God knows how, this guy was a living legend in Thailand, and I had been doing the sport for five minutes. The truth was, he cared about his reputation more than the money, and he wouldn't put me in a fight where I could hurt someone or get hurt myself. It's embarrassing to see now how I behaved, but hopefully, this will ignite something in some of you. It's okay to be the student. It's okay to feel lost and out of your depth. This is the healing journey; it was never going to be easy – so let's stop pretending it is and start baring all, so we can step forward, once and for all.

Another reason I was disappointed that I couldn't fight at the Beatdown was that my best friend was flying over to see me for my birthday, and I wanted her to see me fight. I wanted her to be proud of me, and how far I had come. She didn't care, though; in fact, she said she didn't want to watch me fight, she was worried I would get hurt. My plan had been that my birthday weekend could kick off with my fight, and then we could celebrate after that. However, my trainer was intent on ruining my plan. So, I decided I would celebrate all weekend instead. Screw him.

Catherine arrived a few days before my birthday, and it was so great to see her. That night we took a taxi into Patong with a few other people. Patong is a very interesting place. It was booming. The bars were rammed with people; the Thai women and ladyboys were doing their best to take people into their bars to earn money for the evening. We met up with some friends from back home and ended up having a really late night. I wasn't drinking because I had training the next day, but I did stay out and have fun with them all. It was good to be out enjoying company and not be so focused on the training and discipline. I also felt this was a huge step in my growth again; being able to go out and party without actually drinking, or getting involved in the antics, but being present with people. It was a big deal, and I was proud of myself. I was happy and grateful to be around two dear friends from back home, for the first time in a very long time.

I went training the next day, whilst Catherine stayed in bed. It was Friday morning, so I left her to chill whilst I did my morning and afternoon sessions, before I downed tools to celebrate my birthday weekend.

On the Friday night, I arranged for a group of us to go out to dinner at an Italian restaurant I had been introduced to on an earlier visit. I wanted my friends from home to meet my travelling friends. We all met at my place, and headed off on mopeds – flying down the roads, hair blowing in the wind. It was such a great feeling. My friends from home loved it. We had an amazing meal that night. At one point, I sat back and watched in awe as my two worlds came together as one. They all got on really well, and I loved them so very much. They were all so very important to me. It filled my heart with so much love.

At the end of the meal, the restaurant gave us all free limoncello shots, and as much as I thought twice about it, we all ended up downing the shots. It's fair to say that was the start of the birthday celebrations.

On the way back, we got on the mopeds, two people on each bike. I'm pretty sure we shouldn't have got on the bikes after the shots but we all thought we were fine to drive. We had such a laugh on the journey home. I look back at some of the things that I did when I was travelling, with my head in my hands. My mum would have had a fit if she knew her daughter was riding along with no helmet on at 60 miles an hour, weaving in and out of traffic. It was almost like I felt invincible at times when I was away. Any time things looked a little hairy, it seemed a force would step in to protect me and keep me safe. It wasn't that I was not aware of the dangers. There were signs and warnings everywhere about how many people got hurt riding motorbikes. I personally had known three people that died in Thailand on motorbikes – people that I actually knew; so you can imagine the actual numbers of people that fall off their bikes and get hurt, or worse. Thankfully, I lived to tell the tale, although it's definitely not something I would do now. Believe it or not, I'm actually a very good driver. A little heavy on the right foot, but generally pretty sensible.

The next day, Catherine and I went out on the moped to find a beautiful beach to relax on. We topped up the tan to get a nice crisp glow in readiness for the BBQ Beatdown later that evening. The last time I had been drinking was over Christmas, a month or so earlier. I had decided that I would let my hair down for the BBQ Beatdown and my birthday. In all honesty, if I could have swept my birthday under the carpet that year, I would happily have done so. I was loving my training. I was loving being fit and healthy. I knew I was super close to getting the fight I had been focused on, but my beautiful friend was over from England and she was expecting a good time, so that is what she would get.

On the Saturday night, I got dressed up and put some make-up on. It always used to make me laugh how people reacted when I turned up outside of gym clothes; they always looked shocked. I guess they were used to seeing me in training gear, sweating my bits off with absolutely no make-up on. So when I did make an effort, it was well received.

That night, there were loads of people out to celebrate my birthday. The fight team were all present, most of the trainers were there, and a huge group of the friends I had made whilst I had been over there too. I was so happy that they had made the effort to join me and celebrate. Of course, it meant the night got messier than it needed to, and quickly too. I was getting glasses of wine poured for me the size of tumblers. On top of that, there were shots being passed around, and because it was my birthday, apparently that meant I had to drink them. My friend took a shine to one of the strength and conditioning coaches that I'd become good friends with. She had decided he looked a bit like the cartoon character He-Man – and to be fair to her, he really did. The two of them ganged up on me to start doing tequila shots. Now, I'm not very good at drinking tequila at the best of times, but I was also totally out of practice at this point too. Tequila is something I would normally avoid as it would make me get angry and erratic, so I avoided it for years. The two of them were encouraging me, though. I lost all my willpower to say no at this point. Shots are not a normal size in Thailand either, you don't get a shot glass, you get an inch of tequila in the bottom of a normal drinking glass. Before I knew it, I was absolutely annihilated.

There was no other word for it – annihilated.

Catherine told me a couple of days later she spotted that I was in a right mess very quickly after the shots. She didn't know what she was going to do with me. I didn't know where I was, I barely knew my name at this point, and this was only about 9 in the evening. What a legend!

I said to Catherine that I needed to go home; the issue was, I couldn't walk. I was an absolute mess. Catherine, God bless her, took me home. My beautiful best friend was always there to save me. She told me this story so many times afterwards. She picked me up and put my arm around her neck, and she physically walked me home. The best bit about it was she had to sing to me all the way home because as soon as she stopped singing, I stopped walking. My chosen song for Catherine to sing that night was In Da Club by 50 Cent. So, she was walking me home singing, "Go Shorty, it's your birthday," over and over again. As soon as she stopped, I stopped. "Go Shorty, it's your birthday, Go Shorty, it's your birthday."

Eventually, she managed to get me back to my room, and put me into bed. Apparently, I was gone in an instant. I was completely out of it, but at least she knew I was safe. She then tottered back to my party, and didn't return until the next day! Good on her, I say!

I woke up the next morning, in the early hours, needing the toilet, and thinking – *Where the hell am I? What's going on?* I had absolutely no clue what had happened. I didn't remember anything of getting back to my bed that night. It's actually embarrassing, but thankfully, I was safe. And thankfully, Catherine was there, sorting me out, like the good old days.

I didn't feel great, to be honest; the alcohol had been intense and I had no idea where Catherine was, so I was panicking a little for her safety. On top of that, we were off to Phi Phi that day – the thought of which actually made me feel sick. It was going to be a right old mission! A mission that at that point I was not up for. Minibus, boat, and lots of walking. That was not what I needed; I needed bed, cuddles and comfort food.

I finally managed to track down Catherine and she was feeling very rough too. She'd had a brilliant night by the sounds of it, and I was proud of her. She always made her own way in everything. She wasn't the kind of person to miss out. If she wanted something, she would get it!

Somehow, miracle of all miracles, we managed to get ourselves on the boat; it wasn't pretty, though. I told Catherine I was going to go and sit outside and dangle my feet over the side of the boat. It was such a beautiful day and I thought the sun would help. Catherine on the other hand thought it would be sensible to sit inside. Within about twenty minutes though she ran outside and started puking over the side of the boat. What a pair!

We got to Phi Phi and it was beautiful. Our plans were to stay in a nice hotel and relax for one day and night and then travel back the next day; I had to get back to training. If you have never been to Phi Phi, it's tiny but it's stunning. The only way to get there is in a boat, and there are absolutely no cars on the island at all. You get around on foot or maybe a push bike, if you're very lucky. Phi Phi is actually where they filmed The Beach with Leonardo Di Caprio. There's a beautiful viewpoint where you can go up and see everything. It's incredible. You can go on speedboats, go diving, there are monkeys everywhere, it's absolute paradise. Well, let's say it used to be paradise until the tourism kicked in and then it got completely overwhelmed and lost its way. The first time I ever went, it was pure and untouched. When I went there with the girls, this time, it had been massively ruined by tourism, people were getting drunk everywhere and it had gone totally downhill.

We checked into a beautiful hotel that was up on a hill overlooking the island. That evening we walked down into the town to get some food, and although the place was stunning, I didn't feel like I wanted to be there. I felt hanging. Catherine was hanging as well. All she wanted to do was go to sleep. But the other girl that we were with was really on a mission to find a man, and Catherine and I were being her 'dead-inside' wing women. We really tried, we took it for the team up to a certain point and then we had to tell her that we were done and we needed to go to sleep. We had hit the wall, there was no way we could stay out anymore. So we went back and left her with some random guy she had met along the way.

The next morning, it was actually my birthday. After a good night's rest, I felt amazing, but I was all done with celebrating my birthday – the drinking, partying, and eating. And we still had a long journey to get back home.

Once we arrived, I decided to go to training. Catherine said she would come and watch me train, she had started to warm to the idea of what I was doing. As soon as I got in there, before I even got to show Catherine around, my trainer called me over, "Come, come, come, come."

Catherine said, "Oh shit, you're in trouble. He knows you've been drinking all weekend!"

Thankfully he didn't speak very good English at that point, so he didn't fall for Catherine trying to get me into trouble, instead, he said to me, "You fight."

I said, "Yes, I want to fight."

He said, "No, I got you a fight."

I was so happy. "That's amazing, thank you. When is it?"

"Eleven days," he said, straight-faced.

"Eleven days?" I asked in disbelief. Fight camps are normally many weeks of training and intense preparation, and now after everything, I find out it's in eleven days!

I immediately thought – *Shit, I've just undone all of the amazing work that I've done. I've literally just destroyed my body over a weekend with so much alcohol. What the fuck am I going to do?*

You know, the ironic thing about it, if I hadn't had one drink that weekend, that fight would have never transpired. It's just the way that the Universe works – it urges you to stand in your own shoes, to be disciplined, to be careful what you wish for and what you actually call in. I would have to get all of the alcohol out of my system very quickly to get into the best shape of my life and be able to fight in less than two weeks' time.

Catherine said she was glad she wouldn't be around for the fight, she didn't want to have to witness me in that way. I was excited by the idea of the fight, and I knew it would be an important part of my life, but I was also terrified. There were a few moments of real doubt. I looked at Catherine and I said to her, "I know you're here for a bit longer yet, but I've got to get my head down and work hard here."

She said, "Damn right you do. If you're getting in that ring you have to make sure that you are at the top of your fitness game. Do whatever it takes."

And literally, from that moment onwards, at about two o'clock in the afternoon of my birthday, I went into total focus mode, nothing was going to distract me now. This fight meant everything.

And I was going to do whatever it took to win it.

67

As much as I was excited that I had been given the fight, after chasing it for months and months. I quickly realised that just four days of partying had taken its toll. I had drunk a lot of alcohol, not slept properly, and not eaten great either. All of the things that had become non-negotiables for a while had disappeared. I'd still done a bit of exercise over those four days, despite all of the other activities that had been going on, but it just wasn't enough. It's amazing what you can do, or rather undo, in just four days. I felt guilty for going out and drinking. I felt shame for not sticking to the programme. What had possessed me? I had this dream and I sabotaged it, just like that.

I hit training hard. I had to. Catherine was fine entertaining herself, and, more often than not, she wanted to come and watch me train, as the scenery in the gym was almost as beautiful as most of the beaches. There was a lot of eye candy at the gyms. It has to be said, that place in Thailand had more beautiful people than I had ever seen, and in such a small space. She didn't seem to object to any of it anyway.

That first day I did a strength and conditioning session, and then I did a Thai boxing session. Catherine had never seen me do anything like it before, and so she was shouting at me when I was training to keep my motivation high.

"I'm proud of you!" she was screaming across the room, taking videos so I could see where I was at. That first session was not great for me – I was feeling rough; I wanted to be sick and my form was absolutely diabolical. The thing is with Thailand when you're training, it's all open-air, and the humidity really gets to you – you're not in an air conditioning unit like we are used to back home. You are out there with the elements and sweating buckets on the mats. On top of that, I was detoxing from all the alcohol. I was pissing sweat from every single pore. The more you sweat, the more they push you, and the more they push you, the more you sweat. The more you sweat, the more you need to drink. It's an absolute vicious cycle. And this day, it was exceptionally hot. I was dripping from head to toe, my hair was dripping wet, and sweat was dripping off my elbows. It was really disgusting, but at the same time, I loved it. I had missed it. It was a love-hate relationship – at times it was punishing, but as soon as you stop, you want to go again!

After that first session, I didn't think I was going to be able to do it. I had 11 more days until the fight; 9 more days of training like this. I had to keep my focus. And that was the key thing that I recognised in that initial session. I did beat myself up quite a lot during the session; I felt guilty for going out drinking, I felt resentment that my friends had led me astray. The harsher reality, though, was that it was all me. I had made the decision to party, and I had done that because I wasn't getting my own way by being allowed to fight in the beatdown. I could easily have said no. I could have easily stayed focused. I didn't. I chose to let my hair down and relive the old days. Trust me, if I had a fight in the diary, there's no way I would have ever drunk even a drop on my birthday.

Ricky saw me when I was in this mood of being really angry with myself, and he took the piss out of me because he knew what I was going through. Now Ricky was a very good boxer. He'd done lots of amateur fights. He'd been targeted as one of the members of the team that was going to go to the Commonwealth. He would have been up there with the very best, but injuries and a few other things, stopped him from taking on that path for a while. He said to me, "Look, why don't we do some sparring? Why don't we do some training together to get you ready for your fight?" I really appreciated that. In the back of my mind, I was already thinking of asking Ricky to corner my first fight. I trusted him with my life, I trusted my trainer too, but my trainer couldn't speak to me in English properly. I had lots of people that could corner for me if Ricky couldn't, but deep down I wanted him. So, when he asked me about doing some training together, I was happy, but I also knew I was going to regret it. I knew that he was going to piss me off. He was going to trigger me. He was going to push me to breaking point, but I had no option but to say yes because I knew he would get me to the top of my game. He was going to be my accountability buddy throughout this training camp. And as painful as it would be, I only had to endure this shit for less than two weeks – because for the two days before the fight itself, you aren't allowed to train at all.

My trainer went in really hard on me. It was almost like he'd flipped a switch.

He said, "You're fighting now, this is serious. You're going to have somebody knee you in your stomach. You're going to have somebody punching you in your head. You're going to have somebody kicking you and hurting you. Their target is to hurt you." So he really upped his game to a whole new level – and he was tough beforehand. And now, all of a sudden, he wasn't taking my shit, he wasn't taking my excuses to have a water break. It was literally as if we were doing the fight. He would do five-minute rounds to make sure that I was perfect, and then only give me a one-minute break, and then go straight in for another five-minute round. Now, some of you that watch the UFC, or something like that, might think that's really easygoing – trust me, it's not! Five minutes, when you are being pushed, punched, kicked, and hunted down, especially by a six-foot lunatic – and he was a lunatic – it's not easy going!

That first evening, when Catherine and I went out to dinner, I said to her, "Babe, I have to change my life. I'm being shown so much stuff, I need to change. The old way doesn't work for me anymore." Catherine never said anything, but I wouldn't have blamed her for thinking I was just being dramatic. I could tell she was thinking that I would change for this fight, get it out of my system, and then be back to the Lucy that everyone knew. Good time Lucy. Party girl Lucy.

The next morning, after my first session, I woke up and I went straight back into the hardcore training cycle – a 5k run before training, a 2-hour training session, a strength and conditioning session at lunchtime, followed by a 2-hour training session, and then finish on a 5k or 10k run in the afternoon. I would have to do that every day until two days before the fight, when I would be ordered to rest and prepare.

The second day went well. I worked hard, I felt great, and I was focused.

The following day was when Catherine was flying home. Admittedly, I was a little bit distracted because I wanted to see her off, and it was during my training time. I put her in a taxi and said goodbye to her. It was sad because I didn't know when I would see her again.

Once she was gone, though, I felt a little bit relieved because I didn't have to worry about entertaining her, and I didn't have the distraction of going out for drinks. I could be completely laser-focused. I had about seven days at this point before I had to down tools, so I threw myself into it with everything I had.

Ricky, bless him, was amazing. He was by my side the whole time. We would get up at about five in the morning and go to one of the beaches that were about a 20-minute moped journey away. We would do beach sprints or stair sprints – and those stair climbs were absolute hell! Some mornings we would run up the hill, where the Big Buddha was at the top – it's probably only a mile or two up, but it's a steep fucking hill. It's steep in places, and then it's gradual, and then it bends and goes steep again. From the second you start, to the second you get to the top, there is no letup whatsoever. We did this most mornings, before our first official 5k run of the day. So my training went to a whole new level. Ricky was my biggest cheerleader, mirror and bully all rolled into one. He showed me everything I was capable of, took absolutely none of my shit and mirrored back the pieces of myself that irritated the heck out of me. He would shout at me, "Come on Lucy, you can do it!" Regardless of what had gone on between Ricky and me, I knew there was no way he wanted to see me get hurt. He knew he had to toughen me up. He had to make sure I was ready. So he was chasing me up the hill, screaming at me, and getting in my face. He was pushing my buttons big time. Trust me, I'm not sure anyone else would have got away with what he did. I was humbled by the assistance he gave so freely. I was absolutely exhausted, and in truth, I wanted to cry on many days.

A couple of days into my new training plan, I got a message from the nurse that I had met at Christmas, saying she had arrived in Phuket. I'll be honest, when she messaged I got this feeling of – *Oh God, now I've got gotta look after somebody else.* I didn't really have time for that, but that evening I met up with her for dinner, and I introduced her to a number of people so that I had no issues with her being reliant or dependent on me. She was there for a month, so I'd have plenty of time to spend with her after my fight. To be fair to her, she got it. She knew that I was going to be head down and bum up and very limited on time. I certainly wasn't going to be going out drinking or partying or any of that stuff – which actually worked for her too because she had come over here to get fit and get her head together. She was really supportive and encouraging of everything I was doing.

A couple of days later, I was in my training regime and I was hurting. My body was under pressure – you've got to remember I was in my mid-thirties at this point. My body wasn't quite like that of a 21-year-old, which is the age that most of the other people that were doing this training camp were. The training was really starting to take its toll on me. I said to my trainer, "I'm going to skip my run after my last session of the day."

He said, "No you not," in his beautiful little Thai accent. When I left the gym, he followed me on his moped. Now, if you've ever been to Thailand, you may have seen kids running down the road in their shorts and their trainers, being chased by their parents on mopeds to get them ready for their fights. This is what my trainer did to me.

There was a loop you could take from the gym. It's a long, fucking horrible loop. Whichever way you went, you always ended up with the massive hill. It was just awful. So, I was on the run that evening, and I'd run down a street – which is where all of the gyms were, and where lots of people knew me. When I was running down there, being chased by my trainer, a lot of people cheered me on and shouted my name, and I got a little bit of adrenaline from them, it helped me a little bit. After that, there is this long, laborious, shitty, bland, vanilla part of the road which goes for about five kilometres. It was the worst part, always – it was hot, there were potholes in the road, it was just horrible. On top of that, I had seen a snake there before – and I know I have mentioned before, but I'm fucking terrified of snakes.

So I was on this horrible run, I was already in pain before I began, and I started welling up. I stopped and said to my trainer, "I need to stop."

"Run!" was all he said.

I had no choice so I carried on running and I started crying. I started sobbing my eyes out. The thoughts in my head were horrendous – *You can't fucking do this, Lucy. Why are you setting yourself up to do something you've got no fucking clue how to do? You don't know that you can fight. You don't know that you're strong enough. You're too old, you're too fat.* All of these things were going through my head – constant self-sabotage. I was still running at this point and blubbing like a baby as I did it. People on the street were watching me and watching him chase me on his moped. I know they were used to seeing this kind of stuff over there, but I felt embarrassed. I was so emotional. I just wanted to run away.

I got to a point where I couldn't take it anymore. I stopped, and I looked at him and I said, "Fuck you, I'm not running anymore." And I sat down on the kerb, put my head in my hands, and I cried, and cried, and cried. He didn't know what to do with me. He sat on his moped and he stared. He shouted and pointed, "You run! You fight, You run."

Through my tears, I shouted back, "Is that all you have got to say to me? I can't do this anymore. I can't do it." I was having a full-on meltdown and drama in the middle of the road with lots and lots of people around to witness it. Hissy fit central on a busy road in Phuket. He looked at me with a look that I will never forget.

You know that look your dad gave you when you were little, when he was really pissed off with you? That was the look he gave me. I looked back at him and I had this feeling come through me – *You can fucking do this, Lucy. You're going to get challenged in this fight. You are going to have a moment where you don't think you can do it, but you've got to get back up and you've got to go.*

He carried on staring at me. I stood up and I said to him, "Fuck you," and I started running. I kept saying, over and over in my head, "You've got this, you've got this. You're going to do this." It felt like that sequence in the movie Rocky when he is running up the stairs, and he's running on the beach – only there wasn't heroic music playing in the background for me. I gave myself the biggest pep talk of my life. *If you want to do this you've got to go to places that you've never been before. If you want to do this, you're going to be faced with the best. If you want to do this, you've got to step back up and get it done.*

God did I hate it, though. I hated it more than anything I've ever hated in my life. I hated him. I wanted to push him off his fucking moped into the busy road.

Eventually, I got to the peak of the hill, which felt good for a moment, but then you have to come down again, and there are still hills on the way down! I got this huge rush of energy coming up within me. It was almost like I had broken through the breaking point. Now I liken this to where people say they hit the wall when running a marathon, and although I don't know because I've never run a marathon, I imagine it must be something similar.

I was totally focused on getting home, and nothing else. I wasn't thinking about the fight. I just needed to make it home safely.

Somehow I got back to the gym and I stopped running. I looked at my trainer, and I must have shot him daggers because he simply said, "See you tomorrow," and he scuttled off on his bike. Even though I had got through it all, I just thought – *You fucking arsehole.* It's amazing who and what you can blame, rather than taking ownership of your own creations.

I went back to my hotel and didn't speak to anyone. My girlfriend, the nurse, called and asked if I wanted to go for dinner. I told her I wasn't in a good way. She said she was coming over right away, and she did. She took one look at me and asked, "What's happened?"

"I'm pulling out of my fight," I said.

"What's gone on?"

"I'm going to burn out, my body is hurting. I've got no energy. I'm fucking tired. I can't do this. I don't know why I ever thought I could do this. I'm too old."

She sat me down and said, "What are you doing? Tell me, what are you eating? Are you eating enough?"

I explained to her what I was eating, and all the liquids I was drinking. It's really tough to constantly eat two hours before training, and to squeeze in the right amount of food that you need to be able to have the energy to train and fight.

She said to me, "Look, would you be open to trying something if I give it to you?"

"Right now, babe, I will try anything."

She disappeared for ten minutes and then came back with a bag full of coloured capsules, they were pink, green and purple. She said, "Can you see the different colours?"

I said, in a smart-arsed way, "That's purple, that's green and that one is pink. Of course, I can see the colours."

"Good because some people can't. I need you to take four of each of these capsules every morning until your fight. "

"Wow, that's a lot of capsules to take."

"Lucy, just take the fucking capsules."

She was adamant. I accepted it; I had been told. I was going to take the capsules. Now, in all honesty, she could have given me crack at that point and I probably would have taken it because I was desperate, I was so broken, I was on my knees begging for help, and thankfully this little earth angel came along with something she said would help. I trusted her. Now, thankfully as it turned out, the capsules were nothing dodgy at all. All that was in them was just fruits, veggies and berries. That's all it was. I did what she said, though. I took four right away.

The next day I woke up and I felt like a different person. Literally overnight. I felt energised, and I felt fresh. The night before I had been covered in bruises, and that morning they were almost gone, honestly. From that point, I started calling these capsules magic beans. I thought – *Fuck yes. I'm back.* However, as good as I felt, I had to see if I could get through the training and still feel good on the other side. That would be the challenge.

That day, interestingly I was sparring with Ricky. Now, he's a lot stronger than me. Men are.

Ladies, I don't care what you say, men are stronger than women, and we need to just recognise that they are built differently, not better than us, just differently.

Anyway, I was sparring with Ricky, and we were having a good session. All of a sudden, out of nowhere, I don't know if I caught him first in a certain way, but he threw a fucking bomb at me. A full pelt punch, that hit me hard in my face. Normally, he would hit me when we were sparring, but only to the same level that a woman would hit me, he would never go all out. This time though, he unleashed a full blown punch. *What the Fuck?* – I thought as I flew backwards into the cage wall. It didn't floor me. I stood it, and in that moment I thought – *Fucking hell, if I can take that, no woman will ever hit me that hard. I can do this!* I had newfound confidence, and from the most random accident.

Ricky was upset. He apologised profusely. However, he had actually done me a favour. And as much as a lot of people will think he was out of order – how dare a man punch a woman like that – I'm really grateful he did. It gave me the confidence that I needed. As much as it hurt, I didn't get bruised, and it gave me some gold to bribe him with for many years to come.

I felt like he had given me the key to remember that I could do it. I could get it done.

A couple of days later, in the morning, it was my last training session before I had to rest and prepare for the fight. My trainer was throwing the medicine ball at my abs to make sure that I was tough enough. I had been through a few days of what is known as shark tank. It's intense and really hard. Basically, it involves six different trainers around you, and you have to fight with one of them, and then move on to the next one, and then the next one, and the next one, and so on. You keep going until you've been around all of them, and then you get a minute break and then you go again. And these guys were the toughest; these guys were serious fighters. It was absolutely hideous. I wanted to throw up and pass out. There was so much ego piping up, telling me to run away, to call them all bullies, to sit on the floor and just not do it. I wanted a break, or to have a drink of water, but they just kept pushing and pushing. They knew if I could get through this, I would be able to do anything. And, I did. I survived it all. I never appreciated until that moment, quite how far the human body could be pushed.

At the end of my morning session, my trainer said to me, "No run today." I could have jumped on him, knocked him on the floor and kissed him all over. Then he told me, "You go home. You eat. You stay out of the sun for the next two days. You get your hair done on fight day. You go and get a blessing from the monk. Other than that, you see no one, you speak to no one, you literally eat and rest."

I thought – *Woooah! Nobody's telling me to stay out of the sun.* The rest of it I was happy with, but the sun…oh no no no!

He looked at my brown skin and said, "The sun will drain your energy. You are too brown," and he walked away shaking his head.

Now I'm one of those people that get really energised from the sun, so I fought this guidance somewhat. I went out for a quiet dinner that night and I spoke to a few fighters. I asked them what their take on it all was. They told me to follow my trainer's advice. Just eat and rest.

So that's what I did. Even though I didn't want to.

For those two days, I would go for breakfast, because it was an opportunity to eat, and I would go out for lunch, and then I would go out for something in the afternoon, and then out for dinner too. Basically, any opportunity to eat. Other than that, I was locked in my room, focusing. And the really interesting thing is, this is where I really got connected to meditation. This is where meditation came into my life. I focused on my breath because back then I thought I was a bit shit at meditation. In all honesty, my head was spinning so fast with so many different ideas and distractions, that sitting in my own thoughts was impossible. I would normally have distracted myself, but all distractions had been removed. I had no choice but to focus. I would initially focus on my breath and how that felt. This is when I realised I was exceptionally visual. I started to get visions of myself winning my fight. I saw myself in the ring, bouncing around – happy that I had won, and then with my arms being raised in celebration. By focusing on my breath – I didn't realise that I was doing breathwork, meditation and visualisation at the same time, and how profound that would end up being for my life.

Now I didn't know who I was fighting, I had no clue what size they were going to be or how experienced they were. I just trusted and I kept speaking to God – for the first time in my life. I trusted there was a God and he was going to show me the way. I spoke to my grandad at every opportunity. I kept calling on the people I knew who had passed away. I asked – *Please keep me safe*. I would visualise my hands being lifted in victory. I would visualise myself being excited, strong, and full of energy. I would visualise myself hugging my trainer after I had won the fight. I visualised myself doing the Wai Kru – the dance that you have to do at the start of a Thai fight. I visualised myself being blessed by the monk. I was really immersed in this process, tapping into who I was, and this innate knowledge of what I had been put here to do. I did not know why this fight was important, or what impact would be created from it, I just knew somewhere in my soul it was going to be a big deal.

It made me realise that the more I consciously breathed, the more powerful I became, and the more powerful I became, the bigger the visions; the bigger the visions, the deeper I would go. I would do this for hours, locked in my room on my own. I would come out and say to people, "Woah, you're not going to believe what I've just seen." They thought I was batshit crazy. This was the first time I had connected as deeply as I had. This was my first remembrance of how powerful my visions were and the signs that would come through. I knew before then I was powerful, I knew I was a force to be reckoned with, but this was different. There was a belief coming into me that felt unstoppable. I felt as if anything I set my mind to would be mine.

68

On the day of my fight, I had to go and get my hair plaited. I had long hair, so the last thing you want is your hair going in your face when people are kicking, kneeing or elbowing you – you need to be able to see, to make your next move. My friend, the nurse, said she would take the day off training and come with me to get my hair done and go to see the monks. She was keen to make sure I looked after myself and got properly fuelled up in readiness. In reality, I feel she was more nervous than I was at that point. I was pretty chilled. I knew I could do it. I knew it was done!

The very first thing we did in the morning, was to go and see the monk at the top of Big Buddha. So I drove on the moped, with my friend on the back. We told them I was fighting, so they put a band around my wrist and told me it was for protection. It was a bit of a nothing event really. My friend was really proud of me, though. She thought it was amazing to have been blessed like that. We then went and put some motivational words on the trees, and wrote on some tiles and gave them to the monks to include in their building work, as was customary.

I wasn't satisfied with the blessing, though. I felt something more was needed. As we were driving back, on the way to see the girl who was going to do my hair, I got this real insight that I needed to do something. That's the only way I can describe it because I wasn't aware that I was channelling at this point. I wasn't aware that I was being guided. The way I explain it to people these days, I almost feel as if somebody has their hands on my shoulder and they literally put me in the situation where I have to be. Back then, though, I didn't realise that there was something that was guiding me and showing me the way.

So, on the moped, on the way back, I saw a temple – one that I must have passed so many times before – and I said to my friend, "Babe, I need to go in there."

"What you on about? You've got to go get your hair done."

I just spun the moped around and shot into this temple. I said to her, "I don't know why I need to be here. I've just got to be here."

"Okay, whatever you feel you need to do. Do you want me to come with you? Or would you like a moment to yourself?"

I told her to come with me. I had no idea what I was doing. I just felt pulled to there. We walked in and I felt the need to sit on the floor for a second. There's a really beautiful picture of me sitting on my knees and my ankles. I'm looking really skinny sitting there, and you can see that I'm really contemplating what's about to take place. The next thing I know, a Thai lady who could speak relatively good English, said to me, "I think you should go and see the monk." I looked at my friend and asked, "Are you okay if I go?" She nodded, and so I went off with this lady. She took me into this place where all the Thai families went, and they were giving gifts to the monk. The monk was doing a proper, special blessing. The monk took one look at me and he told me to sit. I sat there for a few minutes, whilst he was doing his thing with other people, and then he called me to him. The Thai lady translated for us both. She told me he said, "This is what you are here for. You are special. A special one."

I told him I was doing my first fight, and that my trainer couldn't bring me because he was too busy, and so my friend had brought me to come and get blessed. He did this whole ritual on me. He kind of sealed me in. He did all of these really beautiful things. And I just sat there and sobbed like a baby. And while he was doing it, the lady was explaining everything to me. He was offering protection, saying how strong I was. He was bringing in an energy of strength and protection for me. He was calling in Buddha to make sure that I was going to be successful in whatever way success looked to me. It is important at this point in the book to remember that sometimes success is losing because you need to know what that feels like, so you have a greater appreciation of what winning feels like, when it happens. Life is here to be experienced; to humble us. We need to remember what it's like to learn the lessons of how to elevate and push ourselves further.

In the end, we were at the temple for about two hours. It was such a beautiful experience. Although, I didn't have any gifts to offer, I gave the monk some cash. I kept saying, "Thank you, thank you, thank you." The monk told the lady, "She's going to do this. She's very special. She's very strong." I blubbed once again as she translated.

It was the first insight into how monks read and feel my energy.

On the way back, I got my hair plaited, then I drove up to the gym. I walked in and I saw my trainer and I told him all about the monk. He didn't really understand what I was on about, but he kept saying, "I'm so proud of you. I'm so proud of you. Now go home. Go home. I see you here at nine o'clock."

The fight was going to be late on in the evening because it's too hot to fight earlier in the day or the evening, so I went back and lay on my bed and asked for help. By doing this I broke a barrier that I had within myself. I smashed through my own glass ceiling. By being forced to stop and sit with myself, I recognised that breathwork, meditation and visualisation were very, very powerful tools for me. I hadn't seen any results yet, but I could feel how powerful it was. I felt so calm, so still. I processed the way that the fight was going to be. I knew I was going to knock her out. I could see the result before it happened. I could see it clearly. I was visualising that I was going to knock her out in round number one. I saw her on her backside. I could see it. More than that, I believed it. I was strong. I could hold my own with most of the men, there was no way my opponent was going to be as fit and strong as I was.

Eventually, the time came when I had to go. My friend picked me up to go to the fight. On the way there I felt fine, initially. Then, about twenty minutes before we got to the venue, the fear kicked in. I walked in and everyone was looking at me, they were sussing me out as a fighter because they wanted to bet on me. Ricky was there for me, he was one of my corner men. I had my trainer there too, and I had my friend, the nurse. There were also about 40 people there supporting and cheering me on.

It was a great night, even before the fights started. There is nothing better than a load of people who love you being there to support you in whatever it is you are doing. It doesn't matter if it's speaking on stage or walking into a ring. I also had the support of thousands of people back home, which felt good. I had hundreds of messages, requests to stream the fight, and messages of encouragement and love. I was focused. It was not just me I was doing this for. I was doing it for everyone back home. I was doing it for those who could not do it for themselves.

I was getting ready, getting in the zone, stretching and doing a bit of shadow boxing and stuff. Ricky was helping me stretch out. I've got some amazing photos of the two of us from that night. One, in particular, is where my legs are in the splits; in another one my trainer is wrapping my hands; and in yet another photo, Ricky is holding me up and he's in my face, shouting in my ear, getting my head in the game. You can see we're so caught up in the moment. It was a really beautiful, humbling experience. I trusted that man with my life. He knew this shit, he had done it before many times, whereas for me this was the first time, so I needed his strength, his help, and his wisdom.

I was third on the fight list. I saw the other fights, and I was focused and ready. I was the only female fight that night. I had my gloves on. I had hot oil all over me – and the oil is really hot, by the way. It's not just standard baby oil. It's special stuff that helps the muscles, and it helps the blows slide off. I also had a cape on. I hadn't realised that would happen, but here I was being depicted as a superhero with my cape on, way before I ever energetically stepped into that role.

It was such an appropriate image because I was about to go out and do something that was going to transform the whole of the rest of my life. I didn't realise that at the time, I was just doing what I was told to do, but looking back it was so powerfully poignant.

I walked out through the curtain, out onto the ring where hundreds of people were watching and applauding. I thanked everybody for being there. And then my opponent came out. She thanked everyone too. We had to do the Wai Kru, which is basically where you face off against each other; you seal the ring and send respect to your trainer. My trainer took my cape off, put my gum shield in my mouth, and I was good to go.

The adrenaline kicked in. My opponent, this girl, was probably twice my size – honestly. She was a big girl, but I also knew I was strong. I knew that I could do this. My trainer said to me, "Round number one, we respect each other. We talk, we figure it out, we get our distance."

In my head, though, I was thinking – *This motherfucker's getting knocked out. I have seen it! Nothing is stopping that.*

The fight started and I went for it, I gave it everything, and this girl couldn't even punch. She was huge, though, one of her legs was probably five times the size of one of mine, but that's not the point, she can't punch, so I'm going to use my hands. I'm going to just outbox her. Twice in the first round, she was on her arse. I honestly don't know how the guy didn't stop the fight. She was scared of me. You could see she was petrified, but because she was Thai, he kept the fight going.

I was in my corner and my trainer and Ricky were shouting at me, "Use your knees. Use your fucking knees!" My trainer poured ice over my head, which was hideous – it's the worst thing you can do to someone at that time, they believe it freshens you up, I believe it's heart attack material! I was truly in the zone. I was confused, though, I asked my trainer, "Why are the rounds so short? We've been training for five-minute rounds, and these feel like they're 30 seconds." My trainer told me that the women's fights are shorter. This was good news, this meant I was super fit and over-prepared.

For the second round – I went back out and I was literally throwing this girl around like a rag doll. She was on her arse, and then she would get back on her feet, then she was on her arse again. I could tell that the guy had not wanted to stop the fight, he wanted to save her embarrassment, and probably for her to win. If there was any way he could have swung it for her, I'm pretty sure he would have done, but I was all over her.

I got back to my corner and I said, "She hasn't even touched me. What are they doing? Why haven't they stopped it?"

All Ricky said to me was, "Get it done."

Round three, and I went for it big time. I got her in a clinch, which is where my hands were around her neck and she couldn't do anything. She couldn't punch me, she couldn't kick me. I launched her to the ground, and I heard Ricky and my trainer telling me to use my knees. Now when you get kneed, it really fucking hurts. Most people get winded and then they have to stop the fight. I kneed her, then I threw her around some more. The ref jumped in and said, "No more, no more. She's taken enough." Whilst waving his hands in the air as if to stop the fight.

I had done it! Months of waiting, and being patient, and hard, hard work. I had faced my fears, stepped into the ring and proven to myself once again that I could do anything. I screamed in the middle of that ring and jumped around like a loon. You can see the look of delight on my face in all of the pictures. Everything that I visualised had happened. Okay, it wasn't in round one as I had visualised, but everything else had happened exactly as I had seen it.

Once again, the butterfly had emerged in all her powerful and colourful glory.

69

The buzz of having your hand raised as the winner of a professional Muay Thai fight, in Thailand, was the best feeling I had experienced in my life up to that point. Wow! I was ecstatic. The Thai people are usually very respectful in victory, they raise their hands and then they get out of the ring in an extremely gracious way. That was never going to happen with me! Not this time, anyway. I was fucking buzzing. The referee raised my hand in victory and then I went off, jumping around the ring like a lunatic, so proud of what I had just achieved. Was it the most graceful victory? Absolutely not! What it was, though, was proof that grit, determination, focus and consistency can win! People watching the fight were laughing at me – the crazy lunatic jumping up and down with sheer delight on my face. The ref didn't know what to do, so he just watched and clapped with the rest of them. Any grace or dignity that I did have, left the ring in that moment. I'm pretty sure my trainer was hanging his head in shame, but I will never change. I love to show how I am feeling, and in that moment, I was so elated and I wanted the watching world to know. I had a huge following on Facebook, and there were hundreds, if not thousands, of people around the world watching, and sending messages of delight and joy. It wasn't just me that won that night, we won. I feel it was the first step of the 'light' winning; another warrior had been activated. The future mission was officially inflight. Although, I was blissfully unaware at that stage what it would entail.

When I eventually decided to stop having my little moment of fame in the middle of the ring, I ran over to Ricky and threw my arms around him. I was on one side of the ropes and he was on the other side, and we bounced up and down with each other in celebration. He leaned in and whispered in my ear, "I could see Mike Tyson in your eyes before you went in there, she didn't stand a fucking chance." I will never forget those words, they meant so much at that moment. Knowing he was proud of me made all of the hard work, the punches, the focus, and the drills worth it. My trainer came over to me and said, "I'm so proud of you." Quickly, though, his praise turned to criticism. He handed me some water and said, "Why do you not use your knees? You should have used knees! You are so strong with your knees!" I just looked at him and then I looked at Ricky and I just thought – *Fuck you! Let me enjoy my moment.* Talk about pissing on someone's fireworks!

I do get it, though. He has trained many, many champions. This was his way of life; up until he was in his late thirties he used to fight every single week, so doing it properly for him was important. There was no celebration. There were no rest days. It was a case of rock up, fight and then come back the following week to go again. Whereas for me, I was just throwing myself in there to see if I could do it or not. This fight was very much a test of my strength, discipline and mindset.

I went over to have my gloves taken off. The gloves they give you to fight in are pretty manky. I wouldn't like to consider how many other hands have been inside of them – yuk! Underneath the boxing gloves, your hands are strapped quite heavily, to protect your bones. My coach helped me get my hands out of the gloves and then cut the wraps off me. I was on another planet. The feeling running through my veins was like nothing else; not even the best orgasm I had ever had compared to this buzz.

Once my hands were free, I was like a crazy little jumping bean. I had all of my team around me, and they were now jumping around with me, and joining in the celebrations. People were talking me through the fight, and all the moves I had made. There were so many people chatting to me all at once, and wanting to share their experiences and the messages of support that people were sending.

Then it started. People began congregating around me, and queuing up for photos, or to just talk to me. Children were waiting patiently to speak to me and ask if I felt they could go on and fight one day. It was really strange. I had never had this kind of attention before. For the first time in my life, I was someone. I was someone that people wanted to be around. I stood there for about half an hour, talking and having photos taken – whilst my team watched on smiling.

As the adrenaline started to wear off, I began to feel the pain in my shins from all the low kicks I had chopped my opponent's legs with. I decided that I had to go and get some ice. As I walked out, the crowds went crazy for me, and I loved it. My ego was piping up at this point, bigger than I've ever known. Everybody was patting me on the back and telling me what a good job I had done. Total strangers were leaning in and taking selfies as I walked past. I didn't know whether to be weirded out or excited at this newfound fame.

There were about 50 of us from my gym that made the effort to go to the stadium that night. I was so grateful for all of their support. Once all the fights were over, everyone decided to go for a drink to celebrate. I was absolutely buzzing and I wanted that feeling to continue forever. I had convinced myself that I was never coming down from that feeling, despite my sore legs. It was such a great night. My trainer and Ricky didn't come with us, but even if they had been there, I don't think I would have spoken to them. I was so high from the fight, I didn't even need to drink. I had one beer the entire evening, not my usual choice, but I thought that with a beer I could sip on it for a longer time. I was so engrossed in the natural feeling of joy and elation and I didn't want anything to ruin it.

At about 2 in the morning, I decided that I was going to bed. The bruises had started coming up on my legs, and I was feeling some other weird and wonderful aches and pains from where I had obviously connected with her during the fight. The adrenalin was keeping me from feeling the full extent of the pain, thankfully.

I got back to my room and I couldn't sleep for ages just running through the fight and allowing the energy in my system to calm down. I was finally all alone. It was time to decompress and process all that had gone on that day. I had done it. I kept smiling to myself, then my grandad popped in my head. He would have been so proud of me. I was his little warrior. I wish I could have called him to let him know I had won. The thing is, he knew. I felt he had been there with me.

I barely slept at all that night. I was too wired. I actually didn't know what to do with myself. How did people that fought weekly deal with this?

The next day I got up and went to the gym to train. My trainer took one look at me as if to suggest I was crazy. He sent me home to rest. Just as I was leaving he said to me, "Oh, by the way, I've got another fight for you, in two weeks' time." He told me that because I was fit I would have no problem being ready in time. This time I wouldn't be fighting a Thai native, my next opponent was from Sweden.

I was really excited at the thought of another fight, and I also didn't want to rest and stop training. I didn't want to lose my edge, but my trainer wouldn't allow it. He took absolutely none of my shit, so I took myself off to the beach for the day.

I sat on the beach, the day after my victory, expecting everyone to still be living in glory with me. However, it wasn't the case. That was last night, this was today, and people had moved on. It was time for the adrenaline crash. I was staring out at the blue sky, and the serene sea. I sat on my towel, with my head in my hands and I thought – *Is that it? Is that all it's about?* Nobody had ever managed my expectations; what goes up must come down. And even if someone had told me, I'm not sure anyone could have got through to me how full-on and lonely that feeling is. I had never anticipated it, but actually, when I looked back, many of my best friends and even my sister were always depressed within a couple of days of their fight. I had never connected the dots. Here I was in paradise, victorious, but feeling so low.

I spent a lot of time in the sea that day, to get the bruises down, knowing the saltwater would really help.

The next day I managed to talk my trainer into letting me train, which he begrudgingly did, and I started pushing myself again. At first, some of it was hard to do because my shins were sore. I had never kicked an actual human up until the fight because when you are training you have pads on your legs. The fight was the first time that I had actually connected shin on shin. Ooooh, it makes me shiver just thinking about it. It's horrible.

For the next week, I pushed myself really hard. I was a week out from the fight when one morning I woke up and I had these awful big lumps under my armpits. I went to my trainer and asked him if he knew what it was. I thought I had picked up some dodgy, Thai disease. Always worst-case scenario with me! Actually, though, it was my immune system crashing. Normally when that happened to me it would target my throat and my tonsils, but this time it targeted underneath my armpits. My body was once again saying to me – *You're pushing too hard*. Typical Lucy, rather than paying attention to it – you'd think I had learnt by now – but I kept pushing. I said to my trainer, "I'm good. I can keep training, I'm fine."

He replied, "We're going to see how you are over the next day or two. And if it's not better, you're not fighting."

There was no way I was going to lose the opportunity to fight, so I did a few things that were a little bit extreme to try and get rid of these lumps. The first thing I did was I went to the chemist and I got some medication – not too extreme. The second thing I did, and definitely the worse thing, was to allow one of the professional fighters at me with a needle. It was a clean needle, to be clear, but he tried to suck out the stuff that was in the lumps and reduce them. I didn't realise it but it wasn't just a lump, or an abscess or boil, it was actually my gland that had become swollen and hard, and it was the size of a golf ball by this point.

The next day I went to my trainer to see what he thought. He lifted my arms up, took one look at the mess in my armpits and told me point blank that I wasn't fighting. I was devastated. I felt weak. I felt useless. I felt like I should have been stronger. Hello Ego!

It was piping. I wasn't getting my own way. Looking back on it now, I feel that I was being massively protected from that fight. I don't know why, or what might have happened, but the lumps cleared up very quickly and they never appeared again, and I trained for many more fights after that.

I felt gutted though, it really hurt me. I was getting all these needs met by being the fighter and I hadn't fully acknowledged that yet, so when I had it ripped from underneath me, it stung.

So, of course, what does Lucy do when things go wrong? She runs away. And that is what I did. I packed up my things and left Thailand, albeit with a view of going back at some point because I did want to do some more fights, but I gathered my stuff and headed off in the direction of home.

70

I had the wedding of one of my best friends to attend at the end of March in Cyprus, and I had promised Kyle I would come to the UK en route to see him. I arrived in the UK in the middle of March and so I had a bit of time to spend with Kyle before then. I'd also decided that whilst I was home I was going to surprise my mum. I'd reached out to my stepdad and asked him if they were going to be home during a certain few days, just to gauge where they were at. I told him I had a delivery that I was sending to mum, but I wanted it to be a surprise for her. So, I navigated things the best I could without giving myself away.

On the way back, I was feeling wounded from the cancelled fight, my ego was seriously dented. I had won this incredible fight, but I felt as if I'd lost. Kyle picked me up from the airport, and it was so good to see him. It felt so nice to be with him and back in my home country, where everyone speaks the language and I could eat whatever food I wanted. It was really lovely to have Kyle to cuddle up with in the evening. He was amazing. He ran me around here, there and everywhere. We didn't have long together, though. We only had a few days before I was flying off to Cyprus for the wedding, so we decided to take a trip back home to sunny Bournemouth, where I would attempt to surprise my mum. Bless Kyle, he drove me from

Hertfordshire down to Bournemouth, and then dropped me off at my mum's because he thought it would have been a bit weird if he turned up for the surprise, having never met my mum before.

My mum and stepdad are somewhat old-fashioned in that they always park their cars in the garage, and so I had no idea if they were even in or not. I stood at my mum's door, holding a big bouquet of flowers. My stepdad came to the door, and he was shocked to see me, but he held it together and said, "Carol! Carol! There's something at the door for you." I just stood by the door, trying not to giggle because my laugh is very noticeable and highly contagious, and I would have given myself away immediately. My mum came out of the kitchen, looked towards the front door, then she saw me and took a step backwards with the shock. Then, she burst into tears. It was the best thing I've ever done.

I had managed to keep it quiet. Nobody knew I was even home. It was the first time on my travels that I went stealth. I'm really good at keeping secrets when I need to.

I spent some quality time with my mum. It was so beautiful. She was so happy to have me back because she didn't want me to go away in the first place. Seeing the look on my mum's face, and for her to feel that she was important enough for me to make a detour to see her, was priceless. It's a memory that I'll treasure until the day that I die.

Much later on that day, Kyle came to pick me up, and we made it back to Hertfordshire. The next evening, I was flying over to Cyprus for the wedding, and I was taking my best friend Catherine with me because when I had accepted the 'plus one', Kyle wasn't yet in my life. Typical Lucy and Catherine style, we decided we would go on holiday for a week, but in the middle of that week would be the wedding.

The two of us set off on yet another mission. It was like we were on our flight to Vegas again. It hadn't been that long since I had last seen her because she had flown over to see me for my birthday, but so much had happened since then. When you're travelling, you meet people every day. You get into all kinds of sticky situations. This book would be the longest book in the world if I were to share all the crazy situations I got into on my travels. Catherine wanted to hear everything, though.

We arrived in Cyprus and got to our hotel, which was stunning. We had a few days to relax before the wedding, and that's what we did – we just had fun. I had decided that I was going to wear a really, really bright yellow dress for the wedding because I was Little Miss Sunshine. My grandad always used to call me Little Miss Sunshine, and so that was who I was going to be. When I later saw the photos from the wedding, everyone else was in normal, muted, pastel colours and then there was me in bright yellow – HELLO! That was how I was feeling, though. There are so many amazing pictures from the wedding with me being silly and pulling faces, and being in my element. I have never looked at myself in a photo before and thought about how happy I looked, but on this occasion I did. I really did. I was starting to undergo the transformation from self-sabotage into being very, very happy. I barely drank on that trip. I spent a lot of time speaking and connecting with different people, especially at the wedding, figuring out where they were at in their lives. At weddings, you have to talk to people that you wouldn't normally talk to. This wedding was amazing. Catherine and I had such a great time and I am proud to say that Laura, whose wedding it was, remains one of my best friends to this day.

I flew home a few days later, and landed in the UK for one last night with Kyle. We had the most incredible night; a night I'm sure neither of us will ever forget. Something happened between the two of us. We reached a certain inner-standing with each other that we never had before. We realised we were very much in love.

The next morning, I was due to fly out. I really didn't want to go. The previous night Kyle and I had talked about him coming travelling. He was sick of work and wanted some time out from his family, as they were going through a pretty transformational period. I never thought he would do it, but he said he was going to quit his job and come meet me to travel. I really wanted him to. I wanted to share these experiences with him. From the way I had recently felt after the fight, to this feeling with Kyle, it highlighted to me that so much of the journey is about polarities. It was bringing into my consciousness that one minute things could be amazing, then the next minute it could be quite tragic, or painful. I guess this is a good lesson to note, we live in a polar world right now. When there is an ultimate high, the chances are that you will have to experience something that brings you down slightly. It's all about balance. I hadn't recognised it fully at that point, but I was navigating it intuitively with ease and grace.

I headed back in the direction of Asia alone, and with a heavy heart. I had decided that I was going to do some hopping around Asia. I had been very Thailand-focused so far, so I thought I would go off and explore some other incredible countries and cities – places that I hadn't ever been to before. The freedom you experience when you are able to explore a new place with just a backpack on your back, and you can go wherever you want, whenever you want, is exhilarating. I had the best time doing it all on my own. I tasted foods that I would never have thought I would have tasted. I experienced things, and met people, that my path would never have crossed. Families would welcome me into their homes. Every experience was incredible. And you know, for somebody like myself, that's what travelling is about. It's about stepping into a culture and embracing every element of it.

In the midst of my travels, I got a message on Facebook, "Lucy, Sanong is missing you." My Thai trainer had sent out a message for me, and instantly my ego started popping up. *It's time for another fight. I need to get back to Thailand. It's time to get fit. It's time.* So I responded saying, "Okay, let him know I'll be back soon. Tell him to book me a fight."

So, following my intuitive pulls again, I navigated my way back there within a couple of days. And I went straight back into training. I felt sharp because I'd had about a month off proper training. Kyle and I had trained a bit, he would hold pads for me and we used to go to the gym, so I wasn't unfit at all, but I hadn't been pushed properly for a month. I had this newfound energy. I felt stronger than I had ever been. I had more discipline than I had ever had. I had more motivation than I had in a long time. The lumps under my arm didn't resurface and any of the things that had previously plagued my journey weren't there anymore.

Within a couple of days of being back, I had a fight booked for two weeks' time. This time, though, I was booked against a girl who had had over 220 fights. She was tough. People were asking me if I was sure that I wanted to do this. In all honesty, by this point, I knew I was pretty good. I wasn't technically there by any stretch of the imagination, but I was strong, with a mindset that no one was going to take me out, and I had a bloody heavy right hand. The more I heard about this girl, and the more people told me about her, the more I didn't care or wish to hear about it. This was about me. This wasn't about the people who sat on the sidelines. This was about the person that gets in the ring, not the opinions of others. All I knew was that I would give it my all. I would figure it out.

I trained harder than I'd ever trained. I had all of the guys from the MMA team helping me, and everybody was really charged up for this one. Ricky wasn't around at this point to spar with me or help me in any way, so I had to rely on the other fighters to help me. I knew everyone had my back. I was so focused during this camp. I knew what I needed to do.

A couple of days before the fight, again I was told I had to sit at home and stay out of the sun. I had to eat and get fuelled up and let my muscles relax. And this was where I started to have very, very powerful visions come through my meditations again. I was starting to see things that I can't explain, or I certainly couldn't explain back then anyway. I was starting to see images and places and people, and I didn't know who they were, or where they were. I just knew that at some point I was going to cross them. You know the feeling of deja vu when you know that you've been there before and that you've experienced a scene before – it was like that. Some people would call that dreaming, but I was wide awake. I was predicting what was going to happen, and I kept hearing the words that there was going to be a massive lesson that came out of this fight. This made me think about whether I should be doing it or not. A massive part of me was scared of what I was about to learn. Maybe my cockiness and certainty needed a little dent in it. I could have easily talked myself out of it at this point, but I did not want to let people down.

I went to the monks for a blessing, and it was such a beautiful experience. I didn't have anybody around me like the time before, when I went with my nurse friend. It was just me doing this on my own this time. I went in and was given the bracelet around my wrist like last time, and then three monks took care of me. They ushered me into a ceremony, a service with just the monks. I sat with them throughout it all. It was like they had taken me under their wing. God knows why me, there were no other Westerners there. I sat in this sacred place, during this extremely special service and I thought that no matter what happened, experiences like these do not happen for everyone. Nobody would ever be able to take them away. The fact that beautiful souls around the world were welcoming me into their homes, their places of worship, and into their cultures was magical.

Looking back, they were showing me that I had to step into being the true Lucy; every step of the way. People were so kind, generous, and loving; it made me remember that I was kind, generous, and loving too. I had got a little bit lost along the way, and I'd forgotten that was who I really was deep down. It was such a beautiful epiphany that I had in those two days, when I was forced to relax and go inwards. I relaxed into this space where whatever was meant to be is what would happen. This is probably not the best mentality to go into a fight with a girl who has had 220 fights, but that was how I felt. I felt relaxed. I felt chilled. I certainly did not feel I was about to go to battle.

It came to fight night and I was walking through the building to get to the back area where I could get ready, and I saw the girl that I was fighting. She was a bit taller than me, maybe by three or four inches, and I thought – *Yeah, that's okay*. And then I saw her legs, and they were like tree trunks. And at that point, I thought – *Oh my God! If she kicks me with them, that is going to hurt – a lot*. She didn't scare me, though. She tried her best to intimidate me. She would come over to where I was getting ready and just stand there, watching my every move. She was trying to get in my head while I had my hands wrapped and when I stretched and warmed up. She didn't know what she was dealing with, though. It was almost like I had a trained warrior inside of me who knew this had to be done. It wasn't a case of if, when, or how. It was a case of – you've just got to do it. I'm going to battle, and I'm going to fight for my freedom. And this is what's going to happen. I felt strong. I felt good. It was time to re-awaken the warrior. It was time to prepare her for war.

After all the preparation, I entered the ring. I did my dance, and my trainer took my headband off. Soon after that, the fight began.

Normally, in round number one in Thailand, you're supposed to be quite respectful of each other and you feel each other out. I'd learnt from the previous fight that it actually maybe was the right thing to do. So that's what I did this time around. I just tapped it out and started to get my reach with her. In the second round, the cheeky bitch elbowed me, or she tried to but she didn't connect. I saw red. Elbow!

It was actually within her rights to do that but it was like a red rag to a bull. If she's going to do it, then to heck with it, so will I. From that moment forward, I was throwing elbows constantly. It was ridiculous because I would never have thrown an elbow if she hadn't first but because she did, I went to war. It was like the red mist descended. The old Lucy appeared, the angry Tasmanian devil just came out of nowhere and I kept going for her face with my elbows – which is really horrible when you stop and think about it. We had quite a brawl actually. It was a good fight. And at the end of the five rounds, we were both still standing, despite all the elbows. She had done this flying knee thing and caught me on my chest, which was actually a really good move. There wasn't any major damage done between us, nobody was cut or bleeding, but it was a proper good brawl.

In the end, when the result came in, she had won the fight. This proved to be an unpopular decision with the crowd. There were so many people screaming at the decision. It was so interesting because the girl was a Thai girl and so the feeling around the ring was that they had given her the fight for that reason. A little Thai lady came up to me and she said, "They wrong. They wrong. You won." I only lost by one single point. And as much as I was pissed off at losing, I had lost to a girl who had fought over 220 fights. She was bred to do this, and here I was having held my own with her after just one previous fight. My ego was dented, but she came up to me afterwards and she was actually really sweet. She said to me, "You're a really tough girl and I'd like to do sparring with you." This is a typical warrior. You go in, you do what you've got to do, at whatever cost, but then you're friends afterwards. This is what I love so much about Thai boxing. There's no animosity. There's no calling each other out. You get in there, get the job done and go home. And it was such a beautiful thing that we did.

After the fight, everyone wanted to go drinking. I went along, but I didn't have one drink. This was a huge step forwards for me. I didn't feel like I needed even one drink to fit in or to drown my sorrows. I sat there for about an hour, then made my excuses and left. This was the first time I had ever done that, and it wasn't because my ego was piping up and I felt let down – which, admittedly, I did – but I actually realised that night that I didn't need that bravado anymore. I didn't need to be the person I had projected I was for so long. I could just be me, whatever that looked like. And if I didn't want to drink alcohol, then I wouldn't drink alcohol. If I didn't want to do certain things, then I wouldn't do it. I would just stand in my own truth and do what I wanted to do.

It wasn't long after the fight that Kyle quit his job and told me he was coming to join me travelling. I was so happy. I honestly never thought he would do it, so this was huge for him. It also showed me that he was committed to us. I'm not sure why I had doubted that; the guy had been waiting for me whilst I travelled around the world. We decided that we would start his travelling exactly as I had done, with a fight in Vegas! We got lucky and managed to get tickets to go to the Mayweather vs Pacquiao fight. I flew from Thailand back to the UK, grabbed him on the way and we went on to Vegas together.

Kyle had never been to Vegas before, so I showed him around. We had the best time. Classic 'old-style Lucy' – despite my recent good form, we got over-excited on night one and got absolutely wasted. We went to the casinos; he liked them, I didn't, but I am always pretty lucky in them. We won everything that night. I was his lucky charm. The more we gambled, the more we won, and the more drinks they supplied us with. It was the first time we had a drink together since the previous November. Every time that I had seen him, since the Dubai trip, one of us wasn't drinking – for one reason or another. We decided that we were going to make a big deal out of our first Vegas trip together.

Initially, the plan was to save the drinking for the Saturday night of the boxing, but we got carried away on the Friday night and got absolutely tanked. We went to bed at about 6 in the morning. I'll be honest, I'm really surprised we didn't do something stupid that night like get married. We were so drunk and crazy in love.

The next morning was awful. We both woke up feeling rough. We were that drunk we both wondered how we had got home, and we had passed out on the bed without even getting undressed properly. As a result, we found it extremely difficult to navigate that night with the boxing. It was strenuous. It reminded me of that time in Vegas with my ex-boyfriend. I never seemed to learn, hey!

We watched the fight and it was good, but we started to feel like we wanted to go to bed because we were so tired. That was too lame, so we decided to try and wake ourselves up by going out and exploring. We made a beeline for the roller coaster outside of the Paris Hotel. If anything was going to wake us up, it would be that! We were walking through the Paris hotel, attempting to navigate our way to the rollercoaster. The hotels are huge over there. You would never, and I mean never, find someone unless you had decided on a specific time and place to meet. As we walked through the Paris Hotel, Ricky was walking toward us.

Of all the people in the world! What were the chances? It's almost impossible. It was the weirdest situation ever. It was so frickin ridiculous. I said, "Hey, what are you doing here?"

Ricky shot back, "What the fuck are you doing here?"

He looked at Kyle with a strange look and then said, "Alright, I'd better go." It was really awkward. I had never experienced awkwardness with Ricky – besides the week on the boat when we totally ignored each other, of course. It wasn't a nice interaction. It started to play on my mind. *Why the fuck had I just bumped into Ricky? Of all of the people in the world, anywhere in the world, I bumped into him.* It felt really significant at the time, but I couldn't work out what was going on. I was with Kyle too, so I didn't want it to affect our time together. He didn't know about my past with Ricky.

I tried hard to enjoy the rest of the night. We went on the rollercoaster, we went for pancakes, and we took a long meander back to our hotel – stone-cold sober too, we didn't drink a drop that night. We got on really well and had a great laugh, neither of us taking things too seriously.

Vegas was the perfect start to Kyle's travels, exactly as mine had been all those months earlier.

We flew back to the UK together, to pick up Kyle's things, and have a little bit of a farewell do for him. We were only back for a couple of days before leaving again. He had arranged a get-together with his crew and I had arranged for my best friend to come along. We went to a pub in St Albans, where Kyle lived. We were ready to have a fun evening, with a couple of Kyle's brothers, some of his friends, and my best friend to keep me company. I was not up for drinking much that night, I wanted to keep a fresh head for our travels, but everyone else had different ideas. Very quickly, the wine was flowing, and then in typical fashion, the shots started being poured. I joined in. His mates liked the fact his girlfriend could keep up with the boys doing shots. The thing was, I actually couldn't. I was out of practice, and it all got too much for me. An argument erupted and it ended in a brawl. I ended up punching Kyle, and then someone else picked me up and threw me at the floor – it was a bloody disgrace. It was far from my finest moment and a perfect example of cross wires mixed with too much alcohol.

Kyle left me that night. Rightly so too. I had been an absolute menace. My best friend was shocked. She had no idea what had come over me. Neither did I. It was like I had been possessed by something. Literally, something had worked through me, and it had been extremely destructive.

The next day, when I went to grab my things, I apologised to his family, never expecting Kyle to ever forgive me for what I had done. We talked things through, though, and he said he wanted to come to Thailand. He knew this behaviour wasn't me, and he thought we could work through it. I felt so sad that I had created this upset. I was deeply embarrassed by my behaviour. I made a promise to him that I would never break from that moment forward; I promised I would never do anything like that again – and I didn't.

It was Kyle's dream to go and fight in Thailand, and I nearly ruined it all for him. My anger and aggression – and all because of me not getting my own way – nearly cost me something I loved. I had to get it together. To this day, I have never drunk another shot.

I had really wanted to go to the Philippines, but after my behaviour, I had to do what Kyle wanted us to do. I was lucky he was even coming with me. I sat on the plane with him, all cuddled up, sobbing my heart out. Why had I done that? What had come over me? If I wasn't careful, I was going to lose him.

We chatted at length on the plane. We decided that if we were going to work, we had to forget what had gone on. They were his words, not mine. I really struggled to forgive myself, though. Kyle was much more forgiving than I was at that point. One of his brothers had really turned on me since the fight. I knew that was playing on Kyle's mind, but he said to me we had to forget it, he'd made his decision and he chose me. He said he was ready to train, get a few fights under his belt, and then do a little bit of travelling.

We got back to Thailand and both started training again. Within a few days of being back, Kyle pulled his groin badly. Really badly. He had pushed himself too hard too soon, and he had been humbled by it. With what I know now, the Universe was asking him to go inwards, to sit with what had gone on; thankfully back then, I knew nothing of this because he would very likely have told me to piss off. He couldn't lift his leg up, so he had a massive hissy fit, "Right, fuck this shit, we might as well go to the Philippines." So that's what we did.

We packed up our stuff and went exploring.

We ended up going on a truly magical mystery tour of the Philippines and Bali. It was incredible. We had such a great time together. All of the drama that had occurred before leaving was very quickly forgotten about. With every day that passed, we became closer and closer. We were back in love, and it felt wonderful to be travelling with someone else.

The only challenge I found on these travels was that I couldn't get vegetables. From my experience – and maybe I was looking in the wrong places – I could only get chicken and rice or meat and rice. I also found the levels of poverty in the Philippines quite challenging. Kyle couldn't cope with it at all, he's such a sensitive empath. We would see these homeless kids on the street, and I would go and get food parcels for them. Kyle would get a bit angry with me because he thought I couldn't fix everybody. I really wanted to take these kids under my wings, and give them a bath, a hug, and somewhere to sleep for the night. Kyle couldn't cope with the fact that I was engaging with those energies.

On the way to Bali, my case got lost again. My case has gotten lost a few times on my travels – but then I have travelled around the world probably about 15 times, so, it's not too bad in the grand scheme of things. When it didn't come off the plane I could see Kyle was worried, thinking I would lose my shit again. He probably would have reached for a helmet if he had one. The thing is, I didn't react at all. This was actually the first time I really realised how much of a transformation I had made. This was in July of 2015 and less than a couple of years ago I would have lost my shit, not just lost my luggage. Not this time, though. Funnily enough, when I checked my bags in, I had said to Kyle, "I don't know why, but I feel I'm not going to see that bag again!" Watch what you wish for, hey?

When it was clear that my bag wasn't coming off the plane, Kyle was more stressed about it than I was. I went into practical mode, "There's nothing I can do here. I'm going to go and have a chat with somebody and see what they can do about it, see if they can locate it, and then let's just crack on with our holiday." Kyle was shocked because he'd seen me get pissed off about things before, and lose my shit – the recent fight was a perfect example, and being argumentative was my default setting. Not on this occasion, though. I had truly learnt from my recent experience, so I was as calm as anything. The argument with Kyle, which had notoriously gotten completely out of hand, had changed me for the better. I had never realised how far I was willing to go until that fateful night. Now, I realised I could not do certain things and expect to get away with it anymore. So, I never did them again.

We got in the taxi and Kyle was looking at me funny. "Are you alright?"

"Yeah. Why shouldn't I be?" I replied.

He started laughing. "You've just lost your bag and you're not even bothered about going to buy clothes or anything?"

"Oh, don't worry about it. It's going to work out just fine."

That moment crystallised the huge transformation that had taken place in me. From the Lucy that had left the UK in September of the year before, to the person I was now, was a catastrophic change. Little did I know that the catastrophic changes were only just about to begin.

Synchronicities and Signs

Have you ever stopped and given consideration to how 'random' it was that you met your partner when you did, and all that needed to align for you to cross paths in that moment? Or that conversation you had on a bus ride with a total stranger that ended up being particularly important for later that day or that week? This is what is referred to as a synchronicity. A force that flows around us, guiding us on our path, leading us to our purpose, passion, and the highest experiences of our life.

This book is compiled of signs and synchronicities, in an attempt to normalise quite how guided and connected we all are. Look at this story. Do you see how everything and everyone is linked? All of the people who were destined to play a magical role in the journey were doing exactly that – the good, bad and ugly? We were all being placed exactly where we were required to be. We had destinations, messages, things we needed to do, places we needed to go, and experiences that needed to flow, so that we could step through it together.

Look back at your life. Are you in awe of how absolutely divinely placed it was? What were the chances you would bump into someone 'randomly' then they would remain in your life to shake you awake? Can you see your pattern? Your path? If you had not been put in that exact place, at that exact time, life would have been so very different. It's so magical when you stop and look at it.

If we have the patience and willingness to allow our eyes to see it and our souls to feel it, everything works out perfectly, in our best interests, always. We don't know the words that get spoken about us behind our backs. We don't always know the paths certain souls may lead us down, intentionally or otherwise. This, though, is where the gold resides. When we resist and force things to go the way we want them to in our minds, rather than trusting the flow, the lessons we learn may be far more intense than is necessary, and all down to our stubbornness.

Trust that whenever you are being re-directed – even if it does not feel like it when it's happening, it's always happening for you – upon reflection, further down the line, you'll see it was actually the end of a chapter. For whatever reason, your souls did exactly what they needed to together. No hate or disappointment is required, only gratitude for playing their part in your masterpiece.

71

After a couple of absolutely magical months of exploring, learning to surf, going to the beaches, walking through jungles, and doing other amazing things across the Philippines and Indonesia, we decided that we would actually make our way back to Thailand. Kyle's groin was fully recovered and he really had it in his sights that he wanted to do a fight. So, as much as I was done with Thailand and I didn't necessarily want to go back there, we agreed to go back. We had been getting on amazingly well, despite all of the craziness that had occurred before we left; we had somehow managed to put it behind us and move into an even better place with our relationship. I was only resistant to go back to Thailand because I knew I would get that spirit back in me and would want to fight again, and this part of the journey was not about me. I wanted to support the man who had so graciously supported me over the last 12 months.

We spoke about returning to where we had both trained before, but Kyle had a bad taste in his mouth after he had pulled his groin there. My very original trainer had opened a gym up in Hua Hin, another part of Thailand that neither of us had been to, so we decided to give that a go. We knew going there would be totally different to what we had known before. It would be a simpler and more basic life – training, running, going to the beach and eating good food. All I wanted was to enjoy myself, and to support Kyle. For the first time in my travelling journey, I lay my own personal goals aside. I was happy to sit back and enjoy the huge transformation that had taken place in me. I was breaking out of the cocoon and blossoming into a beautiful butterfly. I knew that going back to living the fight lifestyle, without actually having to fight, would help me in a massive way.

Meeting Kyle in September 2014, even though I hadn't really wanted to meet anyone at that time, had helped to heal my relationship wounds. I was so grateful to this beautiful, sweet soul for reminding me that, no matter what, it was important to keep my heart wide open to even the mere possibility of love. I genuinely believe an angel placed Kyle in my life at that time. So now it was time for me to support his dreams, to ensure there were no regrets later on in life. What I didn't realise back then, was that all of this kind of stuff can create emotional trauma in other people. So, I could have created a trauma response in him that all women take away your dreams, but I was starting to intuitively connect these things. And while you can't make your choices in life worrying about the effect they have on other people, everyone has to take responsibility for themselves, their choices and the way they effect those around us.

We got to Hua Hin, and it was such a contrast to where we had been before. It wasn't green and pretty in the same way as it was around Phuket, but it had its own charm. Very quickly, we found an apartment where we could base ourselves, it was ten minutes on a moped away from the gym. The only problem was it wasn't that easy to get a moped. We were used to being able to easily rent one for as long as we wanted to, but here we had to hunt somewhere down for us to be able to find even just one moped. This actually worked out fine because Kyle always wanted to drive, and I was happy just sitting on the back taking pictures and clinging on to his abs.

We quickly got into a daily routine of training, except Sundays. Kyle was a really good fighter. He had the potential to be something absolutely incredible in the fight world, but it became clear pretty early on, that there was something not settling quite right for the pair of us. It wasn't that we argued or anything like that, we just didn't feel settled. There was something missing. It wasn't a comfortable feeling for me, so in typical Lucy fashion, I got 'ants-in-the-pants' syndrome and orchestrated a move to Bangkok.

I used to train at my sister's fiancé's gym. They had bought a Thai trainer over to the gym for a year, and he had been my trainer the whole time that I'd been there. We had grown together, and I truly believe that having a Thai trainer train me 2 or 3 times each week was a game changer. He was tough! He picked apart all of my faults and all of the corners that I cut and he wouldn't take any of my shitty excuses. He showed me how to move properly, how to breathe, how I needed to connect, and how I should respect my opponent. He ignited the warrior within me, but to do so with control rather than it coming from a space of anger – which is what it started to be with me. Whilst I had been travelling, this guy had moved back to Bangkok. He had messaged me about my fight, and asked me to go to his gym. I told Kyle how amazing this guy was and he asked to see some videos, to check out who he was and what he was like. Kyle liked what he saw and said, "Fuck it then, let's go there if you think that this could be good." I loved how easily things flowed. If something didn't feel right, we just did something about it. There was a strong level of trust growing between the two of us.

Before we left Hua Hin, we were walking through a mall one night and Kyle picked out a beautiful diamond ring for me. He made me try it on and was about to buy it for me, but I said no. I don't think we ever spoke about it again after that. I didn't say no because I didn't love him, I said no because I felt he had so much more living to do. In hindsight, I recognise how dismissive and cutthroat that may have felt to him. I genuinely saw myself being with him at this point; I would have married him there and then if I'm honest, but I knew we had much more growth to do. I'm not sure if Kyle felt hurt by my rejection because we never ever spoke about it again. Nice one, Lucy!

That night we got home, packed our things and prepared for the three-hour drive to Bangkok the next day. We were excited as we knew the training was going to be phenomenal, and that was what mattered to Kyle. What we didn't realise, was that we were jumping from the frying pan into the fire.

72

When we got to Bangkok, we quickly discovered that the gym was in the back end of nowhere. It was an hour outside of the city, so we could not make use of any of the transport that makes city living so easy. It was truly stunning, though.

We had a walk around and realised we couldn't find any healthy food within walking distance, and we couldn't find anywhere to hire a moped, although we walked miles trying to. In Thailand, if you don't have a moped, you can't get around easily. Everything is too far to get to on foot and the roads are blocked because there are too many cars on the road. With no moped, we would have to walk everywhere, and that would leave us really limited as to what we could and couldn't do.

The area we were in was traditional Thai. The only food available to us was from those little trolleys where people would be selling octopus and a multitude of other weird and wonderful things like that. Chances are, it tasted amazing, but for somebody that was starting to take an interest in what I ate, there was literally nothing that I could find to satisfy me. At that point, the anxiety kicked in, as we both started thinking about what we were going to do. No moped, no food, no life. And we intended to be there for a month or two! We considered going back to what we knew and to a place we were familiar with, but that was the easy option. So, we decided we would give it a couple of weeks, even though we knew it was going to be tough.

On the first day, we walked from our apartment, and it was only about a 15-minute walk to the gym, but it was 30 odd degrees. We had flip-flops on, our bags full of gloves, kit, wraps, shin guards and all the other stuff. It was sweltering even getting to the gym. When we got there, my trainer, Yod, was so happy to see me and he told everyone there all about me. He told me how much he had missed training with me since I had left to travel. It was really nice to get reconnected with him on his home turf. I told him I was here to train with him and I was really excited about it, but he then informed me that he was going to train Kyle and I was going to train with somebody else. I thought it was a bit odd but I understood he needed to suss out Kyle. He pointed to the young man who was going to train me. When I say young man, he was more like a young boy. The kid was such a little cutey, he didn't speak particularly good English, but he was very attentive. He paid attention to everything I was doing during the warm-up and did his best to have a little chat with me in broken Thai. Yod and Kyle started training together and they were getting on great. I could see Yod was quite impressed that he had somebody who actually knew what they were doing. Kyle looked like he was in his element too; finally getting the training he had been wishing for. As much as the food situation stressed me out, I breathed a sigh of relief that Kyle was going to have his day.

I started to train with the kid. He was holding pads for me and I could see he was quite impressed with how hard I could punch the pads. For a girl, I can hit, especially with my right hand; it's like a little bomb when I release it. We carried on training and I could see he wanted to push me harder. We took a break, I grabbed some water and he spoke in Thai to Yod. When we started hitting pads again, he was coming at me harder and harder, stronger and stronger. He was really pushing me to my limits. Exactly what I had been asking for! I thought – *Take it easy on me, it's my first time in ages.* I was out of breath, it was boiling hot sunshine, but there was no let-up whatsoever. He pushed and pushed me. As much as it hurt, if felt good! Kyle and Yod were laughing as they watched on. Yod said how impressed he was with how much I had come on since he last saw me.

The session was hard; probably one of the hardest sessions I'd had in a long time. In the breaks, I was sipping on water and gasping for breath. By the end of the session, I was laid out on my back, dripping in sweat and trying to get my breath back. The young kid came over, gave me a hug, and a thumbs up. He said, "Good," and then he disappeared. Yod started to put Kyle and I through our paces doing some bag work and a few other things, which was great fun. Suddenly, the kid came back and he was in his school uniform. I had my head in my hands, laughing so hard – it was hilarious. I had been done over by a fucking school boy. And yet, it was one of the best sessions that I ever had. The beauty of this kid was that he was still excited and so passionate about fighting. I found out afterwards that he was a Thai champion, he had won lots of fights in his 'younger' years, but he got injured and was just coming back into it. He was billed to be a big thing in Thai boxing, if he could stay away from injuries. I'll never forget that session.

Walking home from training, dehydrated, sweating buckets and guzzling water, all we wanted to do was eat some good food, but we couldn't find anything. And for me, that's not a good place to be. We started to get a bit antsy with one another because I'm one of those people that unless I get fed I'm not great. I own it, and I'm not as bad these days, I can manage it better. However, back in those days, hanger was a real thing. It wasn't that I got angry with everybody, but if somebody picked at me they would know about it.

We ended up having to dump all of our stuff back at the apartment and to walk for ages, which was far from ideal. We were already starving, having trained hard for a couple of hours. We must have easily expended about fifteen hundred calories in that session, and about three litres of water. Eventually, we found a place to eat, it was okay, but not great. We sat there deciding what we were going to do with ourselves. On the one hand, it had almost everything we wanted – it was quiet, it was peaceful, it was beautiful, but, ultimately, we had to eat, especially with the training we were doing, otherwise, we were going to get injured. I had already become quite familiar with that, every time I trained when I didn't have enough fuel in the tank, I would pull a muscle or something would happen in my body to let me know I wasn't in balance. Kyle had it too where he had pulled his groin through pushing too hard. It was good that I was intuitively starting to recognise these things and to consider my body and its health more and more.

We decided to carry on for a little while. The training was phenomenal, but the less food that we ate, the less energy that we had in the tank, the more it hurt and the more frustration kicked in. We did do some amazing classes there, and I feel, looking back, that it was a real shame that we couldn't get our transportation sorted. This place could have been a huge evolution for us individually, and an even bigger evolution for the pair of us. We couldn't last, though. It became too much, too hard. We found ourselves in a position whereby we had to make a decision to move on again. So with a huge, heavy heart, we left.

We ended up going back to the city of Bangkok. We knew there were plenty of gyms and the transport was easy, there were plenty of food options, and it would all be so much easier for us. We tried a couple of the gyms, but got fed up with them very quickly. The standard just wasn't what we were looking for. A couple of the gyms didn't want women training there, which was an interesting dynamic. It was like every step of the way we were being blocked. We tried our best, though. Then it started. Kyle began talking about going home. He was missing home, missing his normality and the structure he was used to. It made my stomach flip. I was nowhere near ready to go home.

Now, I get it. Life was pretty tough. We'd had an amazing couple of months travelling, but then his dream of fighting in Thailand just seemed to be moving further and further away from him. He was missing his friends and his family. Like me, he was a fixer and he knew stuff was going on at home that he couldn't fix by being away. He also talked about missing jumping in his car and going places. He was missing work too because, a bit like myself, he was a workaholic. There were all sorts of different emotions coming up in him. I had mostly processed mine early on in the trip, so I understood where he was at. He was living in a weird space and kept saying to me, "Everything's going wrong." And the more he said it, of course, the more stuff was challenging us. Eventually, he just came out and said, "Look, I'm going to go home. I want to go back to Dubai for a holiday on the way home. You don't have to come if you don't want to."

I felt as if someone had punched me hard in the stomach. He had been so patient with me and he was right, it had been extremely challenging for the last month or so. It did feel as if everything was going against us, and something was calling him home. I knew that if he went, I would have to go too; or at least that's what I told myself. There was so much guilt inside of me. I'd met this guy a year earlier and I'd been on the road ever since. He had quit his job, come over and sacrificed so much to join me, and now I was in the reverse position whereby he was asking me to go with him. I didn't want to, but I was in a dilemma because I really loved him, but I didn't want to do what he was doing. It was challenging. It brought up so much healing for me. I wanted to use my voice and say, "Listen, I know that there are things I've still got to do. I'll come to Dubai on holiday and then I'm going to continue on my way, and if that means it's over, so be it."

I didn't, though. I said, "Okay, fine."

Worst decision of my life, and yet the best decision at the same time.

73

We booked a flight from Bangkok to Dubai, with the intention of being in Dubai for about ten days, then heading back home to England. When we got there it was so hot. It was August – what were we expecting? It was 45 degrees! Nothing can prepare you for that summer heat in Dubai. I've never felt anything like it. On top of that, I didn't want to be there. I was sad that my travels were coming to an end. I wanted to carry on, and with not getting my own way, the trauma started to surface. I would find myself getting angry over the most ridiculous of things. He would ask me to do something and my default response would be anger rather than the loving state that I'd started to step into. I own it now, it was all my own doing, he never made me do anything. I could easily have made a different decision and continued on the path on my own again. Back then, even though I had been brave and left everything I knew and loved behind once, all I wanted was to be loved. I was not at the point of loving myself, so I still looked to others to provide that for me. I held Kyle in higher regard than myself and what was intuitively right for me. After all the growth I had done, I found myself back in a place of fear.

The trip to Dubai was okay all in all. It was really just a sunny holiday, and something I probably could have done without. It was unbearably hot too, and it made it hard to relax. One day, we were lying on the beach, sizzling. We had gotten there really early as we knew by 10 am it would start to get uncomfortable. I was so hot that I ran into the sea to cool down. I charged straight in, and threw myself in expecting it to cool me down but it was like a scolding hot bath. It was hilarious. I was hopping in and out of the sea, not knowing which heat was better or worse and not knowing what to do with myself. I guess it was pretty symbolic of the heat and tension that was simmering between Kyle and I. I didn't want to be there, and he just wanted to get home.

On the second to last night, Kyle got so angry with me that he kicked the TV in the hotel room and smashed it. At that point, I just had to leave. I knew he would never hurt me, but things were getting close to ridiculous at this point. I went down to the hotel lobby to reflect. I sat there thinking – *What the fuck am I doing? I don't want to be here. I don't want to be going home. Why am I doing this? Why am I continuing to follow somebody else's dream?* It was a test for me. Bear in mind I had left my job, gone travelling and done all this amazing stuff to get rid of my fear once, and yet now it felt like the fear was setting in again. The difference this time was I was starting to recognise that it was trauma; the trauma of a man leaving me because my dad had left me. Those old abandonment issues were surfacing. I wanted to cling on to Kyle, rather than let go and surrender. Nowadays, I trust that if I let something go and it's intended to be, it will come back to me. However, back then, I was still clinging to it. With Kyle, I really thought the world of him, but every sign was screaming at me that I needed to end it; I just wasn't quite ready to see it. I had spent a year making this work and I wasn't going to give up that easily.

A couple of days later, we flew back to the UK. On the flight back, I was pissed off. I was angry at him for smashing the TV, I was questioning myself and projecting my anger onto him, but I was angry at myself mostly for not having the courage of my convictions. Although I didn't see it at the time, this angry behaviour that Kyle was showing me was my mirror. It showed me exactly what I had been like a couple of months earlier. I was triggered by someone else behaving as I had done. With what I know now, I realise that we get shown it, so we can heal it. I wasn't standing in my truth and he was. He knew what he wanted – even if that wasn't the same thing I wanted. This was my test – and I was failing, miserably!

74

When we got back to the UK, Kyle went off to Hertfordshire and I was going to stay with my best friend for a little bit. She came to pick me up from the airport. She was so excited to see me, but I was in a right old mood! I got in her car and said, "Fuck this. Get me home and let's go out and have some fun because I'm so fucking pissed off to be home." She wanted to know what had happened and so I explained some of the stuff that had gone on. Yet another holiday romance that clearly needed to be over. We talked while we drove back to Essex, which was where she lived. That afternoon, we went to the pub and got smashed. It didn't take much to get well oiled because I'd not been drinking much over recent months. We created quite a storm in Billericay that afternoon. It was so good to be back with my bestie. I forgot all about Kyle for a while.

By the middle of the next morning, I hadn't heard from Kyle yet, which I thought was a bit weird, but it was Saturday and so I assumed he was busy sorting his stuff out. It got to the Monday, though, and I still hadn't heard from him, so I sent him a message saying, "Are you alive?" He did get back to me pretty quickly, but there was an undertone. My perception was that he was being an arsehole. He was being closed off. Bearing in mind, I had followed him home, so what did he have to be so pissed off about? It wasn't me that had kicked the TV in. It wasn't me that caused that argument. And again I got that thought – *What the fuck are you doing here, Lucy? You're investing your love and your energy in somebody that clearly doesn't give a shit.* At this point in my life, I was a master at pretending nothing was wrong. I told Catherine that Kyle was being hard work, but I never alluded to how much I was actually hurting. I was still too tough for that, and it was my biggest downfall. Lacking that vulnerability, hurt only one person – me!

And ironically, I feel that one of the sexiest qualities someone can possess is their authentic vulnerability.

I packed my stuff up from my best friend's house, after a few great days. It was time to head South, to my mum's house in Bournemouth. After only a few days there, I decided it was time to find myself a job back on the trading floor. It was time to get back to reality! A reality I had hoped I would never need to return to, but I quickly regressed and decided that I needed to find myself a new home back in London and get my life back on track. It was time to get myself a base, earn some money and get back to all my friends closer to London. Many people asked me why I would not stay in Bournemouth. It was simple. I had such an amazing childhood there, but the drugs and all those teenage memories weren't particularly happy.

As soon as my CV was back out on the market, I was headhunted by five of the big banks; The Royal Bank of Scotland, The Bank of England, UBS, Goldman Sachs and Barclays were the interested parties. It didn't take long and I had been certain I wouldn't get a job easily.

Very quickly, I got consumed by the interview process. Emails, phone calls, in-person interviews. It was like a full-time job in itself. For a while, it was constant. The busiest I had been for a year. My fear during this process was that they would think I was a lazy, good-for-nothing for taking a year out, but they were actually really impressed and in awe of what I had achieved whilst I was away. A couple of people said how calm I appeared. I was a different person to the girl who had gone through this process before. I wasn't scared to stand my ground either. I told them I would willingly start early each day, but I would be taking an hour for lunch, to train Muay Thai, and I would be leaving at 5.30 pm at the latest, so I could work on my own business after hours. I'm not sure they were ready for such straight talking, it wasn't the done thing in that world, but it was what I needed to do to survive being back there. Knowing who I was and what I wanted, helped me quickly eliminate Barclays and Goldman Sachs. It was just too much, they wanted too much from me. I intuitively knew that those banks would not be keen on the way I wanted to work.

I continued with the interviews for the Bank of England, the Royal Bank of Scotland and UBS – the United Bank of Switzerland.

I walked into the Bank of England; it's fascinating knowing what I know now that I decided to pursue that one. I walked into the building just outside of Bank Station in the City of London and it sent shivers down my spine. There was an eeriness to it that was uncomfortable, but, in all honesty, I kind of liked it. It was really weird. It intrigued me no end. There was a haunting, chilling energy to the place.

The Royal Bank of Scotland did an in-person interview, then I had to have a telephone interview, and then I had to go back and deliver a presentation. There were so many different interview stages, but I just thought I would ride it out and go along with it. I had a level of trust that it would all work out as it was divinely planned; although that wasn't quite the language I would have used back then.

From the start of the process, I had my heart set on working for UBS. It would be a pretty awkward journey for me to get there each day, but it was where I knew I had to be. I paid lip service to the other banks, knowing that my full intention was to go to UBS, if they offered me a job. I had always wanted to work in their building, it fascinated me – a little bit like I had when I was younger and drove past the Chase Manhattan building when I lived in Bournemouth. I decided during the interview process that I liked the environment and the atmosphere there. I also really liked the guy that had been interviewing me. He was laid back and very excited at the thought of bringing some new energy into the team. I feel there was something about the place that my soul connected with. I had made my mind up, and although I wasn't aware of the power of manifestation, I figured something mystical was happening because as soon as I made my mind up, the other two banks offered me the job and said they needed an urgent response. Decision time! I actually turned the other two jobs down before I even had validation from UBS. And then, literally, within a day or so of me rejecting the other two, I got the UBS offer. And then the penny dropped – *Wow, I literally can get whatever I want!*

When I look back on my career and every other job I had, I got everything I ever wanted. Every time I ever set my mind on something and I was certain about it, I got it. If I wanted a pay rise, I got it. It was really interesting to acknowledge it and then start to recognise it and utilise it for other areas of my life also.

Once the offer was made, it all happened very quickly. I had to go through a quick but intense security check as I was set to start on the 19th of October 2015.

I had moved up to Kent to stay with a friend for the first month, miles away from Kyle. We would catch up once a week, which at the time was enough. Things were still pretty fraught between us, despite him doing his best to try to appease me since we got back. Mentally, I had semi-checked out of the relationship. In all reality, I should have ended it. I should have used this as a fresh start, but I didn't. We loved each other, and we were just in denial that it was ever going to work.

I was actually really happy to be going back to work. I was looking forward to earning a fortune again. Rather than going back permanent, I had decided to do something I said I never would, as it was too risky; I went contracting. This meant I was essentially self-employed and would charge a day rate, but then I was responsible for doing my own taxes. The money was big. It could easily have become addictive, but I had a plan. I knew that I was only going to be there for two years maximum because that is what I had set in my mind. Two years of making money, and in the background building up my client base as a nutritionist and coach; then I would get out of there, and finally spread my wings and fly. It was only going to be a short, sharp stint.

This 'two-year' plan had come about whilst I was staying at my mum's house. I was sitting in her kitchen one day, and all of a sudden I got this download – although I didn't know that's what it was at the time – it was just a feeling that I needed to start a business called Activ8U. I felt I needed to set up an Instagram page and that this page would be my accountability buddy for the version of me that I wanted to create. If I went back to corporate, this time around I would make sure that I exercised, and that I ate healthily. I would have healthy boundaries in place. And in the background, I would make sure that I would create a business that could support me enough to get me out of my contract. So I had the vision to guide me through. I was stepping forwards, but I knew that I had to go back to the old, for a while, to be able to step into the new.

75

When I started back at work on the trading floor, in October 2015, everybody thought I was a total weirdo. Nothing much had changed in that world, but I brought a level of sass and pizazz they were just not used to. I took salads in, lined all my health supplements up along my desk, I had two huge bottles of water to get through each day, and I brought a huge stock of healthy treats that I had made. My colleagues watched me for a few months, in awe of the fact I was a badass at my job, but also so certain about my health and my personal life. Each Thursday, I would turn down the offer of post-work drinks, and stand in my truth. I preferred to get home and go to Muay Thai at Scorpions in Beckenham. And because I was standing in my truth and not getting caught up in the noise of office life, people started to really value me.

In my spare time, I began training as a health coach, as well as starting a degree in nutrition. I created the Activ8U page and was adding value to that each day. I was also prepared to do whatever it took to avoid all of the dis-ease and repetitive sickness that I had whilst working in Corporate previously. I made a commitment to myself that I was going to stay well because I didn't want to go back to having those chronic health issues again.

At this point, I hadn't quite established the connection between my sickness and emotional trauma, not on a conscious level anyway. In my head, it was work that had made me sick. I put it down to the stress, and even the air conditioning. The denial! That was still my belief system at this time, though. The tangible solution for me was nutrition – and so qualifying as a nutritionist and qualifying as a health coach seemed perfect. The other non-negotiable had become regular exercise.

I set standards for the first time in my life. I said I would get into work at a sensible time and leave at a sensible time at the end of the day, and I honoured that. I exercised every day, and mostly during lunch breaks. Often, I'd actually be gone from the office during lunch for about an hour and a half – by the time that I had got there, done an hour session, got showered and then got back. I didn't care. These were my standards. They were just going to have to put up with it

— and they did. They knew how effective I was whilst I was in the office. I would deliver more than the average person because I wasn't average. I could multi-task better than anyone.

Setting my standards was a game changer. And that's the beauty of standards and boundaries. They're uncomfortable whilst you're figuring them out, but as soon as you lean into them fully, your life is greatly improved — and often the lives of the people around you. I was starting to stand in my truth more and more. I just thought that I was growing and getting to know myself a little bit more. I didn't quite realise that I was in the midst of a catastrophic change.

76

As 2015 came to a close, I was feeling pretty good about myself. I was feeling really comfortable and I actually thought I had the balance right. I was earning lots of money, my boss was sound, the job was easy. I figured I could probably stay like this and cruise my way through the rest of my life.

Kyle and I had continued to patch things up, to a degree. It was a weird transitional period for both of us. I was not really committed to it, but I didn't want to let go, and I'm pretty sure he felt the same about me. In November, I moved into my own place in Blackheath in London. This meant that Kyle was able to come and stay with me as often as he wanted to and that made it a little bit easier for us to see each other. The brief time apart had allowed us to reflect on our relationship and so things were a bit better for a while. He would come down from Hertfordshire to London on a Friday night, or a Saturday morning, and stay for the weekend and then go back, but it wasn't like it used to be. I don't think I was prepared to let go of what had happened in Dubai; not that I was brave enough to admit that at the time. And while we did have some amazing times, we also had a lot of not-so-great times. We argued, especially come the end of the weekend when it was time to leave each other again. He was not really a fan of my friends and I never really got to know any of his, especially after the incident with my brawl.

At around the same time I moved into my apartment, the continuous bleeding from my womb started up again. Besides my own sadness at this, it also didn't help things with Kyle. Every day, for 9 months, I lost a significant amount of blood. Some days it was so bad that I couldn't even make it to work, or out to meet friends. I became unusually flakey and it created problems within my friendship group.

At the start of 2016, despite the blood loss, I was probably in the best shape of my life up to that point. I was running 3 to 5 miles every day, training hard with my Thai boxing and strength and conditioning coaches. I was approached about a fight in London. I felt good and ready to go, so I took it. I upped my training to another level, running every day down by Greenwich up to the O2, through Greenwich Park and back. I felt absolutely incredible, even though I was contending with the drain of the blood loss.

The fight came around pretty quickly. I weighed in at just under 57kgs, she was slightly heavier than I was. I was hungry and focused. It had been a while since I last fought and the buzz of the fight preparation felt good. It was the first time I'd actually had to cut weight properly. In Thailand, you could get away with it, but not in the UK.

The fight started fast. Unlike in Thailand, I didn't have to be respectful in that first round, so I went all in and smashed her in round one. Her corner threw the towel in within the first 90 seconds. All that training, and it was over so quickly. She must have been 10 to 15 years younger than me, but let's not forget that at this point in 2016, I was 38 years old. I just channelled the same energy I did in Thailand. I felt so strong. I felt like a warrior. No wonder her corner called it, especially if Mike Tyson was in my eyes again.

77

A few weeks after the fight, I was running along the canals in London during lunchtime, when something stopped me. It wasn't something physical, there wasn't a person there or anything, but something held me by my shoulders. It was so interesting. I looked around, there was nothing there and I thought – *Why did I stop? That's a bit weird.* I turned around and looked at the canal and thought it was so pretty. I grabbed my phone and took a few photos of it, and then carried on back to work. I thought nothing else of it.

A few days later, I was going through my phone, attempting to delete some photos to manage my phone memory storage. I saw the pictures that I had taken by the canal that day and it made me wonder what that was all about. I looked at the picture and I couldn't believe it. I could see a dragon, two angels, and an actual human in the clouds. It blew me away so much that I posted it on my Instagram.

I immediately sent it to a lady who I had done a quantum healing session with, and I said to her, "I think God is in my picture. I need to send it to you, you'll be blown away."

I was introduced to this lady by my nurse friend in Australia. Her brother, who was very spiritually aware, had suggested that this lady had helped him get more connected to his truth. I knew nothing about quantum, other than this lady sounded pretty cool, and every single cell in my body tingled when I heard about her, so I knew I had to connect with her. At this point in 2016, I had only had one session with her, but I knew she was amazing by the way she made me feel, although, in all honesty, it didn't quite make sense to me yet.

When she saw the picture she went crazy, she couldn't believe it. Honestly, when you looked at the picture there was this person in the clouds, as clear as day, it wasn't just wishful thinking. It's worth pointing out that at this point, I was not yet awake to this kind of stuff. I had started recognising a few signs and things, but not ones so directly aimed at me. That photograph was absolutely mind-blowing.

Now, I truly, truly believe that that was the day 'they' decided that they were going to pick me. More of 'they' later.

78

Kyle and I were doing our best to cling to our relationship, and I was also having to deal with the issue with my womb, which was worsening week by week. I would go to the doctors and they would prescribe me some sort of drug to take. It would stop the bleeding for a day, then it would start again. Throughout all of the stuff with my womb, that had gone on for years by now, it felt like nobody took me seriously. I was losing a lot of blood this time around, though, but whenever I went to the doctor, they wouldn't listen to me properly.

It's bizarre that just because a women loses blood each month through her menstrual cycle, it's not considered a problem when she loses blood out of her cycle.

It seemed that the health system in the UK was in as bad a state as I was. It had become a bureaucracy, overwhelmed with paperwork and red tape. It was no longer about health anymore; it had become a business.

On top of everything else, significant mould started to appear in the apartment in Blackheath. Within a very short period of time, it got so bad, I was informed I needed to find somewhere else to live. Yet another bundle of stress to add to my already stressful situation. Looking back at it now, they were all signs trying to get my attention, but I didn't want to recognise them.

I tried to do my best to work through the bleeding, I still trained regularly and went to work as normal. However, it got to a period in the summer of 2016 whereby it was becoming embarrassing. One evening, I was going to my friend's birthday party and I walked down the hill to get on the train to go into central London. By the time I had gone from my apartment to the train station, I had bled through everything that I was wearing. Now, I knew this was happening, so I used to wear a super plus tampon and a super plus towel to do any journey. The train station was a ten-minute walk, but I bled through all of those layers and through my clothes in that short time. I sat there at the train station and sobbed, trying to make sense of what this was all about.

It got so bad that it became very isolating. Some days, I couldn't even get to work because of the blood. Thankfully, my boss gave me access so that I could work from home. I physically couldn't get to see people or I'd let them down at the last minute, and as a result, my friends started to disappear. There was never any pattern to the bleeding, it was unpredictable and so it was impossible to manage. And in my world, it felt like everything was collapsing. Everyone was being removed, they were not putting up with this new flakey version of me, and I was too embarrassed to tell them the truth. My family were miles away, and my boyfriend too, and here I was going through one of the worst periods of my life, pretty much alone. Why was this happening to me? Surely with the amount I was focusing on my health and nutrition, this shouldn't be happening?

One particular day, I was at my apartment trying to get out and to see a friend. I wasn't drinking or anything, I just needed to get out of the apartment for my sanity. I couldn't get out though because of the blood. Every time I stood up, it was like something was falling out of me. It was hideous. I called my mum and cried my heart out. I told her that I couldn't cope anymore, and I didn't know how I was going to get through it. It was truly awful. I constantly felt like I was going to faint and I was permanently dizzy. Once again, my health was being stripped from me, only this time I thought that I was doing all the right things with my nutrition, exercise, and supplements. So what was going on?

After I got off the phone to my mum, my sister called me. I didn't want to speak to her. She tried a few times, so I ended up answering the phone to her, "Kirsty, I'm not in the mood to talk."

"Get a bag ready we're going to the hospital. I'm coming to pick you up now."

Shortly afterwards, she arrived at my place and dragged me to the hospital. She was a real big sister that day, something I was not used to. I was so grateful for her. At the hospital, she said to them, "We're not leaving until she has some answers, so I suggest you sort it out and get a gynaecologist here and find out what's going on with her because she's going to bleed out."

They ran a load of tests on me. Obviously, I was dangerously low on iron and I was dangerously anaemic, but there wasn't a solution. All they said to me was what they usually said – that they needed to operate on me to remove the lumps and that will stop the bleeding. And, of course, they told me to take some pills to stop the bleeding, and then take some other pills to mitigate the damage the other tablets could potentially do. I realised that day that we were all just guinea pigs to the medical industry. They had no clue what they were doing most of the time, they were making it up as they went along.

In the past, I just did what I was told when it came to doctors and medics. Now, though, I knew better. I realised that anything that I put in my body to try and suppress something that was happening, was going to create further problems. Giving me a pill to stop the bleeding, when my body was clearly giving me a sign that it needed to bleed, did not sit well with me at all. I told them I didn't want to take a pill to stop the bleeding, and they didn't like that. They didn't like it because they didn't have any other solution other than for me to take an iron supplement for me to get my iron back up, but then with iron supplements, I would get real bad constipation. It was too much for my body to be able to process. I just wanted them to get to the root cause of what was creating these lumps in the first place because then we could deal with that, and sort the problem once and for all. Clearly, a healthy me was not good a business model.

I found myself in the hospital pondering how I had ended up in this position again. I had a health trauma going on, I was not really happy in my relationship, I had to move out of my apartment, and I was starting to lose my friends. I felt very low, and very lonely, I was ready to get off this merry-go-round now.

Eventually, I got an appointment to go and have the surgery on my womb. I'll be honest with you, it was a nice respite. Much as I hated the idea of having more surgery, the bleeding was horrific. And, it did stop the bleeding. About four or five days after the surgery, I stopped bleeding completely and I started to get a level of normality back again.

79

Soon after the operation, I moved into a brand new apartment in Greenwich, looking out over the Thames, and for a moment things were looking up again.

I made a massive effort to stay on top of my health completely. I was already very good, but I took it to another level. I would sit at my desk with all my fruit and supplements laid out because I was adamant that I wasn't getting ill again. I was done with it. That's when people started asking me for help; they would ask me questions about their health issues, and I would advise them; sometimes from the knowledge of what I had been taught, and other times, intuitively, stuff would just come out of my mouth. They would listen, take the action and the next thing, they would be healed. I was doing my mundane corporate job, but I was learning to help people, to ignite their healing journey and get them back in alignment with their bodies. And doing all that by simply following my own experience and my own healing journey. People trusted me. Okay, many of them thought I was fucking nuts, but they also trusted me, which allowed me to start to trust my own intuition more and more too.

At some point towards the end of 2016, my boss came to me and proposed extending my contract by another year. I still had one year left to run, but he wanted to extend it there and then and lock me in. I thought about it but told him I would rather leave it as it is and maybe discuss it the following year. It would have been easy to just extend it, I was being paid a lot of money, and working sensible hours this time around; I could have stayed there, without question. The thing was I was starting to become a different person. A person I really liked.

When I look back at photos of this period of time, I'm really proud of the person I was. Physically I was in the best shape of my life. I had made a clear decision that I was no longer going to allow any dis-ease into my body. I now recognised that not everything I had been doing over the years had served me in the best of ways, and for the first time ever, I was embracing the idea that the dis-ease in my body had been created by me, rather than blaming unfortunate circumstances, genetics or anything else for that matter. I hadn't fully connected the dots around emotional trauma, yet, but nevertheless, I was getting there and extremely proud of the woman I had become. For the first time in my life, my eyes were opening. I realised that when it came to health, everything mattered – food, drink, alcohol, friendships, relationships, even down to conversations with strangers.

It was a Monday morning, the 7th November 2016, I remember the date very clearly. I'd had a really fun weekend. Kyle had come down to meet me at Waterloo and I had met him under the clock there. We had a really nice weekend together, and for the first time in a while, we were almost back to how we used to be, and enjoying each other's company. I had gone into work that Monday with a spring in my step. It had been my dad's birthday the day before, so I had also spent some quality time with my family.

I was sat at my desk on that Monday morning. It was edging close to lunchtime and I remember thinking that I hadn't heard from my mate Jimbo since Saturday afternoon, when he had called me absolutely smashed. My phone started ringing, it wasn't a number I recognised. I don't normally answer unknown numbers, but for whatever reason, that morning I did. It was a guy called Rich. He was a friend of Jimbo's and I had got to know him over the years, but I didn't know him all that well. It was strange to hear his voice on the end of the phone, especially while I was at work. Little did I know when I answered that phone call to him, my life would be changed forever.

Rich told me that Jimbo was dead.

It was like one of those moments in a movie where the room just spins around the main character while they remain motionless. I sat in disbelief, tears rolling down my face, trying to comprehend what he had just said to me. Jimbo – my best friend was gone.

My heart shattered in that moment.

On the Saturday, I had been waiting for Kyle under the clock at Waterloo, when Jimbo had called me to have one of those crazy chats that we always had. I knew he was away in France with some friends for the day. When I answered the phone, he said, "Babe, I'm on the crazy train." That's what we used to say to each other, back in the day when we were out getting wrecked and having a crazy time together. And although I wasn't partying anymore, we were still very close friends. He loved me and I loved him. He called because he was getting back on the Eurostar at midnight that night and he wanted me to meet up with him, "Come on, Lucy. Come out for old time's sake. I know it's not you anymore, but come on! For me!"

I said, "Babe, I love you, but I'm not going to come and meet you. There's no way. I'll be fast asleep by midnight. Just know that I love you. Get home safe." And the last words he said to me were, "Babe, I love you. To the moon and stars."

I later checked and saw that this conversation was the last time he ever looked at his Whatsapp. Later on that night, he was walking back to the Eurostar and he fell about 15 metres to his death. He died instantly, apparently without any pain.

Listening to Rich, in the office on that Monday, I couldn't contain myself and I burst into tears. The assistant to the man who ran the department came over and grabbed me. She picked me up and took me over to an empty office, sat me down and just let me cry it out. I will be eternally grateful to that woman because she held space for me. It wasn't the words she said but she held space for me to cry and to be sad. God bless her, she went to my desk, picked up my things, and locked my computer. She asked me, "Who do I need to call? Who can come and collect you? We need to get you out of here."

She went and spoke with my boss and various other people and she cleared my schedule for the rest of the day. And I let her do it. For the first time in my life, I really surrendered and let somebody look after me. I was absolutely heartbroken. And the worst thing about it all was that Saturday, the day he died, it was my dad's birthday. He had chosen to leave on a date that would be etched in my heart forever.

I'm grateful to him for the message he delivered me through his passing. I wish he was here. I wish I could talk to him. I wish I could hold him, laugh and joke with him, but more than anything, I'm grateful to him. He gave me the kick up the arse I needed to show me that once again I had become complacent. I had become stuck and comfortable, and, once again, I had been choosing to stay in a rut.

I went home, as instructed. I went through a massive amount of mourning, and I really stepped into victimhood for a while. The funeral was booked for December, on my mum's birthday – so once again another date that would be etched in my heart forever. In true typical Jimbo style, there was no way he was ever going to let me forget him. Not that I could anyway, but he made sure of it with these dates.

The funeral was horrific. It was lovely to have all the gang back together, but not in these tragic circumstances.

Between Jimbo's death and the funeral, I had made the decision that I was going to run away, again. My old programme of running away was resurfacing. Lucy? Run away? Never! I booked a flight; I was going to escape to Thailand.

It's all becoming a little too predictable, hey?

The Universe had no intention of allowing that to be the case, though.

80

A few days after the funeral, I packed my things and I went to Thailand for a few weeks to get my head together. I was going there to get my energy back. I was going there to figure out what do next. Two of my girlfriends, one from London and one from Leeds, were going to fly over and join me before Christmas, so there were going to be three of us. Initially, though, I was going to be on my own for a little bit so that I could recalibrate and get my head together after the shittiest end to the year.

I had a good time on my own, it helped me to sort myself out a bit. It gave me some much-required downtime. When the girls arrived, I was ready to have some company and crank up the good vibes. I know Jimbo would not have wanted me moping anymore. It was my responsibility to live for him too, and my goodness, we definitely did that in those two weeks. We had such a good time. We went off on our mopeds, exploring cool places, and I did a lot of training.

One day, though, something interesting happened. The hotel that we were staying in had a roof terrace and a rooftop swimming pool. I was up there, swimming in the pool. I pulled myself onto the edge, to sit on the side, and my friend came over to me, sat down next to me and said, "Lucy, are you really okay?" It was a strange question to ask out of nowhere. Nevertheless, out of my mouth came this response, "This is where it ends. By this time next year, I will not be in Corporate. I have to get out. I'm going to do whatever it takes to create a business, to give me the money I need to survive, and the financial backing to be able to get out." It came from nowhere. It sounded pre-planned, but it wasn't. My friend looked at me in a knowing way, she knew how determined I was and that I would most likely create this. As I had stated many years earlier, when my parents got divorced, I would never rely on a man for money, well this statement about creating my own business was another one of those moments. It was written in stone and nothing was going to stop me.

A few weeks later, in January, when I returned to work, I worked at my day job, and in all my spare time, I created a network marketing business. I went with a product I was already using and extremely aligned with, in order to empower an empire of people to create shifts with their health, and go on their healing journey. It went hand in hand with my training to become a nutritionist and my passion for health coaching. It made perfect sense that I would align the two as a quick fix to get me a secure income and get out of Corporate as soon as possible.

Through January and February of that year, I put a spotlight on every area of my life. Work was easy. I had realised I had become complacent, so I put things in place to ensure I felt uncomfortable enough to move. I reached out to some of the people who organised events within UBS and asked them if I could run seminars during lunch hours to share knowledge on health and healing. I got permission to do this very quickly, under the guise of reducing sick days in the office. Each month, I would put myself in front of two hundred people who were all keen to hear some simple tips and tricks to keep them well.

The hardest realisation I had from losing Jimbo was that I was in a relationship that was no longer serving me, or healthy. I knew I had to do something about it, but it hurt to look at it. I had spent the previous two and a half years holding on and making it work, and then, all of a sudden, I could not hide any longer. I kept thinking about how precious life was and that at a moment's notice it could all be taken away. I deserved to be happy, living the life I knew I was capable of having. I was evolving on my soul path and my soul mission, but the relationship with Kyle was not evolving with me. My goodness did that sting.

At some point in February or March 2017, Kyle and I sat down and had 'the chat'. I shared with him how I felt that for the first time in my life I had connected to something that was showing me my future path. I explained how I felt; I was about to embark on a journey that was unknown, and yet felt so familiar. I really felt I had something I had to deliver to the world, but it was almost unexplainable – just a knowing, a feeling within. He knew where this conversation was going. He looked sad, I could feel the hurt within him. Then he did something that was totally out of character. He started accusing me of cheating and being unfaithful, and thinking there must be someone else in my life.

Wow! That hurt. Yes, I had distanced myself from him since Dubai. Yes, I probably should have explained all of this a lot sooner; however, I would never have done that. I was evolving, and he knew that on a soul level, but wasn't ready to hear it on a human level. It was awful. That day, when he walked out of mine, it broke my heart, and no doubt his too. It made no sense to me, and it was me doing it, so how could it have made sense to him? Looking back, he must have thought I was crazy – 'There's something I have to go and do, I don't know what it is, though.' I mean that's weird, right?

Within a few weeks I was starting to feel much better. I missed him like crazy, but I knew it was the right thing to do. There was a knowing inside of me that I was going to be going on a journey; and having a partner at home, children, a new house, and all of that stuff would not align to it. We did not speak after he left mine that day. We left each other alone to heal, in peace.

A few weeks later, I remember feeling pretty groggy. It was unlike me. The only issues I really had at this point in my life were to do with my womb and that had been okay since the last operation. This was an unbelievable tiredness and an intermittent feeling of sickness. It was weird. I found myself having to rest a lot more, take time out and sometimes even cancel my training, which was unheard of. A few weeks later, my period did not show up. I thought nothing of it. I felt it was probably the changes I was feeling in my body, it would show up when it was ready, despite being regular as clockwork normally. I did not click. And then, one day, it did.

Oh fuck! – I thought. I spoke to my best friend, and she asked me if there was any way I could be pregnant.

"Kyle and I split up weeks ago – surely not?" I said to her. After Kyle and I split up, I decided that until I knew who I was, I was not going to get involved with a man. It just wasn't fair. The hurt he showed me when we split up was not something I was going to choose again. I needed to know who I was, to be certain about the person I was going to be with.

I did a pregnancy test and it was positive. Oh fuckety fuck! I had to reach out to Kyle. After initially asking if it could be anyone else's – I guess I deserved that – he was amazing. He came down to mine, we chatted and explored everything that needed to be explored. I shared with him that as much as I still stood by my decision of us splitting up, as I had God's work to do, it was now in God's hands to show what the next steps were of this wild ride we were on.

A week or so later, he came down to my house again, we went out for dinner and whilst we were out, I started bleeding. I remember walking back to the table with tears streaming down my face, and seeing a look of panic on his face. He knew, we both knew. He got me out of there, took me back to my house, and the next morning took me to the hospital. After a short wait, I was taken through into gynaecology, where we had it confirmed I was actually having a miscarriage. The heartbreak between the two of us was tragic. A miscarriage, again! I felt failure as a woman. What on earth was wrong with me? The gynaecologist told me that the lumps were already back in the womb, and that was the reason the baby had not survived. It had been suffocated under the pressure of it. I was devastated.

Despite this, I asked this specialist again, the question I had asked all of them over the years, "Why is this happening?" I did not really get an answer that day, just a plan as to what we were going to have to do when I eventually wanted to fall pregnant. I could feel Kyle's disappointment. This could have been our route back together, but God had other ideas. That was the last time we saw each other, for a very long time.

Unknowingly, all of the bombs and traumatic experiences that had been thrown into my life during the early parts of that year, resulted in me getting my head down more than ever. Through the seminars, products, health coaching and nutrition, I had started to create a programme that would go on to change many lives around the world.

Within six months, I was earning such good money that I could afford to get out of my corporate job once and for all. So, that's exactly what I did.

In September 2017, just under two years from when I went back to corporate, after saying I would only serve two years, I skipped out of corporate for the very last time. I had undergone a massive transformational shift. I had become brave. I had started to trust. I felt strongly that I was being divinely placed, and divinely guided.

I was becoming more and more aware that the messages and the messengers were all around, if I had the eyes to see. If you treat everyone you meet as a messenger, rather than creating attachments and expectations to them, you realise that you are all pieces in the divine game of chess that we call life. It's all divinely planned. All of it. Every moment. Every interaction. The more you surrender, the easier it is. The more you resist, the bigger the peaks and troughs are that you have to navigate. When I realised I was being moved around, not because it was necessarily what I wanted to do, but actually because my energy was required in those places. From that point onwards, life became much easier.

When I finally stepped out of that office in September, I felt free. I was able to allow my intuition to flow again. I felt freer than I'd ever felt in my life. I was free to travel without any responsibilities, and with a healthy body, mind and spirit.

PART THREE
THE JOURNEY HOME

81

Leaving Corporate for the final time should have been scary. I had a busy few months lined up, which kept me somewhat distracted but it should have been a lot more scary than it turned out to be. My first trip after the great escape was Dubai. I was invited to speak over there, so planned some cool experiences to enjoy, including a skydive. I loved it; the surrender, the exhilaration, and the view was absolutely incredible. Interestingly, when I saw the pictures that were taken of me on the dive, there were orbs in my pictures. I checked my friends pictures, she had none. I asked to see other people's and they had none either. I found it a little bit weird, until I asked my quantum healer to cast her eye over the images. She informed me very proudly that they were not actually orbs, they were UFOs. Wow!

From there, I returned to the UK for a short period of time to move out of my house. I did not know where I was going to be, or what I was going to be doing, so made the decision to surrender my home again and embrace this life of being totally free. I was looking for less commitment at this time in my life, especially as my relationship with Kyle had fizzled out, so I had no relationship commitments, nothing holding me in one place, and no one depending on me. I felt that this was the time for my soul mission to be wholly and fully inflight.

I knew it had been whispering my name and looking to remind me of my mission since birth, and initially – as a kid – I had listened, until life became complicated and so I had switched it off for many years. Finally escaping Corporate in September 2017 was the leg up I needed to actually surrender and trust fully. I had been trusting my intuition about seventy per cent of the time at this point. Following the Dubai trip, I was able to surrender wholeheartedly.

At the end of 2016, I had booked to go and do Date With Destiny with Tony Robbins, they only did it once a year, and I couldn't get the time off work to do it in 2016. So, I made the commitment that I would do it in December 2017. I took time off work – so even if I'd stayed working, I had booked the time off to go. It was my destiny to be there. It was part of the magical divinely orchestrated plan. Due to the event being held in Florida – and my wandering soul knowing there were so many countries to visit on that side of the world – I had planned a magical trip over Christmas and New Year to take some time out, reflect and see where life took me.

In November, I sorted my house out, got my stuff together, and released all the attachments I had to my things. For someone in the environment I had come from, it was such a weird thing to do. I recognised in that process just how much unnecessary stuff I had. The number of attachments, the amount of old stuff that I was unknowingly tied to.

I'd been convincing myself that I knew what freedom was, that I had been living it for the last two years when I worked in corporate because I went from the attitude of working from 7 in the morning till anything from 7 to 11 at night, to somebody that would rock in at half-past seven in the morning and knock off at half-past five, and I'd take a decent lunch break. I had convinced myself that was freedom. I was getting paid big and working a lot less than I used to, and training in the day too. I was winning, right? Wrong! I was still shackled. I was still trapped in systems that I did not want to be in. Yes, I had shifted. Yes, I had been able to free up a lot of time compared to before, but the reality was, I was still trapped. Due to the nature of creating a side hustle at the same time, I was always busy. If I wasn't doing that job, I was doing this job. I was constantly on the go. It was only really in November that I recognised what true freedom felt like. I didn't have to get up in the morning – although I still did. I didn't have to go to work – my work really did not feel like work anymore. I didn't have to answer to anyone. I didn't have to be in a particular location. The only things I was tied to were working with my clients and ensuring that my business ran smoothly. I had nothing stopping me from being whoever or whatever I wanted to be. I didn't have a routine. I had finally stepped out of it. Now it was the time to choose everything consciously. It was magical.

With the trip planned to Date With Destiny during the first week in December, in true Lucy fashion, I was on a plane by the end of November, heading over to Palm Beach, Florida, where the seminar was being held. *No point hanging around the UK* – I thought. I had also decided that I was going to go to Cuba to spend Christmas and New Year with one of my girlfriends. She was going to fly over from Manchester and meet me there. When she left in early January, I would go on somewhere else, I just was not too sure where. I really wanted to go to Guatemala because of a picture Ricky had sent me some years earlier of a beautiful lake there. As soon as I saw it, I knew I had to go. I was petrified, though, at the thought of going to Guatemala on my own. All the stories I had heard made me think it was scary – guns and all that stuff. Here was my imagination going off again, just like it did when I went to Ecuador. It didn't help that my mum watched all sorts of nonsense on the TV and added to my paranoia by telling me, "Oh, my God, you can't go there. God knows what will happen." Although I had been to South America before and Central America, Guatemala, on my own, was a whole new kettle of fish.

My dilemma was that I didn't plan to come home in between trips, so I had to prepare for all these different trips in one go. For those who have ever been to a Tony Robbins event, you'll know it's bloody Baltic in the room where he runs the events, it's freezing. So despite being in much warmer climates than the UK, you had to prepare to freeze your bits off. You had to layer up and ensure you were nice and warm.

After that I would move on to Cuba, which was going to be a scorcher, and then likely another super smoking hot destination. I'll be honest, I'm not really a winter kind of girl. I love the heat. I love the sunshine. I love the light.

Leading up to the trip, I set the intention that I was going to be well; there are a lot of people who get sick when they go to Tony Robbins' events. I had been to Unleash the Power Within previously and everyone dropped like flies afterwards. I was forearmed and forewarned. I was calling in good health by repeating mantras, "I'm going to be well. I'm going to make sure that everything is in alignment. I'm going to make sure I travel with ease and grace."

On the plane over to Miami, there was a guy sitting in the row in front of me. At one point in the flight, I decided to go for a little wander up and down the plane, as you do when you want to stretch your legs and the plane isn't too busy. I ended up speaking to the air hostesses, and the guy sitting in front of me must have overheard, because when I said that I was going over to see Tony Robbins, this little head popped around, like an ostrich – you know how people do when they want to see who's talking? I finished chatting to the air hostesses and went and sat back in my seat, and within a second of sitting down, I had this face appearing over the seat. "Did I hear you say you're going to Tony Robbins?"

"Yes, I am," I replied.

"I'm going to see him too; how mad is that?"

Anyway, we chatted for a while and then it transpired that he had seen me on Facebook, which was very interesting. He had been following a lot of the work I had been doing. At around this period of time, well before all the lockdowns, I was starting to become very vocal on Facebook. I was talking about higher levels of consciousness, the fact that shifts were coming, and all sorts of spiritual things. I shared my experiences with anyone who cared to follow me, unknowing that I was activating people every time they watched my live videos. I had been sharing the things that had happened on my journey to that point. He had found me somehow on Facebook and followed me. Chatting to him made the rest of the flight really interesting.

When we got off the plane on the other end, he asked me where I was staying and, no surprise, we were staying just around the corner from each other, so we ended up sharing a taxi, and continued to have a good chat. He explained many things to me, including why he was going to Date With Destiny and how he was looking to release things. As much as I was predominantly about nutrition and health back then, I was becoming more and more aware of the connection of our life events to trauma. While I was talking to him, I was connecting the dots of how his trauma had manifested. I didn't even really know what I was doing, but it was just flowing through me. Thankfully at that time, I didn't open my mouth and say, "Well, have you thought about this or considered that?" I sat, held space and allowed the activations to flow through me.

It's incredible how an apparent simple conversation with someone can end up going through a whole process in my physical vessel, that then leads to me identifying why they created whatever it is that is going on with them. I know this sounds a little out there, but it had become my truth. Everything on my path, up to this point, had led me to suddenly being able to feel and know certain things. I can't explain it any other way. The clearer I became, the clearer the messages came through me. Sometimes I cannot believe the information I know about complete strangers, from a brief conversation. Everyone tells you where they are and what's going on, if you are bold enough to listen fully, and be still and quiet enough to not respond.

In the taxi, we agreed to go to the conference together the next day. He was a nice enough guy, lived in Notting Hill in London, and I felt safe with him.

The day before Date With Destiny, whilst in the hotel, I met two ladies. One lady was very glamorous; you could not help but admire her beauty and the way she held herself, gliding through the reception. It transpired she had been a supermodel in her past. Everything about her was so perfect and elegant. She was very, "Yes, sweetie, darling." That kind of behaviour. I chatted with her for a while, and unknowingly, she connected many dots whilst our conversation flowed. Signs and synchronicities had become a normal, everyday standard at this point. The normal 111 or 222 was a thing of the past now – unless my attention was required quickly. The signs had become more profound and more directed at me personally, and they were coming in like lightning.

I was then introduced to another girl from Manchester. She was a babe. We hit it off immediately. Her being from Manchester was a sign in itself. I never really appreciated how important Manchester was going to end up being during this journey. I had missed a number of pointers up until this point. It had been attempting to get my attention that something required my energy there. Laura was really sound – we are good friends to this day – and we have worked through some serious stuff together. It has not always been pretty, but we have kept on keeping on no matter what.

All of the people I met, who were going to the conference, were looking for something. Looking for answers. Looking for healing. We were looking for a process, or something, that we could take forward with us. At that time, Tony Robbins was the person for me. I was a corporate girl, and he was somebody who I looked at and thought – *Show me how you created your business. How did you become who you are?* It fascinated me. That's all I was interested in, what I needed to do to break through so I could create a business and be as inspirational to people as he was. Now, if I'm being honest with myself, my desire was to be a motivational speaker at that time. I saw myself being on stage. I saw myself in a speaking role. I just knew that I had been given the gift of communication. When I spoke, people stopped, listened, and then got fired up to take action. I didn't know how or what I would talk about, but I knew I'd been given the gift of speech. I was in awe of Tony Robbins at that time.

I had been listening to his motivational videos since 2015, when I used to stomp to the train station, or when I would go out running. He got me connected and fired up, and I wanted to do the same for other people. Those kinds of people are good at that. If you are somebody who feels the doom and gloom from the world, or if you are feeling a bit down, listen to something that gets you ready for action. You will feel so much better for it. Allow your energy to start pumping. Create a higher vibration for your cells. That's what I did.

It turned out that most of the hotel were going to the Tony Robbins event, so there were lots of connections taking place all over. It came to the time that we had to go and check in to the event, and the girl from Manchester suggested we go together, so we did. There was a lot of people in attendance, so there were many stages to the check-in process. It took a while. You had to deal with lots of queues at these events. People who have never been can never quite imagine what it's like to organise that amount of people in such a small space. The event I was at had maybe five and a half thousand people. So that's a lot of people to organise and arrange in just a few hours. It was a fascinating thing for me to watch and observe. I remember thinking to myself, this will be me one day. People will be coming to a 6-day event just like this, only I will be reminding them of their spiritual gifts, and how to break through the traumas that were holding them back. I will get them re-connected.

It took us a few hours to get through the queues, then Laura and I went to get some food and get to know each other a little bit better. We found lots of other people too, and eventually, there was quite a big group of us hanging out. We shared lots of insights, our reasons for being there, and stories of our past that bought us to this now moment. This was the first time I started to notice that I was intensely listening to every word people were saying. I really listened for the first time in my life, and it felt amazing. Rather than steaming into the conversations, I sat back a bit, and I was getting the answers to their problems filtering through me. It was like I had an inner book of knowledge that I could tap into at a moment's notice. Again, thankfully, I closed my mouth, and I didn't let any of what was going on in my mind out. It was so interesting sitting there listening and recognising all of these people's traumas and tapping into the deeper meaning of what they were talking about.

I decided to go for a run that night. Now, I don't often go running at night; I'm more of a morning runner. That night, though, I felt like I needed to stretch my legs, get my blood flowing, and my heart beating. It was magical too. Everywhere I went signs were flowing through, from the road signs, to the taxis going past. I felt I had already been on a bit of a wild journey, that had bought me to this now moment, but everywhere I went and everywhere I looked there was no escaping it. I felt it deeply; this was going to be a life changing trip. I felt as if this had been divinely planned for my presence to be there.

The next day was day number one of the programme. And, I'll be honest, most of us were all feeling wretched – jet lag and all the rest – but we were excited for what lay ahead of us. I wasn't taking any chances, and so I was tripling up on all my capsules and other supplements; I was drinking loads of water and I took loads with me, and, of course, I had about 25 different layers to wrap up in. Tiredness, long days, extreme cold and an anticipated lack of decent plant-based food played on my mind slightly. I really did not want to slip into being sick again. That vibration no longer resonated with me. In fact, what used to make me feel secure – antibiotics, hospital visits, operations and such – all attempts to get my attention – were no longer resonant with me at all. I realised I had created it all because I was too scared to open up. What if I owned the fact I had created it all myself? It was still slightly uncomfortable, I'll be honest.

Day number one came and went. It was a straightforward introduction. We were told during the day that we would be put into groups the next day. I wondered, naturally, who I was going to be placed with – clearly, I wasn't going to be placed with the people that I'd already met because life doesn't work like that – and that would probably be too easy anyhow. My control issues started to rise up – that part of me that likes to know what's happening in this kind of situation. *Why not tell us today? You're telling us we're going to know tomorrow. So why not tell us today?* They gave us a colour and a place we needed to be at a particular time the following day; that's where we would meet our team. My ego was still piping – *I want to know now, then I wouldn't have to attend the morning bit, we could catch up on a little bit of rest, maybe just go along to the afternoon part.* The typical, high flying corporate girl looking to cut as many corners as possible.

The next day we got there super early, about 7 am as directed. Tony Robbins doesn't attend his seminars until about 4 in the afternoon, so this felt slightly over the top, but there was a lot of organising of people that was required in the mornings. We were put in groups and introduced to our supervisors – I think Tony calls them Team Leaders. It was actually great. I got to meet this new team of people that I would be with for the next six days or so.

In Tony Robbins' world, there is a hierarchy, exactly what you would expect from a businessman. There are lots of people who are Team Leaders and wear blue t-shirts. They lead the whole team. On top of that, each Team Leader had a couple of people who would help them out. They were known simply as Leader – they wore bright orange t-shirts. The lady who was our Leader, I felt instantly drawn to. I thought she was quirky, maybe even a little bit witchy. She was super straight talking and felt a little mischievous. I liked her. She felt as if she would be someone I could get on with. I felt drawn to her energy. What was even more fascinating, was that she also felt drawn to me. We had a couple of little chats when we were doing some exercises. I asked her opinion on a couple of things and I could just tell that a new bond that was being formed. I felt it; there's no other way to describe it. I liked how outspoken she was. No surprise, she was an Aussie! She introduced herself as Katrina, and she felt like home to me. Another beautiful unknown union in flight.

Over the next few days, as I became closer to Katrina, she told me I needed to be in certain positions on certain days. She was positioning me for the most incredible experience. She was giving a little insider knowledge. I had explained to her what I'd been through and what had happened to me to bring me to this point, and she gave me some great advice on how to get the best out of the conference. She was really, really helpful. An earth angel at a time I cried out for one, again without knowing.

I'll be honest with you, although the seminar was really amazing for what I needed at that time. Did it help me fix my traumas or anything? No, but it brought them to the surface. I didn't realise where my trauma came from; I truly believed my trauma was all around my mum and dad's divorce. Many things had compounded in a short space of time. My parents got divorced. My sister told me she was a drug addict, and all of the aftermath of that. So I felt that that was from where my trauma stemmed, and quite frankly, it would be a reasonable start for most people's emotional trauma. However, while I was at this event, the things he was saying and the way he was coaching people, I started questioning myself.

The work I did that week, made me look back further, and question everything deeper. During the time I was not in the room, I would be asking myself – *What happened before the divorce?* It was a week or two after Date With Destiny finished, that I got the epiphany that it was the conversation with my dad that happened when I was eight years of age that had triggered a massive unconscious spiralling. That moment, and everything that happened since, had then brought me all the way to this moment, and it all started with me sat in the passenger seat of my dad's car. That was the start of everything for me. So, with that in mind, I'm not going to say that Date With Destiny wasn't valuable. It was amazing for what I needed at that time. It helped a lot of things to come to the surface. It made me realise how important men were before I adopted the attitude of – *I'll use them and abuse them.*

So many amazing things happened at Date With Destiny, but I know now it was just a reason to get me to go to Florida to get connected with Katrina. I'm one hundred per cent certain about that. I met some incredible people there, some that I still stay in touch with today. However, I know that this was about connecting Katrina and I.

82

On day four, Katrina asked me what my plan was for the near future. "You're a long way from home. What comes after Miami? Do you go back to work?"

I replied, "No, I'm actually going on a bit of a mystery tour. First, I'm going back to Miami for a few days, and then I'm catching up with someone I met in Vegas."

The previous June, I had been celebrating a good friend's 40th birthday in Vegas. We had a crazy long weekend partying, and celebrating, before I took myself off, as I do to intuitively travel. I ended up visiting some stunning places along the way to stay in the mountains to do some writing in Colorado. It had been calling me for years and it was magical. On the journey back to Vegas, I ended up stopping randomly – never random – at a place about an hour away from Vegas. I was tired and fancied a dip in the pool, some food and a decent rest. I checked in, went to the pool, threw myself in and nearly took the head off a Bradley Cooper lookalike. When I apologised to him, he heard my accent, and with a huge smile, lifted his glasses off, and it's fair to say that was that. We flirted and connected, and I ended up having an amazing night with him and his friends. I laughed like I had not laughed in a very long time. We connected deeply. So much so that he followed me to New York for the weekend before I went home. After a little while, he had been ready to move to the UK to be with me, I felt like my Christmases and birthdays had all come at once. Then, I totally freaked out; which essentially ended what we had. I was good at that, destroying good things. An unknowing commitment-phobe, believing it was everyone else, never myself.

Despite all of that, when I let him know I was going over to Miami, he asked if he could come to see me.

Katrina was laughing at my stories and my relationship antics. "Anyway, I am then going to meet a girlfriend of mine in Cuba for Christmas and New Year."

"Oh my God, I love Cuba," Katrina replied excitedly. She was such a bundle of energy. She was amazing. I just loved it. Her enthusiasm for life was contagious. "Oh my God, you're going to love it. You are reminding me of my own eat, pray, love journey that I went on for several years. Girl, you are making me get the travel bug back! I can't believe you're about to do that."

I said, "To be honest, I've got this dilemma. I really want to go to Guatemala; it's calling me. I've seen this lake that I need to go to, and it's just telling me that I need to go there, but I'm shit-scared. I know I have to go, but…."

"You're not going to believe this," Katrina interrupted. "Well, actually you might. Guatemala is my favourite place in the world. Would you be up for me coming with you?"

A little bit of my ego was thinking I didn't really want somebody with me, but on the other hand, I knew I really needed somebody to hold space for me on that leg of the journey. So I said, "I'm up for it.

Let's see what happens hey?" Katrina was married, so she had to check hubby would be okay with her disappearing so soon after New Year.

Day number five of Date With Destiny was interesting. They put us through a meditative process. I was pretty good at meditating at this point of the journey. I was very visionary. The process he took us through involved sound and drumming up energy in the room based on frequencies. The physical process itself was called Deeksha. Tony explained that there were many trained practitioners in the room that were going to walk round and intuitively go where they were guided to put their hands. He explained to us that shifts could take place within you if we were open to it. I set the intention for the best experience ever! I set the intention that I was going to get somebody to come to me physically, to experience the hands-on. Tony explained that there were five and a half thousand people in the room, and there was no way the leaders and helpers could get around to everyone individually. If somebody was drawn to come to you, they would, but he explained that regardless of that, everybody in the room would be getting the exact effects of the process. Essentially, you did not have to feel hard done by if someone did not physically come to you. He continued to explain the process and get us into alignment.

Eventually, we were ready to start the journey. We were asked to close our eyes, sit quietly, and allow the process to do what it needed to do. All of our experiences would be individual and just as magical as each other. I was asking and manifesting for one of the leaders to come over to me. *Please bring somebody to me. Please bring somebody to me.* It must have been like a red fucking beacon of light on my head, "Come to me mama because I want you! I need your help! It's time to heal once and for all, I am ready!"

A little while into the process, out of nowhere and a complete shock, I had my best friend Jimbo appear in front of me. This is my beautiful bestie who had died the year before. He wasn't physically there in front of me; he was in my mind's eye, clear as day. Tears rolled down my cheeks as I got to see him exactly as I remembered him. I felt the emotions becoming overwhelming, when he said to me, "Sweetheart, you've got to go to India." At that point, I burst into tears, he gave me his sweetest smile and said again, "Babe, I need you to go to India." I continued crying, releasing myself from all of the emotions that had been festering. I was so deep in the process –

fully immersed. With that, I felt somebody coming into my energy field. Just when I did not think I could go any deeper, it hit me – *Oh, fuck* – we are going in! All I can say is that it felt like some sort of activation from my toes all the way up to the top of my head. It wasn't like goosebumps, it was like this energy was rising through my body in a wave. It moved up step by step by. I felt so incredibly activated. It was a combination of the music, the gongs, the energy being sent through me, and the visions I was getting.

Now, as I'm writing this, it dawned on me that this experience was like the Ayahuasca journey I went on, where I was being guided and shown things. I'd never connected the dots until now, which is interesting. The power of storytelling!

Back in the room with Jimbo, I kept asking, "What's the reason for India? What's the reason for India? What's the reason for India?" And interestingly, the process we were being shown was of Indian origin. All Jimbo told me was, "You will know in the next few weeks." So I thought – *For fuck's sake. Fuck off with you all making me keep having to wait.* My ego was starting to properly pipe up at this point. Despite the noise of my mind, I remained deeply entrenched in the process. When the process came to an end, Katrina came over, she could see I had been crying, she held me in an embrace and asked, "Are you okay?"

I sobbed, "My best friend came to me. My dead best friend. He died last year. He told me I have to go to India, and I will find out why in the next few weeks."

She kept hold of me and said, "Okay, so you've got to trust, write this down and make sure that you don't forget about it. Make sure that you immerse in these signs you have been getting."

I told her somebody had come to me during the process and helped activate me, and that it was so powerful. Katrina pushed herself back, and held on to my arms with her hands; she looked me in the eyes and said, "Babe, it was always going to be me."

We both stood there crying and hugging one another because we knew we were soul family. We knew at that point that we were going to go on a magical journey together. There was no denying this bond, and the formation and alignment of souls that was taking place. It felt incredibly important.

83

A few days later, when we got to the end of the event, Katrina approached me and said, "So, are we going to go to Guatemala?" She was just like me, straight up, no messing about, a get-shit-done girl.

"Let's do it!" I replied. "Can you get away from your husband, though?"

"Oh, let me worry about him. He's used to the way that I just have to go off and travel, and I have to do this now."

Katrina is very psychic. She can connect in with dead people very, very easily, and she can help release their souls. She's done some incredible work on this planet and continues to do so to this day. She's a force to be reckoned with. A little pocket rocket, a little like myself. I didn't know this then, but I got to know it as we travelled. She was a very amazing soul. I told her, "I intend to leave Cuba on the 2nd of January and go to Guatemala; you get there as soon as you possibly can afterwards."

She didn't mess about. "I reckon I can be there by the 3rd. Do a day on your own, and I'll come and meet you. We'll keep in touch between now and then to ensure everything's in alignment and you are still keen."

And that was that. I was buzzing because I was going to get to the lake. Katrina had already told me that there was a place in the lake that she had to take me to and that we would go on a journey there. I was totally wide open to anything at this point. My soul remembered hers and I was ready to go on the journey of a lifetime. I could feel it bubbling.

One of the processes that you go through with Tony Robbins is very much about stepping back into the energy that you choose to step into. So, if you're a man and want to be a stepping up into the masculine, or if you're a female, you want to be stepping up into the feminine. This day, Katrina dragged me by my hand and stood me at the front of the stage, she turned me around as the men were going through their process and told me to stand, look and surrender. My goodness was that the best advice she could have given me. I truly believe this was a shifting point in my surrender of the divine masculine energy that had occurred with that incident with my dad when I was 8. I made the conscious decision that from here onwards it was about transitioning to my true essence, that of the true divine feminine.

Katrina asked me before I left on the last day, "What's your biggest fear leaving here?" I knew the answer right away, I said, "I'm about to go to Cuba to meet a girlfriend who is very like I was, in the corporate masculine energy. I'm not putting her down, she's an incredible woman — but she embodies the corporate masculine energy, and I have literally just surrendered to be this little flower, ready to bloom for the first time."

I realised that I feared that if I saw her, I'd step back into the old, and I didn't want to do that. I was starting to feel I could become more vulnerable with men, and I didn't want to get back into that space of looking at men as just 'things'. I knew that Cuba would help me be in a feminine space because of the dancing and the music, but there was this contradictory energy I was dealing with. The men in Cuba are very, very sensual. They are strong leaders, that was what I was looking forward to. They're the ones that kind of throw you around the room. Not in that way!

Katrina asked me what I was going to do about that. I went away and wrote about it and looked at this fear that I had. I didn't journal to the level that I would go to now, it was a very high level at this point, but it made it clear to me that I had become a very masculine male energy in my work and my life. I realised this so much so that I actually called Kyle up and apologised to him. I was crying, and I told him I was sorry for what I had done to him, basically cutting his balls off. I told him I realised what a bitch I had been. He thought I was on drugs, or was in trouble at the time, but once I explained fully, he appreciated my calling, and that freed me up from it all.

Anyway, I left the event and got on a train to Miami to spend a few days grounding after the intensity of Date With Destiny. The apartment I had was incredible; it looked out over the ocean. It had a beautiful infinity swimming pool, with a beach-like area to sit out and look over. I chose it because I knew I would need a decent space after living in a hotel for a week or so. I knew I would be clucking for decent food. I settled in quickly and everything felt great.

It was about 9am that day when my sister messaged me. It was unusual to hear from her when I was away. She messaged me,

"Can you talk?" I messaged back that I could talk. She called me. When I answered, she was screaming, and I mean screaming uncontrollably. I couldn't make any sense of her. "Kirsty, I don't know what you're saying to me. Breathe, breathe." I started panicking myself and thinking – *Fuck, is it Mum? Is it Dad? What's going on?*

She continued to scream down the phone, "How could this have happened? Why is this happening?"

I said, "Kirsty, I don't know what you're talking about. You are going to have to stop, take a breath and tell me so that I can at least appreciate where you're coming from with this and if you need my help." It took her about five minutes to collect herself enough, and then she told me that my half-nephew – my nephew's half brother – had been killed. He'd been hit by a car and killed that afternoon. He had been holding his dad's hand crossing a road when a car had hit him and ran over him. He was killed instantly on the spot.

Absolute heartbreak.

I didn't get it. I was angry. That well-known masculine energy started surfacing. I wanted to fly home. I wanted to fix it all. I stepped into victimhood. I had just been through a magical six-day collapsing of these heavy energies, stepping back into my essence of the feminine energy, and then this happened.

This right here is a great example of why I say to clients that I don't care who you are or what you are, or even how good you think you are, as soon as you think you're on top of something, you're going to get the biggest fucking curveball of your life. And this was my curveball – how on earth was I going to deal with this monstrous one?

I was packing up my shit, whilst talking on the phone to my sister. I had decided I was going home, nothing else mattered. I was on the phone with my sister for three or four hours that day. I held space for her to be able to be angry, even though I was angry myself. It was too early to start learning to accept or forgive; we all needed to just allow ourselves to be angry and raw. Kirsty's son, Josh, his heart was breaking. He was so close to his half-brothers; the one that got killed was a twin. Ironically, the twins were the exact same age as my half twin sisters. There was so much pain all around. Josh was so young to be experiencing this loss, especially as he had not long lost his grandad, and now, his baby brother. The poor little lad didn't know what was going on – he had been blasted with endless amounts of shit already in his little life. My sister was still close to Josh's dad, so she was really feeling the hurt and pain of it all too.

It was the worst day ever.

I was on my own in a strange place, with nobody I could talk to. All I could do was sit on the phone with my sister because I couldn't get there quick enough, even if I wanted to. I felt really unhelpful. I couldn't have been in a worse place if I tried. I told my sister that I was coming home on the next available flight. My sister was incredible in what she said to me – she'll probably never realise how transformational she was that day, in her darkest moment. I was always looking to follow my sister, be with her, and be loved and guided by her. That day, in her darkest hour, she said, "Lucy, what do you think you're going to achieve by coming home? What do you think you can do? Do you not think it's better that you stay there? Do what you need to do. Be the strength for us because you're away from it, and then come home in time for the funeral."

I knew what she was saying, but it felt like she had punched me in the face. Why is she pushing me away? Why does she not want me there?

I spoke to my mum, and my mum said, "Look, she's got a point. What do you think you're going to do by being here? You'll be annoyed for coming home and not being able to do anything." Again, I felt rejected. God wants me there, but clearly, he had other plans for me, or else I'd have been there.

That night, in American time, when everybody in the UK was sleeping, I decided that if I couldn't help by being at home, I would help from abroad. I created a Go- FundMe page to help pay for the funeral. I decided I was going to use my platform for something good. I was going to use my Facebook page – which I had built up a lot of followers on – for something good. So, that's what I did.

The next morning, as soon as the sun came up, I went and did a run on the beach, and then I went live on my Facebook account and explained to people that I needed their help. We raised about six thousand pounds in just a few hours, to put towards the funeral. So in some way, my needs were being met. My need to be needed was being met.

Over the next few days, I needed a distraction, and thankfully I had the guy that I had met in Vegas come to meet me. I had wondered at the time why he was coming, all of a sudden it made sense. I had to go through this on my own, but now was the time I needed some company; I needed to be looked after and held.

We planned to go to dinner, and bless him, he came over from Nashville to meet me. We went out that night, and had a lovely evening. It was lovely to see him again, even though I was heavily distracted by my family back home. I was also overthinking the potential drama of going to Cuba with my corporate friend. This guy was a nice distraction for a short time, though. It was good to be around someone. It was nice to be able to speak about what had happened to my nephew. He lent his ears, held space and reminded me that it was okay for me to feel safe. I will always be grateful to him for that moment. He was definitely someone that came in for a reason and a season. A season I will never forget.

84

The very next morning, he flew home, and I went to Miami Airport, heading in the direction of Cuba. I checked into my flight, but I hadn't organised a visa. Thankfully, they helped get that sorted for me at the airport. I sat in the departure lounge, waiting to board when I got a message from my friend – the one who was supposed to be meeting me. She messaged me to say that she had been turned away from her flight, and the earliest she would be able to get to me would be in a couple of days. Now, one part of me thinking this was great, but also to be careful what you wish for because I was looking for a way to get out of that trip with her; I'm clearly a good manifestor.

The other part of me was thinking – *Oh shit, I'm going to Cuba. I don't speak Spanish. How the fuck? I don't even know where I'm going or what I'm doing. Oh my God, I'm going to do this on my own.* And this was a pattern for me. I had it when I went to Ecuador to meet Ricky, and I really stepped into this fear mode again. I became really pissed off with her. *How could she have been so stupid not to organise her visa?* The irony of thinking that, especially when I had to sort my own visa out at the airport. What a hypocrite!

I sat down, I can vividly remember, it was a green chair looking out over the runway, and my phone started ringing. The number calling was an ex-boyfriend. In shock, I answered it. Obviously, I needed some attention or something. We started chatting, he said he had heard about my nephew and wanted to send his condolences. On reflection, it was very nice of him to reach out and offer an ear. Out of nowhere, he declared that I was the one that got away. What the fuck? I mean, we had only gone out for a little while, and that was years ago; so where did this come from? I'd been out on a heavy night with the girls and walked into a pub, I'd seen this guy and said, "He's coming home with me." It wasn't one of my finest moments as a woman, but that is how we got together. We ended up going on a very karmic journey together – to say the least. It was volatile. It was passionate. It was all driven by aesthetics and looks. And perhaps, if he had called me up many years earlier and had this same conversation with me, I probably would have been putty in his hands, but there was no way I was going there. Not today, Satan. Not today!

I thanked him for calling and told him I needed to go to catch a plane, and then I sat there on my own on this green chair thinking – *What is coming next? How many more times, Universe, do you need to push me to my limits?* My nephew just died. The girl I'm meeting is not turning up. And now an ex-boyfriend is calling me out of the blue and declaring his undying love for me. I didn't have much time for that question to be answered, I was called onto the plane, and I headed off to Cuba, unknowing that I had just passed the first of many tests.

85

After an intense pre-Cuba experience – which I had clearly called in for my greater good – I took a hop, skip and a jump from Miami to Cuba. On the plane, I endured many hours of my ego creating mayhem and fear.

As we landed, the fear and insecurity switched to full pelt. There was no more security for me, no safety net, no more protection. Even being on the plane, where at least some people spoke my language, had at least been a bubble of protection. I didn't know what Cuba was going to be like. I had heard it was very backwards, and I do not mean that in a bad way, just that I thought I would be going back in time to a place and a way of living that I probably hadn't experienced in my lifetime.

Getting off that plane was a real struggle. I didn't want to do it. I stepped off the plane and wanted to get back on it. I've ticked that box, and now it's done, let me go home.

The strange thing about it was, at the same time that my ego was chattering away – pulling fear to the surface – in my heart, I knew that this was going to be a whole new level of revelation. My heart knew that I needed to go on this journey, and I needed to go it alone. I had created all of it. I had manifested my friend not turning up. I had manifested that I was going to have to ask for help and be vulnerable, and step into my feminine. Having been in my masculine energy for such a long period of time, I had realised I wanted to step into my divine feminine, and this was the test I had unknowingly called in, to prove that I actually meant it.

Honestly, the concept of the divine feminine and masculine energies was reasonably new to me. I knew I was kick-ass – a real warrior as far as women go. I also knew I was a control freak – and not in a good way. Now I had an awareness of it, though, I had to do something about it. I kept thinking – *Oh shit, I've been something that I don't want to be, and now what am I going to do about it?* I found that now I didn't want to be around other women that were in a toxic masculine energy. I wanted to be around those who could demonstrate to me what I needed to do. I needed those footprints to lead me so I could walk in them and follow. For the first time in my life, I wanted to follow. I was ready to surrender to someone else, someone who previously I probably would have looked at as weak.

The divine feminine and masculine energies are spoken about a lot these days. On top of that, we hear a lot about toxic masculine and toxic feminine also. Whether you are straight, bi-sexual, or gay, you have both masculine and feminine energies within you. We are made up with a mix, to create balance; and I don't mean a perfect 50:50 split.

Some obvious qualities of the divine masculine energy are assertive, strong, action-oriented, confident and logical. There are many other qualities of the true divine masculine; however, with just a few you can get the idea.

Likewise, the qualities of divine feminine are emotional, focused on feelings, vulnerable, nurturing and loving. For many lifetimes, we have been led to believe the divine feminine is weak. It is all soft, touchy-feely, and focused on healing – and whilst these three qualities are true, the divine feminine energy is extremely powerful – some would say the most powerful.

Both the masculine and feminine energies have been distorted over the years to suppress the true essence and sheer strength of what we are able to create when we work together. We have been led to believe that women do not need men – as we can do it ourselves – hence the huge drive to emasculate our men. I'm not saying for one minute that a man cannot do a woman's work and vice versa, but let's keep it real. Men are stronger than women, and women tend to be more nurturing. We have distorted the roles.

I admit, I had thought divine feminine was weak. I thought it was feeble. I wanted to do all a man could do, remember?

Now though, I was stepping into this really beautiful, feminine essence and it felt good to be back home in what was always intended to be, for this lifetime.

I got off the plane, went through customs and grabbed my luggage. Nobody spoke English. Not even one person. I kicked myself once again for not learning Spanish when I had so many opportunities to do so. This was a recurring theme, so many times I could have made that effort to learn the language, but had decided not to.

I walked through the arrivals area where people are met in by their loved ones. This is my favourite bit about airports. Wherever I have been around the world, I love watching people being reunited; I create little stories in my mind as to where they have been and what their stories were. I am such a hopeless, old romantic at heart. The people who were picking me up were going to be waiting outside, so, unfortunately, there was no welcome party for me. I remembered that I didn't have any cash because of the discrepancies and complications between America and Cuba. There had been a long time stand-off between the two countries, so I couldn't get Cuban money in America and had to get it when I landed. It was interesting, you were not allowed to take Cuban money out of the country. It all had to stay in, apparently. It felt like this was a country that had an invisible prison wall around it. I was led to believe that if you're from Cuba, it's challenging to get out. It was too expensive. No one could afford to first and foremost, then there was the challenge to get money out. It was almost like they had you completely locked into their systems, and that's fine if you're happy with that, but if you want to go and explore the world, or if you want to make something bigger or better of yourself, then it's a very, very challenging process that you need to get through. It may be different now, but back then, that's just how it was explained to me. I felt so privileged and grateful for my English passport.

I asked a security guard where I could get some money. He didn't understand a word I said; he was rude and aggressive which led me to feel vulnerable. I waved some money in his face to communicate, and he pointed me towards a cash machine. When I got there, it was such a challenge. You couldn't just put your card in and get your cash out; there was a weird process you had to go through. I was stuck. I breathed and asked the angels to help keep me calm and safe. Thankfully – ask and you shall receive – there was a girl there, similar age to me, and she spoke near-perfect English and was fluent in Spanish too, so she helped me get my money out. Thank you, earth angel. I was so grateful. I asked her where she was heading and suggested she could get in the car that was coming to pick me up. She agreed, and so we went out to find the car, which was, rather fortuitously, being driven and attended to by two quite attractive men. We both looked at each other and smiled. Things were working out quite nicely. It got even better when they showed us to a really beautiful old-style American car – like something you would see in the movies. It was convertible, light turquoise in colour with white detailing, and they had the roof down, which was pretty cool. It was late at night, so it was perfect to get some of the evening breeze. We crammed the luggage into the nooks and crannies and off we went.

As we drove, she talked to the boys and then translated to me. They asked us both to go out dancing. She seemed keen, I just wanted to get out of my clothes, shower and recalibrate, so they dropped me off at my apartment.

I had a quick look around, and the apartment itself seemed fine, but I soon realised that it didn't have good wi-fi; it had some weird system whereby you had to go and buy tokens, and the tokens only lasted an hour. I couldn't work it out for the life of me. It hit me like a punch in the face – and by this point in my travels, I'd had plenty of them. I'm in a country on my own. I'm in an apartment in the middle of nowhere. I can't get any water, food or anything like that as everywhere is closed now and it's pitch-black outside. I'm supposed to be with my friend but she's not turned up. I had no means of communication and I couldn't even let my family know that I'm safe. I was totally cut off from my world. My ego was piping up big time. I was trying to decide if I should go out and explore, and potentially get into some bother, or worse, I could get lost. I figured it would be better to check the place out in daylight, and so, as it was almost midnight, I took a shower and went to bed.

I woke up the following day, and everything felt brighter and better, as it always does. The sun was shining. I could see where I was and where the apartment was. I had thought the night before that I was in the middle of Beirut and a war zone – I think we all know how dramatic my mind can be in these situations – reminiscent, once again, of my arrival in Ecuador. Once I got outside and looked around, it was beautiful. I took myself for a long walk to explore because I needed to get some water and grab some food, and I wanted to get my bearings and know where things were.

I had no idea what to do about the wi-fi and the mobile phone situation, but I decided that no matter what it cost me, I'll sort it out and worry about it when I got home. I went into a shop, bought a SIM card for my phone, and tried to figure it out. It didn't work, though. I talked to a few people, and they told me there was no mobile data at all in Cuba. Strange! In this day and age! The only way you could connect was wi-fi, but even that was challenging. It felt like my world fell apart at that point. I couldn't get hold of my friend, who was supposed to be flying over in a few days. I couldn't get hold of my family, and they had all the trauma with my nephew going on. And at that point, I had no idea how to even get back to my apartment. All the things I had become heavily dependent on and had taken for granted were gone. I was being stripped bare, raw to the core. I was going to have to figure out a way to make it work.

At that point, to be honest, I wanted to cry and have a tantrum on the floor! I was ready to throw the towel in and go home to be with my family in their time of need. I went into full-on victim mode.

There's no other way to put it. I wanted to cry, but I somehow stopped myself. I sat on a wall, with the sea behind me. A bright pink American-style car drove passed me. As the car went by, the guys in the car wolf-whistled and screamed at me. They looked like they were having the time of their lives, and somehow it gave me the kick up the arse I needed. *You're in a country that you've always wanted to go to. You're in a land of pure love. You're in a country whereby connection is so important. Sort yourself out. Get yourself up and start enjoying yourself. Get a grip girl! You got this.*

So, that's what I did.

I gave myself a little pep talk, and I set off. I walked all day. I went for lunch and sat out in a beautiful Italian-style courtyard. It was stunning. I walked all along the sea. It was a fantastic day. And just like that, my day shifted from the worst day ever, to one of the most memorable; what a contradiction.

On my walk back, I decided to go a different route, and I came across this nice-looking hotel. It was a four-star hotel, so I decided I would stay there for a few days when my time in the apartment ran out. I thought it would be more sociable as there would likely be a few people who could speak English. I noticed, though, that there were all these people hanging around the outside of the hotel and almost hugging the hotel wall. It was bizarre. I asked somebody what was happening, and they said people were using the hotel's wi-fi. The hotel was one of the few places in the area that had good wi-fi. This encouraged me further to stay there. I figured I would be safe; I could speak to people, sit in the sun, and go for a swim.

Ironically, later that night, I sussed out the wi-fi in the apartment, and I got a message from my friend saying that she would be delayed another couple of days. By this time, it would be almost a week that she would have been delayed. I couldn't work out why this was happening and why I was being made to wait even longer. *What the fuck is this all about, please?* I hoped it would all make sense one day.

Without waiting for my time in the apartment to come to an end, I decided to move into the hotel, knowing all of the facilities they had would make life much easier for me. I moved in, and quickly realised that the hotel was haunted, without any shadow of a doubt. There was really weird energy there; it had a strange darkness about it. Clearly, some heavy things had happened there.

I planned a trip for myself as if my friend wasn't coming to join me, and the very next day, I went off on my travels. I booked a flight and went to San Pedro, the place where Madonna apparently wrote La Isla Bonita. I had the most incredible time there. It was a wonderful experience.

One day, when I was sitting having lunch, all the people started dancing around me. I sat by, quietly watching, doing my own thing, and then an older couple started dancing together, and I was in absolute awe of them. I kept thinking – *This is how I choose to be when I'm older. Totally head over heels in love, still connecting, still dancing, with that glint in my eye.* This was me watching my future self in action. The connection, this union; I was being shown it for a reason. I watched, mesmerised. It was reminding me that the divine feminine is as powerful as the divine masculine. Coming together is what this was all about. It activated something inside of me that day. The next thing I know, a hand was beckoning to me to stand up. The older gentleman – probably old enough to be my grandad – took me by the hand and started dancing with me. And we danced and danced and danced. I had the best time ever that day. I had never felt so loved and protected by a complete stranger.

It took me into a space of knowing; this was what I really came here for. I didn't come here to be angry. I didn't come here to be frustrated. I came here to learn, to live, and to remember my soul's true essence. I was a divine feminine wanderer and I needed to bring this dance, this vibration, back up through my body. By the time this man finished dancing with me, I just wanted to kiss him. I was so happy that he had snatched me out of this funk I'd been in. He had ignited 'The Wanderess' again. She was back!

Feeling reignited, I booked a flight to the other side of Cuba. Now trust me when i say this, the flights in Cuba are treacherous. You have to hold on for dear life and pray you will make it there. There have been numerous incidents that don't make for good reading. I was determined to travel Cuba, though, and I felt protected. I had developed an inner knowing that I would always be protected whenever I was on the road – not to the point where I was arrogant or silly with my choices – I just knew I was always going to be okay.

I checked into a beautiful hotel. It was an all-inclusive place, easy for me to get food, to run on the beach, and go to the gym. I also knew there would be a lot of tourists and people who spoke English. It was stunning. I had needed a little bit of this. The only downside was that it was full of couples and I was all on my own. So, I decided that I would use my time to start writing my book – the very one you are reading now. I was going to immerse in the writing process. There was so much to remember just from the last three or four years alone, and I was worried about leaving anything out because so much of it had been magical. Sitting down and writing it helped me to finally see the bigger picture of it all, and how everything had been divinely placed.

I met a really beautiful girl called Jen from England. She worked in Canary Wharf, exactly where I had just left. I spent quite a bit of time with her and her partner, having some wonderful conversations because we had that connection of working in the city.

After I had been there a few days and done some excellent work, my friend finally arrived. I told her I had moved on from where we were initially meant to be, and she came up to meet me where I was, rather than me go back to her. It was really interesting because although she did bring a lot of drama with her – having had her visa stopped, and then her dad got sick, which is why she was delayed a couple more days – it was actually great to have her there. Listening to all her crazy dramas, after I had been on such a beautiful, divine feminine journey, made me realise that everything had happened perfectly – I could observe this and not get involved at all. It could flow over me without getting sticky. I was left to be alone there so that I could step back into my warrior and, in particular, my divine feminine warrior.

We had decided, even before we had arrived in Cuba, that we were going to spend Christmas in this most exquisite little place off the West coast of Cuba which we had seen pictures of. In truth, there was nothing Christmasy about it, but it had an absolutely beautiful beach – a vast stretch of beautiful golden sand, the water every shade of blue imaginable. It was stunning. It was what you would describe as picture-perfect.

We arrived there, and it was even better than we had imagined. We hired a moped to get us about with ease and grace. We knew we would only be there for a few days, so we wanted to make the most of it. Where we were staying, we had these beautiful hammocks on the balcony that overlooked everything, there was the stunning beach we could walk along, and most excitedly, there was this really beautiful sea turtle sanctuary nearby. Anyone who knows me – and my little sisters will tell you – I am a mad turtle fan; sea turtles in particular. I just love them. I've had some amazing experiences with them, especially when I was in the Galapagos Islands. I held a baby sea turtle in my hand and released it back into the wild, which was incredibly beautiful, something I will never forget. I have a massive affiliation with them. I love them. I love how quick they are. I love how they are when they are in the water. I just love everything about them.

We went to the sea turtle sanctuary, and it was incredible. We walked in, and the man who owned it took a massive shine to me, possibly because I looked a bit Spanish. He allowed me to pick all the turtles up, hold them, touch them, feed them and get my hands dirty, which is what I really wanted to do. I just wanted to get close to these animals and love on them. We spent quite a bit of time there. The guy was a beautiful soul, and the conversation I had with him was very much like the conversation I had with the old man on the bench back in Ecuador. We spoke Spanglish, he was speaking Spanish, and I was speaking English, but we somehow understood each other.

A few days later, when it came for us to leave, he stood outside and waved us off, shouting, "Come back soon." It was so beautiful. There was something magical about the whole experience. It was one of the few times in my life I had ever allowed a man to step up and guide me. I was allowing my heart, my intuition, and my healing to come online.

It soon came round to Christmas Day and Boxing Day. To be different, we decided to go to the beach. We went swimming and did lots of wonderful outdoor things. We were determined to enjoy as much nature as possible because we were going back to the city for New Year.

When we got to the city, we hired a bright pink American car to drive us around for the day, which was amazing. We took loads of photos of us sprawled all over the bonnet. It was a day of fun and giggles, and to be honest, it was more fun doing it with somebody else. We had a lot of laughs. We took risks. I wouldn't have got in a car with a man on my own, but with her there, it felt safe – there were two of us to kick him in the head if we needed to. We were both trained, professional fighters in Muay Thai – which was how we had actually met, training in Thailand.

The night before New Year's Eve, my friend was adamant that we had to try authentic mojitos whilst in Cuba. Now I am not a cocktail drinker at all, if you want to get me wasted, then give me rum, tequila or cocktails. On this occasion, though, I agreed, but said I would choose the place where we went. She agreed, and we set off on our mojito mission. After a short walk around, we stumbled upon this place that looked homely, it had all the doors open, and it felt like the lounge of a house. They had great music blaring, and I immediately knew this was where we needed to go. Unfortunately, there weren't any tables, so we were asked to sit at the bar until one became available.

We ordered mojitos, obviously, and I wasn't looking forward to it at all; I just don't like the taste of rum. It arrived, and it had mint leaves in it, but I don't like my drinks with stuff in them. I took my first sip, and it was sensational. Oh my God, it was so different to anything that I'd ever had before. I knew then that this was going to be dangerous – little Miss 'I don't drink cocktails' has a cocktail in her hand that she likes, and it's full of the stuff that she knows will create mayhem. It went down far too easily. My friend ordered us both another one each! I realised she was staring at the guy behind the bar, flirting with him while we sat there. It was so amusing to watch it, especially with the mindset I had these days. It made me laugh, watching the way that women work; previously, that would have been me.

Our table was eventually ready, and we were on our third mojito. The food was a tapas menu – my absolute favourite – we ordered loads of stuff. The food was incredible, and the staff looked after us like princesses – the service was flawless. I had the awareness to stop drinking and to start being sensible about four cocktails in. I was having such a lovely experience that I didn't need the alcohol. The two guys working there gave us a significant discount on the bill, which we were both slightly confused about, until they asked us if we wanted to go out with them that night. We both smiled. They were good looking guys, but this was not who I was these days. I realised where this was all heading, and I wasn't interested. I was happy to go out, but I knew some boundaries needed establishing. Wow! Who was I becoming? Who was this woman? And under the influence of alcohol too!

We went out that night and had a great time, but we were just visiting a few bars and getting into the vibe of the place, not drinking much. The incredible thing about Cuba is the vibe that you get. Even before dark, the music comes on, and that's it; the party starts. It's all about having fun. It's all about lightness, laughter and truly surrendering to the things that make you happy. Now, this was the night before New Year's Eve, so we weren't going to get too crazy, especially as we had a big party planned at the hotel the next night.

I was flying off on the 2nd of January to Guatemala and leaving my friend on her own for a day, so New Year's Eve was going to be our last night together. We had these beautiful little outfits to get dressed up in, and the hotel had given us masks and things to put in our hair. We were so excited. We knew it would be a night to meet people, eat good food, and most importantly, we were going to dance a lot. Nothing could have prepared us for what was coming, though.

The setting for New Years Eve was stunning. There were candles lit everywhere, and the space was set up so beautifully. Music was playing, an incredible barbecue was cooking, various enticing aromas swirled and mingled in the air, and there were lots of different types of entertainment. The hotel had brought in a well known Cuban pop band, who we knew nothing about, but were apparently really big over there. Everyone was going crazy for them, and I mean really crazy. We just threw ourselves into it regardless – when in Rome and all that. As it turned out, one of the guys in the band took a real shine to me. He would come to where I was and sing right in my face. I was laughing so much because this kind of thing always happens to me. I've had it happen in Nashville and all over the world. People somehow make a beeline for me out of everybody else there. It was so funny. He tried to get my number, but I made my boundaries very clear to him.

After we did the midnight countdown, the party really got started. Native Cuban salsa dancing! It was incredible. It went off. I had imagined that even if we had the best night, we would probably be in bed by 1 am, but I ended up dancing with one of the dancer guys until 5 am. We had a beautiful connection, he was such a strong partner and because I had done ballroom dancing when I was little, I really got into it. This guy helped me really step up into my true essence. He activated something within me that I did not remember

I had until that point. My friend was off dancing with somebody else, we would swap partners for a while, but then this guy focused on me exclusively, and we ended up dancing all night long. He was supporting me perfectly, helping me, and what he will never know is that he genuinely unlocked the divine feminine within me. He made me realise that dancing is one of the things that can get me to release my soul. I loved dancing as a child, it always thrilled me, but that evening unlocked something in me – this divine feminine essence that I had been suppressing for such a long period of time. And I loved it. I loved it so much.

Eventually, we went to bed. We had blisters on our feet from dancing.

When we woke up the next morning, we laughed so hard thinking about the craziness of the night before, but it had been a good crazy and not a bad one. Yes, we had a few drinks, but we were knackered and aching because of all the dancing. We were hungry and tired and so we took a little stroll around the city, looking for a cup of tea and breakfast. It was all a little bit too much effort, to be perfectly honest. It started raining, so we went back to the hotel. I was leaving the next day and so needed to get sorted. All I wanted to do was sleep, pack my things and get going. I was pretty much done with Cuba by that point; I'd been there quite a while by this time.

I had loved it, though, every experience. I had changed, and I was welcoming the changes. Cuba had turned out to be an important piece of my puzzle. The men I had danced with had unlocked something in me that was profound.

I was ready for the next part of my journey, though.

What I didn't know at that point was that the next part of the journey wouldn't just be profound, it was going to be absolutely catastrophically life-changing.

86

I left Cuba in awe of what had gone on. How on earth did I arrive so full of dread and fear and be leaving head over heels in love, grateful for every single second of what had unfolded? All I could do was smile. I was still feeling a little bit dodgy from New Year's Eve because although I had a few drinks, I hadn't slept much, or eaten particularly well during the evening, which tends to be important to how I'm feeling. Nevertheless, I felt in awe of how my path was unfolding. I was excited and a little bit apprehensive too. If this happened in Cuba, what on earth was about to unfold in Guatemala?

I was slightly anxious in anticipation because I was going to have to be there for a day all on my own before my girlfriend arrived. And, of course, in typical Lucy fashion, my mind was in overtime, having heard some of the things about Guatemala over the years. The same old internal fears kicked in. I had heard about the guns, the drugs and how it was very easy to get involved in something that you shouldn't be getting involved in. Despite all my travel experience – the same fears came up. I knew, though, that I was capable of getting through it. I had been there. I had done it. I had transformed and grown through so many situations. No matter what, I could face it, feel the fear and step through it anyway.

I also had it in my mind what it might be like when Katrina arrived. We had already been on such a huge journey. Although we had only spent a short time together, we had remembered each other. She had unlocked something in me. My best friend, Jimbo, who had passed, had come through because of Katrina. All of the signs and synchronicities that occurred when we were together were not just a coincidence. I knew she was somebody that was going to be in my life, and I was excited about that, but at the same time, I had no idea what would happen when we were actually travelling together. *Would we get on? How would we slot into each other's routines?*

The flight over to Guatemala wasn't far. The airport was bustling and extremely disorganised, which I was actually really starting to like. I was beginning to feel at home in organised chaos. I made my way through the airport and got a taxi to my hotel. I had purposely booked myself into the best hotel in the area for one night. Katrina was arriving the next day from Washington, and I was meeting her at the airport. Once she landed, we would be getting straight on a bus and out of there. We didn't want to be in Guatemala City. It was not calling me in the slightest, so we used it as a hub – in and out.

Once I got to the hotel, I dumped my bags and went to the gym. I did the most amazing two-hour workout. It felt so good to be back in what I would deem 'normality', after such an adventure without any of it. I'm pretty adaptable. I can sleep in the Amazon in a wooden shack, but I am also very at home with creature comforts. I embraced the moments of peace, being on my own. That night, I ordered room service, had a bath and went to bed. It felt so good to just be.

The next day, I went to the airport to meet Katrina. She was a few hours later than expected because she had experienced some delays and issues at customs. I was ready and waiting for her as soon as she arrived. I waited outside the airport because that's my preference. I'm a fresh air kind of girl, I prefer it to air conditioning any day of the week, even if it means I'm sweating. Waiting for Katrina, though, it was really hot. I felt uncomfortable and pretty vulnerable also. People were coming up to me, asking where I wanted to go, and offering to take me here, there and everywhere. It all felt a bit too much. I had shut myself away for the last 24 hours, only seeing people at my five-star hotel, so it was a bit of a rude awakening. I was excited for Katrina to arrive as nothing seemed to phase her.

All of a sudden, the double doors of the airport burst open, and out blasted my friend. She screamed at me excitedly, "Hiiiiii. Oh my God! Oh my god! It's so good to see you." She's so dramatic. She grabbed hold of me and gave me a huge hug. At that point, all of my fears melted away, and I just knew that we were going to have such an incredible journey together.

I surrendered to her from that point because she knew where she was going, she had been there before. We had made basic plans when we had spoken over the weeks since Date With Destiny, over many messenger conversations. I had shown her the picture of the lake that Ricky had shown me all those years ago, and she was excited to finally be the one to take me there. That was what she called 'my lake'. I was open to it being her lake at that point. It was her lake. I had never been. I had seen it and felt the magic from a picture, but this was going to be my first time actually there.

As I have said many times already, Ricky has been a huge messenger for my whole awakening journey. Unbeknown to him much of the time, nevertheless, he has been such an essential part of everything that happened to me. I had first seen the lake back in 2014, and I had wanted to go there ever since but had been too scared to, not that I ever admitted that, until now.

Katrina guided us in the direction of Antigua – not to be confused with the Caribbean Antigua. We got on a minibus, and once again, as all of the minibus journeys tend to be, an interesting journey started to unfold. It reminded me of the crazy bus journey to Pai in Thailand, when I injured my back. Katrina and I sat in the minibus, bobbing and wobbling around. It wasn't a long journey, probably an hour and a half, but it was great for us to catch up with each other properly. I had to tell her all about Cuba, and she had loads of stuff that had been going on with her since we last saw one another. Katrina is extremely psychic, and with my intuition coming online at record speed, we seemed to be a powerful pairing.

We arrived in Antigua, and instantly, I was in love. It is still, to this day, one of my favourite places in the world. I loved it. It is one of the most mystical places ever. I fell in love with its quirky, charismatic vibes. There is just something about that town that felt like home. It felt like I had walked that land before, a strange but beautiful and inexplicable feeling.

We found our hotel, dumped our bags, and decided to go walking around the town. Every corner that we turned was enchanting – whether it was the organic food, the salsa studios, or the beautiful, tiny restaurants that had so much character, so much pizzazz about them. It had truly remarkable energy. One of my favourite things about it was that you could see the volcanoes off in the distance, smoke billowing out from their tops, and now and again, bursts of lava coming out. It was amazing; a wonderful experience to witness. I never realised back then, quite how Mother Nature uses these beautiful creations as her way of communicating with us.

We spent a few days in this place, experienced some excellent food and did loads of fantastic walks. We visited a beautiful church and found some tremendous farm shops. We had several special days there. I even met up with a girl I had met on my travels, she was living in Guatemala, so she came over to meet us. It was fascinating to speak to somebody who lived there and experienced this place on a day-to-day basis. As a tourist, I obviously looked at things through rose-tinted glasses, but she lived there, so she also knew what darkness took place, and so she did give us a different side to it.

One day, we decided we wanted to climb a volcano – we felt it would be something memorable to take with us from the trip. We knew one of them was pretty active, whilst the others were dormant at that time. We agreed to do the climb as part of a tour with a guide.

We got picked up early in the morning by a large bus fully loaded with people who were up for going through the same experience as us. We decided we were going to climb the volcano and then go on to a spa afterwards. We felt we would deserve an afternoon of nurturing once we had finished the climb and before we moved on to our next destination.

Standing at the bottom of the volcano was incredible. The thought of climbing it was both daunting and exciting all rolled into one. The guide told us all about the last time it erupted, not that many years earlier either. It was enough to make me realise how little notice Mother Nature gives before she bursts. The climb was okay, though. Not easy, but not impossible. The tour guide was great; he kept us going and our spirits up. At some point, we came across people taking the easy way out and making their way up on the backs of ponies – which, if I'm honest, kind of broke my heart.

The whole experience of climbing the volcano was exhilarating. Now and again, I had to stop and take it all in and take some photographs. I love a good view. You could see the other volcano, Fuego, from the volcano we were on. We watched as it spouted its lava, and it flowed out and down the side of the volcano. It made my soul sing. It felt to me as if I was watching the anger, frustration, fear, and resentment bubbling to the surface to be released, to be healed. And while that seems so pertinent to the journey that we're all on in these present days, at the time, it just fascinated me. I couldn't put any rhyme or reason around it. Even though I was well on the way of my healing journey, I hadn't yet gotten to that point whereby I realised every single thing was a messenger. I had read amazing books like The Celestine Prophecy – and I had really loved them – but I wasn't quite at the point where I realised a volcano, a bird, a flippant conversation with somebody could be a profound messenger for your journey.

We eventually got to the top of the volcano. It was breathtaking, literally. I was probably very annoying for everybody else because all I did was say, "Oh, my God. This is amazing. Wow. Oh, my God. Have you seen this?" To be fair to me, it was incredible. Besides the unbelievable view, we were actually in the clouds, and I had never experienced that before. I felt like all the most amazing things I had ever envisaged happening in my life were taking place right now, I just hadn't considered that it would be at the top of a volcano.

Something happened to me on that volcano as I started doing what can only be described as 'weird shit'. I found myself stopping and touching things, kneeling down, closing my eyes, holding my hands in funny positions. None of which I had ever done previously; however, in those moments it felt so right to do so. Even stranger was that I felt like I knew exactly what I was doing, and that I was communicating with Gaia. Years later, after conversations with various different people, I realised I was doing some sort of healing process. I kept saying to Katrina, "I don't know why I'm doing this." She said, knowingly, "Well, I'm sure you'll figure it out one day."

After taking in the views for a while, we headed back down. Halfway down, our tour guide stopped. He pulled out a load of twigs, and he spiked some marshmallows onto the twigs and roasted them over the hot lava. It was such a cool experience. I was off my head on sugar afterwards. What was really interesting for me was that I had never before toasted marshmallows from a bonfire or a fire pit or anything. I was fortunate that my childhood had been spent in nice hotels and places like that; we had never been camping. And here I was, at the ripe old age of 39, having my first ever toasted marshmallow, and I loved it. I guess it's relevant to say that if in your life there are things that you haven't experienced yet, then you aren't supposed to experience them, just trust that. For me, I had to wait until I was nearly 40 before I had toasted marshmallows. Why didn't I have them when I was eight years of age? Because it wasn't meant for me then. And I know that sounds ridiculous. It's a marshmallow on a stick, but actually, there's a very important message in that. Everything happens in divine timing. Even the small stuff, maybe especially the small stuff. The plan is far greater than any of us. It's orchestrated. Divine precision. Anything that you force is not going to happen.

When we arrived at the base of the volcano, I was ecstatic. Other people were moaning about the cold and the harsh climb, but not me. I said, "Oh my God, I've just been up a volcano. I'm so happy right now." It was a significant achievement – a bucket list item. After it was done, I told a couple of my family members that I had gone up there. Their first comment was "What would you have done if it had erupted?" I just don't think like that. I work on the premise that I am safe and protected always. I'm sure some would roll their eyes and think that's arrogance, and I would understand that reaction;

however, I truly trust that we go through what we are intended to. My feelings have always been to take the leap of faith and trust the parachute will open.

We got on another bouncy bus to take us to the spa. The spa was excellent and just what we needed after the morning we had. We met some girls on the same bus and also going to the spa, so we hung out with them for a bit, immersing ourselves in the natural hot spas and watching the volcanoes in the distance as they did their thing. It was a delight of a day.

That evening, we were exhausted. We returned to the hotel, grabbed some food, and then packed our bags as we were heading out early the next day for our magical mystery tour to the lake. I was so excited to be going there. I was filling myself up with so many amazing experiences, it was a challenge to remain present. When one was done, the next one was just around the corner.

87

The following day involved yet another minibus journey. Bouncing, rocking, swaying and bobbing all over the place. Katrina fell asleep because she was feeling a bit rough from the journey. I had my headphones on and sat listening to some tunes and bouncing excitedly about in anticipation of finally getting to see the lake. Katrina had said we should go for a week as I would fall in love with the place on arrival. I was a little apprehensive, though, as Ricky had suggested one day would be enough there. I trusted Ricky as I'd known him longer, and we had similar interests, likes and dislikes, so I decided to play it by ear with Katrina and see how we got on. I didn't want to sign up for a week and then be ready to leave after one day. Similarly, I didn't want to sign up for a day and be hungry to stay for longer.

The bus stopped, and as I got off I was greeted by the lake; Lake Atitlan – the lake I had been thinking about for years. It was very impressive. Off in the distance, the lake looked beautiful, but where we were standing – in the place where the boats pulled up to take you across the lake – it looked a bit skanky. I was thinking – *Surely you could have made a bit more of an effort here, fellas*. Judgey Jane kicked in for a moment. I quickly booted my ego into touch and dropped back into my heart space – *You know what? I know there's going to be some magic out there.* I knew deep in my soul that in the middle of that lake, there was a story to be told. It had been calling me for such a long time. It was time now to surrender and figure out why this enchanting lake had been whispering my name.

Katrina had told me that we needed to go across the lake to a place called San Marcos. It was the place where all the spiritual nut jobs go – her words. The hippies, the mystics, – you know, the quirky lot that your mum side steps in the supermarket. There were many little 'towns' around the lake. Some of them quiet, some party areas, and some more beautiful and tranquil than others. We agreed to spend time in the spiritual area as that was what we were there for. Signs, messages and answers.

We got on a little boat across the lake. I was sitting quietly, looking out across it, taking it all in, when suddenly I felt a massive surge of energy. It hit me in a physical way. It encouraged me to go inwards. I was being shown I needed to switch off the noise and be silent. I could hear Katrina chatting to me, but I zoned it out. I felt like someone had switched the electricity on and somehow I was connected to it. All sorts of information and answers started flowing through me. Insights and visions of things I knew nothing about, and yet all of a sudden I felt as if I knew it all in detail. At that moment, I felt as if I had been selected for something special. I did not know what, I just felt as if things were going to start moving pretty rapidly from here – unlike the boats.

Katrina was chatting away to people. I put my hand over the edge of the boat and let it drag along in the water. I felt energy coming up through my hand and into my body. It was like something was igniting within me. There was some form of activation taking place in my soul.

We arrived at the other side of the lake, at what we were told was the port. Judgey Jane kicked in again. *What the fuck is that? That's not a port! That's a wooden boardwalk, at best.* I honestly thought, at first glance, that I would be lucky if this place even had running water! We had a little wander around, and I was looking at Katrina and giving her 'the look'. What on earth had she bought me to? I had never been anywhere like it, but I remembered this feeling of judgement was often uncalled for; seeing Ecuador at night, and arriving in Thailand. It was that same old feeling, assuming I had made a wrong decision to be there. As much as I recognised it, I had no idea what to do about it, so I took a deep breath and carried on.

Out of nowhere, a cat appeared. Whilst we were figuring out what to do, I sat and stroked it for a bit. It seemed to like the attention. We moved on from where we were, and the cat started following me. I said to Katrina, "Not really a cat person. I've got to be honest. I'm so much more of a dog person."

Katrina replied, "Ahh come on girl, how can you not love it? Look at it, it's so cute."

"I'm a dog person hun. Cats are lovely, but they're not my first choice."

"Love the pussy, Lucy. Love the pussy," Katrina shouted in my direction, giggling as she spoke. We were having a good laugh about it all, even though the place seemed totally backwards. The cat, though, was determined to follow me.

"Love the pussy, Lucy."

"Alright, Katrina, I'm loving the fucking pussy the best I can," I giggled.

We moved on. I followed Katrina because she had been here before and knew where she was going, apparently. The cat followed me. It was walking by my side. "Do you think the cat needs some food, Katrina?"

And all she kept saying was, "Love the pussy, Lucy. Love the pussy."

I was trying to love on the cat, but all I was thinking was – *I hope this cat isn't going to be glued to me for a week because I'm going to get pissed off with it pretty quickly.*

The cat must have felt my vibes because at that point it stopped and just sat down. *Thank God for that!*

It became obvious that San Marcos was absolutely tiny. It's probably only five hundred yards from end to end. There are thin, cobbled streets with little buildings shoehorned in here and there. It's almost like how I imagine a gnome village would be, that's the best way I can explain it. There were these little alleyways that would lead between two properties, and they would lead to other properties built behind them. It was like a rabbit warren of a town.

We stopped in a few places to look for somewhere to stay, and of course – due to our lack of planning, nowhere appeared to have any rooms. I was getting frustrated as I had it in my head that I would be staying somewhere with a view of the lake, but at this late stage we just needed anywhere to stay. We stopped at a little place to grab something to eat and got chatting to the guy that owned the business. He said he had a room we could have. We would have taken anything at that point, so we figured if we stayed there a couple of nights, then eventually something better would become available — preferably somewhere with a lake view! I knew it would happen at some point. It was beyond faith, it was a knowing. I kept saying to Katrina, "We will get what we need. The divine will prevail," — which was my new favourite saying.

After we had eaten, we walked around and asked a few more people if they had rooms, but nobody did. I suggested we go back to the place near where we had gotten off the boat and see what was happening there. The first place we went into, I said to the guy, "I don't suppose you've got any availability starting from tomorrow for maybe five or six days?"

"Oh yeah, you're in luck. I do have one from tomorrow, with a lake view. It's upstairs, though. Is that a problem with all your bags?"

I looked at Katrina and said, "I'll carry the bags on my own if it means I get that view." And so, as ever, the magic of manifestation worked again.

As we were leaving, the cat arrived again. It started purring and doing its thing, curling itself around my legs, rubbing itself against me — which I do find a bit weird, I'll be honest with you.

Katrina was laughing and saying, "Love the pussy, Lucy. Love the pussy." To which I just rolled my eyes in her direction and carried on our merry way. I was so happy inside, I knew I had to be in that location looking at that lake. I had no logical idea why, I just knew without any question that was what was required.

We found our way back to the little room that we were staying in for our first night, and although the room was small and very basic, it did a job. I slept well but woke up the following day feeling like it had been a busy night. In the previous few years, since this journey of awakening had been activated, I had become aware of the fact that most evenings my soul would leave my physical body and disappear off around the world, into different dimensions, to carry out much-required work for the world, and to help it wake up. It sounds crazy, I know. My soul had known there was going to be an awakening, which was why I had gone through everything I had been going through, but I didn't comprehend this on an intellectual level for a long, long time — not until years later when I met people who helped me normalise this stuff. I thought I was just weird and going a bit crazy and so I did not dare talk about it. Thankfully in Guatemala, I was with someone who got it and even did it herself, so we could talk openly about it without judgement. I also had my quantum healer, Debs, to help me make sense of it.

That night, though, I didn't know what was happening, but I felt a magical tingling; there was something that was being activated in my body, that was — and the only way I can describe it — bringing me back online. I didn't know what it was and all I could say is that it felt like an activation — like something was being switched on. It felt like when somebody says something to you and your inner knowing knows it to be true, so you get covered in goosebumps. Well, it was like that, only on the inside. It wasn't a physical thing that you could see on the outside, but it was something that was going on in my physical vessel. It felt really beautiful and very powerful.

The next day we moved to the new hotel, and compared to where we had stayed the night before, it was really quite plush. The view was incredible, it was that view I had dreamed of and I was so happy. We decided that we were going to go and see a shaman and do a cacao ceremony that afternoon. We walked up through the town and eventually found where the shaman was holding the ceremony. There were probably about 20 of us gathered, and while we waited, we all chatted and got to know each other. Eventually, the shaman appeared and he explained a bit about the process, and then he gave us each a cup of cacao to drink. I didn't really appreciate the whole cacao thing at that point, and I didn't get a great deal from this experience either. It wasn't like I had such an amazing experience with it that I thought I must use cacao going forwards, but it was a positive experience. Nothing at all like the ayahuasca journey that I had been on, the cacao was very ordinary, very grounding. What I did realise afterwards, in hindsight, was that there was a really beautiful vibration there. We connected as a group, and it opened up our hearts. There was a warmth that the cacao brought to us. The shaman walked around the group and he shared some profound things. He would speak to certain people, and there were messages that started to come up — things around a young person passing, which obviously was very resonant for my nephew, but I didn't connect the dots at the time and just admired whoever the message was for, holding space, not realising in actuality, it was likely for me.

After that experience, Katrina wanted to do it again, but I told her I wasn't too bothered, I would rather go and do some meditations. I was at that point in my journey where I didn't want to be getting into any form of plant medicine. I wasn't against it, but I was somebody that used to take a lot of drugs and I didn't want to get hooked on that mindset again. At that point in time, I felt as if I was naturally an open channel, I was being guided and I would like to explore that in its natural form first, without any outside substance to influence that.

Later on that day, we decided to go across the lake and check out the 'party town' — as it's known. It wasn't my scene at all and so after about an hour, I told Katrina I wanted to head back. She was happy to stay on and so I got the boat back by myself. As I was crossing the lake on the way back, I draped my hand in the water again. It was a message that I kept getting — I had to put my hand in the water for some reason. I felt as if something under the water was going to feed me messages — again. I knew that sounded bonkers at the time, so I kept it to myself.

At the other end, I got off the boat and the cat was waiting there for me. I let it follow me, but internally I was cursing it. *What is it with this cat? Why on earth is it making a beeline for me all the time?*

It was a nice day, so on the walk back to our room, I decided to sit outside, be present, immerse in the sunshine and take in the stunning view. It was breathtaking. No matter how many times I looked at it, it always took my breath away. Within seconds of me getting through the gate to our hotel, a hummingbird, in all its glory, appeared right in front of my face flapping its little wings. It was only about six inches away from me. I knew this was not normal. Hummingbirds are timid, they do not come close to humans, especially not this close. It was a stunning creature. It was that close to my face that I could see all of its feathers and the integration of the colours. I was in awe. It was a truly magical experience. Once again, I felt chosen. No one would ever believe this happened, so I lost myself in these precious moments. The hummingbird stared at me, then looked away, stared again, then looked away again, before flying off. *Am I losing my mind? Or did that really happen?*

I sat down to process that miraculous experience and the cat jumped straight on my lap. Now, this was a step too far for this cat. I just wanted to be left alone. I stroked it for a bit, hoping it would get the message. "Love the pussy, Lucy, love the pussy" was rattling around my head, so I did my best to love on that pussy. I was confused. Was this really happening? Was someone winding me up here? Or was this really going on? I contemplated if maybe all the drugs I had taken over the years had finally taken their toll.

Later that day, when Katrina had returned from 'party town', I told her about the cat, but I didn't mention the hummingbird to her – it was too strange to explain, and I still wasn't sure if it had actually happened. We were both feeling tired and were ready to call it a day. I said to Katrina that although I was tired, I was feeling intuitively drawn to go and do a meditation at a place called Las Piramides that was just opposite where we were staying. Las Piramides was a retreat centre, although that is not the most perfect description of it. It's a place where people go to get connected and to learn spirituality and all sorts of tools for the journey. It's a very beautiful place that creates an awakening within people; you can go and stay for as long as you want, or you can just turn up and pay for a meditation session, a clinic, or a workshop. Katrina was happy to come along and so we headed off to see what we would find there.

We got there, and it looked very basic from the outside, there was an area with a couple of huts where you go to check-in. When we walked through that area, we then entered a mystical garden. It was really beautiful. We stepped into a big pyramid. It was fantastic. People were hanging around, meditating, and chatting, and many of them were staying in the little pyramid teepees. There were all the facilities and amenities you needed to stay there, and people did stay there for long periods of time.

We looked around, there were pyramids everywhere. There was one huge pyramid where people could go and do meditations, yoga, and other stuff. And then there was a smaller pyramid – a smaller version of the bigger pyramid – I never quite got my head around what they did in there. Then there were copper pyramids that people would go and sit in to enhance their meditation experience.

I didn't really understand what that was all about either, but people said it was great for healing. I trusted that it was obviously not right for me at that time because they just didn't call to my soul at all.

We crossed the beautiful little garden, walking on stepping stones to get to the big pyramid, where the meditation was to take place. We had to take our shoes off before we entered the pyramid, and then we were encouraged to find ourselves a bed or a seat. I like to lie down when I meditate and so I found a place to get comfortable. There was a girl that came in, she was probably a little bit younger than me, and she took the meditation. She started speaking really beautifully. There were certain things that she said that resonated deeply with me and I just found myself closing my eyes and feeling into the vibration. I loved what she was saying and how she was saying it, I felt awe for this woman. I went into a beautiful mediative space, and I was observing myself, listening to the wisdom. As we dropped deeper into the meditation, it felt like she was almost talking directly to me. Some of the things that she was talking about in this meditation, reminded me of the situation that had happened with my nephew. My ego piped up with this sense of longing – *Why can't she be talking about me? Just imagine how helpful it would be, but she's not, she's talking to somebody else. How lucky they are to have her channel all of this information for them.*

I am very visionary in my meditations. I close my eyes and the first thing I see is my third eye. It comes up as a really beautiful, big, brown eye with really long lashes. It's a beautiful shape, extremely dark and mystical in appearance. It's funny, sometimes I shut my eyes to tap into information, and sure enough, the beautiful third eye shows herself. I appreciate not everyone sees this. We all have different sights and images that communicate with us, so do not be disheartened if you have never seen 'your eye'. This meditation was no different. I went in through the third eye and drifted into the cosmos, whilst listening to her words and guidance. At one point, I saw a bright light bobbing around everywhere. I thought it was my mind's eye playing with me initially, but once I was able to focus more intently and surrender to what was going on, I was able to see very clearly that it was Tinkerbell. She was bouncing around and creating such a beautiful playful energy. It made me weep for my nephew.

After the meditation finished, I went over to the girl and thanked her. I let her know what a real gift to the world she was. She thanked me in return, and we got talking for a while. It transpired that she was the daughter of the lady who owned the place. When I was leaving, she gave me a big hug and said she hoped to see us again soon. I really wished I had known about this place. I would have been keen to stay a month if I had been able to. I would have liked to have seen what I was able to achieve under the watchful eye of someone like her. I had never had a mentor in the spiritual world. The journey I had been on had been all my own doing through intuitive pulls. It surprises many people when I tell them that this was the case. I'm sure some do not believe me, but it's the truth. I have had people hold space for me on several occasions and I have had many readings over the years, but that has been it. When I look back, I'm quite proud of the magical journey I have been on as it's been a total lone ranger journey.

After the meditation, we were both exhausted and so we agreed to go back to the room and get an early night. I went to the outside bathroom to get myself ready for bed – there was no en-suite here. I came out of the bathroom and the cat was there, waiting for me. I thought – *What the fuck is with you, cat?* And in my head, I can hear Katrina saying, "Love the pussy, Lucy." All I can think, though, is – *Fuck the pussy. Just leave me alone. Space dude. I need space! You need to learn about space right now.*

The cat followed me back to the room, and there was just no way that it was coming in. So I told it firmly, "Fuck off cat!"

I told Katrina that the cat was following me and waiting outside. I think you might know what she said to me in response.

I nodded off very quickly, but I woke up in the middle of the night and I got this clear message about my nephew, how I had to go to India and that my nephew was attempting to communicate with me. I acknowledged the message but didn't think too much of it. I looked over at Katrina, who was twitching around – as she does in the night – and then I fell back asleep.

The next morning, I woke up and I said to Katrina, "Oh my God. My nephew came to me last night."

Katrina looked at me as if to say 'shut the fuck up', and then actually said, "Your nephew came to you? I was up with him for two hours last night, having a discussion with him about how you will not pay attention to him, and you are too distracted so he can't communicate with you."

My jaw dropped open, and chills ran right through me.

She continued, "He asked me to give you a message. Please stop being distracted. Put your phone down. Focus! The cat is him trying to communicate with you."

What the fuck? What on earth was she on about?

Katrina could see my shock, but she carried on, "He's embodied in the cat to get your attention. He has been trying for days to get your attention, but you're too busy not loving the pussy!"

Instantly, a huge wave of guilt flooded my body. I didn't think it was the best time to tell Katrina that I had been telling the cat to fuck off.

Katrina spoke again, "He gave me the message that the hummingbird was to get your attention – God knows what that means?" With that, I started crying. I hadn't told her about the hummingbird. She continued, "Your nephew is getting your attention by the cat. He is the cat. He wants to spend time with you. He is trying to get close to you."

I felt awful, I had been less than polite to that cat, and all the time it was my nephew trying to get in touch with me. I felt absolutely terrible. It was an unbearable kick in the teeth.

Katrina wasn't finished, "The hummingbird was to get your attention, the cat is how he's trying to communicate with you. I don't know why, but I've got to tell you that there was a boy from India that went to your nephew and helped him cross over when he passed."

That was too much for me. The India connection reminded me of the message I had got during Date With Destiny, from my friend Jimbo, who had passed. He had had told me I needed to go to India. What the heck was going on? All these messages and synchronicities, and all happening so fast. It was intense. I didn't know what to do with myself. I told Katrina that this was freaking me out and I needed to call my sister and find out if the Indian boy had any significance.

I called my older sister and asked how everything was going, bearing in mind what they were having to deal with, and then I said, "Kirsty, can I possibly ask you some really weird questions? Just go with me." She said it was fine, so I said to her, " Did Shane have an Indian friend by any chance?"

Kirsty thought about it for a moment and then said, "Wait, yes! You're not going to fucking believe it, this is weird. On Christmas Day, we were at mum's house and Mark put this movie on, Lion. It was a true story about two Indian kids, and one of them gets killed by a train. I couldn't believe Mark put that film on when Shane had just been hit by a car."

Speaking to Kirsty on the phone sparked something off in me. All the dots started to be connected. My nephew had told Katrina that the boy that had helped him had been hit by a train. Katrina then told me that there was also a little girl that was there, a white girl who had been badly physically abused when she passed. Katrina said that there were three kids together in a little union. Whilst I was speaking to my sister, Katrina was tapping away on her computer trying to find out the true story of the little Indian boy and the train. The little boy's brother was killed by a train, and the boy got lost and separated from his family. The boy ended up in orphanages and was groomed for sexual abuse, but luckily managed to avoid it. Later on, he had a girlfriend called Lucy – of all the names in the world, and the Indian boy was adopted by an Australian family; with all the links I had to Australia, and Katrina was Australian. There were so many signs and dots being connected – even things like child abuse which would become a huge part of my journey later on. Everything was starting to come together, even if it did not make total sense yet.

My best friend, who had passed, delivered me the first message about India whilst I was in Florida a month earlier, saying I need to go to India. That message had been facilitated by Katrina at Date With Destiny. Then my nephew was communicating another message about India to Katrina while we were in Guatemala, which was then being validated by my sister in Bournemouth. At this point, it was hard to argue that there wasn't a divine plan at play. A divine plan so perfectly orchestrated, and we were pieces of that plan moving around and creating the necessary shifts based on intuitive pulls we all receive.

It was all a bit too much for me. I burst into tears and said that I needed to take time out and get my head together. My sister was totally confused, "I don't understand what's going on. Tell me, Lucy, I don't get it. You need to share."

"Kirsty, I'll call you back when I've made sense of it." I put the phone down and was heading out to get some fresh air, when Katrina said, "Are you ready for the next bit of the message now?"

"Seriously?" I shrieked.

"You've got to go and speak to a lady called Chaty in Las Piramides."

"Katrina, this is where I draw the line. I'm not going to Las Piramides. I got a message from a dead child telling me that I need to ask for a woman called Chaty. I'm just not doing it."

Katrina was great, though. She is very persuasive. In fact, she's truly amazing. She allowed me my moment, then literally kicked my butt and walked me over to Las Piramides.

I walked in feeling really nervous. I've got to tell somebody that my dead nephew has told me to ask for someone called Chaty. Beyond random and very bizarre. The first person I saw was the lady who had taken the meditation the night before. She was sat behind the front desk. I tried to distract myself, looking around at the crystals in the shop. Katrina was having none of it, "Ask the question, Lucy. Ask the frickin question." I shuffled over to the desk and spoke to the lady, "I know this is going to sound really weird." She smiled her beautiful smile, which told me that she was probably used to the weirdness. "My nephew was killed in December. He got hit by a car and he transitioned very quickly. He came to me and my friend last night. He delivered two messages to my friend and one of them was that I've been told to come here and ask for a lady called Chaty."

The lady smiled again, "Oh yes, that's my mum."

I couldn't believe it. It was unreal. No way! I shook my head in disbelief and looked at Katrina, who just shrugged her shoulders. In my head I was thinking – *I don't know what's going on here, but this is so weird.*

Then, the girl said to me, "I'm really sorry but my mum is out of town. She'll be back on Thursday."

"Oh no, I'm leaving on Thursday. I have to start the long journey home to make the funeral on time."

"My mum has such a huge waiting list, I don't think you'll be able to see her. I might just be able to squeeze you in on Friday."

"I have to leave on Thursday. I've got to get back for my nephew's funeral and I've been told very clearly that your mum has got a message for me to take back for the family."

I must have looked disappointed because she said, "Let me see what I can do." I left my details with her, and Katrina and I left. We were really hungry by this point. Earlier we had spotted a beautiful place called The Garden Restaurant, so we took a slow stroll up there.

When we got to the restaurant we looked around for a table. I spotted a man and woman at a table and intuitively decided to go and sit next to them. Not long after we sat down, the lady turned to me and she said, "Darling, you know that you've got to go and shine your light, don't you? You know that you are meant for much greater things on this planet. You know that the world needs you to go shine your light?"

I was shocked, these were the words my grandad had used when he was dying. I looked at Katrina, who was looking at me. There was so much weird stuff happening, it was getting silly now.

The lady continued, "Darling, you know that this trip is going to change your life. You are going to find your life purpose on this trip. You really are a very special person."

What the actual fuck?

The lady smiled at me, "Please just keep trusting and just know it's all going to become clear. A very important message is going to be delivered to you in a pyramid before you leave this lake."

Everything she was saying was activating me, giving me goosebumps. I was being activated once again by the words that my grandad had used for me. It was like going back five years earlier. I didn't really know what she was talking about, but I had learnt enough to go with it by this point without being too overly freaked out.

I said to the lady, "You remind me so much of my grandad. All the words you are saying, my grandad said to me when he was dying."

"Darling, your grandad is here with me. He just wanted to use me to let you know that he's with you, that he loves you, and that he's so proud of you."

Oh my God! To hear her say that was powerful. I started crying.

We chatted to the couple for ages, and really connected on a deep level. A couple of hours later, we said our goodbyes. I was blown away by everything that was unfolding. I couldn't get my head around it because it was happening at such a fast rate, there was no time to digest each bit before something else unbelievable happened. I had not known anything like it since embarking on this journey.

We headed back to the hotel, and I went to the outdoor bathroom to wash my face and brush my teeth. When I stepped outside the bathroom, the cat was there waiting. This time, though, I said, "Come on you, let's go." And the cat followed me back to the room and curled up on my bed and slept the night with me.

The next day, I received a message from the daughter of Chaty. She said her mum was due back tomorrow and could see me at 10 am and to bring a pen and paper with me. Amazing! Although the magic was so powerful these days that nothing was actually surprising me anymore. I had woken up that day feeling an urge to do a meditation, hoping that it would help me process the events of the day before, so I headed back to Las Piramides. I was due there the following day to see Chaty anyway, but it was such a beautiful space that I thought it would be the best place to meditate.

The daughter was there again, and we spoke for a little while, and then I went and got comfortable, ready for the meditation. Another woman appeared, she looked like an angel, and she had a really lovely, positive good-witch vibe about her with her long, plaited, grey hair. It was clear she was a powerhouse. I was in awe of how beautiful her skin was. I was in awe of how beautiful she was. There was nothing fake about her, she was completely natural – no makeup or anything, just a flowing, white robe. She walked around a couple of times and then started speaking. I know now that she was channelling, but I didn't know that at the time. She settled everyone down into a meditative state, and then she started talking about life after death.

My ego piped up again, not wanting to believe these messages could be for me. I was thinking – *Oh my God, these messages are amazing. Whoever is receiving them, I hope they get the healing. I hope they get the love. I hope they get everything that they need from this.*

Ego aside, the meditation was amazing. It was extremely profound and loaded with love.

Afterwards, I thanked the woman for the meditation. She was polite and thanked me for sharing. She said she had not known why she went off on one about life after death as it was not the subject she was intending to speak, but she recognised it was obviously what was required. Katrina and I said thank you again, and we headed back to our hotel.

The next day, I had my session with Chaty at 10 am, so I got there with plenty of time to spare. The daughter was there again and she greeted me warmly and said to me, "I hope you have a really good time. Whatever the message is, I hope it comes through for you. I hope you get whatever it is that you need."

I had no idea what I was in for. I thought I would be meeting with this Chaty person for a sit-down and maybe a cup of tea. The next thing, this woman came to meet me, and it was the woman from the meditation. She was Chaty. It turned out that she had returned home early and so had taken the meditation the day before! I was already in awe of her, but now I was blown away.

She walked me over to the small pyramid. We took our shoes off and she began to set the room up. Eventually, we sat down together. I sat cross-legged, facing her. And she said to me, "Okay, Lucy, before we go any further, what brings you here today? My daughter told me that it was quite important that you saw me."

I told her the story about my nephew and that I was going home tomorrow for the funeral. She dropped her head and she said, "It was you. The messages in yesterday's meditation, they were for you. I didn't know why I was talking about life after death. I had no idea. I wasn't supposed to be doing that but I was taken over by something that had to deliver a message."

I sat opposite her and could not help but start crying.

She asked me about the family and how they were doing, and then she said, "Are you ready to tap into some energies and get some messages that are going to help you and your family release whatever needs to be done and get in alignment with why this had to happen?"

"Yes, yes, yes. I'm ready."

"Are you ready to connect to your divine purpose?"

I could have screamed, 'Yes, yes, yes — tell me!"

"I'm going to drop us into a space of meditation and then I'm going to call in my guides and we're going to go from there. I'd like you to get comfortable and I'd like you to get into a meditative state. If you brought some paper and a pen, you might want to write down what comes through. Stay in a meditative state until I start talking, then you can write it down, so you don't forget it." Thankfully, I had remembered to bring stuff with me.

Within seconds of closing my eyes, it felt like a block of concrete had been dropped on my lap. I felt like I was being pushed further and further into the ground. I couldn't move, and then all of a sudden this whooshing started to happen all around me. Whoosh! Whoosh! Whoosh! It felt like a heavy pulsating all around me. I started crying uncontrollably. All of this energy was building up around us and I couldn't move my legs. Then Chaty started channelling, and so I opened my eyes and started to write down the things she was saying. She told me that there was an altar that I had to set up in memory of my nephew so that the energy could be focused there rather than all the treacherous stuff that was going on around the situation. She told me that Shane was one of a twin – which he was – and she said that they had shared a soul. She said that this was very rare in twins, but sometimes it happens. And when it happens, one of the twins has to go early. It normally happens for karmic lessons for the family, or someone else – in this case, the driver. Little Shane had graciously said he would die so that his twin could survive. Shane would bring the healing into the family, but his twin would continue the journey and they would communicate with each other forevermore.

The stuff coming through was profound and I was desperately trying to write it down, whilst crying like a baby. Chaty kept going. She said the reason that the accident happened was that the lady driving the car needed to step through some karma of her own, so Shane had given his life to assist this lady step through her karmic lesson. This was mind-blowing stuff to hear. Chaty reassured me not to be angry about it. It was karma and soul contracts playing out. It felt so heartless to my human, but it connected deeply with my soul.

The channelling went on for ages. I was much calmer by the end, but then she said to me, "You don't have children yet, but you are the mother of many. You've been put on this planet to change the way that motherhood is looked at in this world. You are here to increase the feminine energy and to make a huge difference. You've got no idea how many children you hold. It's your job to go home and prepare your sister so that she can look after the family. And then you can go off and do the job of waking people up globally. You are the person that has been chosen to activate the mothers to come back into their divine heart space. The divine masculine who will support you will show himself when you and he are ready. You have such a huge role to play, it's an honour to have met you."

Wow! That was some heavy stuff she said to me. I was still trying to write it down, thinking I could make better sense of it later.

Chaty asked me to close my eyes and we went back into meditation to complete the process. When I opened my eyes, we were both crying.

This was the most profound and beautiful experience of my life. It was beyond words. This incredible woman was like nothing I'd ever witnessed before. At the very end, she said to me, "You know, you've got to keep looking out for your nephew. He's going to show himself to you constantly. And you also need to bring it up into the consciousness of the family that they will see him and hear him and feel him, if they choose to."

We stood up and walked out of the pyramid. Chaty reached in and gave me the biggest hug. It was a real mother bear hug. And I needed it. I sobbed in her arms.

After that, I went back to the hotel and sat on the beach looking out over the lake. It was the place I went to every single morning that I was there, to do my journaling and rituals. At this point, I had to simply sit and allow everything that had happened in Guatemala to process. I was in awe. I was in awe of what this lady had done to my life. I was in awe of the fact that in 2014 I was shown this lake and here I was sitting beside it right now, having gone through this absolutely massive transformation process once again. I wondered if this journey would ever stop, or was this it now?

Katrina appeared and I told her what had gone on with Chaty and we both sat and cried together.

The next day, I had to go home to the family and the funeral. I had a very long journey ahead of me. I had to go from Guatemala back to Miami, Miami back to London Heathrow, and then from London Heathrow to Bournemouth. That would give me a lot of time to process everything and a lot of time to think. I didn't quite know what to do with myself. On the one hand, I felt alive and activated and on cosmic fire, but I also felt such sadness that a beautiful five-year-old boy had surrendered his soul in such a selfless act to save his brother. It was such a contradiction of feelings and emotions. Duality at its best.

I said goodbye to Katrina, who was staying on a little longer. I got a very early boat out of there. I thought I would be the only one on the boat, but it was packed and it didn't feel safe. I thought it was going to sink and so on the way over I continuously said a protection prayer. This calmed me down and so, just as I had on the way over, I put my hand in the water of the lake. All of a sudden I got this message to pick up my journal, so I did.

A message started coming through me, and this is what I wrote, *"Please close your eyes and let these words run through your body, I encourage you.*

Let them past your ears. Allow each word to touch your soul. If there is one wish this gorgeous family has for each of you, it's that you treasure these thoughts every single day and we learn from this tragedy.

Life is a wonderful gift. Wherever you are in your life right now, I urge each and every one of you to find the good in each situation. Maybe you are frustrated with your lack of progress, maybe your relationship is not what it used to be, the children misbehave frequently, you aren't where you anticipated for your life or maybe you are sick.

Whatever is going on for you right now, our wish for you is you stop, take a deep breath and appreciate the wonderful opportunity you have been blessed with to experience this thing called life, as a human being.

Wherever you are, keep fighting.

One day all of what you are going through will make sense.

For now, trust there is something greater than us that will show us why we each have been chosen.

Hope. Let's make a commitment today to give hope to our next generation. Encourage them to believe there is something far greater than this tragedy. Let's educate them that blame is something we create in our heads and most situations can be resolved with open honest conversations and love. Let's promise to teach them to believe, always. That there really is so much to live for. Let's commit to earning their trust and showing them the way.

Love is the greatest force of all. The World we currently live in is in desperate need of more love. In every situation that you find yourself placed, give love. If someone hurts you or a situation causes you pain, search deep to see where you can return love. It's so easy to lash out, retaliate and blame. We are in a culture where these emotions are the norm.

We appreciate this goes against the grain of society to shower each other with love and affection. Let's be the change we want to see in the World. Let's make sure, God forbid, if something like this ever happens again, that we know and they know they are loved more than anything else in this World.

I ask each of you to dig deep and send love not only to Shane Junior today, but for the young lady who took Shane's life. I imagine she is in a very dark place right now and no one deserves that.

Gratitude. And finally, be grateful every single day you open your eyes. Forget whether the sky is blue or grey, take a deep gulp of oxygen and smile, give thanks for having the opportunity to live again.

Tomorrow is never promised. This life has a plan for you, you will never know when the last time you may take in sweet oxygen is, so our wish for you is that every day you live your life. Do things that Shane Junior is no longer able to do.

Talk to him, make him proud and know that every single step of the way he will be by each of your sides."

I was just watching my hand write all this stuff. And that was the first time I ever acknowledged that I was being channelled. I was scribbling frantically to keep up with what was coming through. It was a right fucking mess! Once the messages stopped, I put my book back in my bag.

I lay back and placed my hand back in the water, and closed my eyes. Suddenly, another message came through – *The Mayans have been guiding you. The Mayans brought you here. The energies of your ancestors are channelling you to bring everything back online. This lifetime is the lifetime that we are all very much going to be coming back online and bringing it all together.*

I had no idea what that meant. At that time, I didn't even know anything about the Mayans, but I wrote it all down and figured that I would do a bit more research on it when I eventually reached civilisation again.

Many people have asked me over the years what I mean by a download, an insight, or a message. The most common question I get asked are – how does it appear and what does it feel like? Most people would like to believe it's a really blatant sign, or a physical being that shows up, and that there can be no misinterpretation; however, it's just not the case. I have never had someone show up and say, "Hey Lucy, here is a business idea for you. We will leave it with you, we trust you to get it done!" and then they disappear. It's just not what happens at all. A download often shows up as an idea that appears, totally out of nowhere; and it's often extremely different from whatever you were thinking about in that previous moment.

Often, I have to grab a piece of paper and write it down, so I don't forget it, and then trust it will make sense, one day. I believe we are all given these downloads each day; it's just most people brush them off, or forget about them for a couple of reasons – they are too busy, or if they do catch them, the download makes no sense and then the ego pipes up and talks them out of taking it further.

My advice – keep your phone or a notepad close by and keep a note of any weird or wonderful things that fly in. They'll make sense one day.

Channeling is a bit different. An example of this is when you are talking to someone and something extremely profound comes out of your mouth, maybe even on a subject you know nothing about, but it comes out so quickly and with passion, you feel certain about it. That is what I refer to as channeling. I believe this to be a force working through you at that moment, to deliver a message to whoever you are speaking to, or engaging with at that time.

Channeling can happen in many ways – writing, speaking, meditating, exercising, or pretty much anything you do. You can feel an overwhelming sense of something working through you that assists in your success. That's exactly what I feel happened to me that day on the boat.

I got off the boat and I looked back across that lake. I remembered the first time I had ever seen it in that photograph that Ricky showed me, and now I looked back over it, after having the most unbelievable transformational journey. I knew that my life would never be the same again. The synchronicities, the signs, the profound connection to Mother Nature – the animals that had been communicating with me so clearly, everywhere I went. I had opened my heart to so many incredible people. Whether it be the man on the beach smoking his weed every morning that I would chat to, or the beautiful, profound conversations with the people at Las Piramides, or the people in restaurants that I talked to. Every single person was a messenger that brought something to the party. And every single message was about what had happened to Shane, and Date With Destiny. I was in absolute awe of it all.

I looked back over that lake and I knew that I would be back. I knew that I had to go back. It was no longer Katrina's lake, it was my lake too. I knew that there was more that needed to be unlocked from this space. I looked back on that lake with so much love. I also looked back on it with an element of fear because now the responsibility of my destiny was on my shoulders and there was nowhere to hide. I knew it now, and there was no way that I could ever go back and turn that knowing off.

88

So, here I was finally leaving the place that I had been so scared to even go to. I was heading in the direction of home with very mixed feelings. I had a very heavy heart because I had to leave early to attend the funeral of my five-year-old nephew. And yet, I also was feeling excited because I was leaving as a totally different person. I had changed in so many ways. I even wondered if my own mum would recognise me. I also had a huge responsibility on my shoulders. Not only did I have the responsibility of delivering the messages to my family, but there was also this extremely important information I'd been given around the Mother Energy, and the Divine Feminine. Apparently, I was going to be the one to remind the Mothers, the Divine Feminine of what they incarnated for. I had no idea how I was going to do it, I was not even a Mother myself, but apparently that was not important.

The minibus journey through Guatemala was the perfect example of the dichotomy that I was living in. As I bounced and bobbed around inside the bus, one moment the bumps would bring out happiness and excitement in me, and then the next minute the heaviness would rise.

I read through the message that I had channelled and written down on the boat. It was unbelievably profound. I kept reading over it. I couldn't yet get my head around where it came from. I trusted, even though I couldn't answer my own questions, and as much as my ego wanted to make logical sense of it, I surrendered and trusted that it was exactly what it needed to be. I had experienced so many virtual slaps from the Universe that resulted in magic, that it was becoming easier to let go and trust.

I travelled for almost an entire day before I touched down at London Heathrow Airport. I got that sinking feeling as soon as I stepped off the plane. After the glorious sunshine I had lived with for the last seven weeks, stepping into the cold, grey, English winter was a shock. I hadn't even figured out where I was going to be staying, I had just got on the plane in the direction of home and trusted that it would all work out exactly as intended. This was the most beautiful part of the whole journey, the realisation that in just a matter of months, since finally leaving corporate, I had gone from being an absolute control freak to someone who was totally comfortable 'winging it'. I actually didn't want to have a plan. The thought of having a plan made me feel sick. And in fact, whenever people said to me, "Hey, we need to plan something," it would repel me. I would think to myself – *Let's just see what happens.* I had started to believe the calls I had been receiving. I knew that 'something' had been calling me, rather than it being my ego wanting to go to a country. It could not be my own doing; there was something far greater than I ever thought possible guiding me to all of this.

I got the coach from Heathrow to the station in Bournemouth, where my mum was picking me up. That journey wasn't great. I started to feel the heaviness of the situation that I had come home for. A funeral, and not a funeral of somebody who had lived a full life and had amazing memories; I was attending the funeral of a five-year-old boy who had been tragically killed, holding his dad's hand while crossing a road.

The first day back to Bournemouth was okay. There were the wonderful aspects of seeing the people you love, after not seeing them for a while. You get to chat, catch up, and be a bit naughty with your food choices. If your mum does not have tea and biscuits on the go, is she really a mum? My mum loves a biscuit or a chocolate bar and sweets. It takes real willpower to be there and resist her confectionary charms.

The next day, though, was the funeral.

89

On the morning of the funeral, I went to spend time with my sister and and her son – my nephew, Josh. He was devastated. He loved his little brother so much. This was too much for his little heart to contend with. I just wanted to take away all of his pain. It was too much for someone so young. Life can be cruel.

I drove my nephew and my sister to the parents of Shane, the boy who had died. He was one of a set of twins from my sister's ex-partner and his new partner. It was a terribly sad scene. The kids were causing mayhem, keeping themselves distracted, but Shane's mum was distraught. Shane's father, my sister's ex-partner, was devastated too. He had closed himself off from the person I had once known him to be. He had been with my sister from when they were both young, so I had got to know him well over the years. It was devastating to see him so broken. He was a shell of himself in that house that morning. He didn't want to speak to anyone. He didn't want to be around anyone. I can't even begin to imagine the guilt he felt. He was the one who was safeguarding the child, holding his hand, at the time when he got killed. And as much as there was absolutely nothing that he could have done, I couldn't begin to imagine the guilt that he must have been feeling.

I did my very best to keep the vibration as high as I could, considering the situation. I observed what was going on before I spoke to Shane's dad and I did my best to give him a lift with my energy. When the hearse arrived at the house, as is the custom in the UK, it was a terrible shock to all of us.

I drove my sister and Josh to the cemetery, ahead of the procession. We wanted to make sure we got a space, without any issues, and Josh had really wanted to make sure that he was close to the front, and so we honoured his requests. It was our job to keep him as calm as possible through what would probably be the worst day of his life.

As I walked into the church, one of the children came over to me and grabbed hold of my hand. Now, I had been given the message that I was going to be there for the children and for the family when I was in Guatemala, but I never knew how that would play out. This beautiful child intuitively held my hand, and so I bent down to speak to him. With that, he pointed at a window at the top of the church, and said, "There's Shane. He's waving." My heart burst open in such a beautiful way and a tear rolled down my cheek. This was an extraordinary confirmation from the divine, of course, coming through a child as the messenger.

Children are so much more open to seeing things than us adults. It is believed that children between zero and seven remember their roots, where they came from and what they came here to do. If you have a flighty, determined, slightly out-there child, trust me – they remember. Nurture them, they will be the world changers. To me, the sight of Shane was a sign from the gods. It was a sign from Chaty, back in Guatemala. It was a sign that I was there doing exactly what I needed to do. My heart swelled.

The funeral itself was brutal and beautiful all rolled into one. It was very connecting, and deeply emotional. It felt like Shane was there with us, the children could see it.

The family had chosen for Shane to be buried rather than cremated, and so after the service, we had to go out and bury the casket. I had never attended a burial before, only cremations, and so this felt so much more intense because it's so much more real with the visuals. I will never forget the sound of the mud hitting the casket, a sound I had never heard previously. It felt so final. As his body was lowered down into the earth, a massive rainbow appeared out of nowhere in the sky. It had been a cold morning, but as far as I remember it had not been raining, just grey. It was a beautiful sign from him. It felt like he was saying – *Don't worry, I've got this. I'm here and I will walk with you all from this side.* It was both beautiful and heartbreaking. We all saw it and smiled, as this beautiful little boy said his final goodbyes to his family – for that lifetime anyway.

The whole experience was extremely distressing. Just 48 hours earlier, I was having the time of my life in Guatemala, receiving messages from anyone and everything, without a care in the world. Here I was, back in the UK, at a tragic funeral.

Following on from the funeral, we went to the wake. Here in the UK, we have a funeral and then follow it up with drinks, usually at a place that was special to the deceased person. The parents had booked a place with a bowling alley next to it. All the kids were running around and playing in the bowling alley, somewhat oblivious to the occasion. They were having fun. We could learn so much from them. I was standing in the main room when the same little boy that had held my hand in the church came over to me again. He whispered in my ear that he was playing with Shane. I followed him over to the bowling and watched as all the kids played together – many of them I imagined could see Shane, and were playing with him too.

Kids don't see what we see, they are still open. It's our programming that stops us from seeing things. We believe that what we see is reality but it's not, it's programming, it's all an illusion based on our experiences and traumas. Kids are untainted still. All I can do is hope and pray that the magical, divine connection that they have at that age continues throughout their life. I am doing all I can to remind the parents to hold space for their little ones.

Shane's dad looked so sad, so I took the opportunity to wander over to talk to him. It's so hard to know what to say and what to do in that situation because so few of us can truly empathise with a parent who has lost such a young child. I subtly shared some of the information I had received from Guatemala without freaking him out. I knew he was nowhere ready to hear the full extent of the information I had been given. I feel he did take some peace from what I was able to share because a couple of days later he messaged me and shared how grateful he was for me attending; and for the information that I'd given him, although he did ask me what I had been having in my herbal teas that had sent me 'crazy'.

90

The next few days weren't easy. Most people were feeling sad and a bit sorry for themselves and the situation. That was certainly the case with my mum, although it didn't last long. Very quickly, she was back on form, "So what are your plans? What are you going to do? Where are you going to go? Why aren't you working? I thought you'd set up a business. Aren't you supposed to be coaching people? What about getting settled, finding a home?" In all honesty, I didn't know the answers to any of her questions. I had sold everything I owned and rid myself of every commitment.

My dad had asked to see me for a couple of days, and so I said I would if I could stay at his house. Now, in all honesty, this was weird for me and my dad; it was great, but a bit weird. My dad and I had only been back in touch for a couple of years at this point. We had a big fallout the last time I had stayed at his house because his wife had accused me of bringing a guy back to the house. My dad had spoken to me about the situation and I explained my side of it. He decided to side with her, for whatever reason – most likely for an easy life. From that point on, though, I made a decision, it was the final straw.

My dad's wife had never liked me. From the moment she got introduced to my sister and I, it was very obvious we were an inconvenience, even though she had known about us. She wanted my dad all to herself. Every time we would go there, she would feed us things that we didn't like. She didn't want to get to know us. It always felt like she was putting up with us to keep my dad happy. Maybe she knew he would leave her if she did not accept us.

On the day that my dad sat me and my sister down in his house and told us he was marrying this woman, I stood up and told my sister to stand up too, and I told my dad and his future wife that we were leaving. I said to my dad, "This will be the biggest mistake you ever make," and I walked out. I was 18 years old. I got in my little Nova – which was my first ever car – and drove us both back from Twickenham to Bournemouth. I was furious. My sister was in shock that I'd behaved like that in front of my dad as I had always been such a daddy's girl. It also was not like me to be like that. Something inside of me knew that this woman was not a very nice lady – and that was when I was 18! The signs were there as to how intuitive I have always been; however, life and distractions stifled my realisations.

As you can imagine, that little outburst didn't do much for my relationship with her. She tried to make sure her and my dad had as little as possible to do with us. My relationship with my dad suffered badly, but we kept it going the best we could – that was until she wrongly accused me of having a guy back to the house. That was the final straw for me. We didn't speak for seven years after that. No communication whatsoever.

We eventually became reacquainted when my dad messaged me out of the blue and said he would like to speak with me. This was a shock in itself because it was normally me that had to make the effort. I was at work at the time, working at UBS in Liverpool Street in London. I told my boss I had to pop out for a while, he said okay and I went out. I met my dad at a Starbucks near Liverpool Street and we had the most beautiful conversation. A conversation that was long overdue. I was still harbouring some anger with him for siding with his wife. It was still very early days in my healing journey – but I had developed a deeper level of empathy with him. He shared things with me that day that I had no idea about. He revealed things that were going on behind closed doors and it opened my eyes and helped heal some things between us. He told me he was going to divorce his wife, he couldn't stand being with her anymore. He told me I had been right all along. Wow! I was shocked. I never expected that. That day, we both agreed to rebuild our relationship together, no matter what it took, we would do it and step through any challenges we faced. I knew she would make it difficult, and this was going to be a whole new level of healing for me.

The saddest and hardest part of not speaking to my dad during those years was that three years earlier he had twins with his wife, and so due to the situation, I had never met my twin sisters. I love children so much, but I had to be true to myself and faking it with his wife wasn't authentic, so I had to step away from that, at the cost of those children. I trusted that they would find out the truth one day.

A few days later, I went over to his house and I met my little sisters for the first time. It was truly beautiful. My heart exploded. It was a Mother Energy like I've never felt before. The girls are so different, even though they are twins. Gabriela is very happy-go-lucky, positive, full of sprinkles and unicorns, and a little naive, in all honesty. Bela on the other hand is a bit more of a deep thinker, she likes to sit back, ask lots of questions and be slightly more methodical, but she's super daring at the same time; she definitely has her big sister's adrenaline junkie spirit within her.

That first time, I was calling my dad 'Dad' and Bela was watching, looking a bit perplexed. After a while, she scrunched her face up at me and said, "That's my daddy, not your daddy." It was adorable. It must have been difficult for them to comprehend; they were three at the time and had had my dad all to themselves up until that point, and then suddenly this woman comes along and says that they are their sister and he's her dad too. By the end of that first visit, both girls were all over me and we were absolutely head over heels in love with one another. I made sure I left before their mother came back, though.

After Shane's funeral, I made the journey from Bournemouth to Weybridge in Surrey, where my dad was living. I was a bit dubious and nervous, to be perfectly honest. Staying with my dad would mean being with my twin sisters, which was cool, but it also would mean spending time with his wife, and I was still holding a huge grudge.

The girls were so excited to see me, especially as I had been away again. They wanted to know what presents I had from my travels. I'm very lucky that I've now got such a special relationship with the girls. I will make sure that I maintain that till the day that I leave this earth. They are such incredible souls, with so much more remembrance than I ever expected from them at their age.

After a couple of days of being there, my dad said something really weird to me. He said, "Lucy, would you consider living here for a little while?" I had no idea where this came from, but he continued, "I just feel that it would be lovely for you to be here for a while and really get to know the twins. It doesn't matter if you come and go, you can go off and do whatever you need to do, but I just think it would be nice for you to be here." After that, he mentioned that he would like me to be the guardian of the twins, god forbid anything happened to him or their mother. It was out of the blue, and totally unexpected. I don't think my dad realised it at the time but his intuition was on point and asking me to stay with him probably saved his life.

My dad's wife was not happy about it when she found out, but she was outvoted by my dad and the twins. And, at the end of the day, it was my dad's house – let's not forget that. She did have one concession, though, I had to sleep on the top floor. That didn't seem to be too much of a problem until I went up there and discovered that the room had no radiators. I asked my dad, "Dad, why are there no radiators in this room?"

He replied, matter-of-factly, "She removed them for some strange reason. No idea."

"Why can't I go in the spare room downstairs?"

"That's her mother's room. Don't worry I'll get you some heaters for your room."

I couldn't be bothered getting into it, although it seemed strange that her mother, who didn't even live in the country, had a room of her own that was never used, whilst I roughed it in the cold in the upstairs room.

I settled in very quickly. The girls loved it. Every day, when they got home from school, I made sure that I had finished with my clients, so I could play with them and have fun. I wanted them to know I was there for them, no matter what.

Some mornings, usually at about 5 am, they would sneak up to my room and get into bed with me. We would all snuggle up and chat away, or on some mornings we would even play dress-up. It was wonderful. One morning, though, when they were in my bed and we heard a knocking at the door. We all shouted, "Come in." There was no answer. The girls motioned for me to go and see who was there, being the big sister and all. I crept out of the bed, "Who's there?" I opened the door and there was nobody there. Weird. The girls were freaked out a bit. "It must have been Daddy," I said, reassuringly. "We'll ask him later."

When my dad did eventually appear, one of the girls asked him, "Did you knock on the door this morning?"

"No, what are you talking about?" he replied.

The girls were spooked. I told them it must have been a ghost, trying to wind them up, but also because I wanted to start to introduce my sisters to the idea that there was more to life than what we are told. To this very day, my sisters still talk about the ghost at the door. Almost every time I see them, one of them will ask, "Do you remember when the ghost came to the door?" It really made an impact in their lives and was not the last time it happened.

A few weeks after I arrived at my dad's, I was in the gym when my phone started ringing. I didn't recognise the number but answered it anyway. Back in those days, I used to answer my phone to anyone, whereas now my philosophy is if you aren't in my phone then I am not speaking to you. I was greeted by a bubbly voice on the other end of the phone, "Hi Lucy, it's Suzy Mitchell." It was a lady from the company I had set my marketing business up with. She said I had been put forward to be a speaker at their seminars and was I interested. The company did two weekend seminars a year – they gathered all of their representatives and distributors together and put on a conference with motivational speakers on stage; it's basically an excuse for a get-together and to celebrate the company's success. I was jumping around the gym with excitement. I could not believe it! What an incredible opportunity. This was the moment I had been waiting for. I was buzzing. I was speaking in Dubai a week or so earlier, so it was all falling into line. I got to go to Dubai, do my speech, get a tan, come back, and then go on stage in Birmingham looking healthy and glowing.

I had it all worked out in my mind. And that's exactly what I did. I had an amazing time in Dubai. It was really hot, which I love, and such a great opportunity to speak in front of an audience. It was a beautiful event. I met a lot of people there, speaking in front of a hundred people or so. It set me up really nicely for the UK event where I would be speaking in front of thousands.

91

Back at my dad's house, things took a weird turn. My dad told me that he was going to tell his wife that he wanted a divorce. He had mentioned this to me a few times over the previous couple of years, but had never actually done anything about it, so I didn't really believe him. I warned him that he should seriously consider whether he was making the right decision and I warned him that as soon as he told her he wanted a divorce she would use the girls against him and go to war with him. I had a strong feeling it was going to be a really messy divorce.

Whilst I was at the gym that morning, he did actually tell her that he wanted a divorce. I was shocked when I found out. I never thought he would do it.

A couple of days after he had announced the divorce, the nanny – who lived with them – mentioned to me that she had received a message from the twins' mother – my dad's wife – saying she needed picking up from the train station. That seemed weird. She would always reach out to my dad. My dad had changed his work habits since the twins had been born, so he could spend more time with them. He would work from home daily, which meant he could pick his wife up when she had finished in London, and also so he could spend time with the girls when they returned from school. It was amazing to see the transformation in my dad. He was amazing with the girls. They were so close to him because he was always there. It was beautiful for me to watch because when I was a child he had been missing in action most of the time, focused on his work. The message from his wife to the nanny was even more strange because it was sent at about 1pm and my dad's wife worked until 5 pm. What on earth was she up to? My dad ended up going to pick her up due to an issue with the nanny's car. When he got home from picking her up, he went back upstairs to his office. She offered to pick the twins up from school, which was absolutely unheard of at this point. Just after she returned with the kids, I was coming down the stairs and I saw a man and a woman walking into the house. "Excuse me, who are you?" They didn't reply. The nanny appeared and told me that these people were the police. I screamed to my dad. "Dad, did you know the police are here?"

My dad appeared at the top of the stairs, "Excuse me, what are you doing? Why are you in here with my children?"

The policemen told him that there had been a third party accusation made against him and it was their responsibility to check the wellbeing of the children. The police eventually left. My dad, though, was absolutely shell-shocked. He was horrified that such a damaging accusation had been made against him. My heart broke for him.

My dad's intuition had been on point to ask me to stay with him. His soul had known at some level he was going to need someone to witness all that was taking place in that house. It was such a great job that I was there at that time because I was able to help him deal with this lunacy of a situation. I could also do my best to protect the Little Beans – my sisters.

The stress took its toll on my dad. One morning I came down early, at about 5 am on my way to the gym, my dad was sitting in the kitchen staring into space. He couldn't sleep, he hadn't slept for days. He just looked at me, looking like he had aged about 30 years overnight and he said, "Lucy, I didn't do it."

"Dad, you don't need to explain yourself to me. I believe you. I know you are telling the truth. We are going to get through this. All is going to be okay."

There had been a lot of speculation and threats coming from the police. They were clearly trying to intimidate my dad. His solicitor thought there was nothing substantial to the claims, though.

Thankfully, we managed to protect the twins from everything that was going on. They had no idea.

Awkwardly, my dad had a family holiday to the Maldives booked, prior to the divorce announcement, and so in order to give the twins some normality, they all went off on holiday. I felt it was essential that he went, and I told him so.

I had been exposed, in recent years, to how corrupt the legal system was, and yet here I was, about to wade into it, to support my dad. It made me slightly nervous, although I never shared that with him. I had to keep strong, focused and I worked constantly with the quantum field to create mine and my family's reality. The pressure was on. Most of us have never understood the principal that what we think, speak and feel creates in our reality. What I mean by that is, you know when have a thought, something like, "I'm going to have a flat tyre," and then, when it happens, you say, "I knew it!" Well, this is in actuality how we work as humans. We are far more powerful than we would ever comprehend. The systems have been designed this way, to keep us from our own real power, because if we could all create abundance, who on earth would go to work and make the rich richer? There's so much that's kept hidden and suppressed from us, to keep us manageable and controlled.

God bless my dad. He was in such an awful predicament. It made me so sad for him. My dad is one of the most gentle, kind, beautiful humans I have ever had the privilege of meeting this lifetime. It was a shame that women prayed on this as a weakness, and, of course, he allowed them to. In fact, he was, and still is, to this day, fucking useless at picking women. The women he attracted were people he could rescue, in order to have his needs met, and then he would give them the earth, but they would end up being controlling and narcissistic.

The family jetted off together, and I stayed to look after the house. One day, there was a knock at the door and it was one of the detectives asking to speak to my dad. I told them he was away and asked what it was regarding. I told the detective that he would need to speak to my dad himself, or even better, my dad's barrister.

When my dad arrived back from holiday, he was pissed off with me for suggesting he should have gone. At this point, I said to my dad, "I actually hope this goes to court. I know it will be awful for you but I want justice to be served so that these motherfuckers can never badmouth you again." As much bravado as I was showing my dad, I didn't really want him to have to go to court. Yes, I wanted these arseholes to show themselves up in court, but I also knew how manipulated the court system was, and they could very easily have found him guilty. It was such an awful situation to be in.

My dad had some important conversations with his barrister, and they asked if I would be prepared to give a statement. Interestingly, I had a session with my quantum healer a little bit before I made my statement to the police. She had mentioned that my voice was going to be a very important part of the trial. She was amazing. She coached me how to be open, honest and authentic, and without the emotion that was obviously involved, due to it being my dad. She brought into my consciousness that this was about my dad's healing from past lives. My belief is that we have all been good, bad and ugly throughout our many lifetimes that we have had. This lifetime, as we attempt to shift into a higher level of consciousness – hopefully for the final time – we must all face the stories of our past and enable the release of the associated emotions that have been holding us back for so long.

A short time later, I went to do the interview at the police station. It was horrible – police stations aren't nice at the best of times, but this one was awful. I was interviewed by a guy, a total jumped-up arrogant prick. He was probably in his mid-fifties, and he had a cocky, know-it-all approach. I figured I would kill him with compassionate kindness, so I made sure I was my normal, bubbly, open, honest, authentic self. I would say things and he would repeat them back to me, and at times he would twist what I was saying and so I would correct him, "No mate, you haven't got that right. THIS is what I actually said."

After we were done, he agreed that there didn't seem to be much foundation to it all, but I said to him, "Well let's see if the legal system works or not. All I know, is that I trust my dad implicitly."

Months passed and we heard nothing. I hoped that was the end of it, but I felt that it was not going to be as easy as that.

92

Before I knew it, the weekend in Birmingham arrived. I travelled up on the Friday from London with a little gaggle of my team. It was a huge event, something we were all extremely excited about, and I was very proud of what we had all achieved in getting to this point. As we were on the train making our way, I looked around the carriage at them all, with tears welling up in my eyes. Since leaving the dark world of Corporate, I had created such a beautiful, thoughtful, giving, caring community. It was such a huge contradiction to where I had come from. Interestingly, I noticed that a couple of people who were travelling with us didn't seem that happy with the team coming together and going on this journey. I noticed it, but let it go, for now. Nothing was going to change the space I was in. I felt so much love, and I wasn't going to allow a couple of sourpusses to change the vibration between us all.

We arrived in good time. Several of the team had a couple of apartments booked, but I was staying in the Intercontinental, which was paid for by the company. Everybody got settled and then we met up to have dinner together. It was a really beautiful and magical evening, but when it got to 11 pm, I said goodbye to my team and headed back to my hotel to get some rest, ahead of the big day tomorrow.

In the taxi, I was silent. I had tears in my eyes, grateful for everything, as we drove down the old familiar roads in Birmingham, a place I knew so well. I could also feel the presence of my grandad so strongly. I just wanted to hear his voice, letting me know everything was going to be okay. I had a few other things going through my head. I had come on my period that night, and I was hyper-aware of the issues I was having with regards my womb and bleeding, so I was feeling really bloated and my dress was already super tight.

When I got to the hotel, a really beautiful Spanish man checked me in. He could see I had been crying and he looked at me with so much love. He asked me if I was okay. I told him I was great, but thank you for asking. And I really was okay. I was happier than I had been in a long time. This event was such a huge opportunity for me and I was overflowing with appreciation – although to other people looking in, it probably looked like I was sad. This beautiful guy, offered to send a glass of wine to my room. You've got to love the Spanish.

I made my way to my room, opened the door and I was further blown away by a gift and message that had been left in the room for me. I read the note and in that moment, I felt so loved. Although it was getting late and I had a busy day ahead of me, I decided to run a bath and lay in it for a while. I even sent my team some pictures of where I was – living my best life.

I immersed in the bath and then switched my phone off, to disconnect from everything and then I sat down and journaled. It was time to be totally present with myself. Tomorrow was going to be a big day, and I wanted to be totally ready for it. I knew there was a message I had to deliver, not necessarily just for this specific event, but something that was deep within me that needed to come out. This event was my first proper opportunity to demonstrate that. I knew that people loved hearing me talk, no matter what it was I was talking about. It was kind of strange but more and more people were asking me to speak, and I felt like tomorrow was a turning point.

The next morning, I woke really early, and with a bump. I must have been off travelling and having fun with my loved ones in other realms. I woke up laughing and smiling, which is a tale tell sign that it had been a really beautiful evening off in the astral realms. Sometimes I wake up and I don't quite land back in my body properly and it feels weird, almost like I'm still outside of myself. When this happens, I have to meditate and allow my soul time to realign with the human vessel. It's rare that it happens these days, but for a while it used to. This particular morning, I felt great, though.

I sat up in bed and journaled for a while, then I meditated and set the intention for the day, and after that I went to the gym. Despite having a busy day ahead, there was no way I was missing the gym. I wanted those endorphins running through me for the build-up of the day. I sat on the floor in the gym, looking in the mirror, and tears began rolling down my face. Happy, proud and sad tears, all rolled into one. More than anything, I would have loved my grandad to be there with me that day to see me. I know how proud he would have been. As it turned out, none of my family were coming. My mum said she didn't want to see me on stage because she knew I would speak about her if she was there and she would get embarrassed – she knows me too well! My dad was in another kind of a predicament, though. He desperately wanted to come, and so did the twins, but in the light of him telling his wife he was leaving her, he wasn't able to.

I arrived at the ICC and my team were already there. I had organised for an amazing guy I knew to come up from London to film the event for us and my team were on standby to guide him in and look after him until I got there. The team were already in the queue, trying to get as close to the front of the stage as possible, so that I would see them when I was on stage and they could show their support for me. God bless them.

The stage was huge and the whole room was enormous. It was actually quite breathtaking, and a little nerve-wracking. How on earth had little Lucy from Bournemouth ended up here, about to walk out in front of thousands of people? Thankfully, I didn't have much time to digest all of it because I had hair and make-up slots that I had to be ready for. I felt like a princess. I was being waited on, dolled up, and guided through places; people were even stopping to speak to me. It was like I was famous. I never expected any of this at all.

And to make it even more surreal, Ed, the cameraman, turned up with his camera, and started following me around.

The day was flying by and it was only about an hour before I was due to be called on stage. My hair and make-up looked perfect – the girls had done such a good job – I hardly recognised myself, but in a really beautiful way. All I needed to do before I went on was to make a quick change into my stage outfit, and then I would be good to go. I have no idea why I picked a red dress to wear on the stage that day. Red was not really my preferred colour, but I had been really drawn to this little number. It was extremely tight-fitting and so not the kind of thing I would normally have opted for, but somehow I was just guided by my soul to wear this outfit, so that's what I did. I definitely had no idea, at that point, that this little red dress was about to go viral and become an iconic image.

I was standing behind the stage, all mic'd up, ready to go on, when I heard the host start to talk about me. I welled up. It was such a beautiful introduction. It blew me away. I fought back the tears and took a deep breath. All of a sudden, my walk-on tune started playing. The lady backstage said to me, "This is what you came for, it's go time." I started to walk onto the stage, when suddenly a huge download came through me like a bolt out of the blue! In 2004, I'd had a reading with a very well-known tarot reader in Bournemouth. She had said to me that I would end up speaking on stage around the world. I laughed at her when she said it to me. I was on the corporate ladder at the time, with JPMorgan, and I really felt that was my destiny. The thought of speaking on stage made me feel utterly sick at that point. I told the tarot reader there was no chance of that happening and I just dismissed it. Well, I was wrong and she was right. And my guides now chose a totally inappropriate time to remind me to forgive myself for thinking she was crazy. It's interesting how these things tend to come through when we least expect them.

I quickly composed myself, took another deep breath and then walked confidently out onto the stage. The bright lights hit me, I remember throwing my arms in the air as the host on stage came toward me, he picked me up and spun me around. I was not expecting that either. It made me immediately panic about the fact that I had no underwear on, and I was on my period. That could have all gone so horribly wrong! In a way, it helped to distract me from the fact that thousands of faces were looking back at me. As the host put me back down, I grabbed the microphone and shouted, "Woo hoo, Birmingham, let me hear you."

Fuck! It was happening.

The speech went amazing. I had a few emotional moments where I spoke about my grandad and when I thanked my team, but other than that it went amazing. I do not remember what I spoke about. Very early on, I ditched the cards and let the channelling commence.

I now realise why I have never been able to stick to a script. There is wisdom that works through me and it does not require a plan at all. I got to the end of my segment and just blew the audience a kiss and then walked off. Most people stay on stage to be clapped and appreciated. As I went backstage, the host said, "You're supposed to let them cheer for you." I just shrugged, I wasn't really aware of what had gone on. I smiled, hugged them, and then went back to try to find my team – easier said than done.

Everyone and their dog wanted to speak to me after that. One of the senior representatives from the company came running over to me to tell me he thought I was phenomenal, one of the best speakers he had seen. He told me I must make sure I do more speaking for the company. Interestingly, he had loved my channelling – not that he knew that was what was happening – but it made me feel a bit better about how off-piste I had gone. It took me about an hour to get back to my team. People were grabbing me, hugging me, and wanting photos. It was all so weird. And although I wanted to give everyone my time, I was super conscious of the fact I had no pants on and I was on my period.

When I eventually managed to reunite with my team, we had such a giggle. They let me know how they felt it went, and they raved and raved. I'm sure they were all somewhat biased, but who cares, I was going to bask in it for a while. We did some filming with Ed, before settling down to watch the final segments of the event.

When everything was finished, we went back to get ready to go out for the evening, to celebrate.

What an incredible day. I had stepped into my essence. I had found the voice from within, and I was living it, breathing it, and all the while, unknowingly, activating hundreds of people while I was doing it. Everything that I had been told would happen was actually happening. And, of course, it had to be in Birmingham too. A place that had already played a significant role in my life. It always seemed to pull me back again.

I stayed on cloud nine for several days after the event.

93

The timing of my living with dad had been perfect. I was already learning that everything was in divine timing, but this truly proved it to me. However, the time was coming closer for me to move on. I had a massive trip planned for June and July. I had a conference booked in Perth, I had to go to Singapore, and I was also being called to go to Vietnam and Cambodia. I was worried about how my dad would be without me around. I worried that the stress of everything might give him a heart attack or something. Besides being a caring daughter, my ego was piping up. I knew that I had to continue to follow my own path, though, all the whilst doing my best to support my family.

The whole time I had been at my dad's, I had been working hard on my business and it was growing really fast. Towards the end of May, I was doing a Facebook Live in my group, when I saw a message pop up from Ricky. It totally distracted me, and it was obvious to everyone watching – many of them sent me messages afterwards asking what went on. When I got off the call, I checked the message properly. He had written, "Fancy meeting up in Thailand next week?" I hadn't spoken to Ricky for ages, but I was actually going to Singapore next week. How did he keep doing that? How did he know? And what was this strange pull that we had with each other? I messaged him back and told him I was in Singapore that week. He wrote right back and told me to change my plans. His exact words were, "Make it happen. Davis, come on! Make it happen." So, as usual, that's what I did. I changed my plans and arranged to meet him in Thailand in a few days' time.

We spoke briefly after that to make some more plans; Ricky told me that he was in awe of my spiritual journey, and whilst we were away, he wanted me to teach him how I had done it. I thought that was interesting on so many levels. Firstly, I didn't really resonate with the word spiritual as such, I was just letting my life unfold as it did, and how could I teach someone something I didn't even realise I was doing? Secondly, it was Ricky who had actually set me on this path, so he knew all this deep inside of him, he just needed to remember it.

A few days later, I flew to Singapore. I had the most profound experience on the plane. It was absolutely unbelievable. I sat in meditation for the whole thirteen hours. I don't eat on planes anyhow, for many reasons, so I meditated, drank water and had some fruit that I had taken on the plane with me. I was getting incredible downloads whilst in the air, I connected with angels, and what I perceived as God came through in the visions — really profound stuff. There were two Aussie blokes on the plane nearby, and every time I would move I could hear one of them say, "She's moving." I giggled and replied, "I'm not dead, you know." We had a chat and I explained to them what I was doing. I opened up to them. They were fascinated by it all.

The plane landed. I began making my way through Singapore airport. It's such a beautiful airport, with the most stunning view. I was walking on the conveyor belt and all of a sudden I got a message for me to stop, sit down and do a live video on Facebook. Strange I thought. Nevertheless, I found a place to stop and I jumped on Facebook. It resulted in a really beautiful, spontaneous live video from the airport. I shared the insights of what I had been experiencing, all the messages that I had received on the plane, and the beautiful divine connection that I had felt. It was one of my favourite lives to that point in my life. Unfortunately, it got deleted a couple of years later when Facebook took my account down. My quantum healer messaged me after I had done the live and she said to me that she had never seen me embody the feminine like I did in that video. It was a really transformational moment, because I had truly surrendered. I felt as if the fight and the resistance had gone. I had trusted that I needed to be on this trip, even though I didn't know what I was going there for. I had opened up to the men on the plane, and that was poignant to me at that time. These guys had asked me what I was doing and I had opened up and shared my message. I was allowing myself to open to masculine energy. Things were starting to flow, perfectly.

I made my way through Singapore airport and got on my connecting flight to Thailand. I was so excited. There was something about Ricky and I that was puzzling. I had randomly met this dude in 2013 and ever since then, we had kept on being in the same place at random times. We had travelled together, I had seen him in Australia since then. He had come over to Thailand to see me. I had bumped into him in the middle of Vegas. It was bizarre. We would always find each other, even though we lived on opposite sides of the world. I loved him so much because he had set me on my path. He is the reason I am the woman I am today. Besides my grandad, Ricky was the biggest piece of my puzzle.

I had decided to stay in the hotel I always stayed in when I went training, Coco Ville. This place had such a special place in my heart, for so many reasons. The strange thing was, even though Ricky had called me over there, I didn't see him for a couple of days. It was as if he was hiding from me. I started training and I would briefly see him and he would wave and that was it. It was really weird. I felt that he was maybe embarrassed because of his vulnerability in asking me to help him with his spiritual journey.

A few days in, I walked through the reception area of the hotel – the very place where I had first spotted Ricky, all those years ago. Ricky walked in and he couldn't avoid me, so he had no choice but to stop. He gave me a hug, sat down and we talked. He opened up, "I am in awe of you, Lucy. I cannot believe the person that you have become and how much you've changed in five years. I'm so proud of you." We had a really beautiful conversation, and Ricky is not the kind of person to dish out compliments freely. He also told me that he had a friend with him who he wanted to introduce me to.

Later on that evening, I got the opportunity to meet the guy Ricky had been speaking about, Hema. He was lovely. I got on really well with him. Ricky explained that Hema sometimes gets these moments where he receives insights. I thought that was interesting. Ricky then told me to tell Hema the Guatemala story. So I did.

It's a long story, to be fair, and it was getting late, so about an hour into the story, Ricky decided that, as he had already heard it, he was going to go to bed. I had a nice evening on my own with Hema. We laughed our socks off, we cried, you name it. I helped him a little bit to break him through a few things. The key message that I got from talking with both boys, was that they still felt that the spiritual journey was weak, and they came from a world of Muay Thai and boxing where they needed to be strong. I kept saying to them that it isn't about how hard you punch, it's about the mentality that you've got within you. It's about the connection that you've got with self. I suggested to them both that as soon as they learnt to connect to their inner warrior, they would be able to box like they had never boxed before, and fight like they had never fought before.

Halfway through the first week, I was feeling really good in training. I felt strong, I felt fit, and I felt amazing. My trainer said I should try for another fight. I told him I wasn't around for long, but if he could arrange one in time I would. There was something within me that always wanted to test myself, and this was one of those moments.

I walked back to the hotel that afternoon, dripping in sweat from the session and excited about the prospect of another fight. I dumped my stuff in my room, which was divinely arranged to be room 222 again. I threw on my bikini and dived into the pool. Shortly afterwards, Ricky emerged out of his room, I had no idea where he was staying, but I had felt drawn to what turned out to be his room the whole time I was in the pool. He got in, I sat on the side and we began chatting. In the middle of the conversation, I got a clear message, "Twin flame." I thought — *What the fuck is that?* I had no idea. I was trying to speak to Ricky but I was being distracted by this constant message that kept coming through, "Twin flame!"

I said to Ricky, "I'm really sorry but I'm going to have to excuse myself and go back to my room to meditate on this message I keep getting."

Ricky said, "That freaks the fuck out of me, but you do what you've got to do."

I went back to my room and meditated on this twin flame thing that was coming through. I've got a deal with my guides that I don't research anything. They will give me what I need, but I will not ever research. It's a bit weird and a lot of people will ask me if what I am saying is my own stuff or research, but it's always my stuff. The only time I will ever research is when they tell me to. Other than that, I'm going to live on my intuition. I'm going to trust. Back then, I wasn't so sure of myself with this, but now I know that this is the way that it has to be. I don't need to look things up unless I'm told very, very clearly. I always trust the messages, and that people will deliver the information that I need. I knew a massive part of my journey was about learning how to trust, learning how to be present, learning how to get the messages, and then integrating them. I'm not here to tell people to do it this way, or to do it that way. I can only say that this is how I did it. It might be the same for you, but it might not, so trust, and you will find the way that it needs to work for you. Now, there are many incredible people out there who research to the max, and I'm not saying that they're doing it wrong. That's their method. This is mine.

On this occasion though, I was told very clearly, without hesitation, that I had to research what twin flames were. I asked several times if I was supposed to research it and the answer was clear. I grabbed my laptop and thought – *Okay, show me where you want me to go.* I typed 'twin flame' into the search engines and the first thing that came up was YouTube, with a selection of videos. Lots of options came up, many of them were two hours long, and as you've probably guessed by now, I'm not that kind of girl. You've got seven minutes of my time to get my attention, otherwise, I'm gone. I found a short, seven-minute video. I clicked on it, and it started telling me what a twin flame was. I listened intently, slightly blown away. I'm almost certain my eyes got wider and my mouth dropped open as I heard what she shared. Wow! Two people sharing fragments of the same soul, but in two different physical vessels. How was that even possible? She then went onto explain that your twin flame is like looking at yourself in the mirror – the good, the bad, and the ugly. All of it would be shown to you from this other person who would have stumbled into your life in an extremely 'random', yet intense way.

The whole point of the journey, whereby twins agree to incarnate at the same time, is mission driven. Yes, you could be in an intimate relationship with that person; however, it was much more about your missions aligning, and your agreement is to mirror back to each other until the awakening occurs. Often you will love them, hate them, care for them and want them to sort their shit out, all in the space of a day. It is about reminding each other of the work you are here to do. Twins incarnate together, collide at a set time in history, to rewrite relationships, love, health, healing and life.

I watched a few more short videos, then sat and processed everything I had seen. That's when the lightbulbs started coming on. You get on so well, are extremely passionate about similar things, then catastrophic events would make you run away – often annoyed with each other. *Sounds familiar* – I thought. You will then find yourself colliding with them in the weirdest of places, to bring back into

PART THREE – THE JOURNEY HOME

your consciousness what you agreed to do. You are normally seven years minimum apart in age. Yep, that's true!

Then, it hit me properly! Ricky is my twin flame! Fuck! Fuck! Fuck!

I'll be honest, I wanted to run. I wanted to pack my bags and run because this scared the shit out of me. This person was put in my life, first and foremost, to awaken me. Secondly, he was there to mirror everything I hated about myself back to me. He had changed me without any shadow of a doubt. Everything I hated about myself, I could see in him, it had annoyed me, made me want to shout, punch and kick him at times. Well, well, well. All of a sudden it made total sense, but it was also something that I really did not want to deal with.

I avoided him for a couple of days, focusing on my training, until one day he stopped me and asked me why I was avoiding him. I couldn't tell him, though. He wasn't ready to hear anything like that. I wasn't sure if he ever would be. Something that I've learnt very clearly is that we're not here to cut corners for other people. We are here to allow ourselves, and other people, to go through our own journey, in our own time. If I told him, he would have gone completely batshit crazy and I would have felt like I was controlling him. As much as I loved him, I did not want him to be my twin flame. He was all of the things I did not wish to see in myself. This revelation was a total headfuck.

I still haven't even told him to this very day. So if you are reading this book Ric, now you know who you are. Surprise!

One day, though, he cornered me and asked me to go to the track and do some circuits with him. I couldn't avoid it, there was just no way, and so I said okay. I suggested separate mopeds because at that time I just couldn't handle being too close to him. We had a great laugh at the track that day. I was off running and Ricky was taking photos of me. That's the funny thing, he's just like me with his photography. He's just like me in so many ways, it's actually ridiculous. That's why we loved each other and got on each other's nerves at the same time. We were the same person, just different souls. It's just so weird when you stop and think about it. As we were leaving, Ric asked someone to take a photo of us both. It's a truly beautiful picture, but the weird thing is that we actually look really alike. That blew my mind even more so. It's so strange. How can two total strangers from opposite sides of the planet actually be so linked?

Later that evening, when I was in my room, I started looking back at some of the old photos of us both. There was one particular picture, where Ricky is cornering me in my first fight in Thailand, and we are both pulling the exact same face. This twin thing went super deep, something I had never noticed before.

More and more the penny was dropping. The lightbulbs were going off. It was like Blackpool illuminations in my head. I could imagine my guides celebrating – *She's finally got it!*

The next morning, I woke up and I had this awful feeling that something had happened to my dad, but because it was the middle of the night in the UK, there was nobody I could speak to. I messaged my sister to see if she was up, but she wasn't. Several hours later, I got a message back from my sister, "Can you call me?" It's never good when somebody says that. I called her and she told me my dad had been assaulted in his own home. The police had to be called.

Two things ran through my mind – the first was that I was furious, and I wanted this situation to be over, and fast! The second thing, was that this was the get-out-of-jail card with Ricky that I had been looking for. I couldn't handle being around him, I couldn't process what I had been told. And as much as I didn't want to repeat my pattern of running away, especially as now I had such awareness on it, I had to go home to be with my dad. I immediately booked a flight, before I spoke to anybody else.

I walked out of my room and, of course, the first person I bumped into was Ricky. I was short with him.

"What's wrong?" he asked.

"I just need to go to the gym. I'll catch you later."

"Is everything okay? You don't seem yourself."

I blurted it out, "I'm going home."'

He looked confused. "I thought you were going to Cambodia and Vietnam, and you were going to come and see me in Sydney."

I had never agreed to the Sydney part, but I just said to him, "My dad's been assaulted, I need to get back to him."

He was shocked but really supportive. He said, "Is there anything I can do to help? Are you sure you've got to go?"

"I've made my mind up. I need to get home. I don't know how long for, but I know I have to come to Perth at some point soon." I hugged him and said goodbye, not knowing when I would see him again, if ever.

I called my sister and told her I was coming home. I told her not to tell anyone because if they knew I was on my way back then they would know a shit-storm was coming. Then, I called my dad to see how he was doing. I said, "Look, Dad, I've booked a flight, I'm coming home. I don't care what you say. I need to make sure that you're okay. I need to make sure that everything is good before I go again." The most beautiful thing about this was, although I was repeating a very old programme of running away from one situation, I was also running to something I hadn't been before. I was stepping into this Mother Energy that Chaty had told me was going to happen. I had stepped into the warrior woman, and it wasn't about me having a fight anymore. It was about me standing in my truth, speaking up, being authentic, and making sure that I lived so honestly that everybody around me could do the same.

That same evening, I got on a flight and flew through the night, landing back at Heathrow the next morning. As I touched down, I knew that a whole new phase of transformation was about to take place. Mumma Bear was home, it was time to protect my family.

94

I grabbed my things, jumped into a taxi and headed in the direction of my dad's house. A massive part of me was very aware that I could easily step into the old Lucy right now. I could be angry. I could be hurt. I could be aggressive. I could have really stamped my feet. What the fuck was going on? I had made the conscious decision that I wasn't going to take that angry and aggressive approach, as much as I wanted to.

I knew there were signs and lessons for all of us in this process. And the biggest lesson of all — that come through whilst I had been on the plane flying home — was that this was about to be my dad's karma unfolding. This was going to be a huge karmic journey for him, and it was not my place to be changing that for him, as much as I wanted to. This was the new Lucy coming through. A Lucy that held space for people to recognise what they had done and what they needed to step into, and to not fall into fixer mode. It was very challenging, though, I have to admit. Imagine knowing how to help someone as close as me and my dad were, and not being able to tell them how to fix it. This was going to be a challenge.

When I finally arrived home, everybody was shocked. They all knew I had a fight planned in Thailand and so weren't expecting me to be there. The relief on my dad's face was unbelievable. I got emotional as I hugged him. I knew it had been the right decision to make. The relief on my older sister's face was clear too – my being there meant that she could go home. The people behind the attack on my dad had created a lot of fear, and that was the real reason I was home. I knew that some clear boundaries needed to be set. I knew conversations needed to be had, but not conversations coming from a place of anger; conversations coming from a space of setting boundaries – what was and was not acceptable.

I wasn't going to be home for long, so I spent the next couple of days making sure that my dad was okay physically. There were a few conversations that we needed to have with the police, and there were lots of conversations that needed to take place internally within our family. My older sister was still in a place of aggression. She was in the protective fight or flight energy, which she had been living for many years – she was a fighter too and that was how she had trained herself to think. Anybody that attacked her family was attacking her directly and she would fight them all if she had to. There was a lot that needed to be dealt with personally as well because I didn't want to step back into those old patterns or mirror my sister.

There was a lot of evolution for me in those few days that I was back. And I loved it. It was the most interesting, challenging, and exciting period I had experienced up to that point. Even though I was dealing with a difficult situation, I was watching the way I handled things and learning how to do it from a space of love, rather than taking the old over-emotional route. What I didn't realise at the time, I was in training for my future work, for when my clients were to go through extremely challenging experiences – which, in fairness, I often invoke in them.

The few days that I was back were truly a gift to me, and, consequently, to my family too. It was an up-levelling of my own personal journey, but it was also an up-levelling of how I communicated. I had to be very careful not to evoke negative emotions from my dad or my sister and bring up their anger again. I also needed to master my communication and question the people that had taken part in this attack. I had to be the neutral in a situation where I wasn't neutral. I learnt how to master my ego very quickly — especially around anger. I learnt how to master walking away and not being dragged into other people's emotional states — whether that be crying, anger, aggression, shame, guilt, or resentment. I was around all of these feelings during the few days that I was home. It's strange to say it, but it was a really beautiful experience.

People often ask me when I'm coaching people, how do I know when to step in, when to step out, and when to poke the bear? And it stems from this situation. This was the start of it. This is where I started to become very aware of how human behaviour works, and what people need to hear from a vibrational perspective. This situation was as challenging as it gets because I was completely entangled in my family and my love for them, so I had to learn to tap into a different aspect of me so that I was getting the vibrational frequency rather than getting entangled in the emotional state and the ego.

It literally took me just 48 hours to get everything to a place of being calm again. There was no bickering, bitching or hurling insults at each other. Not whilst I was there.

It's interesting looking back at this time. I see the old stories — the fixer and the rescuer — just wanting to run and help my dad; however, the most obvious one was the runner. I really wanted to run from all the feelings that had come up in recognising that, in all actuality, the person who had been really pissing me off over the last few years was in fact myself.

Ouch! It stung.

95

Perth had become a really big part of my life since that first visit in December 2014. Although Australia had always been a massive deal to me, Perth hadn't been on my radar until that first visit, but that trip changed everything for me. I now had a group of friends that resided in Perth, so I had something worth returning for. My friend, Hannah — the nurse — had invited me to go to a conference with her in 2016 and something had shifted within me at that event. A lady was speaking, a beautiful lady, called Linda – I can still remember what she looked like and how stunning she was. Her message had hit hard. It resonated with my soul and was without question intended for me. As she was speaking, I looked at my friend and said, "That's going to be me." That was back in 2016, and here I was just two years later, and it was me.

By this point in my life, in 2018, I had about 15,000 followers on Facebook due to me sharing insights of what I was doing on that platform. Every day I would do a Facebook live video, sharing a beautiful message that felt resonant. More often than not, I would not have any idea what I would speak about until I got on there. I would just allow the information to channel through. People loved it. At this time, I was very much about looking after health and healing because I had gone on such a beautiful healing and awakening journey. I was very focused on the physical human body. I would motivate, inspire and offer guidance to other souls, although I did not see it like that at the time. I felt like I was helping my fellow humans. It was weird, I could speak so well. I could make things very easy for people to understand. I never had any formal speaking training, no guidance or even a mentor for speaking or spirituality. Doing it this way, possibly made it much more challenging for me, but clearly that was the intended path, and I embraced it.

By this point, I had learnt to trust more and more that wherever I went, I would meet messengers – in the shape of people, signs, places, and animals – who would help me on the next leg of the journey. I knew that there was more to life than what I had been told. I hadn't just gotten out of my relationship with Kyle and thrown away my career to then be half-arsed about it; I was going after it with everything I had. I knew I had a big mission and I had to fulfil that role, whatever that ended up looking like. I also knew by this point that whatever I thought it would look like, would unlikely be the eventual reality.

I got on the plane to Perth, and it was the first time I'd ever done the direct flight from London Heathrow. It was a 16-hour flight. I was excited. I always get really beautiful downloads whenever I fly; perhaps being closer to God or to what we might call the higher realms, I don't know. It's like there is a more profound link in when I'm flying. This flight was no different. By the time I got off the plane in Perth, I felt so full of love, joy, and happiness. I felt like I was home, and I had never experienced that with Perth before.

My friend, Hannah, picked me up from outside the airport. When we saw each other we went crazy. We hugged, screamed and bounced through the airport. Although we lived on opposite sides of the world and saw each other very rarely, she had become one of my soul sisters. She was somebody I trusted; somebody that I would fly across the world to see. That's really incredible when you think we only met in December 2014 at a random party; random, never random. So if you stop and actually think about those divine connections and how they play out, the divine plan is unbelievable. Every single person comes into your life to serve you, to bring messages and to deliver things to you. Sometimes it is for just a short period of time, it doesn't necessarily have to be forever. Although, sometimes, thankfully, it is forever.

In her car, on the way back from the airport to her dad's house, we were singing along to songs on the radio, dancing and just having a right old laugh. It was funny, because whenever we had travelled together before she had always been holding on for dear life on the back of my moped. Now the roles were reversed and I was the passenger in her car.

By the time we got back to her dad's house, I was pretty exhausted, so we decided to go to the supermarket and get some food for us to make at home. Hannah loved the way that I cook, and so she was pretty insistent that I make us some of the new recipes I had been sharing. I am going to be bold enough to say, everybody loves my food. Whenever I post pictures of it on my social media, I have messages asking for a recipe book. Likewise, whenever anybody comes to my house and they sample the goods for themselves, they get so excited because they taste the different flavours and textures. Everybody asks me what my secret is, no matter what I cook. I'm happy to reveal right here in this book that my secret sauce is love. People don't get it when they're preparing food. They just throw stuff together. I don't create things like that. I create food by giving thanks for what's been delivered to the shop from where I bought it. I give thanks for being able to afford it, and then thanks for all the beautiful colours and nutrients that are going to flood my body from Mother Nature. This is the reason why, no matter what I make – whether it is a quick snack or if I take a lot of time creating a masterpiece – everybody always says that I should open up a restaurant.

That first evening in Perth, with Hannah, I made a beautiful aubergine roll. The recipe came out of nowhere really and I created it in under an hour, whilst we chatted and had a glass of organic red wine. I created a masterpiece for dinner. It was delightful. After dinner, I decided to take an early night to get into the Perth timezone.

The next morning, I was up really early to do my rituals.

Since returning to the UK back in 2015, I had found myself drawn to setting myself up for each day with a series of tasks – what I would call rituals – that I would do each morning after waking up. It had started with water, exercise and listening to a good motivational speech, but over the years, and at this point in my life, it had evolved into so much more. Each morning, without fail, I would get my body set up for success. When I say that, I think of the image of starting a car with zero fuel. It may start, but it will chug along until it gets the fuel it needs to keep it going. We are the same. What I identified is that if I had a good intake of water first thing in the morning, I felt more energised and I had greater clarity. After that, I would take my supplements. The supplements I took back then are the same ones I take today – loaded with real fruits and vegetables to nourish my cells. No matter what happens in my life, those little babies are my consistent. They flood my cells with the good stuff, so no matter what, my body is firing on all cylinders.

In 2018, I changed the order of my rituals around. I began to take time to jot down all of the thoughts that have been going through my mind. This has been one of my biggest saviours on this journey. If you ask me, writing, or what I refer to as journaling, should be made mandatory for the sake of peace on Earth. My clients will be rolling their eyes as they read this. And, in fairness, I do go on about this a lot – but that is because I know how helpful it is. They might moan, and say they do not have the time and make all kinds of excuses to begin with, but when they actually do it, they realise how important it is too.

I like to finish my rituals with exercise. I truly believe we have to move our body, to sweat a little each day. The 3 P's should become normalised in the first few hours of the day – Pee, Perspire and Poop.

That morning in Perth was no different. I did my rituals and then Hannah and I decided to go for a nice long walk along the beach.

PART THREE – THE JOURNEY HOME

From that day on, something strange started occurring. The Universe started communicating with me in an extremely obvious way. Since 2013, it was becoming pretty obvious to me that I was being guided through signs, but this was more like literal slaps from the Universe; and they just kept coming until I 'got it'.

Out of nowhere, I kept seeing signs for Sydney everywhere I went. We would be walking through a mall and there would be pictures, artwork and books about Sydney in the windows. We would be driving along roads and there would be a billboard with Sydney on it. After a few days, Hannah actually said to me, "Have you noticed that Sydney keeps popping up? I've lived here my whole life and have never seen it before. I think Sydney's trying to get your attention." Hannah was unaware at this point that Ricky had suggested that I fly down to Sydney whilst on this trip to Australia. I didn't have the time to go, so it just wasn't worth discussing. Also, I was due back there in September, which was only a couple of months away. It could wait!

Hannah had met Ricky in Thailand, and although she didn't know he was my twin flame, she knew that there was a history between the two of us because we would speak about it openly. People often said things to us like, "Oh, you two should be together." And I would reply, "Yeah, we tried that once, not great." We had good banter about it. Hannah, though, like many others, believed that there was such a deep connection between Ricky and I, that one day we would realise it, move forward from the old and go on an amazing journey together. Most people are in love with the idea of being in love, if you top that with a bloody good love story, people find themselves heavily invested. They certainly were with Ricky and I. They were right to some extent, there was a deep connection between us both, and whether I liked it or not – or would dare admit it at that time – he had changed me significantly. After my grandad, he had set me on my path to what I would call my spiritual awakening. Yes, he irritated the heck out of me, but if I hadn't met him, would I have been here? The answer is probably no. So, I have a lot to thank him for.

It got to the point over the next few days, where the signs were so intense and relentless – Sydney, Sydney, Sydney! Wherever we went, someone would mention it, they would even ask if I was from there; my social media seemed littered with images of Sydney too. The more the signs appeared, the more Hannah became convinced

I was being pulled to Sydney for him. She laughed and told me to 'woman up' and go.

Unexpectedly, as if I had not heard or seen enough, I then received a message from Ricky. "You're in Australia, why don't you pop down again?" I was laughing by this point. Firstly, 'pop down' – it's a 5-hour flight between Perth and Sydney, it's hardly down the road. Secondly, I was starting to recognise the power in all of these beautiful souls who really wanted me to be happy, fall in love and live this romantic love story. They were truly creating something that I was going to have to work through. I remember thinking – *Oh my God, everybody is focussing on this so much that they're actually manifesting it into reality for me.* I explained to him that, as planned, I was coming in September, and there was no way I could do it before then. I had already skipped Singapore to see him in Thailand. He had enough of my time. I was also still processing what I found out over there. In a few months, maybe I would be ready to deal with it all. He was persistent, though, and cheeky with it too. He knew how to play me. He said, "Please come and grace us with your presence, there's stuff you need to do here." As much as I was loving the banter and the attention, I was firm. No meant no.

The more I resisted, the more the Universe kept slapping me hard in the face. It got silly. There were small things like the fact that at the conference I attended a number of the speakers were from Sydney, but I was in Australia, so that's kind of expected. It was the more bizarre, random things that were interesting. People I would get chatting with in coffee shops would be from Sydney. Unexpected conversations in a restaurant with a stranger, who for no reason would explain to me the reason why it is so important that Sydney is situated where it is. It wasn't just a case of connecting dots that weren't connected, it was a relentless barrage of Sydney.

Why on earth was the Universe so desperate for me to visit Sydney now?

The conference itself was an amazing experience. Lots of positive things happened there, and I was truly grateful for the opportunity to stand on stage and realise a dream of mine.

The day after, when I had no obligations and commitments to honour, I went to the beach on my own. I felt I needed some alone time with Mother Nature. I had been around people a lot more than I would normally be, so I took myself off to explore, connect and get grounded, away from the intense energies of all the various personalities around me.

Whilst on the beach, from nowhere, I put my arms out and spun around in the sand. I spun round and round and round until I collapsed on the floor, like a child would do – spinning like a spinning top and then falling down dizzy. As I lay in the sand, laughing at myself, I started singing at the top of my voice. A man walked by with his son and his dog, and he came over to me and said, "It's so beautiful to see somebody at such peace with themselves. Just letting it all go." I thought that that was such a beautiful message to receive because, in all honesty, I had become a little bit frustrated. A few things had confused me whilst I'd been in Perth, especially the stuff about Sydney. As much as I was finding it funny, it was annoying me a little bit. I was feeling unsure about whether I should be going over there. It was June now, and I was going to be there in just a few months. So why all the signs? Admittedly, I had stepped into victim mode about it at times.

Being at the beach cleared my head, though. The beach is one of the spots I choose as my safe space; it very quickly helps the re-alignment of my soul.

I stood up and walked along the shore. I set a really clear boundary with Gaia. I said to her, "I'm not going to Sydney on this trip. I'm going to be there in September. That's not far away, but that's my decision." I then felt drawn to walk into the ocean, even though I was fully clothed in my running gear. I walked in up to my waist, closed my eyes and I said to her, "I will do for you whatever you need me to do. Please let me rest and provide all I can possibly require to thrive whilst on the journey'.

Unknowingly, I had placed a covenant in place with Gaia. I'll be honest, I didn't even know what a freaking covenant was at this point. I had basically created a contract between Gaia and I. She could use my vessel. She could send me wherever she needed to send me; I'd pick up the lessons I would need, and do whatever it was that she needed me to do.

You feed me and I'll feed you.

Simple as that. I was happy to be that vessel.

96

The next afternoon, I said my goodbyes to everyone in Perth and headed to the airport. It was time to head off to Vietnam. Vietnam was another place that had been calling me significantly over the years, but I had ignored it up until now. It's funny when I look back. There was absolutely no rhyme or reason why I feared certain countries and not others.

I had not realised until boarding the aircraft, that it was a full moon that evening. Unknowingly, over the years, I had very frequently ended up flying on a new or full moon. When the moon is in these phases, the energies are quite profound. I know there are many varied opinions on the moon — people ask me all the time if it's a satellite, a hologram, or if it's even real. From my perspective, it really doesn't matter. People see the moon for whatever they choose. The main thing I focus on is that regardless of your opinion, people often use the energy of the moon and focus on it — for better or for worse. It's the same with the sun, sea, positivity, or negativity. If you use your energy at times to focus on something, then anything can be harnessed and used for the good, bad or ugly. It's all about the intent behind it. Personally, I don't have a bone in my body that harbours ill intent. During my awakening journey, I had done the work to remove any such negative tendencies. In going through my dark night of the soul, I had realised so much. I had been utterly delusional about myself and the world throughout my life, and I say all this with zero judgement. We have all been conditioned to be this way through the specific circumstances of our life, and the programming we receive through school, through television and media, and through other people's beliefs — and it all leads to anger, resentment, fear, jealousy and all the other lower vibrational emotions.

By this point, though, everything in my life was to do with love. I wanted everybody to succeed. I wanted to give everybody what I had. There wasn't anything to compete about. It was all about love, and coming from love in any decision or discussion that took place. Although I was still in the infancy stages of my journey, I knew my mission was to bring love back to the world. There are amazing people that have gone before me and attempted with all their hearts to bring love to the world, but they were held back, challenged, and halted because the time wasn't right for the collective consciousness to shift as we needed it to. This was the time. And I knew it. I didn't know how I knew it. Nobody had come down and said to me, "Hey, Lucy, you need to act right now." It was a nagging feeling within my soul. I hadn't been where I'd been – to the depths of darkness – after selling my soul to the devil in my career and lifestyle, to not transmute and transform it all and then remind everyone else how to do it too. I had been selected to go through it all so I could remember what it felt like to laugh, to learn, and to feel vulnerability. I was totally focused, completely on purpose and I wanted to share that.

I boarded my flight to Vietnam, knowing it was going to be a long night of travel. Vietnam had been calling me for a very long time, but I had no idea where I was going. I had not researched anything. That's the whole point of travelling intuitively; however, over the years, many people have thought I'm crazy. And they're right!

Once we were in the air, the plane turned around, so the full moon was shining directly in my window for most of the flight. I basked in the energies of the moon contemplating my mission, excited to see what it was that Vietnam had been calling me for. Once again, the Wanderess was off.

Eventually, several hours later, we touched down. As I stepped off the plane I could not help but smile at that familiar feeling of warmth that hit me. It was unbelievably hot; 40 plus degrees. You could feel the heat despite the air conditioning. I wasn't prepared for it at all. I was wearing jeans that stuck to me like glue in the heat. Bad move! It had been winter in Australia and despite everyone believing Australia is super-hot all the time, winter over there is cold. This transition into the heat was greatly welcomed, apart from. my wardrobe choices.

I jumped in a taxi from the airport to my hotel. The hotel wasn't anything special, but was decent enough for a night or two, until I moved on to the next location when the intuitive pulls come through. This is always my pattern. I pick a location that feels right to fly into, find somewhere cheap and cheerful to stay for a night or two maximum, then from there on I follow the pulls. That level of trust and surrender is where the gold happens. So many times in the past I have wanted to make it make sense, but of course, it's not meant to make sense, and so as a result of trying to make it make sense I missed places or my ego talked me out of it. Once I arrive in a place, as long as it is daylight, I dump my things and go off wandering, looking for what on earth it is that had called me there. A sign would normally appear relatively quickly. People who have travelled on their own will appreciate the fact that we always meet who we need to. You'll be thinking of something, then a stranger will somehow say something that will lead you on to what you did not even realise you were looking for. Travelling the world on my own has been one of the most beneficial experiences of my life. It has opened up so much inside of me; it's given me confidence and trust. It has made me much more street-wise and I have learnt how to communicate with people from all over the world, albeit in broken languages.

Everywhere you walk in the tourist areas of Vietnam, there are young students looking for English people to practise their English with. It's quite a common thing, they're not doing anything bad, they just want to learn and what better way to learn a language than with people who are fluent in it. I had stopped on my walk to take some photographs of something that had caught my eye, when a young boy came up to me and asked me if he could speak to me. We began talking. He told me he was a doctor – which was strange in itself because he looked like a little boy. He explained how he wanted to help improve his language so that he could go and work in the West somewhere one day. He said he could go to work in a hospital but he felt that he had something that he wanted to share with people. I thought it was beautiful. This incredible young man was so vulnerable. What he didn't realise was, and I felt this strongly, he was training to be a doctor and going through everything he needed to go through, but he had a bigger purpose, and I could tell that his soul knew it from the way he spoke. He had realised, on some level, that there was something inside of him that he needed to share with the world. I ended up talking to him for about two hours, so that he could practice his English. His English was actually amazing, he didn't need to practice really, but the opportunity to speak to an English person was helpful to him. I enjoyed the exchange immensely. The only reason we stopped talking was because he had to go to work at the hospital and would be late if he stayed any longer. What a beautiful and kind little messenger I received, and he was one of the first people I engaged with.

I walked on a little bit further, three very sweet, young Vietnamese girls came up to me and asked me if they could practice their English also. They looked so young and appeared to be in school uniform. I spoke with them for a while too. They asked me what I was doing, I explained that I had no idea. They all looked a bit confused. I tried to explain my intuitive healing journey to them. One of the girls asked if we could take a photo together. I still have that photo on my phone. Those girls left an imprint in my heart. Everywhere I go, people leave their footprints in my heart. After we had taken a photo, one of the girls said to me, "Whatever it was that brought you here, we are so grateful because it's like we've been graced with an angel." What another beautiful message to receive. And the feeling was mutual. These beautiful locals had shown me so much, unknowingly.

After I had said goodbye to the girls, I walked for a little while on my own. I sat down and watched people for a while. As I sat there, I kept hearing the word in my mind – Monk. Monk. Monk. It wasn't clear, just something to do with a monk. My first thought was to go and see if I could find a monastery or maybe find a church in the local area that may well be of assistance to me. This is how intuitive travel works. A word, a picture or a vision will appear in my mind's eye, or even sometimes in my physical eyes, and then I follow that and see what happens and see where it guides me. I walked around for about an hour looking for anything to do with religion. I stumbled across a few churches, but it was very clear they were not where I needed to be. So, as I was walking back to my hotel, I stated the intention, "Please bring me more information. If there's something that you would like me to see to do with the monks, all you need to do is show me with much more clarity, and I will do what is required."

I got back to the hotel, grabbed some quick food and went to bed, after all the travel and the walking, plus the heat, I was absolutely shattered.

I woke up the next morning and I had been off with a monk in my sleep. I tend to remember quite a lot of my dreams, or what I like to call superconscious state memories. Interestingly, whilst doing my rituals, I was shown the monk again. This time I could sense that the monk was wearing an orangey red colour, and I was seeing his face much clearer now. Still, though, I had absolutely no idea what it meant or who he was. I mean, how do you find a monk? I wasn't thinking of using the internet, but even if I did, can you do a search on monks? I had no idea how I was going to find out, so I set the intention again, "I'm going to go and do what I need to do because I'm being drawn to a couple of other places. If you want to give me some more information on this monk, then please show me."

Nothing came that day. Clearly, I was meant to just sit with it. So, I went off exploring all of these weird and wonderful places that I felt drawn to. I found a beautiful place, overflowing with trees, plants and wildlife – it's hard to describe because it wasn't a forest or a jungle, just a beautiful park-like area that was so mystical it ignited memories within me. In that space, the elements of Earth, Air, Fire, and Water started flooding through me. It made me sit up as it gripped my attention. What was it about? Why were they showing me this? Everywhere I started to look, from that point on, there would be signs of the elements. Wherever I went, people would be talking about them. Just in the same way Sydney had kept coming up and showing itself to me, now the elements were doing the same.

I found a place to sit, have a drink and try to make some sense of what was going on. There was a map in the cafe and when I looked at the map, I felt really drawn to a specific place. So, I did what I do best, I went to find a little travel agent and asked, "How do I get there?" There and then, I booked a trip to go the next day.

97

The next day, a minibus picked me up and took me to a coach, with a group of other people who were heading the same way as I was. Of course, the person that sat next to me for the journey was from Sydney; just to let me know that Sydney was still going to nag away at me. That person actually delivered a couple of messages and told me a couple of places that I needed to go to. So, I was extremely grateful to them; divinely placed to assist my wandering.

After a fair distance of a drive, we got off at a temple. From the second I stepped off the coach, the elements were everywhere – as we were crossing bridges and driving down roads, on doorways and walls. I journaled about it because it was becoming so prevalent and I wanted to keep a note of all the signs I was receiving. My journaling was quite primitive at that time, not the ten-page rambles that I do every day today. Back then, I would write these little clues, signs and things that people mentioned. I did this to see the patterns or the frequency that things came up, to connect the dots. If a place came up three times, that was the three strikes I required to consider it more seriously.

At the temple, I started getting huge insights. Gods and goddesses were coming to me. More monks were coming in too – all of these different, incredible people were coming to me. Now, when I say that 'they're coming to me', I don't mean they physically arrive, what I mean is that in my mind's eye I see them. I started to see the structures of these people. I could see that there were monks walking in front of me, or that people were praying to the monks in a certain area where I was being guided to. I remember, at one point in the temple, there was a sudden, massive gust of wind – an actual physical gust of wind. It was powerful. I knew something was trying to get my attention in the spot where I was. The element of Air was swooshing around me, to encourage me to look around and see what other signs were there and to lead me onward. Then I would look somewhere else and there would be a fire symbol. The dots started to connect more and more. I am sure it would not have made sense to anyone else. It isn't meant to. When people message me asking me what things mean, I throw it back at them. It's supposed to make sense to you, that's it. That's how this works. It's your higher connection speaking to you in the language it knows it can get your attention. Only you know what things feel like for you.

After we had finished at the temple, I asked the driver of the coach what the relevance of the elements were over here. He gave me an interesting insight. He showed me how a lot of things in Vietnam are actually based on the elements, to bring in the grounding and to make sure that the people are considerate of Mother Nature because these are her elements and they should be respected. I thought what he said was really beautiful. And at that very moment, I got the message about the covenant I had made with Gaia, that unknowing covenant I had put in place dancing on the beach in Perth. The elements were how Gaia was actually talking to me. It was Mother Nature bringing through her language as she was working out the best way to communicate with me. We were figuring out our relationship together, and how to call out to each other. She was bringing in the signs to let me know, to remind me what it was I was to look for as guidance. I hadn't connected the dots until this man spoke to me. He was a messenger. Another one. I know this all sounds weird, it was weird to me too, but this is exactly how it happened.

On the coach on the way back, it was no longer any surprise to me that I sat next to somebody else who was from Sydney. It was actually becoming quite comical. The Universe sure did have a sense of humour. I could almost hear her laughing at me as I rolled my eyes. I wondered how many times she had done her best to get my attention over the years and I totally missed the point. I wondered if that's why she was slapping me so hard now, laughing as I finally got the memo.

As soon as I arrived back at my hotel, I decided it was time to move on. Just like that. I packed my stuff and sorted the route out of there. I had been given a few clues through people during the day, so now it was time to explore where I was required to be. Even if I did not know what I was doing, I always knew I was placed exactly where I was required.

I arrived in Hoi An later that day and although it was very, very busy, it truly had a magical feel to it. It was beautiful. I knew I had to be there. It had all the typical structures that you would associate with Vietnam – the wooden boats on the river, people selling fruit and vegetables. Oddly, it was a thriving tourist trap. It was rare I was sent to such busy places, I preferred the kind of places that were off the beaten track, but I don't get to choose; I tend to do as I'm metaphysically told. I was meandering around, enjoying the sunshine and the scenery, when it started happening again. I had that familiar feeling of people looking at me. I looked around to see if I was imagining it, but I know I wasn't. I seemed to become very familiar to the local people all of a sudden. Very much like when I was walking through Tena in the Amazon rainforest. Large numbers of people started staring at me, stopping me and asking for pictures. It was so weird. What did they know? Did they think I was someone else? I had a lady actually cross the road to come over and ask me for a picture. I had no idea what was going on. I thought they were bonkers but I politely obliged. There are probably loads of pictures of me all over the world, posing with Vietnamese people. There was something that they saw that I couldn't see. I was somehow familiar to them. I mean, I knew that I was very much connected with Asia; every time I went there, I felt like it was home, but this was ridiculous.

I was walking around and three ladies walked by, typical Vietnamese women; holding long sticks across their shoulders and carrying bunches of bananas and fruits in baskets on each end of the sticks. They stopped me and I had a conversation with them for about 20 minutes. I took some pictures with them; we are laughing and smiling, I'm wearing one of their hats, I've got their sticks over my shoulder. It was beautiful. We were just so familiar and at ease with each other. They just knew me. They knew my soul. They knew my heart. At no point did they attempt to sell anything, or push anything, they just wanted to connect.

I spent a couple of days like this, meandering around this beautiful town, chatting to people. The monk kept coming up, again and again, and so I had a word with the Universe. *Tell me who this man is. You've got to show me. You cannot expect me to guess, guide me.* I decided that I needed to go on a bit of a mission and try to find a monastery again, or to see if I can find something to appease this monk who was calling to me.

Vietnam is stunning, I find it so beautiful there, a bit like Thailand was before the tourism changed it so much. Vietnam was very, very hot at that time of year, though. One afternoon, after not being on a pedal bike for many years, I went cycling in 44 degrees of sunshine. If you are prepared to go off-piste in Vietnam you can find some incredible places. It's probably not the most sensible thing to do, but when you're on a mission to find a monk, you do what you've got to do. I was in the middle of nowhere and so cycling was the only option, if I wanted to get about. I cycled through rice fields, down country lanes, along beaches – but I never stumbled across a monastery, or anything remotely like it, the whole time. I could feel it pulling me, in my heart, but I couldn't find it. I won't research things unless I'm told to, but, at that moment, my ego desperately wanted to research and make it easier. I trusted it was not quite the right time.

My life now is an intuitive journey. I am an intuitive, predominantly. Yes, I'm psychic. Yes, I've got other amazing gifts, but first and foremost, I am an intuitive. I know that by doing online research would be like me switching off this gift that I've got and I would be doing myself a disservice. Some people might call that lazy. Some people might call it ignorant, but regardless, I just trust.

I went out for dinner that night on my own, and one of my girlfriends from back home messaged me. She's always been a really incredible messenger through my journey. She once told me that she had a vision of me walking through the ocean and it split to let me through. At the time, I thought she was nuts, but with the wisdom I have now, it makes a lot more sense. Sitting at the restaurant, she sent an image to me, and she wrote, "I just had to send you this." The picture she sent me was one of those inspirational quotes with an image behind it, and the picture she sent me was of the monk. The same monk that I had been seeing in my mind for so long. It was him. I had found him. And it had his name underneath the quote. His name was Thich Nhat Hanh. I didn't know who he was, or where he came from, but he had been calling me to Vietnam for a long time. He had been subliminally sending me messages, showing me that he was looking to communicate. At this point, I felt guided to do a little research on the Internet. I researched where he was, so that I could go and find him, but I was confused; he was living in France at that time. Of course, that led to my ego kicking in, big time. *It can't be him, then. What on earth is all this about? It's a bloody wild goose chase!*

The next day, frustrated by the previous day's events, I asked for a sign; I asked for a very specific sign and within a specific timescale too. *Please show me an elephant by the end of today, to show me if I am supposed to do anything about Thich Nhat Hanh.* I set the intention and then completely forgot about it; I went about my day as normal.

Later on, I returned to my hotel room, and immediately I looked on the bed and saw something unbelievable. The lady that had cleaned my room had transformed my towels into two elephants. Not just one elephant, but two elephants; just to make sure that I got the memo.

There was nothing else to do at that point but laugh about it. It was so blatant, it made me laugh out loud and put my head in my hands. I still didn't know what I was supposed to do with it. I was in a strange dilemma. I felt I was being pulled in two directions. One was toward the monk, wherever he may be, and the other was to Sydney and to Ricky. The two elephants made me think of him too. The twin connection. What was it with twins? Since 2012, when my little twin sisters were born, they were being shown to me constantly. It was all a bit too much to deal with, so I did what I will always do in those moments – I headed to the beach to ground, to connect with Mother Nature, and to collect my feelings.

I spent a couple of days at the beach, conversing with Gaia and immersing in what I now know to be the light activation codes. At one point, during those days, I did a Facebook Live video from the beach. I don't remember exactly what I was speaking about but I do remember the love that I felt at the time. I had never felt anything quite like it before. My phone ended up overheating during the live broadcast, due to the heat, which made me laugh. I do like it when the Universe says 'no, enough is enough, be still and present – I'm taking your phone away.'

After I had finished doing the live video, I sat down in the sand and I felt a level of peace rise up in me that was incredibly overwhelming, but in a good way. I felt so much love coming from back home. I also felt encased in this energy from the monk and the twins.

It was just love. That's the only way to describe it.

My time in Vietnam was coming to an end because I had to go to Cambodia. I had been significantly drawn there at this point, although, as usual, I didn't know what for. As much as I love old ruins and things like that, it wasn't really my bag at that time. Buildings were buildings to me, back then. I was more of a nature person; however, I had learned to trust whatever the pull was and I just knew with every cell in my body that I had to go to Cambodia. At the same time, I felt strongly that I would come back to Vietnam, but for now, it was time to move on. It was time to let go of all of my unanswered questions and surrender.

I'd had a magical time in Vietnam. There had been so many messages, people, and things that had crossed my path – so much gold, more than I could ever remember. That was the beautiful thing about travelling. Never rule anybody out. Literally, just immerse in everything, in every experience, because then you receive what is intended for you.

I packed up my things and said goodbye to Vietnam. I had so much gratitude for the place, and a nagging feeling that I may return one day.

I was off again, to somewhere new. Cambodia was calling. I wondered what mystical experiences would unfold under the magical energy of Ankor Wat.

98

When I got to the airport in Vietnam, I thought it would be a case of simply checking in and getting on my plane to Siem Reap in Cambodia. I'm not sure why I was under that illusion, as that had not been the case for me for some time, so why would this be any different? There was always a messenger to meet, or some reason why I was at a specific place at a specific time. I was starting to realise that nothing was straightforward anymore. Things started happening everywhere I went. It was like I was a chess piece being moved around graciously.

I had checked in fairly easily, my luggage had gone through without any issues, everything was in order with my visa and I had a little bit of time to spare, so I went for a stroll around the airport. Primarily to stretch my legs, but also to find some food. The airport wasn't very big; however, I was quickly learning that the Universe did not need much space to create huge shifts. She will place whoever, or whatever, is required for you in order for you to get the message. It's actually quite amazing what can happen in a very small space. I hadn't eaten for a few hours and I was getting a little bit peckish, it was fast approaching 8 pm by this time and I knew I probably wouldn't get the opportunity to eat when I landed in Cambodia. I was walking through one of the shops and an extremely handsome man caught my eye. His energy and aura were bouncing off him. He was walking around with an inner confidence that captivated me. I looked at him and smiled to myself because I was in awe of the fact that this person was shining so brightly, and then I just carried on looking for something to eat. I hardly acknowledged at the time how handsome he actually was on a physical level – my goodness how I had changed!

A short time later, I was in one of the shops trying to find something healthy to eat – which in itself wasn't easy. I picked up some nuts and some dried mango, and then out of nowhere, the guy with the amazing aura was standing right in front of me.

"What's your name?" he asked me, excitedly. Beaming his beautiful white teeth at me, whilst his gorgeous brown eyes twinkled in my direction.

I smiled at his enthusiasm. "Lucy," I replied. I noticed he had a beautiful jade Buddha around his neck. I chuckled to myself because the more I experienced these things, the more I realised how quickly now people were coming to me with information. I knew this guy was a messenger for me – the jade buddha confirmed it. I immediately felt that he was a sign, or that he had a message to deliver. It wasn't any surprise to me to discover that he was from Australia too.

"It's not easy to find anything healthy to eat around here, is it?" he asked – reading my mind in the process.

I showed him my dried mango and nuts and we laughed.

We started chatting as we walked around the shop together and then he asked if he could come and sit with me whilst we waited for our flight because, of course, he was on the same one. I mean, where else would he be going?

We chatted for a while and I told him a brief version of what I had been up to. He was in awe of my journey. I asked him where in Australia he was from and he said, "Sydney." Of course! So, once again, Sydney was calling me – not that it had ever stopped. The more I spoke to this guy, the more signs he was giving, and the more messages he was delivering. It got to a point in our conversation where I threw my hands up in the air and said, out loud, "Fine, I'm booking a fucking flight."

For a moment he looked at me as if I was crazy, then burst out laughing. "Do you want to explain to me where that little outburst came from?" he asked, laughing. I gave him a very short version of what had happened. How I'd been in Thailand with Ricky, how I had been told very clearly that he was my twin flame, and then I had run away. How since then Ricky had been asking me to go to Sydney, and the Universe had been bombarding me relentlessly with all things Sydney, Sydney. Sydney was driving me potty! I then explained that when he had also said he was from Sydney, and with the Buddha hanging around his neck, and Ricky messaging me that day asking me to come to Sydney – it had reached the point where I had no choice but to surrender.

He turned to me and said, "Lucy, you've got to book that flight. You can't not. What if something magical is about to happen?"

It was a beautiful moment, sitting there with this gorgeous soul who was being so vulnerable and open with me, encouraging me to follow the signs of the Universe, to follow my heart. He was such a beautiful soul, he was sent to remind me that love is all that matters.

He made me book the flight whilst I was sitting there with him. It was a classic Lucy travel story. A total stranger delivering the final blow to make me get on and listen to the calls that Mumma G had been waiting for me to act on. It was hilarious, and as soon as I booked the flight it was almost like I could hear Mumma G breathe a sigh of relief. I messaged Ricky, "Okay fine, you win, I'll be in Sydney on Friday 13th July." He just sent back a smug smiley face. It actually really annoyed me that I was going back. I love Sydney, but I just couldn't quite get my head around why I had to go two months before I was due to be there anyway. It made no sense. Not at that moment anyhow.

Josh, the handsome guy with the jade buddha, gave me his details and we agreed to meet up when we were in Cambodia. We were keen to explore together. It was also clear we both found each other attractive. There was a chemistry between us that was quite electric, but as much as I would have liked to spent time with him, I was too focused on what I was there to do. We boarded the flight and went our separate ways. I had a decision to make. Did I want to spend more time with this incredibly handsome man or take the time to process things and get my head together, before going back to Sydney to deal with my twin flame?

The flight to Siem Reap was only an hour. It was a little propeller plane. There were some children on the row opposite me and they were totally freaking out. I had a chat with them to reassure them that we would be okay, and then I slipped into meditation for the rest of the journey. I decided it was time to ask some direct questions and ask for guidance from my guides and the Universe. *I have listened, now it's time for you to guide me with the who, the what, the where and the when. Show me all you would like me to see for my healing journey. Remind me of everything I have done to hold myself back. It's time to be free. Show me what is required. So I can remind the collective.*

I was reminded during my meditation that my key role was to be love and to embody love. I felt I already knew this, so I was confused. My ego started piping up and I began thinking about Sydney. Why was I being called back there just months before I was due to go? Was this all just a silly game?

I landed at the airport in Cambodia and headed for the long customs queue. I could see that almost every person was being stopped and interrogated by the stern-looking security men – many people were being sent away to fill in forms. I was not in the mood for this; I was tired and just wanted to get to my hotel. Now, normally when I travel, regardless of how the security people are with other people, they are always fine with me. So fine, in fact, that more often than not, they send me their love as I'm walking away. I don't know what it is. I just have this really amazing interaction with people whenever I travel, and this was no different. This bad-tempered man, who had been so stern with everybody else, was smiling at me and asking me questions. It was absolutely amazing. It made me smile. Proof that your energy precedes you.

Whilst I was waiting for my luggage, Josh, the guy with the buddha around his neck appeared. He said, "Oh my God, that was hard work getting through customs. What a nightmare."

I shrugged my shoulders and said, "Well, not so much actually," and I started laughing, which made him laugh too. Apparently, my laugh is super contagious.

"It's because you're a woman!" he joked as he threw his arms up in the air and winked at me. He knew I had a certain way with people that went beyond that. He knew it, because he had it too.

I picked up my luggage and waited outside the airport at the spot where my hotel had advised me to wait for my transfer. I looked around for a guy with a sign with my name on it, but there was nobody there. I thought that it was weird; they had told me that they would be there before my flight landed so that there would be no way that they missed me. I had a little walk up and down and asked a couple of people if they were from my hotel, but they all said no. I sat down on a bench for a minute, and then quickly thought that sitting here wasn't helping, I needed to do something. I had ants in my pants. I wanted to get to the hotel, have a shower and go to bed. I went over to a little kiosk shop in the airport and bought a SIM card. I set it up quickly and called the hotel and asked what had happened to my transfer. They had completely forgotten to pick me up. They were so sorry, but they said they would send someone right away, they apologised profusely before hanging the phone up too. It was going take them about 40 minutes to get to me. I had told them not to worry about the time and that I would sit and wait. Thankfully, I had my mango and nuts, otherwise, I probably would have been hangry by this point in the evening. You see how divinely orchestrated it all is?

I had to go and buy the food. I had to connect with Josh. I stopped and thought about all those coincidences and quickly realised that I must also need to be sat here in this now moment. I wondered what was coming next. I thought about why I had agreed to wait rather than just getting a taxi to the hotel.

I sat back down on the bench where I'd sat previously, and within seconds, a local Cambodian man came and sat next to me. I smiled and said, "Hi," not expecting him to speak English.

He smiled back and asked, "Why have you come to Cambodia?" His English was amazing.

I explained to him that I'd had this pull for many years to come to his precious country, but I hadn't had the confidence until this moment. I explained I had also been a bit scared due to the stories I had seen Princess Diana do about the landmines and other things like that going on in Cambodia.

He asked me, "Why now?" and started laughing. He was cheeky and had a great sense of humour.

I laughed back, and replied, "Good question! What on earth am I doing here?" We both laughed at each other.

"If you could do anything whilst you're here, what would you do?" He asked. I sat and pondered the question. I had not been expecting this. It had come out of nowhere, but I quite liked being put on the spot like that. I tend to do this a lot to other people and so having it thrown back at me was fun.

"I'd like to go to Angkor Wat and feel into the energies and stuff like that."

He looked at me with a more serious look upon his face. He spoke slower this time, emphasising his words. "No, no. If there was one thing that you could do here, what would it be? What do you want to see?"

I didn't really get where he was coming from. I sat and pondered for a few minutes, then blurted out of nowhere, "I want to meditate with the monks." It literally fell out of my mouth without any previous thought about it. I had never considered doing that here, so I had no idea where it came from, but I liked it all the same.

He started laughing. "Nobody has ever said that to me before."

I said, "Well, I'm just not anybody," and we laughed together. "I don't know why, but I really would love to meditate with the monks."

"If I could organise it for you, would you want to go?"

I said, "Yes, absolutely. That would be amazing." I didn't even have any alarm bells ringing that this total stranger who sat next to me on a bench might be trying to kidnap me. I can see it sounds dodgy now, and when my mum reads this book she will have kittens no doubt. For some reason, though, I trusted him. There was something in my soul that trusted his. Like an old, long lost friend that I had just got reacquainted with.

"How long are you here for?"

"I don't really have a timescale. All I know is that I'm here for the next few days until I figure out where I'm supposed to be."

He said, "Leave it with me."

We exchanged phone numbers and then he went off on his merry way. I turned around a few seconds later and he was gone. He seemed to have disappeared into thin air. Had I had a conversation with a ghost? Did I imagine that? At this point in my life, nothing would surprise me; there was so much weird stuff that was occurring on a daily basis – and to be honest, I actively encouraged it.

A few minutes later, my hotel transport arrived, in the form of a bright blue tuk tuk. The driver apologised profusely, to the point that I had to tell him to stop. On the way back to the hotel, I told the driver about the conversation I had with the man on the bench. He looked at me as if I was crazy. It did make me question myself, momentarily; some random dude asked what I would love to do and then all of a sudden he's going to magic that up for me? Why would a total stranger do that?

As we pulled up at the hotel, my new Cambodian phone started ringing. I knew that the only person who had that number was the old guy at the airport and so I answered it. I motioned for my tuk tuk driver to take the call and asked him to make sure the guy on the end of the phone was the real deal. He gladly took my phone and began speaking in the local language.

After a couple of minutes, he handed me back my phone, covered the mouthpiece up with his hand, and told me that he felt the guy arranging the monk trip was a good guy and I had nothing to worry about. I picked up my phone and began talking to him myself. "Hello again," I said.

"Not tomorrow, but the following day, I'm going to pick you up at four in the morning and I'm going to take you to a monastery, and the monks have agreed to let you in to meditate with them."

I was so excited about it. "Thank you so much." I arranged to meet him outside the hotel in a couple of days' time.

This was so cool!

The tuk tuk driver smiled at me and said, "You're really lucky to have met him." I wondered what he meant by that, but I had come so far on this whole journey that I surrendered and thought – *Okay, I'm going on a magical mystery tour.*

I got to my room and it was beautiful; a tropical paradise. The shower was outside and had wildlife growing through it. It was like having a shower in a rainforest. It was incredible. I loved the feel of the place. It had been a while since I stayed in a really beautiful luxury place, so I felt completely at ease.

That night the fun started. The energies of Angkor Wat began talking to me; even that thought was not starting to sound as weird as it might have done just a few months earlier. As I slept, I had one of the most profound astral travel experiences I'd ever had.

I didn't even know that was what it was called at the time, but I know a lot more about it now. Astral travelling is where we go when we are in a superconscious state; some people would call that sleep state. What happens during astral travel is that your soul elevates out of your physical body, which means you can be in two places at once. It means your soul can go on and do other things. It can go and see people, and sometimes this will show up in their dreams. Some people's souls go off and do healing or grid work – anything magical it's drawn to do. Most people don't remember this process taking place, but I would estimate that 99% of humans do this every single night; it's just that they don't remember it. If you have ever been asleep and you felt like you're falling and you suddenly jolt yourself awake. That's a sure sign of astral travel. It's a sign of you coming back into your body, and probably freaking the heck out of yourself when you see your body lying asleep, wondering if you have passed over. I'm very lucky because by working with my quantum healer, I learnt all about this and she helped me to connect with it. I started to write down all my experiences so that I could remember them and connect the dots. These days, it's very rare if I'm not attending some galactic meeting, or my soul is off being a busybody somewhere.

That first night in Cambodia, my astral experiences were profound. There was something in my soul that resonated with the vibrational pulls that were coming from Angkor Wat. I actually ended up astral travelling to Buckingham Palace. I have no idea why. I was not, and never have been a royalist, so this was a weird experience. I embraced it, though. I was walking through the corridors in Buckingham Palace, and although I couldn't see her, I knew Princess Diana was guiding me. I could hear her voice. I could feel her energy. She was guiding me around the place. She would give me directions, "Keep walking, turn left, go right." I ended up in a huge room. It was what I would imagine you would expect from Buckingham Palace; it was what I expected anyway. Very red and gold. It was an absolutely enormous room, but there was nothing in it, just one chair, and even that was just a normal chair, not a throne or anything like that. Sat in that chair was Prince Harry. Princess Diana kept saying to me, "The only person that can help you with this is him." And she was referring to Prince Harry. I couldn't make any sense of this as it unfolded – *What the heck have I got to do with Prince Harry?*

I started talking to him, and he said to me, "All you need to do is find the real me, and I will help you."

I remember coming back into my body and waking up the next morning and thinking that I was literally losing my marbles. *I've been to Buckingham Palace. I've spoken to Prince Harry. I've had Princess Diana on my shoulder guiding me. I'm literally losing the plot.*

It was perfect timing, though, I had a session with my quantum healer booked for that day – it was no coincidence! I knew she could help me make sense of this. I had booked a session with her a few days before, knowing that I was much more on her timeline as she was based out of Melbourne, so we were just a few hours' time difference. As soon as we got on the call, I told her everything that had happened to me the night before. She giggled the whole way through my story. When I had finished she said, "Well, it sounds as if you're about to go on a big journey. You need to trust that if you are called somewhere, that you should go, knowing that you are going to be okay. You will get the messages you need. You will have the support and guidance. All you need to do is listen and trust. You will be looked after."

I took great comfort in her words. Then she said to me, "Princess Diana is with you. And it looks as if she's going to be sticking by your side for a little while."

There's not much I could say to that. I made a clear connection to Princess Diana and the landmine campaign she had staged in Cambodia but everything else seemed a bit strange. I had no idea what Princess Diana wanted from me. I guess I was about to find out.

99

I spent the rest of the day sitting by the pool by myself, taking it easy and getting myself ready for an early start the next day. I had no idea at the time the amount of light codes and activations that were taking place by me being immersed in the sunshine. Each time I look back over the journey, with the wisdom I have now, it blows me away how my soul knew exactly what was required, and thankfully I trusted it. I was so excited to be meditating with the monks. The guy who was taking me to see them had also said he would take me to a few other sites that day and so I knew I would need as much energy as possible.

The next morning, I was woken up very early by my alarm. I was like a bear with a sore head because I wasn't used to having an alarm anymore, I'd stepped away from that. I grabbed some water and made sure that I had a few snacks in my bag because if I get hungry, it's not pretty.

While I was waiting for my guy to pick me up, I decided to be sensible and so I told the hotel what I was doing and gave them my number. I told them if anything happens to me, they know who to go and find. They were great about it.

Not long after that, the guy turned up at the hotel. He explained he had come with a driver so that he would be able to speak with me more directly and explain stuff to me as we were travelling. We set off on the first journey which he said would take about an hour. On that journey, he explained that he had arranged for me to meditate with three monks, but that one of them was a very senior monk. He told me to start setting my intentions for what I wanted to achieve from it, and that some people had very profound experiences with the monks. He felt that they probably wouldn't speak with me, but I could meditate with them. I was happy with that, that was all I had wanted anyway.

I set a very clear intention that day. I decided that I would ask for guidance on the soul mission I was embarking on. I asked my soul to remember what she needed in order to create what was required. I had been told I had a mission, to embody love and to be love, but it still seemed so aloof, I wanted more specifics. Everyone always spoke about purpose being some huge, grand thing that we had to go searching for. I was looking for clarity on mine, more details; this is why I totally get it when people today ask me about their purpose.

The car journey there was profound. He explained to me that Cambodia was the prison with no walls; which I'd never heard of before. The local people weren't really allowed to leave, they were kind of trapped by the system there. He told me all the history of the place and some of the dark things that had gone on. He told me all about the landmines and the genocide; as he told me, my heart ached for the Cambodian people. He delivered so many messages to me on that journey, unknowingly. I had never researched anything about Cambodia, I had trusted what I needed to know would come to me. It's just the way that I work. I started to recognise, bit by bit, why Princess Diana had come here in the first place and possibly what she wanted from me. I could hear her in my ear saying, "Thank you, thank you."

We arrived at the monastery and I got out of the car. The monks came to greet me immediately and they spoke to me, not that I knew what they were saying. They were very kind and loving. The tour guide was staring at me with his eyes wide open because he had warned me that they would not communicate with me at all. It wasn't like that at all, in fact, the main monk seemed to come alive when he saw me, his face lit up like he'd remembered me or had seen something in me that maybe he hadn't seen for a while.

I was shown into the most beautiful temple. It was breathtaking, and so was the view. We sat meditating for about an hour. I kept getting lots of colours coming through, and lots of different messages. I kept hearing the names of places too, places I had never heard of before. Unbeknownst to me, the tour guy took lots of pictures of me meditating with the monks and immersed in this beautiful experience. I'm so thankful that he did that because I love those photographs so much. I look so happy, calm and peaceful in the company of them all.

After we had finished meditating, the main monk did a little blessing on me. Once again, the tour guy was flabbergasted at the way the monks were interacting. I was invited to sit outside with the monks and have some water and enjoy the scenery. It was all such an honour. They offered me some sort of biscuit to eat also. I was truly humbled in their presence.

As we were leaving I asked the tour guy to thank the monks for me and I gave him some money to give to them as a gift and a token of my respect. The main monk began talking to the tour guy, for him to interpret it back to me. He told him about my energy and the vibration I was giving off. He said that when he first saw me he knew something that I was unaware of. He went on to explain some of the beautiful visions that he had been getting through the meditation, visions of me walking through rice fields. This was really fascinating because I had just been in Vietnam walking through the rice fields.

I listened intently as the tour guy described what the monk was telling him. My soul was absolutely buzzing, and it was only about 6 in the morning by this point. As we were leaving, the main monk told the tour guy to tell me that if I ever wanted to come back that I would always be welcome. His exact words were, "We'll always remember her, there's no way we will forget her."

Once we were in the car, I asked him where we were going to next. He said he had originally planned to take me to a few places, but now that he had seen what went on at the monastery, he thought he needed to take me somewhere else entirely, and that we needed to visit a certain village. I trusted him and his intuition by this point. He had delivered so much already. I smiled and said, "Let's go."

100

We went on another magical journey as we wound our way through the roads and streets on the way to a beautiful fishing village. We had many more profound conversations on the way, he shared more of his local wisdom and stories. He was a fascinating man, to say the least.

We arrived at the village, which was beautifully quaint. We got on a boat with a random guy. For a moment, my ego kicked in with the usual scenarios of doom, thinking they were going to drown me in the middle of this river. Despite my inner chit-chat, I got on the boat and they took me to this whole other world, a place that I'd never seen before, not in this lifetime, anyway. It was a beautiful scene with lots of people selling fruit and vegetables from boats on the river. This wasn't just a simple river that floats through a village, this was an enormous river, it felt more like a sea or the ocean. And the boats they would sell from were huge floats. At one point, we got off our boat and climbed onto one of the huge floats for a drink, so that I could see the view from above. It was beautiful. When we sailed passed the homes that were floating on the water, all the family and children would come out and wave to us. It was magical. I felt like my tour guy was showing me a part of my past to remind me that this is where I had come from; my roots from some point. I had been here before, and maybe forgotten it.

When we got back on land, my guy said to me, "Do you want to see a water buffalo?" I was up for anything. I had experienced the water buffalo in Vietnam, so I was more than happy to go along with his suggestion. Whilst I was bouncing around in a cart on the back of a water buffalo I wondered how I had ended up here. A random – never random – conversation with a stranger at the airport and I had gone on this incredible journey, culminating in bobbing about in the wilderness on the back of a buffalo surrounded by water, reeds and the most incredible locals.

It was still early in the day, on account of our ridiculously early start. So my guy asked me if I now wanted to go to Angkor Wat. Obviously, I said yes, with a glint in my eye.

On the drive there, my guy told me even more about the local history, and even more about the tragedies and genocide that had happened here. He mentioned a couple of other places to me, they sounded like the places that I'd been getting through my meditations and through the words that Princess Diana had given me. Although the stuff he shared was horrific and not a vibe I wanted to spend too much time in, I wanted to know more of this stuff from his perspective, and not from the history books. Again, typically Lucy; do not bother giving me the information you have digested from text books, it doesn't really resonate with me. Share your stories. Let me know what really went on from your perspective. That is what lights me up.

We arrived at Angkor Wat. It was such a glorious day. We dressed up respectfully, covering our shoulders, as we had done at the monastery. We went on a tour of the place first, and my guy was showing me around and pointing out certain things. It was an incredible place, filled with mystery and magic. In all the rocks and the trees, I could see animals and faces – things that I would now know and call the 'ancestors'. I could see signs and messages everywhere I looked. At one point, it felt like blossom was falling all around me, but there was no blossom at Angkor Wat. Every now and again, I felt drawn to stop, touch or stroke the rocks and the trees. At other times, I felt the need to stop and just sit and allow the energies to flow through me. I had no idea that what I was doing was feeling into the frequency and the vibration. I was just intuitively drawn to do it. Each time I would connect physically with a stone, a message would shoot through me. I wasn't sure what I was actually doing, but now I know better – it is the stones sharing their wisdom.

We walked for hours and hours. At one point we came across a beautiful stallion with a guy riding it so majestically. Now, I am horse mad, so this was amazing to see. My tour guy said to me it was very rare to see something like that there. It felt like the world was presenting itself to me. Some people would not have even seen the horse that day, it was not their sign. It was definitely mine, and I was embracing it.

We came to the main part of Angkor Wat. My guy said, "I'm going to take you up all the levels, but when we get to a certain point, you've got to go alone." He explained to me that all of the levels in the temple were to do with different levels of consciousness. There is the start of the journey where you start to recognise things. Then, as you go up you start to relinquish your material goods, you start to question things and see things slightly differently, until you get to the top level, which they call Nirvana. Nirvana is where you are so enlightened that you are truly at peace. You recognise all of the signs, you recognise all of the synchronicities and you feel at one with everything.

We started walking up through the different levels. He was explaining to me as we climbed. I love photography, and he enjoyed photography too, so we got some amazing pictures that day. In a lot of the photos, there are orbs floating all around me. The energy was profound. I was picking up lots of different things. I would say them out loud as we were going. I would say, "I feel as if people have their hearts broken here," and then he would tell me a story that explained what I was feeling. I was learning that my intuition and my feelings were picking up extremely accurate information. It was crazy, but crazy beautiful. This was the first I consciously tapped into the energies and then had someone explain what and why I was feeling that. It's a lot of what I do today.

We got to the sixth layer going up to the seventh layer and the stairs were really steep leading up to it. My guy turned to me and said, "You're on your own from here. I'm going to go wait over there." He pointed to an area down below in the shade. "You take your time. It's important you take your time with this bit. If you feel drawn to be out in one minute, do that, but if you want to be out there for an hour, I'll be waiting. I'm not going to go anywhere."

I started walking, and, not for the first time on this journey, I felt like I was walking the Green Mile. I had a bit of fear. I felt as if I was a lamb being led to slaughter. It was a really weird and lonely feeling. I felt out of my depth, I really did. *What am I going into here? This is what they call true enlightenment. What does that even mean?*

I meandered my way up the steps, around the top floor, and the energy felt peaceful. All of a sudden, I got a massive urge that I needed to sit down and meditate. So, I plonked myself down right away, kicked my shoes off, got myself into a comfortable position, and surrendered to my meditation. I said, "Okay, what do you need to show me?"

Immediately, I was shown, in my visions, in my third eye, a lot of hurt, a lot of pain, and the fact that I needed to release it and bring in some light. Now, I was aware that my name in Latin means 'the bringer of light'. I was aware that my grandad kept telling me that I had to bring the light and I had to be the sunshine. In my visions, they showed me places that I had never been to, and I didn't fully understand what they were showing me but the main concept was that I was a beam of light going into these places and helping to lift the vibration.

I sat in meditation for a while. I have no idea of the time because I was off elsewhere. Suddenly, though, it went very cold and very dark. It had been scorching hot sunshine all day. I opened my eyes, stood up, grabbed my shoes in my hand and walked over to what would have been a window, but was now just an empty space. I looked around and saw that a massive black cloud had come over the temple, and it was literally only above this temple. I thought – *That's fucking weird. What have I done?* And then, it started to absolutely piss it down with rain, and I could see everybody scrambling for cover. Then the lightning started!

There was no place for me to go and so I stayed there and watched as the storm raged over the temple, while everywhere else was clear blue sky and sunshine. I walked around the Nirvana floor and I kept getting these beautiful insights. Every now and again, I would stop and feel the need to touch the stone, getting a fuzzy feeling of being home. It was so incredible.

I eventually worked my way back to the starting point. I looked up and all around and I thought – *Wow! That was absolutely magical.*

By the time I got to the bottom of the stairs, it was glorious sunshine again. I could see my tour guy in the distance, he was waving to me to let me know where he was. He came running over to me, "What did you do up there?"

"I've got no idea," I replied, laughing and shrugging my shoulders. "All I did was go into meditation, then I was shown all of this amazing stuff and then the thunder and lightning came."

"I think it's best we get you out of here," he said and motioned for me to follow him. He led me back to the car, and on the journey back I told him what had happened to me up there.

As we got to the hotel, I remembered some of the words that had been given to me in the meditation, they were in his native Khmer language I felt – they definitely weren't English. I asked him if he would write them down for me so I wouldn't forget them. I figured they may be important for my journey. When I repeated the words I had been given, I could see he was moved. He handed me the words he had written down on a scrap of paper and said, "Don't lose these. There are messages here. You need to get on a flight to Phnom Penh."

"I'm so sorry, my geography is terrible. Is that in another country?" I asked, sheepishly.

He smiled and wrote the name Phnom Penh down for me. "It's here in Cambodia." He took me by the hand, looked me in the eyes and said, "I wish you good luck on your journey. Please come back."

I thought that was such a lovely thing to say. And with that, he left.

So, that night, I did a 'Lucy' and booked a flight for the following day to go to Phnom Penh.

101

The next morning I woke up early to catch my flight. It was only domestic, so pretty easygoing in the grand scheme of things, other than the fact I had no idea where I was going or what I was doing. It had all happened so quickly, but I was pretty used to it by this point. One day you wake up, a place pops in your mind, you allow that to manifest a little, maybe a couple more signs show up, and then boom! You find yourself on the way to the airport with only a flight to a location booked, absolutely nothing else to go off. There is never much notice or planning that goes into these adventures – which at first I really couldn't get my head around – but as the years have passed I have learned the reasons why it needs to be that way. When you follow your intuition fully, you do not get warnings, the messages come out of nowhere and then it's about how long it takes for you to choose the path to follow it – or not – as would be the case for many people. In my case, I do follow it, and have done for many years. And nowadays I go pretty quickly too.

I had checked my bags in and, due to it being a domestic flight, I only had a short wait until we were going to board the plane and head off in the direction of Phnom Pen. I had huge amounts of gratitude for this beautiful place where I had been for the last few days. What a magical experience I had lived through. I wondered if anyone would ever believe what had gone on. I also gave huge gratitude for the amazing man I had met. He had transformed my life in those few days. How random to meet someone at the airport on a whim, who totally changes your life, and your perspectives for the better. I felt extremely lucky. He had been sent to me by God, I was certain of that. He showed me things I would never have seen or believed. He shared wisdom I would never have received if I had not been at that airport that night and my transfer had not arrived on time. I felt so loved in that moment. I knew the plan was so divinely orchestrated that each and every time we perceive things are going wrong, in fact they are slotting pieces of the puzzle together perfectly. I hoped I would get called back to this wonderful, magical place. I knew I could just book a ticket any time, but that wasn't the way I travelled anymore. I had to trust the calls.

I naturally assumed that as it was a short domestic flight that the plane was going to be very little, but it wasn't, it was huge. I had both sides of the plane to myself because they had positioned people strategically throughout the plane to balance it out. I had never been on a plane that was so big and yet so empty. There were about 20 of us in total. I didn't complain, though. We took off, I had a little lie down and the next thing I knew, we had landed. I love those flights, the ones where you take off, fall asleep, and then wake up coming into land.

I picked up my luggage and made my way through the airport and to a taxi. I had booked a nice hotel for myself in this location. My intuition was on point to book it. It was slap bang in the middle of a really busy city. I had booked it for the convenience of getting around. This was an in-and-out trip as far as I was concerned. I just made sure it had a gym and a rooftop pool so I could keep myself in full alignment. I had no idea why I was there other than the two names scribbled on a scrap of paper, but something in my soul told me it was going to be hectic and that I would need some time to be present and still at the end of each day. This hotel would be a haven for me.

It took a while to get to the hotel. Primarily because there was a lot of traffic on the roads. And secondly, the taxi driver took me to the wrong location. He took me on a magical mystery tour of the city and took me to the most dead-end places. I looked around and feared for my life at points. Yes, my mind was back in overtime. Thankfully, I had a Cambodian SIM card, so I was able to show him on my phone where to go, he realised where he had gone wrong and set off in the direction of the correct hotel. His mistake would cost me a fortune but I didn't care, I just wanted to get there safely.

As we drove through the city, I felt a sense of overwhelm. Everything was fast. Everything was busy. It was like dropping into Hong Kong or central Bangkok. There was too much going on all around. I was thinking about what had brought me there – the messages and names I had received in meditation, not to mention the whole Princess Diana and Prince Harry thing. It was crazy really. Here I was in this strange city not knowing what I was there for, or even if the names of the places I had received would even mean anything. I had trusted implicitly that this was the place to be.

Eventually, we got to the hotel, and thankfully it was as beautiful as the pictures I had seen when I booked it. I felt really grateful that I was able to choose such a nice place to stay when I needed to. I went into the reception area to check in, not expecting them to give me my room straight away as it was still early morning, but thankfully they did. I pulled out the piece of paper – the one my guide in Vietnam had written the words I had channelled down on – and I handed it to the reception lady. "Could you please do me a favour? Can you order me a taxi to these places?" She saw the names and said it would be fine. I told her I was going to dump my bags and I would be ready to go in 5 minutes.

When I came back down, she had arranged a tuk tuk to take me to the locations I had asked for. The driver was waiting outside and he beckoned me over as soon as he saw me. I climbed on board, ready to go on this adventure – albeit an adventure that I knew absolutely nothing about. I surrendered and trusted more than ever in my life in that moment. I sat with my little backpack on my lap, my phone in my hand and the piece of paper, showing him the locations to which I had been shown to go. Once he had read the paper, he nodded and set off in the direction of the first location. I was bobbing around in the back, minding my own business, and I started to notice that a lot of people were staring at me once again. I was getting used to this happening more and more as I travelled, and so I wasn't overly concerned. It had become one of those things. I observed it, but it didn't freak me out anymore. The scenery was beautiful in parts of the journey. I love to take photos, so I thought I would get my phone out and start shooting some of the scenery. Suddenly, the driver slammed his brakes on, to which I jolted abruptly forward in my seat. The driver got out of his chair, climbed into the back with me and whispered to me, "Put your phone back in your bag and sit on it. I've got a gun under the seat if I need it." My heart sank. I did exactly what he told me to do. I thought – *Where the hell am I? What kind of place have I come to?*

For the rest of the journey, I didn't even look around me, I just looked forward and kept focused on the road ahead. The guy started chatting to me in his own language. He didn't seem to have a care in the world, but all the time I was thinking – *Mate, you've got a gun under your seat. I can't pretend that I don't know that now. Once you see it, you can't unsee it.*

We began heading down a road that was off the beaten track. I didn't have any idea where we were going, so I didn't know if this was right or wrong. He could have been taking me anywhere. He started to slow down and began pointing to something. He pulled into a parking bay, where a row of other tuk tuks were parked. He motioned to a place across the road and said, "Place number one is here. I wait for you."

I thanked him and started walking towards the entrance of this place. It became very clear very quickly that this was the killing fields. I gasped out loud when I realised because I just knew that this was not going to be a nice experience. I had never been sent anywhere dark on my journey, until now. This was the first time that I was on my own in a country where I didn't speak the language, in such a dark and heavy place. I felt very vulnerable and I didn't want to do this. With that, the familiar feel of Princess Diana's presence came back. I knew it was her. It was very interesting. It was a warming and caring energy but strong and assertive at the same time. "Come on, you've got this. I'm here, I'll be with you, but you've got to do this." It was a very sweet, loving, nurturing energy I felt, accompanied by the words, "This is what you have to see. You have to see this side of it. You have to know the truth. You have to know what's been going on behind closed doors."

I walked in through the entrance and put on the headphones that were offered. They provided narration and guidance as to what I was doing and where I was going. I felt an incredibly overwhelming sadness as soon as I stepped in there. I can't explain it. I just wanted to cry. From the minute that I got in there, I felt as if my heart was being pulled. It felt sore, it ached, it hurt. I had never quite appreciated quite how sensitive I was to the energies until this point. I did not connect the dots at the time, but now I look back, it's obvious I was picking up on all of the souls' heaviness. There were maybe a dozen spots that the narration guided you to as you take a walk around the site. There are actual signs scattered around that you can read too. I took the time to read them, but, to be honest, I just wanted to know why the heck I had been sent there.

I stopped at one particular spot, next to a tree. There were lots of ribbons attached to it. You could see holes in the tree and also stains on the bark. The sign next to the tree, and the narration, told me that it was where they used to beat babies to death. Absolute heartbreak ran through me. I stood there and sobbed like a baby. In that moment there, standing by that tree, I felt all the pain and all the hurt of the atrocities that had taken place in that spot. I'd never felt anything like it. It was tragic. It was horrific. It was a level of tragedy that was just unimaginable. I started to feel sick. I walked on a little bit further, hoping that this was as bad as it could get, and then I came to a place where they executed the children and the mothers. The pain inside was awful. It felt as if I could hear, see and feel everything that had gone on there. It was horrible. The sadness of this place and the fear that these poor people had felt was running through me. I just wanted to be held. I wanted to hold them and apologise for all they had to experience. Being there in that heaviness was horrific.

Nowadays, with more experience, I get visions and I get shown what has happened at certain locations. Sometimes I can hear the conversations that took place there too. Back then, though, the feeling in me was more physical, like a tugging at my heart. As I stood there, beside these horrendous landmarks, the hurt and pain in my physical vessel was something that I'd never experienced before. Every now and again, I would feel on my shoulder, the reassuring touch of Princess Diana. She would say to me, "Keep stepping forwards, keep stepping forwards." Had she been a real person saying that, I likely would have punched her.

I got to a particular spot, where a river ran down the back of the site, and I stopped for a while to gather my thoughts. I sat there and sobbed, and asked out loud, "Why? Why? Why?"

And a voice came up in me, out of nowhere, "Because you wouldn't believe it if you didn't see it." And it was true. I would never have believed people could be this cruel.

"But why me? You could have sent a man here to do this. Why me?"

And it was at that moment, much to my disgust, that I realised that this was far bigger than I had ever imagined it could be. I realised that there was a master plan at work that was bringing everything to the surface. The good, the bad, and the very ugly. It was cemented into my being at that moment and everything I had felt as a child about being here for a big mission was coming true. I really was here for the greater good of humanity. It was not just a dream I had told my ex-boyfriend about in a haze, it was really true. All of a sudden it was there in front of me. They were giving me everything I needed to see in order to be able to realise it. Everything in my life up to that point had happened for a reason, even the shitty stuff, especially the shitty stuff. They were helping me to bring in the warrior energy so that I could step up and step forwards. They had turned me into a fighter. They'd got me to meet my twin flame. They had helped me to heal myself. They had got me to this point on my journey, to make sure that I had gathered all of the information I would need, so that I could legitimately, in my own voice, use my words to share what had been going on.

Most people go to these places because it's a tourist attraction. I wasn't there for that reason. I was there because I had been intuitively guided to go there. I thought about all the dots that had to connect for me to actually get there. I sat by that river feeling confused. I was realising the totality of my mission, but I was also in victim mode because I just wanted somebody to hug me, love me and tell me that it was all going to be okay.

I composed myself and carried on walking around the site. I went to some other horrific places where the energy felt very heavy and dark. At the end of the walk, there was a tall building and in all of the windows they had piled up thousands of actual human skulls, one on top of the other. I didn't want to go in, but I got the clear message that I had to. I felt sick again and thought I was going to throw up. Tears were rolling down my face as I walked in. I really didn't want to go. Other people were walking in and out nonchalantly like they were visiting a shop. It felt so dark to me, though. There were skulls in there from babies that were a month old; there were skulls in there from 90-year-old women and everything in between. It was heartbreaking. They had somehow preserved the skulls in this building so that people would remember, but most people weren't recognising the symbolism and the poignancy of it. How could this have been allowed to happen? I felt so passionate about it, yet everyone else just seemed to walk around as if it was normal.

I stood in that building and set the intention that I was going to send love to all of these beautiful souls, who had sacrificed themselves. I took the opportunity to stand in the middle of this building, shut my eyes and to see love and light vibrating through the roof, the walls and out to each and every soul that was in that space. That's all I could do. I felt helpless.

I walked out of that building and I burst into tears again. I thought – *What the fuck am I doing here?* I couldn't wait to get out of there.

As I was heading to the exit, all of a sudden I got a message to do one more lap. I said out loud, "No way, I'm not doing it." It came through, "Do one more lap, but don't look at anything. Just do one more lap."

For fuck's sake!

Begrudgingly, and hurriedly, I raced round the circuit one more time. I was not interested in being there a minute longer than I needed to.

What I didn't realise back then, and I'm very aware of it now, is that when I am present in an area, or when my bare feet walk on the land, I cleanse the place. I also have the ability to release souls. On top of that, each time I finish cleansing a place, I'm guided to walk around it, so I can seal the area where the work has been done. So, I now know what was happening when I was guided to complete that second lap.

I finally walked out of the exit and burst into tears again. The tuk tuk driver came over to me and helped me into the vehicle. I asked him, "The next place we go to, is it like this?"

"Oh, no no. It's a museum," he replied, and he gave me a bottle of water and a chocolate bar because he obviously thought that the sad, little lady needs cheering up. I sat in the back of the tuk tuk on the way to the next location, absolutely furious. I thought – *Fuck you, Princess Diana. Fuck you God! How dare you take me to this place? Who do you think you are? I don't want to go to these places. I don't deserve this.* I was in victim mode massively. My ego was piping up big-time. I felt scared. I felt vulnerable. I was on my own. I was with a guy with a fucking gun under his seat! The driver turned his music up, I think he hoped it would raise my spirits somewhat, it didn't.

102

Thirty minutes later, we arrived at the next place. It was a pretty bland building with huge white walls. It looked like it could have been an old school or something like that. The driver said again that it was a museum. I figured there was no way it could be worse than the last place and so I gave myself a pep talk. Princess Di popped up again with her gentle guidance, "You've got to do this. Keep walking forwards." I said out loud, "Fuck you. I don't want you hanging around me anymore." I was so pissed off with her!

I paid the fee at the entrance and walked in, wondering what this museum was about. I entered through some gates and again they gave me headphones to narrate the way around the place. It became instantly very clear that this was an old prison, but not just any prison, it was the place where all the people were held during the mass genocide – Tuol Sleng.

The first few settings were interesting. Nothing much to see. Then I got sent into a prison cell, and it was awful. You could feel the fear and the panic where people had been killed. It was hideous. I burst into tears again and I thought – *For fuck's sake, this is supposed to be a museum.* And in all fairness, it was a museum, but it was a museum of the mass genocide that took place under the reign of Pol Pot.

It was tragic and devastating to feel the terror and despair in the place. I walked around and tried to make amends with God for my earlier outburst. "I know I slagged you off before but can we be friends again, I kind of need your protection right now!"

The prison was darker than the killing fields. It was a huge place. There were five or six enormous buildings, each with two levels to them. It must have housed thousands and thousands of people, and many of them had died horrendous, tortured deaths there. At one place, they were showing pictures of people that had been caught up in the atrocities, people who had lost their lives. One picture really caught my eye, it was a 25-year-old English lad, he had been working on a boat on the ocean when his boat was captured and he was taken in and questioned. The process that was explained to me was that people would be taken in and interrogated, and they would be forced to admit that they had done something. Once they had a forced admission, then the government could 'legitimately' kill them. This English lad had been clever because during his interrogation, when they had taken notes on his forced confession, he actually gave answers so that his parents would know what had happened to him. Unfortunately, he was murdered. His story really pulled on my heart-strings, though. It saddened me, knowing his plight.

I wrote a note in the visitor book. "RIP, you beautiful souls. I commit to you that we will change history by getting to the bottom of all this, once and for all. Lucy, UK." The date was the 7th of the 7th. I remember it clearly, as I wrote the note. Over the years, I always seemed to travel or be somewhere poignant on the 7th of the 7th. I took a photo of my message because I never wanted to forget that was what I had to do. Get justice. How ironic those words would become in a few year's time.

I walked out of the museum feeling even more heartbroken than when I had walked in. I thought that it was going to be okay after I'd come out of the killing fields, but it wasn't. All of a sudden, I understood why Princess Diana had made me go there and why the names of these places had come through in Siem Reap. My journey so far had been very exciting, there were so many things that I'd experienced and I'd had a good few years of having positive steps take place. And while I had my ongoing health issues, most of my journey had been beautiful and positive. It had been mostly all love and light, which is what most people ask of on their waking journey. Yes, some of the realisations hurt when you recognise bullshit about yourself, but there hadn't been many polarities, I hadn't witnessed much real darkness in the grand scheme of things. But, experiencing what I had on this day was a whole different level. This was bigger than little old me, fighting the good fight on my spiritual journey – this was about humanity. This was about mankind. This was planetary.

I climbed into the back of the tuk tuk and asked the driver to take me back to the hotel. I told him I didn't want any music or to talk, I just needed to sit in silence. It was only a short journey, no more than ten minutes, but nevertheless, I needed to process what had gone on.

We arrived at the hotel, I got out and gave him a tip and then ran to my room. I sat on the edge of my bed and sobbed like a baby for hours.

When I had cried myself out, I messaged my friend Donna. Donna was a beautiful lady who worked with me at this period of time. I'd met Donna in 2017 when she had come to an event that I was running. Over the years, she'd become a very, very good friend of mine and when my business was really starting to take off, she ended up coming to work with me as the customer relations manager. I just had to tell her how sad I was feeling and that I couldn't do anything work-wise for the rest of the day.

I also messaged a girl called Ellie. She had given me some very profound messages over the years. One of the first messages she delivered to me, she had said, "Lucy, I keep seeing you walking between two oceans. It's almost like you are walking and the ocean is dividing as you're walking. Wasn't it Moses that did that?" I thought at the time that it was a pretty profound image she had of me, but didn't think too much of it. I messaged Ellie that day because she was probably one of the only people at that time that I could share this crazy stuff about Princess Diana without her thinking I was totally batshit crazy. When I told her what had been going on, she made me feel better. She made me realise the size of the mission that I was on, and that it was okay to feel vulnerable, and it was okay to cry.

After I spoke with Ellie, I took the rest of the day to relax by the rooftop pool and to process everything that had gone on. It was beautiful up there, and although I was still feeling vulnerable and angry, I was able to switch off. After a while, I decided to sit in meditation and integrate the day's experience more fully. During this meditation, it was the first time God came through properly. Yes, I know that sounds crazy, but it's exactly how it happened. I was told very, very clearly that it always had to be me to do this stuff. It had to be me because I wasn't polluted by religious beliefs. It had to be me because I stood my ground on the trading floor against the men. It had to be me because I had become a warrior. And all of these things that had gone on in my life were tests to see if I was the right one. I began to cry. The profundity of it all. The realisation. I didn't know what else to do with myself, so I just sobbed. I felt like I had been hand chosen for this mission, and what a huge mission it was. I knew there was lots of other people out there doing similar things, but the realisation that you were picked, that's pretty special. I knew I was important. I felt at that moment that maybe I was a little bit more special than other people, and I really didn't want to feel that. I wondered if it was a test for my ego because my perception of God is what came through and he told me very clearly.

As overwhelming as this revelation felt to me, I also felt incredibly privileged to have had the insights that I'd had. I sat there for a few hours until the sunset. As the sun started to set, I said out loud, "I'm going to do whatever work you need me to do, but please, no more levels of darkness like that. At least prepare me. Give me some warning. Don't just slam things like that in my face, and let me have company. I know I can't ask to be given an easy path that's all love and light, but I can at least ask for more information."

I didn't pull any punches with God, or whatever it was that I was perceiving to be coming through me. I stood my ground. But I made that promise to myself. I would do whatever it takes and whatever was asked of me, but I would require more information. I would make sure that I asked the right questions. I was already a good question asker, but that was the point where I became a master question asker. I share this with all of my clients now; if you want to get to a level of peace, if you want to get to a level on your journey where you don't make assumptions, then you have to become a master question asker.

I left the rooftop and went to my room and I stayed there the whole night. I didn't speak to anybody. I didn't even go for food. I just had ice cream and went to bed. I really just wanted to get the heck out of there as soon as I could. It had been awful, but I had needed it. I needed it for my growth, although I hated it. That day had probably been the most awful and yet profound experience of my life up to that point. It was the shock and surprise more than anything. For anyone that knows me, they know I don't like surprises.

I spent the next day by the pool. I still didn't want to go anywhere or see anyone. I journaled and wrote the entire experience down in vivid detail because it was really playing on my mind and I wanted to get it out of my system and write it down so that I would never forget it.

103

Very early the next morning, I got picked up to go to the airport to fly to Singapore. I was staying with a girlfriend who I had known from back in the day when I used to work in investment banking. She wasn't very awake to the spiritual journey, although she had been watching my videos. When I arrived, she joked that she was fearful of what was going to happen in her house with lights flickering and weird shit happening because she had seen the change in me and knew that I had become more connected and spiritual. Knowing how she felt, it gave me the opportunity to become more grounded and human, especially after the events of the past few days.

My friend had a nanny who looked after the children, so we actually got to spend some quality time together. We went out in the evenings and watched some of the England matches in the 2018 World Cup. We did have a lovely time, but after my experience in Phnom Pen, I couldn't get my head together. I struggled. I struggled with the thought that I could get put in situations like that again, and my mind was working overtime.

When it came to leaving Singapore, I was kind of glad to be moving on, and I was finally heading to Sydney, after all the calling and the signs that had gone over the last few months. Ricky was messaging, asking me if I wanted him to pick me up from the airport, but I just wasn't ready to see him at that point, so I told him to give me a few days to settle in. I told him I would explain everything that had been going on but that I wasn't really ready to talk about it just yet, and he seemed okay with that.

Ominously, I landed in Sydney on Friday the 13th. From the minute I landed, it was clear that I had to be there. From the taxi man on the way back from the airport and the things that he was talking to me about, to the signs that were on the street, to the music that was coming on the radio. I knew with every cell in my body, this was going to be once again, another huge journey.

It was buckle-up time!

Arriving in Sydney felt really good. I went straight from the airport to my apartment, which was right near Darling Harbour. It's always my preference to stay there whenever I visit Sydney. I don't really know why. I could stay in many other locations, Sydney harbour, Manly, Bondi or any number of beautiful places, but for some reason, I'm always drawn there – perhaps it's to do with the name – Darling. When I look back to the first time I ever went to Sydney, I stayed in Darling Harbour on two occasions that same trip, so there's obviously something about it that resonates in my soul. Even though back in 2000 when I first went there absolutely none of this made sense.

By the time I got to the apartment, I was pretty exhausted, even though the time zone wasn't too different. I feel it was more the integration process that I was going through that was giving the experience of tiredness. I had gone from a really intense magical mystery tour of Cambodia to integrating into a beautiful family unit in Singapore for a few days, and it was such a huge contrast, one I was not used to. Even around my own family, I did not hide the person I was turning into. And in this instance, I went from being very 'out there' to suddenly being very 'normal'. That normality had stopped me from integrating and processing what had happened in Cambodia; so this was my opportunity to do that.

Typical Lucy, when faced with exhaustion, at this period in my life – I decided to go out for a run. Having been on a plane and in airports all day, where the energy is very stagnant, I needed to get some blood flowing in my body again and get grounded. I ran around the harbour, which is really beautiful. Then I ran all through the city, down into the famous Sydney Harbour, with the Opera House and the Harbour Bridge. When I got there, I found a grassy area nearby, where I could sit and look out over them both, it's a truly beautiful sight – and just moments from the area where I had spent that infamous New Year's Even watching the fireworks. I sat down and decided that I would stay there and reflect for a little while. Those last few weeks had been a wild ride. I kept having to pinch myself to see if I was actually dreaming or if it was real. Had all those magical, mystical experiences really happened or was I living in some sort of Virtual Reality experience?

As I sat there, my phone was going crazy. People that I hadn't seen in a long time knew I was back in Sydney and they wanted to catch up. It was so lovely and made me feel very loved and appreciated. I made some plans to go out to dinner that night with some friends in Darling Harbour – a great bunch of people who I knew I could just have a laugh with. I wanted to give myself a bit of time before I saw Ricky, not that he was intense or anything, but I knew he would ask me deeper questions and I wasn't ready to level up yet.

I sat on the grass verge, for a while, observing people, it was still relatively early in the day. I love watching people, and on that day, I saw people walking and running, there was a couple arguing, and families taking their kids out. It was almost like I was sat on the top of a mountain, like a Buddhist monk, and watching with detachment. I was becoming fascinated with human behaviour, the interactions and the idea that every single person was a messenger to each other. Seeing how people had become such powerful messengers to me made me realise that we all were to one another, it was just that some people couldn't see that, yet.

After a while, I decided to run back to my apartment, and pick up some food and bits from Woolworths – which is the supermarket over there. It always fascinates me because Woolworths was such a big thing in the UK when I was growing up. My nan used to take me there when I was little for some pick 'n' mix sweets, but then they all closed down in the UK around 2008, and it was the end of an institution. So, it makes me giggle every time I go to Sydney or Australia and I go to Woolworths for some fruits and veggies; it takes me back to being a kid in England.

As I entered Woolworth's, there was a girl sat outside and she reminded me of my sister. She was clearly a drug addict and it took me back to a place where I was back in my younger body watching my sister in pain and my family hurting. It was the vacant lost look in her eyes that was haunting. I remembered it so well with my sister. I went into the shop and grabbed some stuff for her. Admittedly, it wasn't the stuff that I would normally recommend people eat, but it was the kind of stuff that she would have wanted to eat. She would be able to eat quickly, getting the sugars and salts that she needed. She was so grateful, she looked at me with tears in her eyes. I know people had done this for my sister back in the day. It put a lump in my throat. When she said thank you to me, it felt like I jumped into her soul and I could feel her pain. I don't share this because I want any gratitude or recognition for it, I share it because she was my sister. She was the mirror of my sister reminding me of how far I had come on this journey. What I also realised at that moment is that I always needed to remain humble. I was living a pretty good life at this point, I was free from all the shackles that had held me back for all of these years, but seeing that girl was really humbling and it reminded me that love was needed. Wherever I was, I could distract myself with travel. I could distract myself by going to different cultures and having these amazingly magical experiences, even when there were dark experiences like in Cambodia, but I always needed to remember where I came from. I realised that although I was starting to help a lot of people and I was doing all of these magical things, family was still important. I needed to remember to check on those at home.

I got some beautiful lessons that first morning in Sydney.

I walked the rest of the way back from the shops to my apartment. The sun was shining and as I was walking I was observing everything around me. I was looking at the architecture. I was looking at the statues, I was looking at the signs and the symbols on the street. I was seeing things differently, noticing intricate things I hadn't noticed before. I had been to Sydney so many times, but I never quite got it.

I never really paid that much attention. I had fallen in love with the memories of my soul.

I got back to the apartment and I had to do some work. I had put it off for long enough, it was time to catch up. I had a few hours before I was due to go out with my friends and so it was the perfect opportunity to get on top of things so I could enjoy my night out.

We had a fun night that Friday evening. It was just what I needed. I only had one glass of wine the whole evening, whilst they all had cocktails. We went to a restaurant on the harbour and had a beautiful meal. It got to about 11 and everything was starting to get a bit wild, so I made my excuses and left – it had been a long couple of days. I walked back on my own, the apartment wasn't too far from the restaurant. I have always felt very safe in Sydney. On the walk back, I was thinking about things and asking myself – *Why the heck am I here?* I could have done this trip to Sydney in September when I was originally due to be there. There were no clear answers, so I just trusted that it would all become clear.

I had a seminar booked for Monday. One of my friends had booked it for us both, it was some kind of spiritual workshop and it sounded okay, so I had agreed to it, but I knew nothing else about it. The old Lucy would have needed to know all the details and been in control of everything, but I just shrugged it off and figured I would find out what I needed to when I needed to.

On the Saturday morning, I went out for a beautiful long run, then went to the gym, for a swim and a sauna. In the afternoon, I walked around exploring the city, ending up in Hyde Park after taking a boat across to Manly for a few hours. It was an amazing day of solitude. I love being outdoors in Sydney. I just love Sydney so much. It is one of my favourite cities in the world – for me it has everything. It was where my heart had been since 2000. Whenever I go back there, I choose to immerse in everything, trying new things, meeting new people. Every time I go, there's something new to discover. They have got some amazing restaurants, cafes and incredible vegan places to eat. I absolutely love it.

Later in the afternoon, I got back to my apartment and I decided that I'd make myself a little snack because I knew I wasn't going to eat until much later on. I had promised my friends, after my early exit the night before, that I would go out with them again that evening.

I was trying to figure out what I was going to wear and I started to feel as if I couldn't really be bothered to go. Now, this is very unlike me. I was only going to be around my friends for a couple of days, so I wasn't going to be able to spend much time with them; this feeling of not being bothered was a bit strange. I went through the motions and got dressed up and put a bit of make-up on, but when it came to leaving my apartment, I couldn't physically get out the door. It was like there was an energy field stopping me and I couldn't get past it. I realise that it sounds absolutely ridiculous. Surely I could just walk through it! But, there was something blocking me. It was like there was a resistance up against my chest and my shoulders that was holding me there.

I decided to sit down and wait for it to pass. An hour passed and I still couldn't get out the door. It felt like someone had sucked the life force out of me, it was a very draining feeling. After several more unsuccessful attempts to get out, I messaged my friends and told them I was really sorry but I was going to have to let them down. This was totally unlike me. I didn't let people down back then. If I said I was going to be somewhere, I'd be there 5 minutes early. My friends were shocked, but, by this point, they'd had a few cocktails, so they were good. They sent me messages saying they would miss me and they kept sending me videos of themselves having fun. It made me smile.

The whole thing was bizarre. It made no sense to me at all. I took my make-up off, got into something more comfortable and I went to bed.

The next morning, I still couldn't get my head around what had gone on, but I went about my day as normal. I went out for a beautiful long run and walked back, just to change things up a little bit. It was a beautiful winter day in Sydney and I immersed in it fully. When I got back to the apartment, I started to think about the event on Monday and how I still didn't know anything about it. I trusted my friend, but it would be helpful to at least know where I'm heading. I checked my emails and discovered the course was being run by a lady who was quite well known in the spiritual world, she had written some books and run a lot of workshops and courses. I messaged one of my girlfriends who lives in Perth and asked her what she knew about this woman. She wrote back immediately, "Oh my God, she is absolutely amazing. You're going to love it." That was validation enough for me. I thought I should check the ticket to see where the event was taking place. I looked at the time on the ticket and then I checked out the venue which stated – The Sydney Masonic Centre!

Oh my fucking God! How had I not checked this before? It was Sunday evening. I'm due to go to the event tomorrow at 6pm. I can't let her down now. I don't let people down, remember? I got on the phone to Ellie, the girl who I spoke to about the darkness in Cambodia. I got on the phone to Debs, my quantum healer, over in Melbourne. I spoke to a few other friends and asked them all to hold space for me whilst I went into the Masonic Centre. A couple of people told me not to go at all. Others told me to protect myself with everything I could – crystals, angels – the lot. Debs, my quantum healer, just said to me, in her beautiful Australian accent, "I've got you sister." And then, I told Ricky. Ricky told me very straight that he was not happy about me going there at all.

I listened to everybody's advice and came to the conclusion that If I was meant to know that it was at the Masonic Centre sooner – so I had enough time to pull out or get a refund – I would have looked at it a week or so ago; but, I didn't. At that point, I trusted that I was meant to be going and that something needed to be seen or heard. I asked everybody to hold space for me as I went in there the next day.

The reason I had such issues with the Masonic Centre was because I had been exposed to the Freemasons – their methodologies, rituals and their beliefs – several years before. Growing up, one of my uncles was a Freemason and I'd heard the word banded about for many years before I understood what it was. As far as I was concerned, it was a group of men that got together and did a funny handshake and women were not allowed. That's all I knew growing up. Through my awakening journey, though, I was shown how inverted religion, the Freemasons, and other similar kinds of communities had become. The Freemasons were the ones that fascinated me the most. It didn't make any sense. I learnt that initiates had to go through a massive process to be accepted. First and foremost, you needed to be nominated by somebody to join. Secondly, there was an initiation process that people needed to go through to get in. And it was only once they'd been through a number of these different initiations that they were actually accepted into the community. It intrigued me that there were these closed, secret societies that existed. Why did they need to be secret?

What benefit were they bringing? How were they impacting the world like that? When you dig deeper and research it more and more it becomes clear that the higher levels of Freemasons are very influential in the way the world is run, and not necessarily with the very best intentions for ordinary people. Now, I genuinely don't think all Freemasons are bad. I believe that there are many lower-level Freemasons out there that are extremely intentional with love and they truly believe they are doing the right thing, but at the higher levels, things appear to get very dark.

It's a subject that can be researched further if people are interested. For me, I had to know what was going on for a massive part of my awakening journey, but because I had, I was scared to go into the Masonic centre. I was scared of the symbolism I was going to see. I was scared of the vibration I was going to feel because, by this point, I was becoming very sensitive to the energies around me. If somebody had been hurt significantly in an area or a place where I was, I would know about it. So, how would I process that in a roomful of 300 people at this workshop? Did I even want to be giving my energy and my money to go into a place like that? The answer was quite frankly, 'No'.

On the Monday morning, I was a little bit edgy. I was even starting to question my friend Kylie as to whether she knew what she was getting us into. Bless her heart, she was at the start of her awakening journey at that point, and she thought it was going to be a really beautiful event. I took a deep breath and just trusted that everything was going to work out the way that it needed to. I had about six beautiful souls around the world who would be sending me good vibes and protection, so I knew I was going to be okay. I was loaded up with crystals and trusted that my guides were going to keep me safe.

We walked in there, and I prayed to God out loud, "Please look after us. Please help us get through this okay. Show me everything you need me to see so that it can help the journey. Get me in and out of here as quickly, and as safely as possible."

I sat down next to my friend, and all the people that we got chatting to were lovely. I thought – *I'm here with good people, so let's just see what unfolds.* The lady who was running the event came onstage and she seemed nice enough. She started chatting for a while, and some of the stuff she was saying was quite resonant with me, so I relaxed a little. Then she decided to do a chanting exercise, and as soon as she started doing it I felt sick. Kylie looked at me and mouthed, "What the fuck is this?" The woman on the stage looked like she had been possessed. My whole body closed down, it was like it decided that nothing was getting in here. I wasn't prepared to give this my time, love or attention. I sat there clutching a couple of crystals. I closed my eyes as if I was getting really into it. I set the intention that I was going to be safe, that I was going to get through it, and that nothing that this woman was doing was going to invert my space. I visualised a spinning light all the way from underneath my feet to the top of my head. I protected myself like a warrior. Anything that tried to hit me, was going to get blown straight back to them.

The lady carried on with her weird chanting, and looking possessed, and then she started singing, and something in my soul told me this was not right. Cheekily, I did a little voice recording of what she was saying, just so that I could remember the words because although I had no interest in what she was doing, something inside me needed to know what the words meant.

Kylie looked at me and motioned for us to get out of there. For a girl just at the start of her journey, her intuition was bang on point. We sneaked out and once we were outside we started laughing. "What the fuck was that all about?" I asked.

"I have no idea, but that woman was possessed," Kylie replied, and we laughed some more.

"Next time, I'm picking the event," I said, and she agreed.

I looked at my phone and I had messages from Ellie, Debs, and about a dozen missed calls from Ricky. I said my goodbyes to Kylie and headed home, answering my messages as I walked, to let everyone know I was okay.

I called Ricky back eventually. "Why the fuck have you not been answering your phone?" he asked. And it's not like Ricky to be like that.

"Alright Dad, calm down, I'm fine," I joked.

"I'm in the city, let me come and pick you up."

"I'm good. I really appreciate you caring, but if you want to come and pick me up, do so tomorrow. For now, let me walk, let me process what's just gone on. But know that I'm safe and I'm good." It wasn't what he wanted to hear, he wanted to be able to help me, but I needed a bit of space to myself and so reluctantly he agreed to meet me in the morning.

As I walked back to my apartment that night, I tried to make sense of what had gone on. This woman was a very well-known spiritual author and teacher. She had travelled all around the world doing this stuff. I had no idea at this point. I thought spirituality was good. I knew that other areas of society had been inverted, but not spirituality. Surely not? It didn't make any sense to me, so I kind of put that on ice for a while and allowed myself to process it. I wrote it up in my journal and settled down for the night. Ricky messaged me asking for the postcode and address of where he should pick me up from in the morning. I actually didn't know it or have it to hand so I couldn't send him it right away. He messaged again later on asking the same question but I fell asleep and forgot to get back to him. Whoops!

The next morning, I woke up and Ricky was getting a bit impatient with me, understandably, as he was coming to pick me up shortly and he still had no idea where I was. I eventually sent him the address and all the details, and all he sent me back was some laughing emoji faces. That was strange and not at all the kind of thing that Ricky would normally do, but I didn't think too much of it.

An hour or so later I got a call from Ricky to say he was outside. He explained to me where he was parked and I told him I would be a few minutes while I sorted some stuff out and handed the keys back. As I stood in the apartment, about to meet Ricky for the first time in a month or so, I was thinking about what I had learnt since I found out he was my twin flame. I had run away because it had all been too much to take in, but he had been on my case ever since about seeing him again. It was like his soul knew, yet his human did not. It was going to be weird for me, knowing this twin flame stuff. However, I knew at some point I was going to have to face him, and this was the time. To top it all off, of course, Ricky knew nothing about it.

I stepped outside the apartment and Ricky was there waiting, bless him. He helped me carry my stuff to the car, and he was laughing and smiling. I thought that clearly someone had got a good vibration going on today. He threw my stuff in the back of his car and then as I climbed into the passenger seat, he said, "You're not going to fucking believe this."

"Try me," I said, figuring he couldn't surprise me any more than the things I had been through in the last month since I saw him.

Ricky continued, "On Saturday night I was here. My mate lives here."

"I was on the 8th floor," I said.

"And I was there on Saturday. We went out for a few drinks on Saturday afternoon and then we ended up going back to his place, ended up staying there, drinking all night and partying. When you told me your address I couldn't believe it."

I laughed. "Oh my God!" All of a sudden it made sense why I couldn't get out the fucking apartment on Saturday night.

Ricky and I had been together just a matter of seconds and already the craziness was starting up.

104

We started driving towards Ricky's house, which was about an hour and a half outside of Sydney. He was asking me questions about what had been happening in my life since we last met, and I was asking about his family; we were having a really good catch-up. And then out of nowhere, he said to me, "Lucy, if you could live anywhere, where would you live?"

"Oh, you know I'd live in Sydney tomorrow if I could," I replied.

"No, I mean what kind of place? By the ocean?"

I thought about it for a while and then said, "My dream home is living in the middle of nowhere, surrounded by horses, with easy access to the beach, a beautiful swimming pool, a gym. A place where I can just do me before I go out into the outside world."

Ricky didn't say anything, he just started laughing at me, and I thought he was a bit rude. He asked me if I was hungry – which I was, I always am – and then he told me he had found this really nice vegan place that he thought I would like.

We sat down in this lovely restaurant and we both ordered chai lattes, which is our thing to do together. I thought it was lovely that Ricky had considered what I liked and had thought about me when he chose this place. We finished up and I had learnt my lesson when he said he was paying. I went to say that I would split the bill but then I just said, "Thank you so much. That's really beautiful of you. I'll get breakfast tomorrow." He smiled.

We carried on the drive to his house, and soon enough we pulled up next to these gates. Ricky said, "This is my house." We drove down the drive and it was a house surrounded by horses, in the country, with a gym and a swimming pool. In that moment, I understood why he had laughed when I was describing my dream house because I had essentially just described his house. Unbelievable!

His house was amazing, such a beautiful place. It was exactly the place I had seen in my visions before, but in those visions, I hadn't known where it was or whose it was, or what I was going to be doing there.

Ricky asked me if I wanted to go training with him. Again, this is our thing. Whenever I see him, that's what we do, we train. We go running together, we go training together, we push each other in good ways. At that time, he was training under a couple of really good guys, so I went boxing with him. We had a really good session. It had been a while since I had trained with Ric and it felt good to be back.

Afterwards, we grabbed some food, even though we were dripping with sweat and in our training gear. We had a good laugh together while we ate and reminisced. Ric and I get on really well. We can communicate about anything, any subject – apart from talking about ourselves and our relationship. We're not very good at talking about anything to do with us at all. This was proven in the car on the way back to his house when he made a snide comment about what happened in the Galapagos Islands. I turned myself to face him, even though we were in the car and I said to him, "Maybe we need to talk about this because there's obviously something underlying." I wanted him to know that I was serious, that I wanted to speak about it, if he was open and willing. He went a bit coy at that point, clearly feeling a little uncomfortable, and so I said, "You know that I didn't know a lot of stuff about you back then. I didn't know that it would upset you so much for me to pay for dinner, there wasn't ever any intent for me to hurt you." I know he heard me that night, but I don't know if he processed it or actually really took it in because it wasn't the last time that subject came up. Either way, I got to say that I was sorry. I got to explain from my perspective how that night had happened and from that moment forward, I forgave myself for the Galapagos situation, even if he couldn't.

The next few days were pretty much the same. I would get outdoors, train, ground, do headstands and cartwheels out on his front lawn. I did my journaling and continued writing this book. I took some time for myself whilst Ricky worked and then in the evening we would hang out. I was focused on a seminar that I was doing in October, I really wanted to help people. I knew I had a gift in my hand. I knew that I had been on an incredible healing journey and I was ready to share what I had learned to help other people do the same. So that's what I focused on when I was writing documents and PowerPoint slides for the seminar – but I just couldn't think of a name for it. My main business was called Activ8U but I needed a name for this workshop and anything else that would come off the back of it, but nothing was coming forward at all. I got to the point where I said out loud, "Come on, work with me! Give me the name!" But, it clearly wasn't the right time at that point because nothing was flowing other than 'Living Intuitively', which was the name of my Facebook group at that time.

One day, Ricky took me to another boxing trainer, a guy called Rodney who had become a good friend of his and someone he believed I would really like. And I did. He is a great guy. He spoke to me about aliens, spaceships and crazy conspiracy stuff that was going around. It was amazing. We got on so well. And to top that off, he is a phenomenal trainer, one of the best people I've ever had the privilege of working with. He helped me become methodical. He made me slow down, showed me breathing and moving my feet properly. He encouraged my head and shoulder movement. As much as I was a professional Muay Thai fighter, I'd never been trained in boxing properly. He made me much lighter on my feet and he made me really learn the movements that you're supposed to use, rather than the sheer power I had. You can get away with things in Thai boxing because you need to be solid to block but with boxing it's different. Rodney made such a difference in my life, we connected on a whole different level.

On the way driving back, it felt as if something had changed between Ric and I. It was almost like something had come in and cleared the air between the two of us. We were getting on really well anyway, we were extremely good friends by this point, but there had always been an undertone of stuff that had never been spoken about because we were too stubborn, similar, closed off, scared of commitment and all that stuff. We were literal mirrors of each other. Our approach was to block it all and hope it would not surface. We covered it up with our friendship, but there was always an elephant in the room.

Ricky suggested we grab some food, even though we were both dripping in sweat. I told him that I wasn't going into a restaurant in the state I was in, so he went into the back of his car and pulled out a grey hooded sweatshirt. I measured it against me and it was long enough to be a dress, so I put it on and whipped off all my wet underclothes. Ricky looked at me as if I was crazy. "Come on, let's go," I said and marched ahead into the restaurant.

After the meal we both really fancied a massage. It was a bit random but it was exactly what we felt we both needed, so we found a local place and we had the most amazing massage.

We drove back to Ricky's and we were both in a really good place. It felt like even more of the unspoken stuff between us had melted away. There was this understanding going on between us and he was igniting this thing within me that actually made me think that maybe I was ready for a relationship – not with him, but he was helping me to see how life in a relationship could be.

The next day, Ricky went out with his family. He's one of six boys who all work together. Every so often, like any business would, they get together, go out to dinner, brainstorm and throw ideas around. As he was leaving, he said to me, "I'll leave my car with you, so you can do whatever you need to do today."

"Thank you, that's great," I said, but knowing he had one of those big ute truck things, there was no way little old me would be manoeuvring it out of the driveway. I was home alone that day and night. I did my usual stuff – my routine, workout and writing. I had some really profound insights that day. It was almost like the divine had recognised I was opening my heart more and more and so it thought it's time to provide some gold. That day, the name of the event I was running came through to me out of the blue. I was sitting grounding on the grass outside the front of this house. Two random dogs appeared from nowhere and adopted me. I sent Ricky a photo of them and asked him whose they were. He replied, "What the fuck are you talking about? They are nothing to do with me. Where have they come from?" It was hilarious. Animals do that to me, they follow me and then adopt me. So I was sitting with these two dogs, doing my work and out of nowhere, the name 'Self Love Club' dropped in. I sat there and thought — *Nah, it doesn't resonate with me. It's not for me.* Boom! It came in again. *Sorry. That's not for me. That's ego. I don't know what it is. I feel like I've seen it on a mug or something, but it's just not for me.* And it came again and I thought — *For fuck's sake!* This is my message. Three times it came. Three times. Three signs. You can't ignore that.

I grabbed my laptop and I searched 'Self Love Club' and as expected the search returned pictures of tattoos on the back of girls' arms or pictures of coffee mugs with the slogan on it. And, to be honest, even the word 'love' still made me feel a bit cringe at that point. I knew it was important and I knew it was a vibration that we needed to go to; but, self-love? What even was that? It sounded rude, it felt self-indulgent.

I sat with it for a while, but I kept coming back to — *No man is ever going to come to 'Self Love Club' because it's so feminine, it's so pink.* It really didn't resonate with me at all. By the evening, I was getting a bit impatient with myself because I didn't like the name and yet it just kept coming through constantly. I decided to get out for a while and get away from thinking about the name. Ricky had told me about a lovely restaurant that did amazing Indian food, and they had an incredible aubergine dish, so I thought I would pay them a visit. That was easier said than done because Ricky lives in the middle of nowhere and the car he had left me was massive. Nevertheless, I fancied a challenge, so I got in the truck and drove over to the restaurant to pick up my food. It was easy enough, there were no issues driving or parking and my food smelt amazing. What I hadn't accounted for was that by the time I headed back to Ricky's it was pitch black outside and I had no idea where his house was. Somehow, I found my way to his road but I couldn't see which his house was. I was looking for his gate, but I couldn't find it. I got as far as a roundabout and I knew I had gone too far, so I had to turn back and try again. I was kerb-crawling slowly along his road determined not to miss the house again.

Finally, after a good while of driving up and down the road, I found his house. By this time, I was starving as I had the incredible smell of the food in the car teasing me. I messaged Ricky and told him what I had been up to. He thought it was hilarious, but not surprising.

I ate my food, it was delicious, and then I realised I needed some stuff from the supermarket! This was going to be more challenging because it would involve parking his monster truck in a multi-storey carpark, but I decided to face my fears and take on the challenge. It went perfectly. I was becoming a bit of a dab hand at this malarkey.

The next day, after Ricky got back from work, I wanted to run the name of the seminar by him and so I asked him, "What do you think about the name Self Love Club?"

"In what context?" he asked.

"Well, it's for the name of my seminar that I'm running in October, I've been told it has to be Self Love Club."

He nodded and said, "Yeah, that sounds quite nice for you girls."

"That's the point. Would you come to a seminar that's called Self Love Club?" I asked him, knowing already what his answer would be.

"Nope. Absolutely not" he said, shaking his head.

"And there lies my problem because I have to help the men as well. This can't just be about the women."

I was feeling frustrated because the more I pushed against it, the more my guides kept on giving it to me in different signs and synchronicities. I eventually surrendered.

Oh well. Self Love Club it is then!

It was coming to the end of my time in Sydney. We had gotten on so well, I was really glad I had followed the intuitive pulls to go back and experience this. We had trained together and hung out a significant amount of time. We'd had a great laugh and it felt like the air had been cleared. I had no idea why he wanted me at his house when he first invited me, but it now made sense. It worked really well. I was in a great space of gratitude for him because he had shown me that I was able to be in a relationship, which was something that I didn't think I was capable of anymore, it had been a while. And now I felt ready for it. I felt as if I was ready to go on a journey. It was time to find the man.

On the way back from our last training session together, he said to me, "I want to take you out on the Friday night before you fly home. I want to take you somewhere really special, to my favourite place in the city."

"Wow, that's very kind of you. Thank you," I said.

"I'll drive us in and we can get a taxi back. Dress up, though, it's going to be special."

I made a special effort that night and when I emerged from my room, Ricky was visibly taken aback. "Oh my God, you scrub up all right." I realised Ricky had never seen me dressed up nice. Our entire relationship had been about training together, rolling and running around in the Amazon, that kind of stuff. It was probably one of the only times that he had ever seen me in heels, up to this point.

We drove into the city that night. We got stuck in traffic on the way and so spent the journey playing old-school dance tunes on the stereo and having a dance and a giggle, reminiscing about our younger party days.

We eventually arrived at the restaurant and it was beautiful. It looked a bit like Batman's cave. The food was stunning, and so was the wine – we sampled quite a bit of it that night.

On the way back, knowing it was our last night together, we were reminiscing and thinking about the fact that two complete strangers had met in Thailand, and here we were five years down the line. In the last two months alone, we had spent almost four weeks together. I turned to him in the car and said, "Thank you. Thank you for everything. Firstly, I never thought we would ever be in this position where we could be civil with each other after what happened in the Galapagos. So I thank you for forgiving. I thank you for showing me that maybe I'm ready for a relationship. I never thought that this was possible, that somebody would actually let me just be me."

Ricky appreciated what I was saying and we continued having a beautiful conversation all the way home. When we arrived at his house, he turned to me and said, "Why don't you just stay? What's the point in you going home, you're coming back here in September anyway."

Typical Lucy, though, I spoke before I thought. "Well, I've got to speak at a seminar, and then I'm running my own seminar on the 1st of September, and don't forget I've got all this stuff to organise with my health."

Ricky came straight back with, "Well I can take you to the doctors and to the hospital." He was being so sweet, so open and vulnerable and it spooked me again.

"No, no. I've got to run the seminar…. I've also got to speak at that Social Media event," I answered from my ego and from fear. I completely missed the memo. I chose to reject his vulnerability and closed down once again.

The two of us just couldn't get to a place of total vulnerability with each other. We mirrored and triggered each other's insecurities. We were both scared of commitment.

The next day, was my time to leave. I sobbed my heart out at the airport. My soul knew that she shouldn't have been leaving, but my physical was concerned with running the seminar and the fact I had people relying on me. I had to show up. And then of course there was all the hospital stuff I needed to attend to. They were all excuses, though. I should have stayed on, and I knew it in my heart. It was too late by then.

I sat on the plane feeling sad. Typically, I was sat on the side of the plane which swept around to see the Opera House and that beautiful view. I sat there looking out the window, sobbing my aching little heart out. I cried for about 5 hours of that journey. I knew I'd made the wrong decision, but in true Lucy fashion, I wasn't vulnerable enough to say so. That journey was a fucking long journey. I considered every option. *What if I had said that? What if I did this? What if that had happened?* I went round and round in circles and it was painful.

When I stopped in Singapore for a transfer to a different plane, I got to the point where I told myself – *Enough is enough. Just stop this shit. Let it go. You didn't make that choice. You weren't vulnerable enough. Now let it go! Move the heck on! At least I would be back with him in a month.*

I had messed up with Ricky again. How many more times would this cycle repeat itself? I knew that if I wanted to be happy and be in a relationship, I was going to have to make some changes in myself. I didn't realise that the Universe was going to hit me so hard in order for me to learn that lesson, and how quickly that was about to happen.

105

I went to hell and back on that plane! All of which was my own doing, which made it even worse. Why could I not think before I speak? Why could I not realise what is being asked of me? Why could people not say exactly what they want – spell it out clearly, so I could get it?

I got back in the UK to August rain and it heightened my depression even further. *Why had I decided to come back from the place where my heart was? What was I scared of? Why could I not let this stuff go?*

Why could I not open up to love? So many questions. The great irony was that I went to my dad's house from the airport — as all my stuff was there and I planned to stay with him for a while — so I was faced with the very reason as to why I had found it so difficult to love and trust in the first place.

I had to pull myself together and get focused very quickly because I needed to call the doctor and find out why I had been losing so much blood over the last few months. I realised that I needed to sort my health out now and I had to leave Australia behind me, emotionally and physically. I also needed to get ready for the seminar that I was running on the 1st of September; and it wasn't like I had long to wait to go back to Australia as I was due to land there again on the 13th of September.

The doctor called me, and because they were well aware of this issue from my past, they didn't even bother to run blood tests on me, they just immediately booked me an appointment with a specialist. The only problem was that the nearest appointment was in November. When I called the doctor back and told him how far away my appointment was, he told me to have some blood tests in the meantime, and check where my levels were, so that's what I did.

A few days later, I got the blood test results back and, indeed, many of my levels were quite low. He told me to take certain supplements and offered me some pills to stop the bleeding. I could have easily taken the pills, but I didn't. In my mind. If you're bleeding, there is something wrong and action needs to be taken. I couldn't get my head around stopping my body from doing something when it was clearly signalling to me that there was an issue.

As a result of not taking the tablets, the bleeding continued.

That weekend I had been asked to arrange a one-day event for the people who I worked with in the marketing business. There were about 30 of us set to attend. I had found a really beautiful location at a golf course about 20 minutes from my dad's house in Weybridge. Donna, who was becoming my assistant, helped me to arrange it all. As soon as we first drove into the place, we both knew that this was where it needed to be. Naturally, there was a beautiful golf course but also the drive up to the clubhouse had beautiful grassy areas, stunning woodland and incredible views from the terrace of the clubhouse. The food was supposed to be really good there too, so we agreed to run it there.

Besides the bleeding, which had become something I was getting used to living with, things had been going okay for me upon my return. I was still chewing the fat on the situation that had happened there, but I was getting on with things. It was only a couple of weeks before I was going back there, I had a real focus to crack on. I felt extremely connected and passionate about life.

On the Saturday – the day of the event – I was really excited. The location was perfect and the crowd that gathered were enjoying themselves. I was the only person speaking at the event that day, and so I was on stage almost the entire time. At some point, early on in the event, Ricky kept flashing in front of my face – just an image of him. I kept thinking – *What the heck? What's going on?* This kept happening throughout the morning. I got to lunchtime and was sitting outside having some food; his face started appearing again in my mind's eye. I said to one of my friends, "Something is going on with Ric because I keep seeing him flash in front of my face as I'm speaking and I don't know what to do about it."

"Maybe you're just missing him," she joked – taking the piss out of me.

I smiled at her, but said, "No. It's more than that. It's definitely something more than that." Sydney was 9 hours ahead and this was just after midday, so it was nighttime in Sydney. I thought – *Oh screw it. I'll message him once I'm done here and check that he's okay.* All afternoon, though, I kept getting these chilling feelings going through my body, and as much as I kept focused, I couldn't shake it off. It bothered me the whole afternoon, but professional Lucy just about held it together.

We had an amazing day in the end. I put the weird Ricky stuff behind me and made sure the day was a success. A couple of the girls suggested going for a celebratory drink afterwards, and as they lived quite close to me, we found a beautiful pub in Weybridge that overlooked the river. As I sat there having dinner, I kept getting the feeling that there was something wrong with Ricky, so I messaged him and asked if he was okay. I didn't expect to hear back from him for a while as it was the middle of the night there.

I went to bed later that night and fell asleep immediately. At about 5 in the morning, I woke up in a panic. I felt that I had been with Ricky in my astral travels, but I didn't really remember the details because I had woken up with such a shock. I looked at my phone and I had a message from him. The message read, "Lucy, I had a heart attack last night."

I was stunned and shocked.

The message continued, "I can't make any rhyme or reason of what went on and what happened to me, but you were there."

My heart dropped. I had never felt like that about anybody. It was like when my grandad died or when my mother had her cancer scare. Ricky felt like family to me. I sobbed. I couldn't even respond to him at that time because I was too upset. *What on earth was going on? Why did I not stay?*

His messages continued to tell me that he was doing okay now. He was still in hospital but was hoping to be released pretty soon. I asked him to call me and he did. He talked me through everything that had happened.

He had been at home on his own. He had been on a bit of a journey with himself, reflecting on things and had started to experience breathing difficulties in his room, so he thought he would go outside to get some fresh air. He managed to get himself outside, but then it started to get worse, the feeling of his chest closing made him panic. Thankfully, he had taken his phone outside with him and had managed to call his brother. He mumbled enough down the phone for his brother to panic and get straight over to him. His brother found Ricky out cold on the grass. He quickly scooped him up into the car and whisked him into the hospital as quickly as possible. When the medical team saw him, they had to bring him back. All Ricky remembered was that I was there with him.

Now, at this point, I already knew that my soul and his soul were intertwined and interconnected, and that's why his soul called me and made the choice. He remembered making a choice to come back. He went on a journey where he saw all that he hadn't achieved and made the decision to come back and get it done.

I listened to everything he was telling me. He had been through a shocking experience. He could so easily have decided to check out at that point. As heartless as this may sound, I had to sit, listen and digest the energetics around this situation. He was a messenger, the most important living messenger in my life at that point. This was significant what he was going through. He was scared, I could hear it in his voice. I wondered if somewhere in his soul he had remembered. His heart attack had happened on the Saturday night going into Sunday morning, and I was speaking with him on the Sunday afternoon. I knew he needed to rest and recuperate and so I told him I would leave him for a few days to concentrate on getting better, but that if he needed me I was here, anytime.

I couldn't believe what I had just heard. I had a seminar that I was due to be speaking at on the Tuesday and Wednesday, so I decided to take the Sunday off doing work, so I could process everything that had just been shared, then spend the next day or so taking time to get ready for the seminar. I used that seminar as a distraction to what was happening with Ric on the other side of the world.

106

The seminar I was attending wasn't my seminar. I was speaking at an event for the company whose products I was selling in my business. I was so excited to have been picked for it because it was a couple of days' retreat at a really beautiful hotel in Windsor – dinner, cocktails – you name it, it was all thrown in. Now, as much as that wasn't really my scene at that point, I was really looking forward to being around like-minded people, who could potentially share some gold that would assist my business growth. The seminar was around social media and business and, at this point, it was my life. I was so excited, despite the fact I was running pretty low on energy due to the blood loss. I felt as if my tank was pretty low all the time.

In the days leading up to that event, I had been to the hospital twice because things had changed within my body. I was getting really dizzy and weak, but every time I went in there, they would discharge me with more pills. Even the day before the retreat in Windsor, I had to go to the hospital because of the bleeding and the masses of clots that were falling out of me. It was very scary.

At that point, I did succumb to taking the tablets to try and stop the bleeding. I was left with no choice, they categorically told me I needed to take them. Then, as usual, they sent me away. They didn't scan me or anything and so I thought I must be just being a hypochondriac and nothing was that serious. That's a dangerous place to be in — where there is something seriously wrong with you, but you are made to feel like it isn't that serious and so you carry on regardless, assuming you are being dramatic. That's the dangerous thing about the medical system; you get a five-minute appointment and the doctor has to diagnose you correctly in that short amount of time, which is never enough and is the reason why doctors are always running behind schedule. I think it's unfair to expect a doctor to be able to serve you in the best way that they can with a five-minute appointment. On top of that, the hospitals and doctors have to do so much paperwork to get you to be seen by a specialist, it's no wonder they would rather not refer you. I'm not meaning to get at the medical industry when I say this, but through this experience, I was being shown the limitations that were in place.

So, thinking everything was okay, I went off to Windsor. It's only a 45-minute journey from my dad's house, but by the time I got there I had gone through a super-plus Tampax and a super-plus towel — which was massive, like a nappy — but I bled through them all nevertheless. It was absolutely horrific. I dashed into the building and briefly said hello to people, and then ran to my room to sort myself out. I was in total despair around it, but I had no choice other than to get on with it.

The afternoon was all about coming together, introductions to various people and setting the tone for the next few days. The next day was going to be much more in-depth, I was going to speak, and several other people had presentations and speeches to make. The location was beautiful and the grounds were stunning. I went out walking barefoot by the river to ground as much as I could. Even though I had this trauma going on, I was able to do some of the things that I needed to do to make me feel a little bit better. And they did. They got me through that first day.

That evening we went for dinner. It was really beautiful, the food was amazing and many people were drinking cocktails but I didn't want to drink at all, I wanted to keep a level head because of what was going on with my body. I stayed out until midnight and then went back to my room, eventually getting to bed at about 1 am.

I must have been asleep about an hour when I woke up and I felt as if my womb was falling out of me. I ran to the bathroom and sat on the toilet. The amount of blood and clots that started falling out of me was scary. I sat on the toilet for an hour, constantly bleeding, crying my eyes out. It was horrific. I didn't know what to do. I was scared. If I went and got back into bed, it was likely that I would bleed everywhere, so I just sat there on the toilet – there was nothing else I could do. I was too scared to leave that room, but I was exhausted. I looked in the mirror and I was yellow. I honestly thought – *Am I going to die in this hotel room on my own?*

I sat there for about an hour and a half, and I felt so exhausted that I just had to clamber back into bed. I wrapped myself up in whatever I possibly could find to make sure that I was safe down there; I was conscious of not wanting to make a mess of the hotel room. I managed to get back to sleep for about an hour and then I was up again. Same thing. Bleeding heavily. The only word I can use to describe what was going on is gushing. Blood was gushing out of me. Again, I sat there and sobbed. *I cannot do this. I cannot go and speak.* It was 6 am by this time, I had the whole day of work ahead of me, and right there and then, I couldn't possibly leave my room. I messaged one of the girls and I said I was having a bit of a nightmare with my period – because I didn't want to go into too much detail – and that I would be a bit late. We were supposed to be meeting up at 8 am but I needed to call my doctor at that time. I needed to be seen by someone immediately. I called the doctors as soon as the surgery opened and pleaded for an appointment later that day but they could only offer me one the following morning, so I took it. I was starting to feel really scared. I had no idea how I was going to get through the day. I didn't know how I was going to drive home. I had lost so much blood, it was crazy. It was like the whole of my insides were collapsing.

I managed to pull myself together enough to get dressed. I was popping my supplements, tripling down on them – anything that might help. God knows how I did it, but I went into the event and held it together the best I could. It came time for me to do my speech and as I started speaking, my voice started getting really croaky and I was finding it difficult to speak. The last time I lost my voice was in 2014, just as my healing journey started. I was lying on a beach in Thailand with tonsillitis. I recall it so well because I remember thinking if I'm going to get sick and take time out, where better to do it than on a beach where I could sweat it out?

Nowadays, I know that the dynamics around losing your voice is because you're not speaking your truth or because something is attacking your voice. Back then, though, I didn't quite have that awareness and I was also in the midst of a major issue. My physical body was under so much pressure because I had lost so much blood and I also hadn't been eating the best. Although the food at the event was amazing, normally if this situation was happening to me and I was at home, I would be loading up on the deep leafy green vegetables, legumes loaded with iron and all of the bright reds and bright purples to replenish my blood. But here, I was at the mercy of the hotel so I could only do so much. I felt really weak when I stood up and extremely dizzy – like you get when you stand up too quickly but it passes in a few seconds, only this dizziness wasn't passing. It got to the point that afternoon where I couldn't speak anymore, which was awkward because I was sat on a panel giving feedback to others. I had to write it down and let somebody else read it because my voice wouldn't work. It was my body saying to me – *Get your butt to the doctor.* I had thought I was a hypochondriac on the Monday and being dramatic about nothing, but now, on the Wednesday, I had lost so much blood, I knew I was in trouble.

Once the event finished, people decided they were going to stick around and have a drink and a chat, but I had to get home, so I made my excuses and headed back to Weybridge. It took me just over an hour to get home. By the time I got there, I felt so weak that I had to go lie down in bed. The only problem was that I was still on the very top floor of my dad's house and I was struggling to even get up the first flight of stairs. It felt like somebody had a blowtorch on my legs and my bones. It was so painful. I managed to climb to the top of the first flight but I had to sit down and rest for a while before I could attempt to take the next set on. I sat there for a while attempting to catch my breath and thinking – *This is really weird. I'm fit and healthy. I run ten kilometres a day. I train Thai boxing most days but I can't get up a flight of stairs. What on earth is going on?*

At that point, I knew that something was really wrong. Through sheer will and determination, I made it to my bedroom, and I lay on the bed and tried to keep myself calm. That night I managed to eat quite a lot of green veggies and load up on red foods just to make sure that I was getting the iron content for my body, and replenishing the blood through the colours of the foods that I was eating. Thankfully, I was trained in this stuff, so I knew what I was doing to a point, even though I was not in a good way.

The next morning, I got up early and went to see the doctor. This time, though, it wasn't my usual doctor, this was a lady doctor I hadn't seen before. She looked at everything with a fresh pair of eyes. She scrutinised the notes of everything that they had been doing over the previous couple of weeks. After a while of sifting through the notes, she turned to me and said, "Lucy, I don't know how to tell you this, but you need to go and get a blood transfusion."

"No I don't. You must be wrong, I was only in hospital on Monday and they said I was fine," I replied, trying to convince myself and her in the process..

"I'm looking at your blood test results. They should have given you a blood transfusion on Monday. I have no idea why they didn't."

In my mind, there was no way I was having someone else's blood inside me. I had worked so hard over the last few years to get myself into alignment with my gifts and let the divine flow through me. The thought of having someone else's blood inside me made me feel all of that would be blocked out. I was adamant that there was no way I could have a transfusion. And actually, the thought of somebody else's blood actually made me feel sick. *What if they had diseases? What if they had HIV?* My mind was going all over the place with this. I knew intellectually that all the blood gets screened and it's perfectly safe, but in that moment where you are faced with a choice, it doesn't make it easier. I said to her, "I'd really rather not have a blood transfusion."

She looked at me sternly and said, "I don't think that's going to be an option for you, but what I would like to do first is run some blood tests."

I was okay with that, at that point. *I mean, I'm bleeding out, I've had blood tests all week. What the fuck – take some more! Why not have the lot* – my ego piped up.

I went from her room, straight to have some blood tests done. This was on the Thursday morning. I was due to be flying back to Sydney on the Sunday evening. I asked how quickly I would hear back from them with the results, but they weren't sure and suggested I should go home and rest. The way I thought of it was that if I didn't hear back from them before I flew off on Sunday then I would just deal with it when I got back.

I went home to start packing for my trip to Sydney and to spend some time with my little sisters before I left. At around 4 pm that afternoon, I began doing a Facebook Live, something I aimed to do every day at this point. I was in the swing of the live, on a roll, chatting away to my followers, when all of a sudden my phone started ringing. Now, when you're live on Facebook and your phone starts ringing, the live broadcast just freezes. I saw the call come in and it threw me off a bit and I even considered declining the call and carrying on with my live broadcast, but something made me pick it up as I knew it was my doctor calling me.

The male voice on the other end said, "Lucy? This is Dr. Webber, and I'm one of the partners at the surgery."

"Oh, hello. Nice to speak to you. I haven't spoken to you before," I replied.

"I've got some updates for you on your blood tests," he said, but he sounded as if something really tragic had happened.

"Okay…" I said, picking up on his demeanour.

"Lucy, can you get to the hospital please?"

I said, "What do I need to go to the hospital for?"

"Lucy, you need an urgent blood transfusion. Your haemoglobin levels are dangerously low," he repeated that phrase again. "Dangerously low." He continued to tell me that I had extremely low oxygen in my body – way under 50% at the time of the blood tests. They figured that I had lost about three and a half pints of blood in a matter of days. I said to him, "Is there another option Doctor?"

He sternly said, "Absolutely not."

I responded, "I'm flying to Sydney on Sunday. Can I do it when I get back?"

"Absolutely no way. This is serious, Lucy. I don't think you realise how serious this is. If you get on a plane and take off, your body will attempt to equalise and you won't have enough oxygen in your body to do that. The outcome will be the plane will not be able to turn around and get you to the ground quick enough to be able to revive you."

My heart sank.

He said again," Can you get to the hospital soon? I'm happy to call an ambulance for you and get you blue lighted. This is very serious."

I told him I would get a lift there from my dad right away. To remind me how serious this was, as he was going he said, "They're expecting you at the hospital. I've arranged everything. If you don't go to the hospital, I'm going to make sure that there is a block on your travel. Because if you travel, it will put not only yourself, but everybody else on that plane in danger."

Crikey. He was serious. I didn't know if he was actually able to block me from travelling but he scared me enough to realise that I needed to get to the hospital and quickly. At this point, I was still getting on that plane on Sunday. I went to speak to my dad for his opinion. I knew he would support me in whatever I choose to do. "Dad, I've just had a phone call from the doctor and apparently I've got to go to the hospital for an urgent blood transfusion."

My dad dropped what he was doing, looked at me and asked, "Oh my, that's serious. Are you okay? What are you going to do?"

"Dad, I really don't want to have somebody else's blood."

"Can you have mine?" he asked, knowing we had the same blood type.

"I don't think it's quite that simple, but thanks," I said.

He asked me to explain everything that the doctor had said to me, so I repeated verbatim what the doctor said. My dad looked at me, and I'll never forget his words of wisdom, "Lucy, do me a favour. Go online and check what level you need your haemoglobin to be at in order to fly." I did just that and I realised that my levels were at almost half of what was considered advisable. And with that, I realised I wasn't getting on any plane without having a transfusion.

I packed a bag and grabbed some food because I had no idea when I was going to be back. It was already late on Friday and so I knew I would be there at least a few hours. I was so ignorant of what a blood transfusion entailed, I thought it might take an hour or so to put some blood in me, then I would be good to go.

Dad said he would drive me there, but he needed to check with his wife what was happening with the girls. A minute or so later, the front door slammed shut and the car pulled off – his wife had purposely driven off and left him to look after the children, knowing I needed to go to hospital. I thought – *What a fucking bitch!* I didn't want my dad to drag the kids out in the car and so I said I would get a taxi. He was so apologetic, but it wasn't his fault, he has shocking taste in women.

I called a taxi.

I arrived at the hospital. Thankfully, my doctor had called ahead and organised it all because as soon as I walked in, they took one look at me, got me a wheelchair and wheeled me into a private space. They put me on a bed and instantly linked me up to various monitors, and inserted cannulas in my arms. I was feeling a bit worried about the way they were treating me and the severity of all the devices they were attaching to me. A short time after I arrived, a beautiful male nurse came over to me. He was incredible. He was so flamboyant and over the top, which I was so grateful for, he raised my spirits. He said, "Sweetie, what have you done? Now don't you worry, we're going to get you sorted."

I grabbed his hand and said, "Can you help me? I need to be out of here by Saturday night or Sunday morning."

"You're asking for a lot, Sweetie," he said.

"Seriously, you've got to help me. I need to be on a flight to Sydney."

"Well, then we best get this show on the road," and with that he took control and got things moving. I'll never forget him. He made me feel so comfortable. He talked me through everything that was going to happen. He told me that the blood had been kept on ice, which would mean it's too cold to go into the body at that point. They need to bring it out of the chiller and warm it up so that it was the perfect temperature, so as not to cause any issues with the human body. Who knew that a blood transfusion could give you a heart attack and potentially kill you if the temperature was wrong? All of a sudden it became even more serious than before. He told me it was going to be a long process, and that they planned to give me three bags of blood. He then went on to explain that each bag can take up to five hours each. I worked it out and all I could think was – *Fuck, I'm here for the duration.*

Within a few hours, they moved me to a private room on a ward because they knew they would be working on me throughout the night. They had run some blood tests when I'd arrived and when they got the results back, they saw that my levels had dropped to a precarious low. My oxygen had dropped to less than 40% and I was in danger of my organs starting to shut down. Hearing this caused some panic in me, and yet at the same time, I had also grown so much that I was somehow trusting the fact that this was happening for a reason. Clearly, there was something I needed to learn from this experience and I was open to it — even though I wanted it over, I knew I had no choice.

I had messaged a friend when I first arrived at the hospital and asked her to bring me some bits and bobs in. Just at the right time, she turned up. She had bought me some shakes and some of my fruit and veggie capsules, plus loads of fruit. She was shocked when she saw me. I asked her to take some photos of me, so I could see what I looked like. They are frightening to look back on. It was all such an eerie, surreal experience. Just five days earlier, in this exact hospital, I was told I was fine and to go home, and yet here I am on the edge of God knows what.

A nurse came in and said that they were going to start administering the first bag within the next hour or so. Now, thankfully, nobody told me at any point that a blood transfusion can kill you. I was completely ignorant and just happy to crack on. In my head, this was a simple process, I would get the three bags done and I would be on my way. I didn't think this was a life-saving moment or that these people were working around the clock to save me, I just thought it was a basic transaction. I couldn't quite understand why doctors and nurses kept coming in to check on me, and why they kept asking me how I was — all the whilst looking stern and apprehensive. I was later told that the initial period of a blood transfusion can be very dangerous.

My friend was asked to leave before they started the transfusion. Once it was underway, I relaxed and set some intentions. I put out a golden infinity — a figure of eight on its side in gold between my heart and the blood. I was constantly thanking the blood donor — whoever that was. *Thank you.* I was connecting myself to the blood, using the beautiful golden infinity, and purifying it. I had a thing in the back of my mind that there was something wrong with the blood, so I thought that all I can do is energetically protect it, energetically protect myself, and energetically purify it. Now, I'm sure some people wouldn't bother doing any of that stuff or think it's total nonsense, but it does work. It changes the intention, it changes the vibration of things. I was in such a space of gratitude at this point, I wasn't thinking — *Oh, poor me, this is going to kill me. Poor me, I'm going to miss my flight.* I was the absolute opposite — I was grateful for this blood. *This blood is going to make me feel better. I'm going to be more energised. This is going to help me get back on track.* I was living fully in that space. I even tapped into the person who donated the blood, I know what their soul looked like. And I kept sending them love and thanks.

The staff maintained their vigilant checks and monitoring of me, still with concern and anxiety on their faces, but I was oblivious. I had to lay with my arm in a certain place which wasn't very comfortable, in a hospital that had a really heavy and dark energy – as most hospitals do – and all I wanted to do was to be at home, with the twins getting ready to go on my flight on Sunday. I wasn't letting that go. Ricky needed me, and I needed to be there for him. That was all I was thinking about as I lay there whilst that first bag of blood was being delivered.

I found out afterwards that there was a bit of a major panic on that first night with me, but my version of events is quite different.

107

I dropped into a space of what I thought was meditation. And in that space, my beautiful grandad came through holding my hand, telling me I was going to be okay. He told me if I wanted to be okay, I would be okay, to trust the process. I was so emotional seeing him in my mind's eye or in whatever realm I was seeing him in. I said to him, "Grandad, I can't die. I've only just got connected to my purpose. I can't die." He gave me a really sweet smile and a knowing look as if to say, "It's all going to be okay." And then I looked past my grandad and there was a figure of a man and I thought – *Who is that?* Then I recognised the vibration and it was Archangel Michael. He was stood tall and proud. He didn't say a word, just stood there and watched. I thought – *This is a bit weird. What's going on here?* Then I felt a gentle, warm feminine presence by my right shoulder – they were administering the blood into my right arm – and it was behind that. It was a beautiful golden glowing presence – and it turned out it was Archangel Gabriel. I looked at my grandad and said, "Grandad, what's happening to me? Am I going to be okay?" He didn't say a word. He just looked at me. And that's when I started saying – or at least I thought I was saying it out loud, "You can't take me. I'm not ready to go anywhere. I've just got connected to my purpose.

I promise you, if you make me better, I will do whatever is needed. I will do whatever it takes to help whoever needs to be helped. I will share my story. I will guide people so that they know that this kind of stuff can happen." I also promised that I would stop giving the medical industry a hard time because although they had showed me the many flaws in their system, they were saving my life at this point.

After a while of being in this space, I must have drifted off because one of the nurses came in to check on me and she snapped me back into reality. I looked at her, smiled and said, "Thank you so much." Because I knew that I was back in my body and I knew that I was going to survive, but I also had the realisation that the reason this was happening was because I still had a little bit of animosity towards my dad and I had to let it go.

For the last hour or so of the first blood transfusion, I sat there and I looked really deeply into the limitations that I had where my dad was concerned, and I found it. I found where it was and how it had manifested in me. And I was able to have empathy for myself, but also to fully forgive my dad. I feel that is why my stepmother had to be such a bitch that night, I had to have that bit of resentment and anger still in me. It was almost like a little bit of a power struggle between me and her, but now I got it. And in all honesty, that was the gift of it. I had finally got it. I finally decided – really, truly, deeply decided that I was going to forgive my dad for everything. I thought I had done the work. I thought I had released it all, but I hadn't fully.

Once the first bag of blood was finished, a nurse came in and asked me how I was feeling. She looked really worried, but I said, "Yeah, I'm good, I'm good."

"Great. We're going to disconnect this bag and then we're going to need to run a blood test on you in a little while, and then we'll administer the next bag."

"Do I really need another one?" I asked, hopefully. In my mind, I was thinking that another bag means another five hours and with all the messing around in between, it was going to be a long night. "You know I've got a flight tomorrow?"

She looked at me and smiled, "If we can get you there, we'll get you there. Just be patient, though, this is your health. This is much more important." All I could think was – *They don't get it. They don't know Ricky has had a heart attack and I need to be there for him.* It was my ego speaking. And, once again, I was putting somebody else above my own needs.

My beautiful friend came back in to see me on the Saturday, bringing more fruit and goodies to keep me going. I was popping my vitamin and mineral capsules like they were going out of fashion. One of the nurses came and told me that I couldn't take them, she didn't even ask what they were. I told her in no uncertain terms that I would be taking them. I think she thought it was some sort of actual medication but they were just fruits and vegetables. A new doctor came in the room and looked at my details and then asked me, "How are you feeling, Lucy?"

"I feel great. I'm ready to go home," I replied.

He looked at me and shook his head, "Not quite so fast, you know, we've got another bag to administer."

"Oh God, really? Another 5 hours!" I was thinking – *Flight to Sydney!*

"Lucy, just so you know, the second one can usually be administered a lot quicker. Just go with it. I've got to run more tests on you after this bag because I don't want you to be leaving here and you getting poorly again. We need to make sure that we do it properly."

I really appreciated his explanation and his concern. At that point, I once again accepted that I needed to be there, so I leant into the process once more. They linked me up to the next bag of blood which started flowing quite quickly. After about an hour, I needed to go to the toilet, so I asked the nurse if it was okay. She said as long as I took it easy, I should be fine. She offered to walk me there but I felt strong enough to go on my own. On my way to the toilet, I realised I was in the gynaecology ward. I looked around and saw a ward full of women who all looked really depressed. I decided to walk in with a huge smile across my face and said, "Hey, ladies, how are you?" All the women suddenly snapped out of their sad little bubble and started talking, not only to me, but also to each other. It struck me later on, that I went in there because I had to see the trauma that these women were going through – many of them had had hysterectomies. At 33, I was told I needed to have a hysterectomy as the course of treatment for exactly what I was going through now. The doctors had started discussions at the hospital about considering it as an option this time too. I was on a mission to get out of there and heal, though.

I needed to ignite the determination in me to heal. I had promised myself – *I'm going to do all I can to save my womb!* I had no idea how at that time, I just trusted that through an intuitive healing journey, it was possible. I chatted to the women for a while, and asked them questions. I feel that I cheered them up somewhat, I felt empowered and it ignited a fire in my belly to prove this healing could be done.

I went back to my room and sat there thinking about those women, whilst the remainder of the blood was administered. I decided I would do whatever it took to make people know that they have another option when it comes to their health and healing.

The doctor came back and he said to me that he needed to send me for a scan, and then some more blood tests. When I went for the scan, they found the lumps, which I already knew were there.

After the tests, I went back to my room to wait for the results.

A bit later on, late Saturday afternoon, the doctor came in. "Lucy, I've got some good news for you. Your levels are up to a place that we feel is more than acceptable, but we'd like to keep you in a little bit longer." I sat up on my bed and I looked him straight in the eyes, and I pleaded, "Please, can I go home tonight? I know you need this bed for somebody else. I feel really good. Please, can you let me go home tonight?" I must have just pierced his heart because he smiled and said, "Let me see what I can do." And with that, he turned on his heels and walked off. One of the other nurses in the room winked at me.

Within the hour, he came back and he said that I could go home. By this time, the night staff had come on, and the lady who had been looking after me on the first bag of blood re-appeared and she came in and said, "I hear you are going home."

I was so happy to see her again. I replied, "Thank you so much for looking after me. Honestly, I'm so grateful to you, and please know that I owe you my life. And I'll never forget you."

She looked at me with a bemused look, and she said, "Oh, I didn't realise that you knew that."

"What do you mean? Knew what?" I asked.

She sat down next to me on the bed and said, "Well, on Friday night, we thought we'd lost you. We really thought we'd lost you. We thought we were going to have to bring you back, but then all of a sudden, you came back. It was touch and go for a while there."

I had no idea. I was blissfully ignorant to it all. I thought I was just off in a meditation seeing my grandad and the two archangels, but I could see now that it was a lot more poignant than just a meditation. I had almost died. I had to consciously decide to come back.

So, within five days of each other, my twin flame and I had very near-death experiences.

108

It's fair to say I had been humbled in a way that I had never anticipated experiencing this lifetime. I left that hospital with tears in my eyes, feeling so grateful for everything that those strangers had done for me. I'd shunned the blood. I didn't want it; however, thankfully, my stubbornness subsided and the medical industry had saved my life and I was experiencing a whole new level of gratitude and appreciation.

That's the funny thing about when you have a near-death experience, something inside of you changes. Your lust for life changes. Your perspective on things change. Your desire to live and be present in every moment with those you love, changes. In a short period of time, I had gone from being a highly strung badass who worked on the trading floor – with very little self-respect and worth – to somebody who I actually had really started to like, and I could now even be brave enough to say that I loved her.

I looked in the mirror in the toilet, on the way out of the hospital, with tears in my eyes. I had so much awe and love for the person that looked back at me. It was that exact moment that I made the decision that my life was about to change, forevermore.

I got out of the hospital, to see my dad waiting for me in the car. I hopped, skipped and jumped my way over to him, dived in the car and gave him a massive hug and a kiss, and I said, "Get me the heck out of here, please, and fast."

It was only about 20 minutes back to his house. We seized the opportunity to have a beautiful conversation on the way back. He kept asking me, "How have you managed to get out so early?" I couldn't really explain it but all I knew was that from the minute I arrived there, I had been telling every doctor, every nurse, and anybody that was prepared to listen, that I was getting out of there on time because

I was going to be making that flight on Sunday. My dad thought I was crazy, "You've just got out of hospital after having a blood transfusion and you're actually going to take that flight?"

"Well, they haven't told me that I can't," I replied. That was my philosophy, it had been the same for some time. If somebody tells me that I can't do something, I weigh it up and see if what they are saying is reasonable or not, and then I go with my gut.

I called Donna, my beautiful assistant, who was due to be flying to Sydney with me on the Sunday, and I said just a few words, "Babe. We're on!"

She was shocked. She said, "Lucy Davis, are you sure you should be doing this?"

"Don Dons, I've never been more certain of anything in my life. We are going. I will see you at the airport tomorrow," I said assuredly. We were flying at 9 in the evening, so we both agreed to be there at around 6 pm. That gave me the day to equalise, process, get my food back on point and find some balance after the craziness of the previous few days.

I called my mum to let her know that I had survived the ordeal and that I was out of the hospital. At that point, I refrained from telling her that I was going to Sydney. My mum has a very different opinion on how life should be lived. She is a real worrier too and although I love her for that, I figured that she didn't need a night of stressing about me getting on a plane the next day, so I conveniently left it out of the conversation. I wasn't sure when I would get to tell her, I decided to play it by ear.

I got back to my dad's house and I wanted to be on my own. It had been a really weird couple of days, a really long night in the hospital, and there was a lot to process. I made my excuses, went upstairs to the top floor, and I sat on the side of my bed with my eyes closed, with my feet touching the ground. I found myself shaking my head in disbelief. *What the fuck has just gone on?* The last time I was in that same room, on the Friday, I was doing a Facebook Live. I was living my best life, or so I thought – okay, admittedly I looked a bit yellow because my body was deprived of blood, which is a pretty essential component – but in my mind, I was all good. Then, just like that, I'd been sent to the hospital where I had to stay overnight, I had been pumped full of somebody else's blood and I'd had a near-death experience. And now here I was, sat on the edge of that same bed. I felt so grateful, and I realised I now had to give back as much as I possibly could. These people had saved my life. They didn't ask for anything from me. They just saved me. And now it was my turn to give back.

I lay back on the bed and tears started rolling down my face. I felt very reflective, very grateful and extremely humbled by the experience. I had nearly died! How do you even comprehend that?

I decided the best thing that I could do was to go to bed and get some well-needed rest. With everything that had gone on, being in survival mode, I completely forgot to consider that my two little sisters would have been very worried about me. I also knew that now I was home they were going to give me an early morning wake-up call, so all the more reason to get my head down.

The next morning, as expected, I got woken up by the Little Beans. They jumped on my bed at about 5 am. They were cuddling me, stroking my hair and asking me constantly if I was okay. There is no love like a child's love. The innocence of their questions, and their begging me not to go back to hospital again was so sweet. The absolute innocence and the pure, unconditional love that they gave me that morning, made me sob. And of course, when they saw me crying they didn't get it. "Why are you crying? Why are you sad?" they asked. I told them I was crying because I was happy and grateful. And I was happy, more than I could ever explain to them. I was so grateful and humbled that I had been given another opportunity. These beautiful little girls hadn't been in my life long enough. I hadn't been able to show them everything that I needed to show them. I had only got to know my purpose for a little while, and that's why I had to keep fighting. That's why I had to come back. I had work to do, and these little beautiful girls were a huge part of that.

Even though I had a decent night's rest, it took me quite a while to get going. I felt much more energised than I had done before the weekend, but everything I had been through wiped me out. There were a couple of points in that morning where I honestly questioned whether I should be flying. The blood was still working its way around my system. I did think maybe I was being a bit silly, but this trip had been booked about six months earlier and it was important. It was already an important trip before Ricky had his heart attack but now it had taken on a whole new level of significance.

It's so interesting how the divine plan unfolds. It was fascinating to see how it had all worked – I had always known that I was going back to Sydney, and that Donna was going to be coming with me because she was attending an important seminar over there. Then, I had been taken out just a few days before I went. I had received the most incredible medical help and support that saved my life. What if I had stayed in Sydney with Ric when he had asked me to? Would this situation have happened? Would it have been worse? Better? Who knows? It needed to happen the way it did I guess, or else it would have happened a different way. Ultimately, there was this incredible paradox – I made choices but at the same time I had no control over the life that I was leading. Wow! It's too much to comprehend sometimes.

I got myself together that day, albeit slowly. I said goodbye to my family, and I headed to the airport. I'll never forget the look on Donna and her husband Barry's face when I saw them. They looked shocked. It was clear they were worried about me. I must be honest when I say that I looked terrible that day but I convinced them I was okay. Twice Donna asked me, "Are you sure you should be doing this?" And even Barry said, "Have you considered maybe going in a few days' time?" I had it in my mind that I had to get back there. With everything that happened to both Ricky and I over the last week, we needed to talk about this. This alignment was crazy. We both had to sort our shit out, and fast!

Donna said goodbye to Barry and we went to check in together. Everything went very smoothly and very soon we were the other side of customs and security, sat down having a drink. Donna very diplomatically said to me, "Luce, can you just do me a favour?"

"Yeah, of course. What do you need, babe?" I asked, innocently.

"Would you mind writing down your dad's, your mum's, and your doctor's numbers for me please?"

"Dons, what's going on?" I asked, more suspiciously this time.

"Lucy, God forbid something happens to you when we take off or when we land, I need to know who to contact."

It pierced right through my heart. I hadn't realised the responsibility I'd been putting on Donna at that point. I didn't have any idea. In that moment, I felt really selfish. How could I have expected somebody, who had become one of my best friends, to potentially have to deal with me not making it out the other side? I said to Donna, "Would you rather us go back? Would you rather us not go?"

She looked at me and said, "Lucy, you've made the decision to be here. I support you, whatever decision you make." I'll never forget those words. I love Donna, so much. She would support me in anything that I did. There was a love between Donna and I, which was just so unconditional. Like a mother, daughter, and a best friend, all rolled into one. It was a real family kind of love. We both agreed to carry on as planned.

We boarded the plane and clung on to each other like limpets as we took off. I was so nervous. I spent the take-off programming myself – *I am well. My blood is equalising. I have enough oxygen for me to be able to deal with this.* I kept affirming this to myself over and over and over. When the plane eventually got up to the peak height it needed to be at, Donna and I looked at each other, we burst into tears and hugged each other. We had made it. I was alright. Nobody else on that plane knew what we were dealing with and what could have potentially gone on. When I look back, I do realise how selfish I was. Anybody could have been flying back to see a loved one, to say goodbye to someone special, or any number of important circumstances, and I could have halted that journey, or made it very difficult for people. It was selfish of me, I just didn't think whilst in the middle of the situation I was in.

Thankfully, it was irrelevant anyhow because we made it up safely. Now, we needed to make it down again! We were soon going to be landing in Dubai in order to change planes to fly on to Sydney. When the pilot announced that we would be starting our descent, Donna clung on to me again. She said to me, "If you feel bad, you tell me, and I will run and I will get somebody to help. You just need to talk to me."

I looked at her and I said, "Don's, we're going to be okay. I know I'm going to be fine." I had the confidence by this point. I was good, although, I did feel a little bit light-headed and I was having some popping in my ears, which is something I hadn't had for many years.

As we finally touched down in Dubai, Donna and I burst into tears once again. We had made it. I had made it. The doctor had said to me that if I was going to experience any problems then it would be around take-off and landing. As far as I was concerned, I was home and dry! We had an hour and a half to wait before our next flight, so we walked around Dubai airport as if we had won the lottery. We had the biggest smiles on our faces, and we had so much fun.

The second leg of the journey went even smoother, there were no problems at all and I felt fine, although we were both so tired from all the high emotions, we passed out and slept most of the way there.

109

We arrived in Sydney and grabbed our luggage with ease. We were both really hungry, so as a reward for our successful travels, we found a place that did a sourdough toast, with avocado, tomatoes, onion, garlic and a bit of chilli on top. It was amazing. There was none of our usual intermittent fasting, or eating fruit before eating anything else – I was hungry. It was a case of 'let's eat' as quickly as possible! And my God, that food tasted so good.

After we finished eating, I had to pick up the hire car. I had ordered one to get me around while I was there. I was going to drop Donna off at the place where she way staying, and then I was going to drive on to stay at Ric's house. The car-hire guy took a shine to me, he started chatting me up. Donna laughed. This always happened, wherever we were. She has a running joke, she says that wherever we go together she needs a big stick to beat the men off. In this instance, the flirting worked because he upgraded our car to a really beautiful little SUV. I hadn't planned on doing too much driving on this trip as I knew my priority was to heal, especially after everything that had just gone on, but having a nicer car would help the comfort.

One of the last things that the doctor had said to me when I was leaving the hospital was that I was going to have to go back and see a specialist. He stated, quite firmly, that I was going to have to consider treatment for my issue and although the transfusion had been a success, the underlying issue hadn't gone anywhere. Medics are just so full of positivity! I had originally gone over to Sydney with a specific mission – to run a seminar in Sydney, but I decided on the plane that I was going to cancel that, and instead, I was going to focus on my health and healing. I made the decision that I was in charge of my health, not the doctors. I was really grateful for what they had done, but I wanted to be in charge of my own health going forward and I was going to do whatever it took to make sure that I didn't need to go under the knife. Even my mum had suggested that it might be time for me to start thinking about a hysterectomy. There was absolutely no way that was going to happen.

I dropped Donna off at her place and headed off to Ricky's house. When I arrived, he wasn't there, but he had left the keys for me to let myself in. I settled in and went to sit outside, immerse in the sunshine and do some journaling whilst I waited for him to come back. A few hours later, he arrived home. He saw me out in the garden and walked over.

"Hi," he said.

"Hi," I replied. There was no hug or kiss forthcoming from him, which was out of character. We sat and chatted for a while, I explained to him about what had gone on in the hospital, when out of nowhere he retorted, "You always have to go one better than me, don't you?"

I wasn't quite sure how to take it. Was he joking? Did he actually think I had a blood transfusion to try and compete with his heart attack? I could tell by the look on his face that he wasn't joking. I thought – *You absolute fucking arsehole! Who on earth thinks like that?* In my mind at that point, that was it. I was done with him. Once and for all. I turned away and tried to ignore him. Thing was, I was in his house, so there was only so much avoiding I was going to be able to do.

After a few hours, he asked me, "Is there a problem?"

I turned to him and said, "It's really interesting because the situation that I've been through has made me really humble. I'm so grateful for everything right now, whereas you seem to be angry and closed off." He was embodying a totally different energy to me. I'm not saying I was right or he was wrong, but we were at two completely different places.

It was so strange for it to come to this, and so quickly too. When I left in August, I was heartbroken leaving him. I felt he had reminded me that I could have a relationship. He had reminded me of my potential. And just a few weeks later, I'm sat here with him and I didn't know who he was, I didn't recognise him. And, quite honesty, I didn't like him very much.

I made my excuses, went for a drive and took myself off into a national park to immerse in nature.

Over the next few days because I was ignoring Ricky, I used it as an opportunity to realign and get super healthy. I went to the supermarkets, bought nourishing fruits and vegetables to feast on – after I was out the other side of the water fast I had put myself on. It was a time for a new level of love I had never been able to achieve before. I got into a really good place – in spite of Ricky pissing me off.

During that time, the name Self Love Club kept coming into my consciousness. It felt like it was being pumped into me from the Universe. It became clear that everything I had been intuitively doing over the last few years, my entire healing journey, was something that I needed to share, and Self Love Club would be that vehicle and instrument to do so. I had a seminar booked for the end of October, this was going to be the first Self Love Club event the world had ever seen. I still wasn't quite in resonance with the name, but it was slapping me around the face constantly, so it seemed I had no choice but to accept it. I felt that men wouldn't like it at first, but trusted they would eventually get it. I knew somewhere in my soul they would step into the space of recognising that the only way they were going to awaken, and the only way they were going to go on their ascension journey, was by loving themselves.

So, Self Love Club it was!

Interestingly, Self Love Club started flowing through as Self Love Soul School at some point too. I had no idea what that meant or why they were giving me another name.

One afternoon, I was fasting, and so an open vessel to receive downloads. I was sitting outside, and information was channelling through me like an absolute train. I went back inside and grabbed a piece of paper and drew out the entire plan for what Self Love Club Hangs was going to look like. Now, the reason I was told it needed to be called Self Love Club Hangs was because we were basically going to get together and hang out for a few hours. It wasn't going to be too formal. It was going to be an interactive thing. People could ask me questions, and hang out whilst remembering what self love meant. The entire plan came through me in a couple of hours. I knew exactly what I needed to do, and exactly where I needed to take it. And at last, I was really comfortable with it. Actually, I was super excited about it.

PART THREE – THE JOURNEY HOME 579

It all came together so quickly, which meant the rest of the time I could focus on myself. I took a technology detox, removing myself from my laptop and my phone. I did lots of driving, wandering off to weird and wonderful places. I walked the earth barefoot, swam in lakes that I was warned not to go in, I ate great food – when I wasn't fasting – and I immersed myself in the simple pleasures of life.

Despite our differences, Ricky had mentioned the name of a Chinese herbalist lady to go and see while I was over there. Initially, I was so pissed off with him I ignored it, I decided I was not going to listen to anything he had to say. My stubbornness knows no bounds sometimes. I think it's called cutting your nose off to spite your face. I deleted the number when he sent it to me. After a few days of thinking about it, though, I decided I wanted to go and see her and so I messaged him, "Could you please re-send me the number of the Chinese herbalist lady?"

"Why? What have you done with it?" he abruptly answered.

"I've lost it, I think," I said, bending the truth somewhat.

I decided I wanted to see her because I was still taking the medication to stop the bleeding, and I wanted to get off them. I was taking probiotics to look after my gut whilst on the medication, but the goal was to be free of the tablets completely. When I met her, Ricky was right, she was amazing, such a beautiful soul too. She asked me a lot of questions and did acupuncture on me, predominantly focussing on my womb. She had pins all over me, then used a hot lamp, whilst she twisted the pins, carrying out all kind of energetics on me. She asked, "Are you open to taking some of my medicine?"

"I'm already on medication, I don't want to take anything else," I answered.

"Herbs I mean," she said, smiling.

"Will your medicine, get me off my medication?" I asked.

"I'd like you to take the herbs for two days, and then I would like you to stop the medication that was given to you by the hospital," she stated.

And as much as I was happy to hear that, I was also scared because I didn't want my bleeding issues again, especially when I was all the way away from home. I trusted her, though; she knew her stuff and I had to get off my medication at some point. She told me to go back in a day or so for some more acupuncture, and to see how I was getting on.

So, the next day I started the herbal medication immediately and I decided not to wait the two days before coming off my own medication. Most normal people would stop them and keep them aside for a rainy day, but I just threw them in the bin, and I decided that this was the day that my bleeding was going to stop from this issue. There was going to be no more bleeding relating to it from here on.

I went out walking to avoid spending time with Ricky. I had an appointment with the acupuncturist in the evening and by the time she saw me and asked me how my bleeding was, I realised not only had it stopped, but I hadn't even noticed or given it a thought! That gave me the confidence to continue on with her medication for a few more days, as instructed by her. She also gave me this other stuff to make as a tea. And she said to me, "Take the medication for a couple more days, then start adding in the tea, and then when the herbal medication runs out you can use the tea for a few more days."

I got a bit nervous at the thought of this. I had managed to come off my hospital medication by transitioning onto the herbal medicine, but now she was asking me to come off that too. Nevertheless, I surrendered and trusted her. She was amazing. She managed to get into my womb and release the energies that had built up in there, and she gave me the confidence to believe that this was where it stopped. I already knew, from my own training, that I needed to get to the source of the issue that was creating these womb issues within me, but this lady had helped me navigate off the medication that the doctors had given me. I'm not judging the doctors for that, they were doing their best with what they knew. Something had shifted within me, though. I was going to make sure that I healed. I was going to be that person that could say, "I don't need your operation. Thank you, but give it to somebody else who does."

I felt that this was my time to heal and nothing was going to stop me. Especially Ricky. I was still irritated by him and I didn't want to allow him to hinder my progress.

As soon as Donna had finished at the seminar, I drove down to pick her up and we agreed to go into Sydney for a couple of days together, before she headed off home. She was shocked to hear how Ricky and I had been together, but we agreed to forget about it all and go have some fun.

And we had the best time.

We checked into a hotel, and decided to go and do loads of cool stuff together, so she could explore the city. As I've said many times before, Sydney is one of my favourite cities in the world, so I agreed to show her around all my favourite places.

One night, Donna and I were getting ready to go out for the night. We were glammed up and ready to go, when I got a message from Ricky saying, "Are you intending to come back here at any point?" I initially ignored him, but then a little later thought it was rude to just ignore somebody, so I relented and wrote back, "Yeah, I'll be back to get my things." That was all I put. Shortly afterwards he wrote back, "Lucy, is there a problem?"

"I'll speak to you when I see you," I replied, but it must have bothered him because he called me right away.

"Lucy, what's going on?" he asked.

I lost it. "What the fuck do you take me for?" What the fuck do you take me for? Some sort of cunt?" And it was almost like me using that word broke something within him because he started laughing and he said, "Have I really been that bad?"

From there, I got the opportunity to explain how everything was from my perspective. I shared what I had been witnessing. And, credit to him, he listened. I never thought he would, but he did. I agreed with him that I was going to enjoy my time with Donna, and then I was going to drop her off at the airport, and then I would come to his and we would sit down and have a conversation.

Donna and I had a magical few days together, before we had to say goodbye. I dropped her off at the airport and I was sad. Sad because I was saying goodbye to my friend, and she would be flying halfway around the world on her own, for the first time. And I was sad because I knew I was going to have this conversation with Ricky, and I didn't know what to expect. I forgave myself for losing it with him, and I was proud of myself for pulling back and not losing it properly, like maybe I would have done in the past. I was sad, though, because after what I had been through recently I had stepped into a space of humility and a total admiration and love for the world, whereas Ricky appeared to have gone the other way, and I didn't like who he had become. I really wanted to run away again. I wanted to jump on the plane with Donna and leave without any more discussion with him. Quite frankly I didn't care if I ever saw him again.

When I got to his, he was being really nice. He offered to make me a hot lemon and ginger with some honey in an attempt to appease me. We sat down on opposite couches, which meant we had to look at each other. Awkward! We started talking. I told him that he wasn't the person that I left a few weeks earlier, and that it broke my heart that he had changed so much. It broke my heart that he always thought that there was a competition between the two of us. I knew what was going on – although I didn't tell him; we were twin flames, so naturally there would be that competitive edge. It was bloody hard work not telling him. Grasping the situation didn't make it any easier for me because I did know we were twin flames, and sometimes I just wanted to slap him. So many people have since asked me why I never told him. Surely it would have made things easier? I'm not sure. It's not my place to change the destiny of someone. I feel we all evolve in the direction that is intended for us. My belief was that he had to figure it out on his own.

I told him I was going to be leaving soon and flying to Brazil. I had explained a little about Brazil when I had arrived. The plan was, I was going to work on healing myself completely, so that I didn't need to be operated on. I had mentioned to him when I arrived that he should do the same thing. He should go to Brazil and heal. And fuck me, did his heart need healing! I could see energetically that if he didn't change, he was heading for another heart attack. However, things had changed for me, and I didn't want him coming to Brazil, not with me anyway. In truth, I didn't want to see him again once I left his in a few days time.

"I want to go to Brazil when you're there," he declared.

I thought – *First and foremost, I didn't invite you to go with me. I just said you should go there and do the healing work.* I wished I had never even mentioned it. I didn't want to be near him, especially in the place where I was going to do my healing. I had already decided before I arrived at his house, during a conversation with Donna, that I didn't want him in my life anymore. I was done with him. I wasn't going to make any more effort with him after I left Sydney. As far as I was concerned, that was the point where our relationship was over. I didn't want to be spoken to like he spoke to me. I didn't want to be hanging around with someone who behaved the way he did. We'd had five great years together. We had learnt so much from each other, but I was done with this twin flame bullshit. I was fed up with being this person's blame game.

I just shrugged in his direction, without really knowing what to say. I didn't want to be mean, it wasn't in my nature, but my goodness was he pushing my buttons – showing me my healing.

Ricky persisted with the idea of coming to Brazil. He wasn't getting the hint at all. So I tried to be diplomatic to dissuade him, but it wasn't working, "Maybe you should just see what the hospital says about your heart before you go making any decisions."

The penny finally started to drop, he let go a bit and actually started making a bit of an effort after that. He asked me to go training with him, to go out for dinner. It was too little too late, though. I didn't want to be around him. I couldn't wait for the plane out of there.

It was such a contradiction. The last time I had left I cried because I wanted to stay so badly, but now I was sad because this was potentially going to be the last time I ever saw this person. He didn't know that and I didn't want to have a big showdown. I wanted to go quietly, and if the Universe caused our paths to cross, then I'd have to deal with that when that happened.

I said goodbye to him and his dad. His dad is so cute and he gave me a rose as I was leaving. It was such a sweet gesture; but it was bittersweet for me. I sat in the car on the way to the airport looking at the rose and thinking – *I can't believe what a journey we've been on together. Two strangers who bumped into each other five years earlier, almost to the day. And now here we are and it's the end of the road.*

110

A couple of days later, I touched down in Rio, Brazil. I had no idea what was about to unfold. My girlfriend, Katrina – the lady who had come to Guatemala – was joining me. As I arrived, I checked my phone and I had a message from her saying she was going to be about an hour, so I decided to take my time getting through the airport. I got my luggage, got through customs without any problems at all and grabbed somewhere to sit, to wait for her.

Eventually, she arrived. It was so good to see each other – it had been about seven months since we were last together, and we knew because of the times we had seen each other previously that we were in for one heck of a ride. I had changed a lot since I last saw Katrina too;

I had been through what can only be described as a series of life-changing events. So much had changed in that period. I was a very different person. I was starting to have boundaries, to speak my truth more than I already was – and I thought I was already pretty brutal – but I had gone to a whole new level. The difference was that I was speaking honestly, from a space of love, and I felt really comfortable doing it.

We had decided that we were going to stay in Rio for a couple of days. I had never been to Brazil and Katrina had never been to Rio. So we felt it would be good to spend a couple of days there before heading up to Abadiania.

I have to be honest, Rio disappointed me. In my mind, I had the carnival vibe. I envisaged bright, loud, boisterous, colours with lots of music and dancing. I expected clear blue skies and bright sunshine, but it was grey, cold and not what I imagined at all.

On the first night that we stayed in Rio, I had a pretty profound situation happen. As I've previously explained, I astral travel, more often than not. A lot of times I don't remember it, but the majority of the time I do. That first morning, when I I woke up, I was in a state of panic. I had the most bizarre out-of-body, remote viewing, astral projection – and I didn't like it at all. I shouted across the room to Katrina, "Oh my God. Ricky is going to die."

Katrina looked over at me and she said, "What are you talking about?"

"Ricky's going to die," I replied again. I took her back on the journey that I'd been on. That night, after I had dropped into super consciousness, I had gone to Australia. I was sat in a room with Ricky and a doctor. From the images I was seeing, I assumed the doctor was some sort of specialist. He was sat behind a large desk and looked extremely formal. I was observing the room, attempting to figure out if this was past, present or future, when the doctor turned to Ricky and said, "You are going to have open heart surgery." I watched open-mouthed as this unfolded. I saw Ricky's willingness to go along with what the doctor had said. He was keen to 'get this sorted'. I had known he wanted to be okay enough to do another fight and to be well, without concern, but open heart surgery seemed extreme. The doctor then said to Ricky that he needed to have open heart surgery very quickly, he was an urgent case.

The view quickly changed; we were no longer in the doctor's room. I was no longer listening to the prognosis, I was viewing the operating theatre, looking down at what was going on in the room from above, almost as if I was glued to the ceiling. This is what people call remote viewing. I had only done this type of thing a couple of times. I still found it ever so weird when I did. I was observing this entire scenario as if it was happening in that moment, yet no one would have known I was there.

The doctor started to perform the surgery on Ricky. It was pretty horrific to watch. I wanted to reach out and help, but I was not able to. I was merely a spectator, with zero power. After a little while, the doctor started to get a little bit more aggressive with the nurses and everybody that was helping him in surgery. I felt him slip into panic and was projecting it onto them. All of a sudden, Ricky started flatlining, which sent everyone into a spin – including me. What the heck was going on? Everyone was panicking, attempting to bring him back. I felt helpless. Someone grabbed a defibrillator and told everyone to stand back as they attempted to reboot his heart. It was heartbreaking. They couldn't do it.

I was crying as I watched this scene unfold. The doctors stood back from him and they decided that was it. There was no more they could do. He wasn't going to come back.

When I woke up in my bed in Rio, that was what I remembered, so I shouted out to Katrina to attempt to make some sense of it all.

Despite the fact that the last time I saw Ricky I had wanted to slap him hard across the face, and never see him again, I grabbed my phone and messaged him. "Hey, babe. I don't know if you're seeing the doctor today or not, but I'd really like to speak to you before you do, if that's okay." I had reached out to him; however, I had no idea if he would respond or not. He may have picked up on the fact that I was pissed off with him. Regardless, I had done all I could, so I put my phone down and I went about doing my morning stuff.

After I had done my morning rituals, I checked my phone again and I had a message from him saying, "I've already been to see the doctor. Give me a call. It sounds like it's urgent."

After breakfast, I called him back. We kind of danced around the pleasantries and then, in true Lucy fashion, I went straight in, "So, what did the doctor say?"

Ricky sounded a bit worried. "He said to me that I need to have open heart surgery."

My heart sank. It was almost like I was watching my astral experience play out in real-time. And, as much as I think it's a really cool thing, to be able to tap into these situations, in this instance it was heartbreaking. I took a deep breath and asked, "What are you going to do about it?"

He said, "I'm going to have to have the surgery."

"Do you not think you should try some other things first?" I was trying to steer him away from the surgery without having to tell him why I was all of a sudden so interested in what he was doing with his life. The problem was Ricky had known me for 5 years, we are twin flames – and even though he doesn't know that – we know each other inside and out.

"Lucy, if you know something, you've got to fucking tell me – I thought we were friends?" Ricky doesn't normally swear at me, this time he did.

I stood in my truth, breathing deeply first, so not to lead him, "I feel that maybe you should look at other options first. Maybe you should get a second opinion or something before you just go along with that."

He said, "Lucy, they have run so many tests and, unfortunately, it's definitive. They've told me that that's what I need to do, so if you know something, you've got to tell me. What's going on?"

I said to him, "Maybe you should consider coming to Brazil before the surgery." Maybe that was a good idea after all.

I didn't know what to do here because as much as sometimes I would love to shake people, so they get the memo, it's not my role to do that – I believe it's actually a disservice to someone to tell them what to do. I am not here to tell people their fate or destiny. By doing so you can change it, I believe it's very important to hold space and ask good questions to help people evolve. The thing is, I also didn't want him to die, I wouldn't be able to live with that on my conscience. Eventually, I said to him, "Look, I was shown a vision last night. I knew that you were going to be told you needed open heart surgery."

He began to get impatient with me, "Lucy, if you know something, you've got to tell me. I'm supposed to be one of your best friends."

At that point, I couldn't hold back any longer, "Babe, if you have open heart surgery, it's very likely that you're going to die."

He went quiet. It was heartbreaking. It was a message that I wouldn't want to deliver to anybody, let alone somebody that was me in a male body – I knew how much it would hurt. I was basically telling myself – *Stop being so fucking stubborn! Sort your shit out, else you're going to die.*

After a while, he said, "Thank you for sharing that with me." Then he went quiet again. I could sense he was contemplating, so I remained quiet until he was ready to speak. I wanted to speak. I wanted to say what I wanted, but this was not about me.

"What are the options?" he finally asked.

I said to him, "Look, I'm going to be in Abadiania to do the healing work in a few days. I would like to set the intention that we send you some healing from Brazil and see what happens for you. Would you be open to that?" I knew he did not like to be told what to do, so I had to be very careful with my words.

He said, "Lucy, at this precise moment in time, yes I absolutely am. I don't know what that means. I don't know what that looks like. But yes, I'm in! What do I need to do?"

"I need a photo of you, in white. Can you organise that for me?"

"What on earth do you need that for?" He asked. "For your wall? Are you missing me?" He retorted in his smart-arse manner.

I laughed. At least he hadn't lost the cheekiness that I had got to know so well over the years. I went on to explain the healing process that would take place in Brazil, as I understood it to be, without having been through it myself.

The next day, Katrina and I took the journey up to the Christ the Redeemer statue. It was one thing that both of us agreed we had to do whilst in Rio. It was very cloudy that day and quite depressing, but we went anyway. We were so glad we did. We saw so many beautiful monkeys and other beautiful animals on the way there and back. Afterwards, we went back to the hotel, as we had to get ourselves ready for the trip to Abadiania. To get there, we had to go to the airport, fly to Brasilia, then it was an hour and a half in a car from the airport.

Back in the April of 2018, I was getting continual messages about a man in white who was calling me to Brazil. In the initial callings, it's extremely basic information that comes through. It's very minimal.

I then piece things together based on signs and synchronicities. Back in 2018, they came pretty slowly; these days, it's a different story. When I started receiving these messages about the man in white, I reached out to Katrina — between us both, we were usually able to connect the dots. After a couple of conversations back and forth, Katrina said to me, "Oh my God, it's him. It's John of God." Apparently, he was a very known healer around the world. He had become quite famous in a short space of time due to the work he had done alongside Oprah Winfrey. I knew nothing about him. I had never heard of this man, let alone known his work. I was just getting started in this world of healing, transformation and spirituality, and although I was on a rocket, I really knew next to nothing.

Katrina sent me a short YouTube video, knowing I would not watch anything that was too long. It gripped my attention. He looked like a normal man, dressed in white. He was shown walking in, then surrendering to the entities who worked through him, and then the next thing, he was holding someone's head back and scraping their eyes with a scalpel without any anaesthetic, or anything to stop the bleeding. It was absolutely crazy. I could not believe my eyes. There was no way this could be true. And if it was, what on earth was his soul calling mine there for?

I must add at this point, I was a handful of years into my journey. I knew there was darkness, I was shown it in Cambodia, but I never knew how deep it went. I didn't know a lot of the stuff that I know now, about how these entities and darker energies work. Looking back, I truly believe this is why I had to go there. I'm one of those people who has to see things for myself to believe it. Other than that, it was just hearsay.

This man had been calling to me and I was getting used to following those pulls. I didn't know what he wanted; he was a healer and there was nothing wrong with me back in April 2018. I was healthy, in really good shape as far as it went, so I planned to go there in the knowledge that this man had a message for me. That was it.

Early the next morning, Katrina and I travelled to the Casa for John of God. It opened up at around seven thirty am for people who had travelled from all over the world, searching for healing. The Casa was a bit like a hospital. It was very white, clean and clinical. There was a number of beautiful outdoor spaces, with grass areas to sit and meditate, and chapels to go in and pray. It was very humble, but loaded to the brim with high vibrational energy from the people it attracted and the entities that worked out of there. Every Wednesday, Thursday and Friday, people would queue up for hours to see this mystical healer. I didn't know anything about John of God before I went, other than that video Katrina had shared with me. There were amazing stories whereby people would arrive in a wheelchair and walk out of there freely. Even before we got in the Casa, we heard some of the magical stories that people shared about their visits. I felt it was amazing to be around so many believers. I felt that was half of it. If you could believe it, you could see it. That was the problem with most people, though, they could not believe it, and hence were unable to achieve it.

When you arrive at the Casa, there are forms to fill out and processes you have to adhere to. If you have never been before, you would take a certain ticket, then join a certain queue. Likewise, if you were a returning person, then you would take a different ticket and join a different queue. Everyone would then sit in a waiting area with hundreds of other people, and wait until your group was called. Once you were called, you would line up in an orderly fashion, in silence, and walk through an area where a number of healers were meditating and praying for the attendees' healing. There were maybe 50 to 100 people in the space where people would walk through. The energy was pretty profound as you walked through that place; a sea of white angels holding space for people. As you walked through, following the person in front, you would eventually reach the spot where John of God sat. He would look at you, scan your body and then he would tell a translator what was required for you. There were a handful of treatments he would suggest; psychic surgery, massage, crystal bed, waterfall or meditation. Depending on what he saw, he would recommend the path of treatment, then the person would go off and do that before coming back. Whichever entity was working through him on that day would guide the vessel of John of God to advise the people who were in the queue. He had a number of different entities that would use his vessel to carry out this work. It was all a bit weird to me this, at this point in my journey, but I couldn't deny what I was seeing – although it all seemed a little bit too good to be true. Whatever went on here, it was absolutely fascinating to watch the belief in people's faces, and feel it in their hearts. People were desperate. He was their last hope.

I was told by Katrina before I arrived, that there was a way to help others who could not attend. I was told by the staff all I needed to do was take the image of Ricky with me and hand it over before he scanned me, so we knew what he was doing for him, and then I would get told my journey. I was in a queue with all of the first-timers, watching as people went through. Some people were told that they needed to go into surgery in the afternoon. Some people were told they needed a massage. Some people were told they needed to go to a nearby waterfall to cleanse. I was fascinated. I wondered how he determined what to say to people. There appeared to be no rhyme or reason to who was being told what. I was a little bit nervous. I had walked through the people meditating, and was patiently waiting my turn for an audience with this man. He would sit in his chair, a bit like a God, and barely look up at people to tell them what was required for them. It was eerie that everyone was wearing white; he encouraged people to wear white, so that the entities can see you much clearer and the high vibration of white would assist the healing process.

It came to my turn. He glanced in my direction, then took the picture of Ricky that I held out to him. He looked at it, threw it into the basket by his side, and he said in Portuguese, "He will have surgery this afternoon." He then looked back at me, continuing in his local language to the translator, "You will go for a massage now, meditation this afternoon and surgery tomorrow at 8 am." And that was it. I was moved on, with the help of a translator, to go and take the steps to get a massage, before going back to hold space for people that afternoon. It was all over so quickly. I was a little flustered that I would be later involved in the group to hold space for Ricky.

I went up the road, to the place where they told me I had to go for a massage. In my mind, I had hoped I was going to get a nice deep massage, which as a professional fighter, I loved. There was something extremely freeing about having someone work deeply into your muscles. I luckily found somewhere that could fit me in in time for me to head back to be in meditation for the afternoon. I went into one of the rooms, which felt very clinical, with the old-fashioned green curtains that they use to be pull around you in the hospitals. I was being massaged by a man, which I did not have an issue with.

He seemed nice enough. The massage started and I could barely feel it. It was more like being stroked than massaged. Although not unpleasant, it almost felt pointless.

Afterwards, I asked what the purpose of the gentle massage was. He explained to me that it was to prepare the body and allow the entities to start working through my system in readiness for the psychic surgery the next morning. It all seemed a little bit weird. The old Lucy would have laughed out loud at this point, and my ego was starting to play up a little bit. I thought that maybe this was all a load of shit, but I went with it anyway. I had nothing to lose. I felt I had to be here, and despite some of it seeming somewhat unbelievable, I wanted to believe. I wanted to believe all of this worked not only for myself but for the masses out there. I felt a responsibility for mankind in some sort of weird way. John of God, or the entity that was working through him, had clearly observed something going on in my body when I had been in his presence. I knew something was going on and I wondered how he knew, which he must have done as he had me scheduled for psychic surgery the next day.

Interestingly, the day before, I had started water fasting again. I had done some in Australia, to reset my body as I knew the power of how it worked in regard to healing, so I had mentioned to Katrina that I would be doing that to catapult the results. She agreed that she would do it also, during the actual healing days. I was totally dedicated to my healing journey here in Brazil and I didn't want anything to get in my way. I meant business. I wanted rid of the growths in my womb, I wanted those lumps gone. They had been plaguing me for years, and although I'd had them cut out of me many times before, I had decided that was going to be the place where I said goodbye to them forever. Water fasting opened me up to quicker, much more intense results.

I guess now may be a good time to share that over the years I have spoken about diets, fasts, and all sorts of things, many of which I never really stuck to. I have done a fast, twice a year for 4 days since 2015, but this one in Brazil was a whole new level. I had a level of focus that I had never experienced before. I had a choice to make. Do I remove everything that could be creating these issues and heal, or do I roll over and lose my womb, before I have ever had children? I made that decision with every cell in my body. I wanted to heal.

I deserved to heal. I wanted children, even though I was single at the time. I knew all of this was to make me stronger, more grateful, and to remind the world what was possible for them.

I had about an hour before I needed to go into meditation, so I met up with Katrina. She was skipping meditation that day. She had not been guided to go, so was not going. I had no choice, I was told. As I sat with Katrina, I started to overthink the meditation, knowing it was likely to be for four or five hours, my ego piped up – *What if I'm too hot? What if I'm too cold? What if I can't sit still? What if I can't stay in meditation for that long? What if I need the toilet?* My mind was on overdrive. Honestly, it exhausts me even thinking about how my brain used to work.

I went for a walk back to my Casa to grab my things and to message Ricky, so he knew what was going on and what to expect. As I walked back down the road to the Casa, I was thinking about how Ricky was my twin flame, and so essentially, he was me. I was going in there to hold space for him, which essentially meant going in there to heal my own heart. If ever there was a head screw, that was it.

The time came for the meditation and healing session. We were all queued up outside of the room, and in a very deep space of contemplation and silence, before we were shown into the room. A gentleman said the Lord's Prayer and then we were guided into meditation. I dropped in really easily, and then proceeded to go off on the most magical journey. I saw myself running through fields of really long grass, and through expansive spaces. I was so full of life, love and vitality. It was incredible. I remember there being a lot of sunshine and bright lights. I remember Ricky being there smiling back at me and saying thank you. I took from that he had received the healing he required, for now. In the blink of an eye, the man said, "Okay, it's time to come back into your body now. Thank you so much for your service today."

I couldn't believe it! We had been in there for over four hours and it felt like no time had passed at all. I was shocked. All of that worry, fear, and overthinking – for what? Absolutely nothing. I laughed at myself.

I left there feeling incredibly grateful, and extremely emotional. I decided to continue the contemplation in their gardens, which had been created to be a peaceful area, whereby people could sit and meditate and look over the stunning views. They also said this was an overflow area. If people wanted to join the healing meditation, yet there was no room inside, they could come out here and direct the healing inwards to the Casa. The valley view was stunning. There is a rumour that the Casa itself is on a live quartz crystal that is in the earth. I could well believe it. There was a vibration to this place that was unexplainable. There were healings taking place every single day that were so far out there, that you often had to check yourself to remind yourself that you were still on Earth, and not some magical off-World. I continued to sit and immerse in the energy for a little while longer. I didn't want to be on my phone. I didn't want to be connecting to anybody, although I really wanted to hear what Ricky had to say, or if he had felt anything during the healing because I had seen so much beautiful, bright light being sent to him.

After maybe an hour or two, I got up and went back to my Casa. It was at this point, I messaged Ricky to ask him if he was okay. Katrina and I went out for a walk, so she could grab some food; I was water fasting, but it has never troubled me being around people when I'm choosing self love for me.

Perhaps many of you reading this would question if a fast is self love, but for me, it's self-explanatory. I love myself enough to do whatever it takes to heal. Giving myself some time out from digesting food and the constant workout we ask of our bodies to process day to day is love for self, in my book. We had a lovely evening. We chatted about everything that had gone on so far. and speculated somewhat on where Ricky was at, and then she reminded me of the do's and don'ts after surgery. She had been here before, so she knew it a lot better than I did.

"Just to remind you, when you leave surgery tomorrow, you will not be able to speak to anyone for 24 hours. You will not be able to go outside in the sunlight. All you are allowed to do is lie down. You can stand up if you need to go to the toilet, but that's it."

I nodded.

She then continued, "Remember, for 40 days after the surgery there is to be no pepper, chilli, alcohol or sex." I smiled.

"I remember the days two of those would have been an issue for 40 days, interestingly now it will be the other two that I struggle with." We both started roaring with laughter. It was true, I had gone from the promiscuous party girl to virgin Lucy, since splitting up with Kyle.

I had no interest in going out drinking or having sex at this point in my life. I had gone a year without. My sweet soul had changed. I was so proud of her.

111

I got back to my room, checked my phone, and I had a message from Ricky. While we were doing the healing on him, it had been his nighttime. He had felt like he had been flipped over, turned and spun around in all sorts of weird and wonderful ways all through the night. I laughed when I read it. His dog had been going crazy all through the night too, barking at something that did not appear to be there. Now, dogs and animals generally are very sensitive to spirits, so what I took from it was that the dog had witnessed the spirits, the entities working through him. Ricky said he was feeling good and that he was going back to the doctors that morning for some more tests. I felt relieved for him that it was over, for now. Time to focus on my own journey that was incoming the next morning. I was a little nervous, but mainly excited. I journaled my thoughts and emotions, before writing an intention for the next day.

The next morning, I woke early, did my rituals, and went outside to ground, before meeting Katrina to walk over for our surgery. We had to be there early, which wasn't a problem. I said goodbye to Katrina for the next 24 hours, then got into the headspace where I saw myself fully healed with two beautiful children. The process started as it did the previous day. I walked through the meditating people, then we were led to a room where maybe 40 other people were sat with us. We sat in the room, and once again the Lord's Prayer was read, then we were told to drop into meditation and focus on the area that was required for healing. I sat in that room and focused so intently on my beautiful womb. I imagined it healthy and free from any growths at all. I had one hand on my womb, the other on my heart and I said to my womb constantly, "I love you so much. We must heal this together. Know that I love you. I forgive you. I forgive myself for everything." As I sat there, I began to really realise the fact that my promiscuous behaviour when I was younger had not helped the things going on in my womb. The surgery was a really beautiful experience. An opportunity to connect with myself deeper than ever. It took no more than 15 minutes. That was it. It was so quick.

Afterwards, I felt a bit emotional. I had no explanation for that. I was sat in a room of strangers focusing on my womb, so why would I cry? I went to stand up and as quickly as I stood, I was crippled over in pain. I let out a yelp. I was in agony. It was like I'd had actual surgery. It took my breath away. I had to sit back down before I could attempt to stand again as it was so painful. Interestingly, it was a pain that I recognised from my previous surgeries. How on earth did that happen? I thought to myself.

I eventually built up the courage to stand up again, I did it very slowly because I knew it was going to hurt. I remained slightly bent over so that I wouldn't stretch my womb too much. We were told that we had to take some herbs regularly, that were being handed out. They were in capsules, and apparently, they would help us with the pain and help the entities to continue to work through us. At this point I did not care what they were, I just needed to lie down.

I was in a lot of pain as I hobbled along. I was breathing like I was about to give birth, when a beautiful lady came out of nowhere, and scooped me under her arm and said she would help me walk back to my Casa. I'll never forget her, she was a beautiful black lady whose aura shone like diamonds. She signalled to me that she was going to walk me back without speaking too much as she knew I was in 24 hours of silence from here. That lady was an earth angel. She saved me that day. I probably wouldn't have made it back without her. It was only about a two-minute walk to my Casa – if you were walking properly – it took me about 15 minutes that day. It was so painful. This lady was so patient. I made a mental note to help anyone in need from here.

When I got back to my room, I lay down and stayed there for a long period of time. The next time I checked, it was dark. I didn't go to the toilet. I do anything. I lay in meditation, saying to my womb, "We've got this. I give you permission to heal. I forgive you. I forgive the human. I forgive everybody that's ever used it." I hadn't been told to say this. It intuitively felt right to embody a deeper love than I have ever felt or experienced. I was pumping energy into myself, imagining my womb being clear. I saw myself having two wonderful children. I saw the love connection that I was entitled to. It was absolutely magical and very mystical. I could feel exactly how love was intended to be.

I had been told I was to remain in silent meditation for 24 hours, but after that time, I still wasn't ready to come out of it, so I stayed in there a lot longer. I messaged Katrina and said, "Look, I'm going to stay silent for longer, so please don't be offended if I don't speak to you. I'm okay, just need to do this for me." She was in a Casa up behind me and she would pop by and wave to me and then she would just go back to her place, just so that we had some human interaction.

Whilst I had been in surgery, I had received several messages from Ricky. The first one said, "I need to speak to you urgently." The second one said, "I hope you're okay." The third one said, "Lucy, you've been offline for ages. It's really unlike you. Please, can you just let me know that you're okay?" And then the last one said, "I'm booking a flight to Brazil." This was all too much for me. I was in a space of pure, divine love – a love like I'd never felt for myself before, and I didn't want him to ruin that. I had remembered who I was. I remembered my passions and my purpose by this point. There was an energy flowing through me that I couldn't explain. I loved me more than anything else on this planet. I sent a message back, "What's made you book a flight to Brazil?"

He wrote back, "Can I call you?"

I replied, "No, because I want to stay silent."

He responded, "Lucy, I have gone from an urgent open heart surgery case to a mild case. I truly believe that what is going on over there is going to heal me. I'm coming. It's my priority to come."

Despite my reservations, I was delighted for him. I was happy that he had got the insights that he needed to get, so that he could actually step through this journey. It looked like he too had made a choice. I was delighted that something had shown him that spirit had his back, that it wasn't a weakness, and if you allowed it to take place, it was actually a strength. At the same time that I had this blissful feeling for him, I didn't want him here because I was in such a good space. I didn't want his energy coming over here and creating shit with me again. I knew this was ego, I knew it was fear, I knew it was my healing. In all reality, I should have been excited to embrace the next round of mirroring he would shove in my face. In typical Lucy fashion, I didn't say anything. I did not put myself first because I want to help everybody, and sometimes that means dealing with things that you don't want to deal with, or speaking to people that you don't want to speak with.

PART THREE – THE JOURNEY HOME

Ricky said he was due to arrive in a couple of days. It was quite incredible the further shifts I had in those few days. I was starting to become stronger again. I had much more focus than I had in a long time. The fasting had been working really well. I was in a regular routine of meditating in my hammock, followed by a walk, then going into the Casa to meditate. Then, I would lie on a crystal bed, then back to my Casa for juices.

On the day that Ricky arrived, I had come back for a juice and to go to the toilet and out of nowhere, I had a panic. I felt something falling out of my vagina. It felt like it had felt when all of the blood had been coming out those weeks earlier. I shut my eyes and prayed. I wiped myself after I finished going to the toilet and there was no blood. I stood up to flush the toilet and at the bottom there were what can only be described as growths. I burst into tears. I knew in that moment that what had been plaguing me had finally dropped out. I had finally healed myself from the inside out. I sat back down on the toilet and sobbed like a baby. I knew I was going to do it, but this was actual proof that it was done. It was so hard to process. All of the efforts had paid off.

I wanted to shout it from the rooftops. I was ecstatic. I was so excited to tell Katrina and Ricky too, but his impending arrival was slightly clouding my celebrations. I didn't know how I felt about Ricky at this point. I kind of wanted to see him and didn't want to see him at the same time. I didn't know whether he was going to be judgmental of the place where we were. Quite frankly, I didn't know what version of Ricky was going to turn up. I guess that's where the insecurity came from, and that showed up in fear. I had gotten used to the loving, caring fun Ricky that I knew so well, but the Ricky I had last experienced in Sydney wasn't really very nice.

Thankfully, when he finally arrived, it was the humble, old Ricky that I had got to know over the previous five years.

We had a good chat. I explained to him what had been going on. He was always really keen to hear what I had to say about the mystical experiences I went through. I explained some of the visions I had been getting, which were most profound. It's amazing what you see and hear when you switch off your distractions. When you sit in meditation for 24 hours and don't speak for a few days, you learn a lot about yourself. You open the channel to downloads and insights that may not have been able to come through in normal life. One of the most beautiful things I was experiencing there was that I was waking up naturally between four or five every morning. My Casa looked out onto the most stunning, beautiful undisturbed vista. So each morning, I would go from my bed to the hammock and get snuggled up with my duvet. I would lie there for hours meditating and watching the sunrise. It was a truly magical experience and an extremely mystical place. Those moments, on my own, in that vast open space, I will never ever forget. I often allow myself to wander back there. One day, I know I will return.

I showed Ric around the place and in typical Ricky fashion, he said he wanted to go through the process immediately. There was no time to wait, and I got that, I really did, but things were different in this space. I believe I knew him quite well at this point – well he was me after all – and I knew I was impatient, so I would need to manage his expectations of what would happen. In fairness, he was open to all of what I talked him through. He felt different to the Ricky I had left just a few weeks earlier, thank goodness. Maybe it was a good thing he was here. Maybe we could heal the rift in our friendship.

112

On the Wednesday, a week since I had first gone in, Ric and I went in together. He was in the first-time queue and I was in the returning queue. When he got to John of God, he was told that he needed to have surgery that afternoon, so he had to prep himself to go in and be silent, and not move for the following 24 hours.

In the same sitting, as I approached John of God this time, the entity was very different. He took me by the hand and told me how very special I was. I felt flattered. I was then told I needed to be a healer in the meditation room again that afternoon, and then I would have more surgery at 8 am the following day. Once again, I was holding space for Ricky to go on his journey, this time, though, he would see me sitting there as he walked through the room of meditators. Weird!

We had a really good laugh about all the rules they told us about – no speaking for 24 hours, no black pepper, sex or alcohol for a month. There were some strange rules that applied. Ricky seemed a little apprehensive about what was going to happen over the course of the coming 24 hours, so I attempted to ease that burden somewhat, by saying, "I'm going to be holding space for you this afternoon. Know that you're going to be safe. Whatever you need to do, you're going to be safe. This is it Ric, it's healing time, be open to receiving it my friend."

The time came for us to go in. We hugged and said our goodbyes. I went off into the meditation room, got myself settled and I felt the pressure was on for this one. My twin flame was here, in person, it was time for this to happen. I had healed, and I was so grateful that I had healed, but now it was time to pass that gift forward to someone else to heal. And who better than my twin flame?

When I was in meditation, even though my eyes were closed, I felt Ricky's energy walk past me. I knew it was him. It was so familiar. I felt an overwhelming feeling of love. It was like a love that you have for a brother, or a child. It was so strong.

In my meditation that afternoon, I was shown a beautiful scene where I was walking as a monk. I was walking down a path and everything I touched came back to life. I was shown the power of healing that was within me. I knew in that moment, if I did things in a certain way, that I was being shown they would come back to life. It would bring them back on track. I was shown very, very clearly that I was going to help heal hundreds of thousands of people, even millions of people. All of a sudden it all made sense. The desire to serve, to help all of these people came flooding back through my memories as a healer. This vision totally validated my journey. It made so much sense. I felt so extremely grateful in that moment.

That evening, I went back to my Casa and had another magical experience in the astral realms. I went to the version of myself that was fully healed. I was living happily with my husband and children. I was shown the beautiful country where I was going to be living – and it wasn't England. I couldn't quite place where it was at the time, but it definitely wasn't England. I was so happy. It was all over my face, and my family's. We were so content. It made my heart swell to a new level. The man was not at all who I thought I would end up with. It was really interesting. He was tall and very handsome, but he was not what I would normally go for. It intrigued me so much who this stranger was. I was excited to meet him when he was ready to come in.

The next morning, I woke early and headed over for my second psychic surgery. What a totally different experience! This time around, after the surgery, it felt like electricity was running through me. A far cry from being crippled over in pain previously. This was a much better experience, I felt so alive. I wanted to talk to everybody, despite not being allowed to. I wanted to go and have some fun, which was interesting as I knew the rules had to be followed. I wondered what healing was actually taking place this time, it was bizarre. Despite my desire for connection, I had to stay in silent meditation. I didn't want to stay put as I was buzzing with energy, and I did not know what to do with myself. After about twelve hours of attempted stillness, I got up and grabbed my journal to start writing my thoughts, emotions and feelings down. Something had other ideas, though, I ripped a piece of paper out, placed it sideways and started scribbling all over the page. I had no idea what was going on. I had no idea what was coming out of me. I was being channelled, and this continued for some time.

Eventually, I felt I probably should get back to meditating, so I lay back on my bed and I ended up falling asleep. I woke at about 4 in the morning. I went to the toilet, grabbed a glass of water and spotted the paper that I had scribbled on the evening before. I picked it up and thought – *What the fuck is that?* When I looked closer at it, it was a business plan. That previous day, in a trance, a daze, or whatever you would like to call it, I channelled a business plan as to how I was going to help get people to the place they needed to be for ascension. It made absolutely no sense to me at that time. Some of the items on there were so far out, but the more I looked at it, the more I received clear messages. I was given really clear information for the Self Love Club seminar I was about to run at the end of October, just a couple of days after I got back from this journey. I was shown that if it was done right, Self Love Club would change the world. It was going to take time, and patience was going to be required, but it was going to change the world. If I could stay consistent, and make sure that I set up certain seminars, people would travel from all over the world to receive the healing. Even though it was from me speaking, rather than hands-on healing, they would get what they required to go on their journey.

In this same business plan, I was shown five locations around the world whereby I would be setting up healing centres – and this was in 2018 before healing centres were even a thing. They showed me the dynamics of the centres, the locations, the people that would come, and the kind of set-up that would be required to ensure the greatest results. They gave me the countries, they gave me everything. This piece of paper was full of information and activations. I was shown that I was going to start doing courses and producing certain products. They showed me I was going to be travelling the world and speaking at lots of different events. I was told my voice was one that people would want to hear. I was blown away. I was so excited, I was bouncing off the walls! I really wished that I wasn't restricted to being quiet and staying in the Casa because I wanted to go and tell the world what was coming.

113

Eventually, when my time was up, I went outside and grounded. I leant on a wooden post looking out across the vista. I was contemplating everything I had been shown, feeling extremely grateful for having been chosen as someone who would help people. After a few minutes, I heard, "Davis." I turned around and saw Ricky standing on the top of my Casa. "We need to chat," he shouted, and then climbed his way down and came over to join me.

When he eventually reached me, he gave me a huge hug and held me close to him for what seemed an eternity. He told me he felt amazing and he was so glad he had come over to heal. I let him speak and share his journey. He mentioned he had seen me as he had walked through and felt so grateful we were on this mission together. It felt sincere. It was nice to have him there. It was nice to be back together. Once he had finished, I shared what had gone on in my most bizarre healing session. He listened wide-eyed as I shared about the business plan that had channelled through. He was visibly excited for me. I told him about some of the other visions and the astral viewing I had been doing. I shared a beautiful vision I had about me getting married. I thought he would be so happy for me, but as I was talking, I noticed his energy shifting towards me. It was an uncomfortableness. I decided to ignore it, I was happy, I felt as if I was being shown the blueprint of my future life, and my goodness after the previous few years, I felt I deserved a little bit of guidance and respite. His discomfort was not my issue.

He suggested that we went for food so we could continue chatting. I was actually really hungry by this point. I fancied a coconut and a juice. I was almost ready to eat again. Whilst we waited for the food to arrive, we continued chatting. We spoke about his diet, his heart, and eventually, we got on to our role models of love through our childhood. I suggested that maybe the role models of love we had experienced growing up weren't the role models that we needed. I then directed to him that maybe he needed to find somebody who demonstrated real love, so he could remember what that felt like. My reasoning was when it came to matters of the heart he had clearly built a brick wall around it. He wasn't impressed. Although I had been talking about both of us, he had clearly taken it as an attack. His energy had initially shifted when I had mentioned the marriage thing, but this conversation created an eruption. He got really pissed off with me. He told me in no uncertain terms that it was none of my business, and, in all honestly, he was right. It wasn't any of my business. I shouldn't have said what I did, but I'm also glad I did because it was the unspoken truth that we both needed to hear. The reaction was also what I needed for my healing – not that I identified that at the time.

From my perspective, how can we learn how to love ourselves through people that don't know how to love themselves? That's where my troubles started. I didn't know how to love or to be honest and truthful in relationships because my dad didn't know. I was mirroring my dad. At around this time, back in 2018, I was very much the kind of person that would verbal diarrhoea all over you and tell you everything I thought that you needed to know to help you evolve. Whereas now, I ask questions so you figure it for yourself – much to many people's disgust and disappointment, I hasten to add. What I've learnt, particularly where men are concerned, is you can't tell them the answers, they won't appreciate it. I know I've pissed off so many men off over the years by taking that approach. So, I learnt to help people to use their initiative and to do the work themselves. Unfortunately for Ricky, I was still in my verbal diarrhoea phase and I know I pissed him off. To break the tension, I told him I was going back to my room.

The next day, he seemed to be okay with me. We went to the waterfall and spent some time in meditation together. There was a little chapel within the grounds of the Casa where the energies of saints would channel through. I really loved this little chapel. It only housed about four or five people, but every time I went in there, I got a really profound message from Saint Rita. On this occasion, when I went there with Ricky, I was getting so much information coming through about him, his heart, and myself, that it was too much. I couldn't process it all, so I had to leave. The channel in me was wide open and the information coming through was so profound. When we left there, I told Ricky I needed to go and sit in meditation for a bit, as there were some things that I needed to process on my own.

I found a quiet place to sit and went into meditation. While I was meditating, there was a fly constantly buzzing around me. It would land on my right arm, my right hand, my right forearm, or my right shoulder. Always on my right arm, though. I thought – *What the heck? What's this fly got to do with anything?* I continued meditating and I got a clear connection to Saint Francis of Assisi. Now, this incredible entity had helped with some of the healings whilst I'd been over there in the Casa. He had been quite prevalent in what I was creating apparently. In that meditation, he told me that if I ever needed him all I had to do was call on him. He said he would be there for me no matter what. He told me he would be with me in London at the seminar we were going to be running at the end of the month. It was so beautiful.

Saint Rita was another one that came through. I didn't know much about Saint Rita, in all honesty. There was something really beautiful about her energy – it was a powerful divine feminine, motherly, grandmother, fun, loving energy. It was almost nun like, as well. She offered her support, along with Quan Yin, who had also been coming through a lot over recent months, especially in regards to the divine feminine vibration that I had started to embody.

The next day was going to be Ricky's last day. I decided during the evening before that I wanted to be on my own. I didn't know what was happening within me, but something was shifting. Something that I had not experienced before was channelling through me and I chose to sit with it to embody it. It was like all of my gifts were coming online. My manifestations were coming through quicker than ever and feeling a love that I had never experienced before was becoming the normality. It was an unusual and uncomfortable period of growth; I was collapsing all of the old masks and stepping into my truth. I had to let go more and more.

Whilst on my own that night, something truly magical happened. I had attended a seminar in Sydney back in September, after my blood transfusion, one that Ricky had organised for me. It was with a well-known healer who was from America, but was married to an Australian lady, and so was quite well known over there. I had mentioned to Ric on a couple of occasions that I would like to chat with this guy, and Ric had noticed that he was running a seminar a couple of days after I arrived. I went alone, Ric decided he didn't want to come. That night, the guy spoke to me as one of the first people during that seminar. I explained that I had just arrived from England, having run away from a potential operation as I wanted to heal. He had been blown away by my story and listened intently as we chatted about what I could do to heal. At the end of the seminar, he announced that one person would win a scholarship to go and study with him in Bali. I remember thinking what a cool opportunity for someone to win. I would have loved it! Well, that night in Brazil, for the first time in a couple of weeks, I decided to check my emails and there was an email from him. "Lucy, we have been attempting to get hold of you, we would like to offer you the scholarship to go and work with him in Bali!" What the actual fuck? I never won anything in my life! I was absolutely buzzing. What a result to be selected out of hundreds of people to go and learn, and for free!

The next morning was Ricky's last day. He was being picked up in the afternoon. When I woke up, I was buzzing! I excitedly told Katrina about the prize trip to Bali, and she was so happy for me. I then saw Ric and was so excited to tell him, but he didn't want to speak. He was clearly in a mood with me. What the heck had I done now? My ego kicked in. I thought – *Fuck you! You're supposed to be my friend. You're supposed to be happy for me. You're supposed to be excited for me.*

What I didn't realise at the time, was he was still pissed off with me for the conversations we had a few days earlier – I only found this out later. I couldn't be doing with his moods, though, so I went over to the Casa to do a meditation. While I was meditating, he must have snapped out of it, as he sent a message asking me if I wanted to go for lunch. I didn't see it, though, because I was deep in meditation.

By the time I looked at my phone, I had a stroppy message from him saying, "I haven't been able to find you, so I'll see you next time."

For fuck's sake!

I walked out of the Casa and went over to find him. He was in a weird mood. He said we should get some photos together, so we took a few pictures, then the taxi came to pick him up, and off he went. It was such a weird vibe between the two of us. I thought we had shared some of the most beautiful, profound times with each other on this journey, but once again, he'd snapped into someone I didn't like. It was becoming something of a cycle.

When he left, I thought I'd leave him to it for a few days. I'd let him reach out if he wanted to. I wasn't aware of what I had done, so I just carried on as normal. He was off to Norway, to go and hike a rock he'd always wanted to go to – which was probably a tad strenuous after what we had just done, but there was no telling him. When I didn't hear from him for a couple of days, I thought I would do the decent thing and message him to check he was okay. A little while later, he sent me a rant, having a go at me about some of the conversations we had and a few other things. I breathed deeply, then messaged back to say, "Thank you for your comments. I'm going to sit with this for a couple of days." This was a huge shift for me. Back in the day, if someone attacked me for something, I would have attacked them back. Trust me, my tongue was venomous when I needed it to be. This time, though, I didn't. I realised that it wasn't important. What he had shared with me was how he was feeling about himself. I would get back to him in my own time. I wasn't going to rush it. I wasn't going to create an issue.

Instead, I decided to enjoy my last few days in the Casa. I did lots of the meditations that were for other people because I wanted to give something back. I also did some healing for myself by going on the crystal beds and spending time talking to people who needed an ear. I sat outside and journaled a lot. It was amazing to feel so connected and alive. Following the rules that had been laid out was really easy. I didn't want to drink alcohol. I didn't want to eat the pepper or the chilli. I didn't want to have sex because if that meant that this healing journey was going to stop, then I wasn't interested. I was fully invested in making this work. I deserved to be fit, strong and well – by the grace of God.

This period of solitude, focusing on self, was a game changer. I could have decided not to invest in myself at this time; my nan was very poorly and she didn't have long left on the earth plain. We all knew that was the case and bless her little heart, because she had been something of a wanderer, she understood why I had to go. Whenever my dad went to see her, I would video call her and show her Brazil – a country that she had not made it to in her life. I felt so privileged to be able to share this experience with her.

The day before I left Brazil, I sat down with my laptop and wrote a response to Ricky's message, and all of the points he had raised. I opened my response with love. I decided that going forward, everything that was thrown at me, no matter how challenging, was going to be met with love. I thanked him for everything he had said, let him know that I had sat reflecting on it and that I trusted the email would be received in the manner intended, with no animosity. I sent it over to him, not expecting a response, and very quickly, I got an email back from him – I was shocked. His tone had changed completely. He had gone from being angry and aggressive to acknowledging that I was changing. His email back to me was actually very sweet.

After I read it, I made the decision that I was to move on now. I replied to him, and laid my cards on the table – hoping he would acknowledge the twin flame energy between us. I wrote, "Listen, there is clearly a connection between us both, we are always going to trigger the heck out of each other. I support you on your journey and I'd really appreciate it if you could support me on mine."

He sent me an email back, but I never responded. As far as I was concerned, that was us, done.

114

The day I said goodbye to Brazil, was a sad day. I had loved it there. I'd only been physically in the presence of John of God twice but I had seen some incredible things. I had been witness to somebody going in there with cataracts and him removing them by performing a physical surgery in front of everybody. No anaesthetic, nothing. It was mystical. It was magical. There was no denying that he was a very, very talented man. There was no denying that he had a gift.

I was sad to be leaving. I felt safe there. I felt more myself than I had ever felt in my life, and I didn't want to leave it. I didn't want to lose that feeling. I didn't want to step out of that bubble that had been created. But, I knew I couldn't stay there forever. I had to get back to reality. I had a seminar to run in just a couple of days.

During the time that I'd been there, I had used the business plan that I channelled to totally reshape what I was going to talk about at the Self Love Club seminar in a few days' time. I had looked at all of the content that I'd put together, changed it all – pulled some out, put some in – and was handed a number of things I had to do to set the seminar up. I was even told what I had to wear.

First though, I had to navigate the journey home. We had to fly back to Rio to get our connecting flights. In the airport, I had to go to the toilet before we boarded. Katrina decided to come with me. I sat in the cubicle, and I received a massive download about spending time in a monastery. I shouted over the cubicle to Katrina, "You're not going to fucking believe what they've got me to do next. I've got to go and spend some serious time in a monastery." I started roaring with laughter.

Katrina laughed, "You in a monastery? You're going to self-combust, girl."

I thought it was hilarious. The monks had been showing up a lot, but now I'm being told I need to go and spend time in a monastery!

I stepped out of the cubicle and Katrina was rolling her eyes at me, "What's next with you?"

"I wonder which monastery I'm going to get taken to? I'm excited." I said, as my mind wandered off to what may be coming next.

"Well, as always with your journey, as soon as they give it to you, you know it's going to happen. It's just a case of when."

And so, out loud, I said to them – my guides, the divine, the powers that be, "You show me which monastery you want me in. Take me where you need me to be, and I will be there. If you want me there for a week, I'll be there for a week. If you want me there for a month, I'll be there for a month."

With that, we got on the plane to Rio.

Once we landed, we said our goodbyes, went our separate ways and very quickly I boarded the plane heading toward home, knowing that in a couple of days I was going to run a seminar. It felt so weird to be heading back to normality and no longer to be in the bubble of the Casa.

I arrived back in the UK, and I was buzzing. I felt different. I wanted to scream from the rooftops about my healing journey. I called my doctor and asked him to organise a scan for me. Interestingly, my doctor's appointment had been pulled forwards and so I was able to get seen much quicker than I expected.

Interestingly, the day that I got back to the UK, I was told very clearly that I needed to wear a particular necklace when I was doing the seminar. It was a quartz heart that I had actually bought in Brazil. I was also told that I needed to do the Lord's Prayer at the beginning of the Self Love Club – now this wasn't resonant with me at all, but I got told it had to be that way. So clearly there were a couple more tweaks I needed to make to the seminar – they were leaving some of these ideas a bit late, though!

On the Monday evening, I travelled up to London with a couple of my girlfriends who were going to help me get set up for the event. I had also been told that before I started speaking at the event I was to keep everybody out of the room, and there was to just be me in there. I was clearly shown how to set the room up. There were certain crystals that needed to be in a certain way, and I needed to call in the entities from the Casa. I did everything, exactly as I was shown.

That night, when I was alone in the room, a fly started buzzing around me and it landed on my right arm. I thought – *That's weird. I'm in a hotel room, there are no windows. Where the heck has that fly come from?* And then I thought back to the Casa, and I realised it was linked to that. I asked the question, "Are you linked to the Casa?" I got a clear answer, "Yes." I said, "Are you somebody who's going to help me?" I got a clear, "Yes." And with that, I got an energy come through me that I remembered as that of St. Francis of Assisi. It was a beautiful moment.

I let everybody into the room. And on that night, pure magic was created. Everybody in the room laughed, cried and went on a huge healing journey. I had no idea the power of what they'd given me in Brazil. I had done the very first Self Love Club. It was the very start of something incredible, but most poignantly, it was the culmination of a journey that had started on that sunbed in Dubai just five years earlier.

What a journey.

What a ride.

And not only that, but I was now walking around with a new guide, who went by the name of St Francis of Assisi.

Epilogue

If you have reached this part of the book, these final pages, I want to truly thank you from the bottom of my heart for coming along on this journey with me.

And what a ride it has been.

In divine serendipity and grace, and in the completion of a perfect circle, I am writing these last few words overlooking the beautiful beach of my hometown, Bournemouth. The place where it all started, is the place where this part of the journey ends. I was told a few years ago that I would complete the first book looking out over the ocean. At that time, I thought that it would be Sydney, but God clearly had other ideas. I'm really glad it brought me back here to Bournemouth, though, as so much magic has taken place since I returned; those stories, I'm sorry, are for another time, and another book completely.

I know I'll be moving again soon, they've told me that too. Who knows where or when? That's just the way my life goes these days, and I wouldn't have it any other way.

I trust that having come this far on the journey with me, that you have seen my life mirrors yours. That's all I am here to do — to help you remember who you are. The very fact that you are holding this book in your hands should be divine validation enough that you are a hugely important part of God's plan. You wouldn't be here, in this now moment with me, if you weren't.

I have only shared my story so that you can connect the dots with your own story. You have a story to tell, you have stories to tell. They may not be like mine, that's not important. What matters is that you start to see the patterns in your life, that you can identify your emotional traumas, that you learn to trust yourself, to like yourself, and ultimately to love yourself.

You too receive the signs and the messages. There is nothing that I have that you don't have. If you see it in me, it's in you — even if you don't experience it, yet. The Universe is mirroring you back to yourself all day, every day. Every encounter, every experience, every person, every trigger is showing you your healing. Everything is happening FOR you, not to you — and when you can grasp that, then your whole world will align in a beautiful way.

I wish that upon turning the final pages of this book, you will have felt the shift within yourself From Head To Heart.

Living from our heart-space more and more is the path that we all must take if we are to become the very highest and best versions of ourselves and to live our most meaningful and purposeful lives. Especially, if we are to now go out and create the world we want to live in; the world where our children, and our children's children, can live in peace, love and harmony once again.

The old world is crumbling before our eyes, and all of the darkness too.
We are the ones who bring the light.
I'm so excited to meet you there.

With all the love in my heart.
Lucy xox

About Lucy Davis

Lucy Davis was a high flying Director in the investment banking system, deeply entrenched in the material world of money, luxury holidays and partying as hard as she worked. When a series of traumatic events caused her world to come crashing down around her, she reluctantly surrendered to what was happening and found herself on a catastrophic, profound, and magical journey of self discovery and healing that would take her all around the world, and help her to rediscover her innate gifts that had been buried for decades.

Living purely by intuition, Lucy was guided to create 'Self Love Club', a brand comprising of courses, workshops and seminars that would take her once again around the world several times, sharing her wisdom, experience, and helping hundreds of thousands of people to recognise their own happiness, embrace their talents, find their purpose, and ultimately to learn to live in 'Self Love'.

In recent years, Lucy has been a frontline campaigner fighting for freedom and human rights; she is a passionate advocate of saving and helping children all over the world.

As part of her mission, in 2022, Lucy founded 'Soul School' – a project she was divinely gifted originally in 2018. No longer content to wait around for the old systems to crumble, Lucy decided to create 'Soul School' in order to build the new world – a space of love, peace and harmony, where individuals and families can go to re-educate themselves and rise in consciousness together.

LUCY DAVIS
FROM HEAD TO HEART BOOK CLUB

As a special thank you for walking this journey with me, I would like to invite you to join an exclusive club where we can continue this journey together. I will keep you updated about my life, and you can ask any questions that you may have about the book and any of the stories within it. It's free to join, there's no obligation, it's simply a way for us to stay connected and continue walking the paths of our lives together.

www.lucydavis.com/bookclub

With love
Lucy xox